Handbook of Cannabis Therapeutics
From Bench to Bedside

THE HAWORTH PRESS®
Haworth Series in Integrative Healing
Ethan Russo
Editor

The Last Sorcerer: Echoes of the Rainforest by Ethan Russo

Professionalism and Ethics in Complementary and Alternative Medicine by John Crellin and Fernando Ania

Cannabis and Cannabinoids: Pharmacology, Toxicology, and Therapeutic Potential by Franjo Grotenhermen and Ethan Russo

Modern Psychology and Ancient Wisdom: Psychological Healing Practices from the World's Religious Traditions edited by Sharon G. Mijares

Complementary and Alternative Medicine: Clinic Design by Robert A. Roush

Herbal Voices: American Herbalism Through the Words of American Herbalists by Anne K. Dougherty

The Healing Power of Chinese Herbs and Medicinal Recipes by Joseph P. Hou and Youyu Jin

Alternative Therapies in the Treatment of Brain Injury and Neurobehavioral Disorders: A Practical Guide edited by Gregory J. Murrey

Handbook of Cannabis Therapeutics: From Bench to Bedside edited by Ethan B. Russo and Franjo Grotenhermen

Handbook of Cannabis Therapeutics
From Bench to Bedside

Ethan B. Russo, MD
Franjo Grotenhermen, MD
Editors

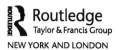

Routledge
Taylor & Francis Group
NEW YORK AND LONDON

First Published by

The Haworth Press, Inc., 10 Alice Street, Binghamton, NY 13904-1580.

Transferred to Digital Printing 2010 by Routledge
270 Madison Ave, New York NY 10016
2 Park Square, Milton Park, Abingdon, Oxon, OX14 4RN

For more information on this book or to order, visit
http://www.haworthpress.com/store/product.asp?sku=5741

or call 1-800-HAWORTH (800-429-6784) in the United States and Canada
or (607) 722-5857 outside the United States and Canada

or contact orders@HaworthPress.com

PUBLISHER'S NOTE
The development, preparation, and publication of this work has been undertaken with great care. However, the Publisher, employees, editors, and agents of The Haworth Press are not responsible for any errors contained herein or for consequences that may ensue from use of materials or information contained in this work. The Haworth Press is committed to the dissemination of ideas and information according to the highest standards of intellectual freedom and the free exchange of ideas. Statements made and opinions expressed in this publication do not necessarily reflect the views of the Publisher, Directors, management, or staff of The Haworth Press, Inc., or an endorsement by them.

This book is a compilation of articles previously published in the *Journal of Cannabis Therapeutics: Studies in Endogenous, Herbal, and Synthetic Cannabinoids,* 1(1) (2001): 5-70, 85-88; 1(2) (2001): 15-20; 1(3/4) (2001): 5-16, 103-132; 2(1) (2002): 3-57; 2(2) (2002): 51-79; 2(3/4) (2002): 5-34, 49-81, 103-131, 159-173; 3(1) (2003): 3-51; 3(4) (2003): 163-174; 4(1) (2004): 29-78, published by The Haworth Press, Inc.

This book has been published solely for educational purposes and is not intended to substitute for the medical advice of a treating physician. Medicine is an ever-changing science. As new research and clinical experience broaden our knowledge, changes in treatment may be required. While many potential treatment options are made herein, some or all of the options may not be applicable to a particular individual. Therefore, the author, editor, and publisher do not accept responsibility in the event of negative consequences incurred as a result of the information presented in this book. We do not claim that this information is necessarily accurate by the rigid scientific and regulatory standards applied for medical treatment. **No warranty, expressed or implied, is furnished with respect to the material contained in this book. The reader is urged to consult with his/her personal physician with respect to the treatment of any medical condition.**

Photographs by Ethan B. Russo. Medicine bottle from the collection of David Watson, HortaPharm, Amsterdam.

Cover design by Kerry E. Mack.

Library of Congress Cataloging-in-Publication Data

Handbook of cannabis therapeutics : from bench to bedside / Ethan B. Russo, Franjo Grotenhermen, editors.
     p. cm.
    "A compilation of selected articles from the Journal of cannabis therapeutics . . . from 2001 to 2004"—Introd.
    Includes bibliographical references and index.
    ISBN-13: 978-0-7890-3096-2 (hard : alk. paper)
    ISBN-10: 0-7890-3096-9 (hard : alk. paper)
    ISBN-13: 978-0-7890-3097-9 (soft : alk. paper)
    ISBN-10: 0-7890-3097-7 (soft : alk. paper)
    1. Cannabis—Therapeutic use—History. I. Russo, Ethan. II. Grotenhermen, Franjo. III. Journal of cannabis therapeutics.
    [DNLM: 1. Cannabis—Collected Works. 2. Phytotherapy—methods—Collected Works. 3. Cannabinoids—history—Collected Works. 4. Cannabinoids—therapeutic use—Collected Works. 5. Plant Extracts—therapeutic use—Collected Works. WB 925 H236 2006]
RM666.C266H36 2005
615'.7827—dc22
                                2005029271

CONTENTS

About the Editors   xiii

Contributors   xv

Foreword   xvii

Introduction   1
Franjo Grotenhermen

PART I: HISTORICAL NOTES

Chapter 1. The Therapeutic Use of *Cannabis sativa* (L.) in Arabic Medicine   5
Indalecio Lozano

Introduction   5
Materials and Methods   6
Results   6
Conclusion   10
Update   12

Chapter 2. Cognoscenti of Cannabis I: Jacques-Joseph Moreau (1804-1884)   13
Ethan B. Russo

Chapter 3. Cognoscenti of Cannabis II: Simeon Seth on Cannabis   17
David Deakle

Chapter 4. The Medical Use of Cannabis Among the Greeks and Romans   23
James L. Butrica

Introduction   23
Absence of Mention   24
The Emergence of Cannabis   25
Appendix I: Passages Discussing Wild Cannabis Possibly Misunderstood As Discussing Domesticated Cannabis   40

Appendix II: Cannabis in Veterinary Medicine   41
Update   42

**Chapter 5. A Homelie Herbe: Medicinal Cannabis
in Early England**   **43**
    Vivienne Crawford

Introduction   43
Cannabis History in England   45
The Modern Era   49
Update   51

**Chapter 6. Future of Cannabis and Cannabinoids
in Therapeutics**   **53**
    Ethan B. Russo

Introduction   53
New Indications for Cannabinoid Pharmaceuticals   56
Cannabinoids and Neuroprotection   57
Spasmodic Disorders   58
Forbidden Territories   58
Update   63

**PART II: PHARMACOLOGY
AND PHARMACOKINETICS**

**Chapter 7. Clinical Pharmacokinetics
of Cannabinoids**   **69**
    Franjo Grotenhermen

Introduction   69
Pharmacokinetics of Δ^9-THC   74
Absorption   75
Distribution   80
Metabolism   84
Course of Plasma Concentration of THC
    and Metabolites   86
Elimination   88
Time Effect Relationship   94
Pharmacokinetics of Other Cannabinoids   99
Metabolic Interactions   101
Conclusion   103

**Chapter 8. Clinical Pharmacodynamics
of Cannabinoids**   **117**

Franjo Grotenhermen

Introduction   117
Mechanism of Action   119
Cannabinoid Receptors   121
Endocannabinoids   122
Pharmacological Effects of THC   125
Toxicity   125
Psyche, Cognition and Behavior   127
Central Nervous System
   and Neurochemistry   128
Circulatory System   130
Some Other Organ Systems and Effects   131
Pharmacological Activity
   of THC Metabolites   133
Pharmacological Effects
   of Other Cannabinoids   135
Tolerance and Dependency   138
Therapeutic Uses   139
Hierarchy of Therapeutic Effects   140
Basic Research Stage   141
Drug Interactions   143
Conclusions   144
Update   165

**Chapter 9. Cannabis and Cannabis Extracts:
Greater Than the Sum of Their Parts?**   **171**

John M. McPartland
Ethan B. Russo

Introduction   171
Materials and Methods   172
Results and Discussion   172
Cannabinoids   173
Terpenoids   178
Flavonoids   187
Conclusions   190
Update   201

PART III: ENDOCANNABINOIDS AND CANNABINOID RECEPTORS

Chapter 10. The Endocannabinoid System: Can It Contribute to Cannabis Therapeutics?   **207**
Vincenzo Di Marzo

The Endocannabinoid System   207
Endocannabinoid Pharmacology: More Than
    Meets the Eye   209
Levels of Endocannabinoids in Tissues: Physiology
    and Pathology   211
New Drugs From the Endocannabinoid System: Curative
    or Palliative?   216
Update   225

Chapter 11. Cannabinoids and Feeding: The Role of the Endogenous Cannabinoid System As a Trigger for Newborn Suckling   **227**
Ester Fride

Interactions of the Endocannabinoid System
    with Hormones Regulating Food Intake   228
Endocannabinoids in Food Substances   229
Developmental Aspects of the Endocannabinoid-CB_1
    Receptor System   230
Blockade of CB_1 Receptors in Newborn Mice   231
Mechanisms of the CB_1 Receptor Blockade-Induced
    Growth-Stunting Effects   233
Conclusions   234
Update   238

PART IV: MEDICINAL USES

Chapter 12. Marijuana (Cannabis) As Medicine   **243**
Leo E. Hollister

Introduction   243
Indications with Evidence for Medical Efficacy   245
Indications with Sparse Evidence of Efficacy   253
Discussion   257
Conclusion   258
Update   263

Chapter 13. Effects of Smoked Cannabis and Oral Δ⁹-Tetrahydrocannabinol on Nausea and Emesis After Cancer Chemotherapy: A Review of State Clinical Trials   **265**

Richard E. Musty
Rita Rossi

Tennessee	266
Michigan	267
Georgia	268
New Mexico (1983)	270
New Mexico (1984)	271
California	272
New York	273
Discussion	275
Update	278

Chapter 14. Hyperemesis Gravidarum and Clinical Cannabis: To Eat or Not to Eat?   **281**

Wei-Ni Lin Curry

HG, Its Medicalization, and the Survivors	282
Cannabis, Pregnancy, and HG	288
Two Women's Stories of Using Folk, Alternative Medicine	293
Conclusion	297
Update	302

Chapter 15. Therapeutic Cannabis (Marijuana) As an Antiemetic and Appetite Stimulant in Persons with Acquired Immunodeficiency Syndrome   **303**

Richard E. Bayer

AIDS in the United States	303
Cannabinoids as Antiemetic and Appetite Stimulant in AIDS Wasting Syndrome	305
Case Reports (The Patients' Perspective)	306
Recent Clinical Research on Cannabinoids, Immunity, and Weight Gain	308
Cannabis and Harm Reduction Strategies for Persons with AIDS	308
Conclusion	311
Update	313

**Chapter 16. Cannabis Treatments in Obstetrics
and Gynecology: A Historical Review**   **315**
Ethan B. Russo

Introduction   315
The Ancient World and Medieval Middle and Far East   315
European and Western Medicine   318
Modern Ethnobotany of Cannabis in Obstetrics
    and Gynecology   331
Recent Theory and Clinical Data   334
Discussion and Conclusions   338
Update   345

**Chapter 17. Crack Heads and Roots Daughters:
The Therapeutic Use of Cannabis in Jamaica**   **347**
Melanie Dreher

Ganja   348
Cocaine   350
Women and Crack   351
Conclusions   357
Implications   358
Update   360

**Chapter 18. Cannabis in Multiple Sclerosis:
Women's Health Concerns**   **363**
Denis J. Petro

Introduction   363
Treatment Options: Acute Episodes, Disease Modification
    and Symptom Management   364
Cannabis in Acute Treatment and Disease Modification   365
Cannabis in Symptom Management   367
Impaired Mobility: Spasticity   368
Tremor   369
Nystagmus   369
Postural Regulation   370
Fatigue   370
Pain   371
Bladder Dysfunction   371
Sexual Dysfunction   372
Discussion   372

Conclusions 373
Update 377

PART V: SIDE EFFECTS

Chapter 19. Cannabis and Harm Reduction:
A Nursing Perspective 383
    Mary Lynn Mathre

Introduction 383
Cannabis Was a Medicine in the United States 385
Cannabis As a Harm Reduction Medicine 386
Cannabis As a Social/Recreational Drug 389
Cannabis Prohibition Causes More Harm Than the Drug 393
Conclusions 396

Chapter 20. Chronic Cannabis Use in the Compassionate
Investigational New Drug Program: An Examination
of Benefits and Adverse Effects of Legal Clinical
Cannabis 399
    Ethan B. Russo   Paul J. Bach
    Mary Lynn Mathre   Juan Sanchez-Ramos
    Al Byrne   Kristin A. Kirlin
    Robert Velin

Introduction 400
Previous Chronic Cannabis Use Studies 400
A Brief History of the Compassionate IND 401
Methods 403
Results And Discussion 404
Conclusions and Recommendations 442
Update 447

Afterword 449

Index 451

ABOUT THE EDITORS

Ethan B. Russo, MD, is Adjunct Associate Professor in the Department of Pharmaceutical Sciences at the University of Montana and Clinical Associate Professor in the Department of Medicine at the University of Washington. He is board certified in neurology with a special qualification in child neurology. He frequently lectures to undergraduate and graduate students in the fields of pharmacy, psychology, sports medicine, interpersonal communications, and physical therapy, among others. He has had a lifetime interest in medicinal plants.

Dr. Russo has written numerous peer-reviewed articles on ethnobotany, herbal medicine, and cannabis, and has lectured internationally on these topics. He has published numerous peer-reviewed articles on ethnobotany, herbal medicine, and cannabis, and he has lectured nationally on those subjects. He is the author/editor of the *Handbook of Psychotropic Herbs; Cannabis and Cannabinoids: Pharmacology, Toxicology, and Therapeutic Potential; Cannabis Therapeutics in HIV/AIDS; Women and Cannabis: Medicine, Science, and Sociology;* and a novel, *The Last Sorcerer: Echoes of the Rainforest* (Haworth). For four years Dr. Russo served as editor of the *Journal of Cannabis Therapeutics*.

Franjo Grotenhermen, MD, has worked in the fields of internal medicine, surgery, and integrative medicine. Since 1994 he has been researching medical uses of hemp at the Nova Institut. He is also a member of the working group on quality of life for cancer patients at the Department of Internal Medicine at the University of Cologne.

Dr. Grotenhermen is founder and executive director of the Association for Cannabis as Medicine (ACM) in Germany and of the International Association for Cannabis as Medicine (IACM). He is author and co-author of a number of books, book chapters, and articles on the therapeutic uses, pharmacology, and toxicology of cannabis and cannabinoids; most have appeared in German.

Handbook of Cannabis Therapeutics
© 2006 by The Haworth Press, Inc. All rights reserved.
doi:10.1300/5741_a

CONTRIBUTORS

Paul J. Bach is affiliated with Montana Neurobehavioral Specialists, Missoula, Montana.

Richard E. Bayer, MD, FACP, is board certified in internal medicine and a fellow in the American College of Physicians–American Society of Internal Medicine. He lives in Portland, Oregon.

James L. Butrica is a professor in the Department of Classics at The Memorial University of Newfoundland in St. John's, Newfoundland, Canada.

Al Byrne is affiliated with Patients Out of Time, Howardsville, Virginia.

Vivienne Crawford is a former lecturer in Renaissance literature. She holds postgraduate degrees in English and American literature from Harvard, as well as degrees in philosophy from University College, London, and the University of Canterbury, New Zealand. She recently completed a BSc degree and clinical training in herbal medicine.

Wei-Ni Lin Curry, PhD, was affiliated with the UCLA/Folklore Program and Archives, Los Angeles, California, studying women's folk healing and birthing traditions.

David Deakle, ThD, PhD, was the James DeKoven distinguished professor of New Testament and patristics at Nashotah House, Nashotah, Wisconsin. He is now a retired Episcopal priest in Portland, Oregon.

Melanie Dreher, PhD, FAAN, is dean and professor, University of Iowa College of Nursing, Iowa City, Iowa.

Vincenzo Di Marzo, PhD, is affiliated with the Istituto par la Chimica di Molecole di Interesse Biologico, Consiglio Nazionale delle Ricerche, Via Toiano, Napoli, Italy.

Ester Fride, PhD, is an associate professor, Department of Behavioral Sciences, and head, Laboratory of Behavioral Biology, College of Judea and Samaria, Ariel, Israel.

The late **Leo E. Hollister, MD,** was affiliated with the Harris County Psychiatric Center, University of Texas Medical Center, Houston, Texas.

Handbook of Cannabis Therapeutics
© 2006 by The Haworth Press, Inc. All rights reserved.
doi:10.1300/5741_b

Kristin A. Kirlin is affiliated with the Department of Psychology, University of Montana, Missoula, Montana.

Indalecio Lozano, PhD, is affiliated with the Universidad de Granada, Facultad de Letras, Departamento de Estudios Semíticos, Granada, Spain.

Mary Lynn Mathre, RN, MSN, CARN, is the executive director of Addiction Recovery Systems, Pantops Clinic, Charlottesville, Virginia, and president and cofounder of Patients Out of Time, Howardsville, Virginia.

John M. McPartland, DO, MS, is affiliated with GW Pharmaceuticals, Ltd., Porton Down Science Park, Salisbury, Wiltshire, United Kingdom.

Richard E. Musty, PhD, is associated with the Department of Psychology, University of Vermont, Burlington, Vermont.

Denis J. Petro, MD, is a neurologist in Arlington, Virginia.

Rita Rossi is project coordinator in the psychosocial research department, Butler Hospital, Providence, Rhode Island.

Juan Sanchez-Ramos is affiliated with the Department of Neurology, University of South Florida, Tampa, Florida.

Robert Velin is affiliated with Montana Neurobehavioral Specialists, Missoula, Montana.

Foreword

The human race prides itself as the only animal through evolution to become a rational being and therefore able to make decisions and take action based on logic and analysis of available data, rather than simply by instinct, other genetic factors, and experience, accumulated mostly through conditioning, as found in other animals. But is this human pride justified? My involvement within the limited field of cannabis therapeutics certainly shows that humans still value instincts and antiquated ideas, some based on a total lack of rationality much more than on reasoned facts. In June 2005 the U.S. Supreme Court declared medical use of cannabis illegal on the federal level, although some states have allowed its use in certain medical conditions. Was there scientific and medical logic behind this decision?

Cannabis sativa is a part of the medical-cultural heritage of many lands. It is mentioned in Assyrian clay tablets as a drug for treating neurological conditions, and it was used for a variety of medical problems in China and India when Northern Europe was still governed by barbarian tribes. Even as late as the end of the nineteenth century cannabis was described by Queen Victoria's physician as "by far the most useful of drugs . . . in some painful conditions," but during most of the twentieth century it was regarded as a nuisance—an illegal drug which did not quite fit the official view of a dangerous narcotic. Yet during the past forty years, science has accumulated a vastly increasing bulk of knowledge of this drug. Its chemistry was clarified during the 1960s, and its psychoactive principle, Δ^9-tetrahydrocannabinol (Δ^9-THC), was identified. In spite of its mild psychotropic effects, in the United States in 1985 THC was approved as a prescription drug against vomiting and nausea caused by cancer chemotherapy, and in 1992 as an appetite enhancer, most often used by AIDS patients.

Over the past twenty years, the mechanism of action of THC was shown to be quite unique. This plant molecule activates two receptors, CB_1 (found predominantly in the central nervous system) and CB_2 (found mostly in the immune system). These receptors are part of the endocannabinoid system, which is involved in myriad physiological processes. It is activated by specific ligands called endocannabinoids, the best known being anandamide and 2-arachidonoyl glycerol, both derivatives of a fatty acid, arachidonic acid. Although completely different in chemical structure from the endocannabinoids, THC binds to the same receptors and elicits the same physiological responses. The endocannabinoids and THC enhance appetite, reduce pain, and affect many of the symptoms of diseases, in particular those associated with the central nervous and the immune systems, as well as impacting a long list of additional body processes. But THC is not the only cannabis constituent with physiological activity. Cannabidiol (CBD), a nonpsychotropic cannabinoid, has been found to be anxiolytic, antiepileptic, and antischizophrenic in animals and humans. We know very little about the activity of the dozens of additional but mostly minor cannabinoids that are present in the plant. Many sufferers of various diseases claim that the effect of using the total plant is better than the effect of THC alone. In part, this may be due to the different modes of administration— marijuana is, of course, usually smoked, while THC is administered mostly orally. However, I believe that the combination of CBD with THC may represent a better drug than THC alone. As these are the main plant cannabinoids, a cannabis plant with a standardized content of CBD and THC may represent a valuable therapeutic drug. Unfortunately, the present irrational bias against the plant may block the introduction of this type of medicine in many countries.

The use of neurotransmitters and neuromodulators as medicinal agents is certainly not new. Many modern drugs are based on them. There is every reason to expect that cannabinoid-based drugs will eventually also be introduced. So why block a valuable medicine? The only reason I can think of is lack of reason in the face of compelling scientific evidence.

This book is a compilation of many articles published originally in the now defunct and difficult-to-obtain *Journal of Cannabis Therapeutics*. The chapters deal with the history of the medical use of cannabis, the pharmacology and pharmacokinetics of THC and other cannabinoids, the endocannabinoid system, and with the various medicinal uses (including the side effects) of the drug. It is, in my view, an excellent overall presentation of the expanding topic of cannabis therapeutics.

Raphael Mechoulam, PhD
Medical Faculty
Hebrew University
Jerusalem

Introduction

Franjo Grotenhermen

This book is a compilation of selected articles from the *Journal of Cannabis Therapeutics: Studies in Endogenous, Herbal, and Synthetic Cannabinoids,* which was edited by Ethan Russo and published by The Haworth Press, Inc., as the official journal of the International Association for Cannabis As Medicine (IACM) (http://www.cannabis-med.org/) from 2001 to 2004.

Just a few years ago, only small clinical studies and case reports on cannabis or individual cannabinoids were available to support their therapeutic potential for most indications. By 2000, only the antiemetic properties of cannabis and THC in cancer patients undergoing chemotherapy and their appetite-enhancing effects in AIDS wasting had been documented by clinical studies with more than fifty subjects. This situation has changed considerably in recent years and will progress further in view of a wide range of ongoing research on medicinal cannabis, much of it initiated by the British company GW Pharmaceuticals, the Center for Medicinal Cannabis Research (CMCR) at the University of California, the Institute for Clinical Research in Berlin, and several other groups. The *Journal of Cannabis Therapeutics* accompanied and supported this initiation of new clinical applications of cannabinoids since its first issue was published in early 2001.

In 2003 the Ministry of Health, Welfare and Sports of the Netherlands made cannabis available in their pharmacies. In 2005, Sativex, a cannabis extract produced by GW Pharmaceuticals, was approved in Canada for the treatment of neuropathic pain in multiple sclerosis—the first formal regulatory acceptance of cannabis for medicinal use since its disappearance from the pharmacopoeias of Western countries in the early-midtwentieth century. In view of the enormous therapeutic potential of cannabinoids, it can be expected that more official regulation by other countries will follow. However, it is difficult to predict where the journey will lead. Besides natural extracts, synthetic agonists to the cannabinoid receptors and inhibitors of endocannabinoid degradation are additional foci of interest and may exert similar effects. For researchers, the patients and our desire to give them access to a valuable and effective treatment represent the goals of our work—a treatment they were often denied for nonmedical reasons. Throughout the world, patients and their personal experiences put medicinal cannabis on the agenda, and it was the intention of the *Journal of Cannabis Therapeutics* to strengthen this force. Anyone who may benefit from using cannabis medicinally should be able to employ it without fear and, if possible, under the guidance of a physician. This is a clear and simple demand, and we hope and expect that civilized countries will heed it.

Including all articles published in the journal during the more than three years of its existence would have been beyond the scope of a single book. Thus, we selected contributions that present a broad overview, allow a good approach to the subject, and are of lasting relevance. Although the emphasis is on selections that deal with the medical use of the cannabis plant, we have also chosen articles on the pharmacology of cannabinoids and the endogenous cannabinoid system, historical reports, and side effect issues.

I would like to thank Dr. Lester Grinspoon of Harvard University who originally proposed the idea of publishing a journal on cannabis therapeutics; the late Dr. Varro Tyler, editor of The Haworth Herbal Press; Bill Cohen, president and publisher of The Haworth Press, Inc.; and Ethan Russo, who allowed the journal to become reality.

PART I:
HISTORICAL NOTES

Chapter 1

The Therapeutic Use
of *Cannabis sativa* (L.)
in Arabic Medicine

Indalecio Lozano

INTRODUCTION

The modern medical and pharmacological literature which deals with
the therapeutic properties of hemp (*Cannabis sativa* L., Cannabaceae)
tends to ignore the valuable contributions of Arabic scientists on the subject. The tradition of the plant's medicinal use was adopted by these scientists from the cultures of the ancient world, having been used for more than
a thousand years as a textile and medicine in Arabia, Mesopotamia, Persia,
Egypt, China, India and extensive areas of Europe (Levey 1979; Escohotado 1989-1990). The role played by the medical, pharmacological and botanical literature of the Greeks in this regard is well-known, dominating
medical circles in Asia Minor, Syria, Egypt and their neighbouring regions
up until the arrival of Islam in the seventh century. The *Materia medica* of
Dioscorides (AD first century), translated into Arabic by Istifān b. Bāsīl in
the days of the caliph al-Mutawakkil (d. AD 861), and the *De Simplicium
Medicamentorum Temperamentis ac Facultatibus Liber VII* of Galen (d.
AD 199) similarly translated by Hunayn b. Ishāq (d. AD 873), were by far
the most important sources for Arabic physicians, and were a decisive stimulus in the development of their knowledge of the plant.

To date, there are only a few works that deal with the history of the therapeutic use of hemp in Arabic medicine (Hamarneh 1972; Levey 1979; Lozano
Camara 1990), and even these only tangentially. The current renewed interest
in research into the curative potential of the plant justifies a review of the subject in light of new Arabic documental sources.

MATERIALS AND METHODS

Medical, pharmacological and botanical literature written in Arabic has been systematically and exhaustively consulted, as far as possible, from the eighth to the eighteenth century. Over the same period, lexicographical, agricultural, literary, legal, historical and geographical sources that were likely to contain data on *Cannabis sativa* (L.) were also examined. The great majority were published texts, though some manuscripts were also examined. Of all the texts reviewed, more than fifty contain information on the plant, although due to limited space not all of them are mentioned in the references of this chapter.

In the Results section, we have focused our attention on the discoverer or pioneer of each therapeutic use, and only the most significant contributions of later authors have been cited. Thus, not all the sources that mention these uses have been included.

This chapter arises out of a background of historical philological studies on Arabic-Islamic medicine, and thus it neither can nor seeks to tackle any debate on the pharmacological mechanisms involved in the therapeutic uses documented here.

RESULTS

Temperament of the Plant, Parts Used and Modes of Preparation and Administration

Arab scientists explained the curative properties of hemp according to the principles of the humoral theory they learned from the Greeks. As is well-known, this theory assumes that each of the simples possesses a characteristic, "temperament," determined by its degrees of "heat, cold, wetness and dryness." Similarly, they largely accepted the opinion of Galen (1821-1833, VI pp. 549 f. and XII, p. 8), who talks of the desiccating and warming power of hemp. However, there is no lack of prestigious authorities who had quite the opposite opinion, stating that cannabis is naturally cold (al-Tabarī 1928, p. 376), or even composed of hot and cold parts (al-Antāki, n.d., I, p. 219; al-Qūsūnī 1979-80, I, p. 56 f.). There is even greater controversy over the definition of the degree of heat and dryness possessed by the plant, with Arab physicians citing properties from the first to the third degree. This is not surprising, if one takes into account that they could find no reference to help them in the works by Galen and Dioscorides, and that the concept of temperament and its degrees do not permit empiric proof in the sense understood by current scientific methods.

The part of the plant that was most used in therapeutic treatments was the seeds, and to a lesser extent the leaves. Methods of preparation differed according to the ailment to be treated, using the oil obtained from the seeds and the juice from the leaves and green seeds.

It was administered externally in the form of ointment in the nose, or orally, or in drops into the ears. Only very rarely is the actual dose which should be used in each treatment' mentioned. It seems that it was commonly used as a simple medicament.

Treatment of Ear Diseases

The first mention of the curative power of hemp in Arabic literature was by Ibn Māsawayh (al-Rāzī 1968, XXI i, p. 124) (d. AD 857), who refers to the oil obtained from hemp seeds and applied in drops into the ear as having the virtue of drying out the "moisture" *(rutūba)* generated by this organ, a curative property which later physicians attribute to the juice of these seeds. In the period in which Ibn Māsawayh lived, the works of Galen and Dioscorides were translated. From them, Arabic physicians learned the use of the juice of green hemp seeds in the treatment of earache caused by an obstruction in the ear (Galen 1821-1833, VI pp. 549 ff.; Dioscorides 1957, p. 304). Continuing this tradition, in the tenth century Ishāq b. Sulaymān (1986, II, p. 133) stated that hemp seed oil relieved earache caused by the "cold" *(bard)* and the moisture in the organ, and also talked, for the first time, of its power to unblock any obstructions there. In the thirteenth century, the botanist from Malaga, Ibn al-Baytār (1291 A.H., II, pp. 115 f.) prescribed hemp seed oil to cure "gases" *(rīh)* in the ear. In the fourteenth century, Ibn al-Jatīb (1972, p. 69) from Granada recommended the use of this oil mixed with gum resin of *Ferula galbaniflua* to relieve "hot pain" *(al-waŷa' al-hārr)* associated with tinnitus aurium. In the sixteenth century, al-Antāki talks of how the leaves of "Anatolian hemp," as he calls it *(al-qinnab al-rūmī)* (Lozano Cámara 1996, pp. 152 ff.), kill the "worms" which develop in the ear, and adds that they have unblocking properties; if you fill the ear with them, all the foreign material which is lodged there will be expelled.

Vernucide and Vermifuge

In the ninth century al-Dimašqī (Ibn al-Baytār 1291 A.H., IV, p. 39) was the first author to mention the vermicidal and vermifugal properties of the plant, noting that it has the power of killing the "worms" *(al-dīdān)* that grow in the body. Between the eleventh and twelfth centuries, the anonymous author of the *'Umdat al-tabīb* (1990, Il, nº 2149) asserted that anyone who has tapeworms should eat hemp seeds, as their shells fill up with the parasites and are then expelled with them in the feces. Between the fourteenth and fifteenth centuries, al-Firūzābādī (1952, I, p. 203) stated that if the seeds of the plant were ingested or applied in the form of ointment over the stomach, this would kill ascaris *(habb al-qar').*

Treatment of Skin Diseases

Ibn Māsawayh (al-Rāzī 1968, XXI i, p. 124) is the first author who refers to the use of hemp in the treatment of pityriasis *(ibriya)* and lichen *(hazāz)*, and suggests that the affected part of the body should be washed with the juice from the leaves. In the eleventh century, Avicenna (1294 A.H., I, p. 434) recommended oil from the seeds for the same purpose. Al-Firūzābādī (1952, I, p. 203) asserted that hemp seeds can be used to treat vitiligo *(al-bahaq)* and leprosy *(al-baras)*.

With regard to the treatment of skin diseases, and halfway between dermatology and cosmetics, al-Rāzī (al-Bīrūnī 1973, I, p. 33) (d. AD 925) was the first to prescribe the use of hemp leaves as a substitute for *Melia azedarach* (L.) (Meliaceae) to stimulate hair growth. According to Ibn Ŷazla (Lozano Cámara 1989-1990, pp. 171 f.) (d. AD 1100), the leaves should be macerated in water and then applied to the roots of the hair.

Purging Qualities

The first reference to the purging properties of hemp was made by al-Dimašqī (Ibn al-Baytār 1291 A.H., IV, p. 39), who stated that the juice from hemp seeds, administered through the nose, purges the brain. In the ninth century this use was also cited by Ṯābit b. Qurra (1928, pp. 21, 97), who included hemp among the simples that can purge the upper part of the liver and eliminate any obstruction produced in this organ. He prescribes that the hemp seeds should be taken with honey mixed with vinegar.

Diuretic Properties

The pioneer of the diuretic power of hemp seeds was Isḥāq b. 'Imrān (Ibn al-Baytār 1291 A.H., IV, p. 39) (d. 907 A.D.). In the opinion of Isḥāq b. Sulaymān (1986, II, p. 133), this property is due to their warming power.

Antiepileptic Properties

Between the tenth and eleventh centuries, al-Maŷūsī (1877, II, p. 116) talked for the first time of the use of hemp in the treatment of epilepsy and prescribed that the patient should be given the juice of the leaves through the nose. In the fifteenth century, al-Badrī (Lozano Cámara 1989-1990, p. 174 f.) provided a spurious tale in which hemp leaves were presented as a remedy that gave an immediate cure to epilepsy.

Carminative Properties

The carminative properties of hemp seeds, already known by Galen, were mentioned for the first time by Ishāq b. Sulaymān. Al-Maŷūsī (1877, II, p. 116) wrote that the leaves have the same property and added that they could be used to treat gases generated in the uterus, intestines, and stomach.

Treatment of Abscesses and Tumours

Between the eleventh and twelfth centuries Ibn Buklāriš (n.d., nº 679) prescribes the juice from hemp leaves to cure abscesses *(jurāŷāt)* occurring in the head. One century later, Ibn al-Baytār stated that if an "oily wax" made with hemp seed oil was applied to hardened tumours *(al-awrām al-ŷāsiya),* the tumours would dissolve.

Liquification and Purging of Humors

Ishāq b. Sulaymān first mentioned that hemp seeds increase the liquidity of the corporal humors. Al-Maŷūsī (1877, II p. 116) attributed the same property to the leaves of the plant and said that they could be used to purge phlegmatic excretions from the stomach. Ibn Habal (1362 A.H. II, p. 185) (d. AD 1213) indicated that hemp seeds were good for evacuating bile and phlegm.

Treatment of the Hardening and Contraction of the Uterus

Ibn al-Baytār (1291 A.H., II, p. 116) prescribed hemp seed oil for treating the hardening and contraction of the uterus.

Painkilling Properties

The use of hemp as a painkiller was not limited to the treatment of earache. Ibn al-Baytār (1291 A.H., II, p. 116) recommended hemp seed oil for soothing neurological pains *(waŷa' al-'asab)*. Around the same time, al-Qazwīnī (1849, p. 293) (d. AD 1283) noted that the juice could be used to soothe ophthalmia.

Antipyretic Properties

Al-Fīrūzābādī (1952, I, p. 203) claimed that hemp seeds were an effective remedy in curing febris quartana *(hummà l-rib')*.

Antiparasitic Properties

Al-Antākī stated that the boiled leaves from "Anatolian hemp" killed lice and nits if used to wash the part of the body where these parasites were present.

Antiemetic Properties

The same al-Antākī attributes antiemetic properties to the seeds from Anatolian hemp.

CONCLUSION

Arab scientists were several centuries ahead of our current knowledge of the curative power of *Cannabis sativa* (L.). They knew of and used its diuretic, antiemetic, antiepileptic, antiinflammatory, and painkilling virtues, among others. For this reason, it seems reasonable to suggest that the data to be found in Arabic literature could be considered as a possible basis for future research on the therapeutic potential of cannabis and hemp seeds. This would seem to be particularly necessary if we take into account that currently the traditional use of the plant among Arab-Islamic peoples of the world has almost completely disappeared due to the legal restrictions which prohibit its cultivation and use.

BIBLIOGRAPHY

Al-Antākī. n.d. *Tadkirat uli l-albāb wa-l-ŷami' li-l-'aŷāb al-'uŷāb.* Beirut: Al-Maktaba al-Taqāfiyya.

Avicenna. 1294 A.H. *Al-Qānūn fi l-tibb.* Būlāq.

Al-Bīrūnī. 1973. *Kitāb al-saydana.* H. M. Said and R. E. Elahie (Eds.). Karachi.

Dioscorides. 1957. *Kitāb al-Hašā'is fi hayūlà l-tibb.* C. E. Dubler and E. Terés (Eds.). Barcelona.

Al-Fīruzābadī. 1952. *Al-Qāmūs al-mu hīt.* Cairo.

Galen. 1821-1833. *Claudii Galeni opera omnia.* C. G. Kuhn (Ed.). Leipzig.

Hamarneh, S. K. 1972. Pharmacy in Medieval Islam and the History of Drug Addiction. *Medical History* 16: 226-237.

Ibn al-Baytār. 1291 A.H. *Kitab al-Ŷami' li-mufradāt al-adwiya wa-l-agdiya.* Būlāq.

Ibn Buklāriš. n.d. *Al-Musta'inī fi l-mufradāt al-tibbiyya.* Ms. al-Jizāna al-'Āmma of Rabat, N. 481.

Ibn Habal. 1362 A.H. *Kitāb al-Mujtārāt fi l-tibb.* Haydarabad: Dā'irat al-Ma'ārif al-'Utmaniyya.

Ibn al-Jatīb. 1972. *Kitāb 'Amal man tabb li-man habb.* M. C. Vázquez de Benito (Ed.). Salamanca: Universidad.

Escohotado, Antonio. 1989-1900. *Historia de las drogas.* Madrid: Alianza.

Ishāq b. Sulaymān. 1986. *Kitāb al-Agdiya.* F. Sezgin (Ed.). Frankfurt am Main: Institute for the History of Arabic-Islamic Science.

Levey, M. 1979. Hashīsh. In: B. Lewis, V. L. Ménage, Ch. Pellat and J. Schacht (Eds.). *The Encyclopaedia of Islam.* Leiden-Iondon: E. J. Brill-Lurac & CO.

Lozano Cámara, Indalecio. 1989-1990. Un fragmento del Kitāb Rāhat al-arwāh fī l-hašīš wā-l-rah. *Miscelánea de Estudios Árabes y Hebráicos* 38 (i): 163-183.

Lozano Cámara, Indalecio. 1990. Acerca de una noticia sobre el *qinnab* en al *Ŷami'* de Ibn al-Baytār. In: E. Garcí Sánchez (Ed.). *Ciencias de la Naturaleza en al-Andalus (Textos y estudios I).* Granada: C.S.I.C.

Lozano Cámara, Indalecio. 1996. Terminología científica árabe del cáñamo. In: C. Álvarez de Morales (Ed.). *Ciencias de la Naturaleza en al-Andalus (Textos y estudios IV).* Granada: C.S.I.C.

Al-Maŷūsī. 1877. *Kāmil al-sinā'al-sina'a al-tibbiyya.* Būlāq.

Al-Qazwīnī. 1849. *Kitāb 'Aŷā'ib al-majlūqāt.* F. Wüstenfeld (Ed.). Göttingen.

Al-Qūsūnī. 1979-1980. *Qāmūs al-atibbā' wa-nāmūs al-alibbā'.* Damascus: Maŷma' al-Luga al-'Arabiyya.

Al-Rāzī. 1968. *Kitāb al-Hāwī fi l-tibb (t. XXI: Fi l-adwiya al-mufrada).* Haydarabad: Dāirat al-Ma'ārif al-'Utmāniyya bi-l-Ŷami'a al-'Utmāniyya.

Al-Tabarī. 1928. *Firdaws al-hikma fi l-tibb.* M. Z. Siddiqi (Ed.). Berlin.

Tābit b. Qurra. 1928. *Kitāb al-Dajīra fi 'ilm al-tibb.* G. Sobhy (Ed.). Cairo: al-Mat ba'a al-Amīriyya.

'Umdat al-tabīb fī ma'rifat al-tibb. 1990. M. 'A. al-Jat tābī (Ed.). Rabat: Akādīmiya al-Mamlaka al-Magribiyya.

UPDATE

Ethan B. Russo

This chapter remains the best short source on this subject available in the English language. The authorities cited in this publication made lasting contributions that heavily affected the Indian branch of Unani medicine, further outlined in a new book chapter (Russo 2005).

This document highlights the extent to which the medical lessons of the past continue to have a great deal to teach us in twenty-first-century Western medicine. Such recognition may do much to reduce the clash of cultures.

REFERENCE

Russo, E. B. 2005. Cannabis in India: Ancient lore and modern medicine. In R. Mechoulam (Ed.), *Cannabinoids as therapeutics: Milestones in drug therapy* (pp. 1-22). Basel, Switzerland: Birkäuser.

Chapter 2

Cognoscenti of Cannabis I: Jacques-Joseph Moreau (1804-1884)

Ethan B. Russo

Jacques-Joseph Moreau (de Tours) was one of the earliest pioneers of modern psychopharmacology (see Figure 2.1). Born in 1804 in Montrésor, France, Moreau pursued medical studies in Tours and Paris, subsequently studying psychiatry under the tutelage of Jean-Étienne Dominique Esquirol, whose eclectic approach to healing the mind included the prescription of therapeutic travel. As part of his duties, Moreau accompanied patients to the Orient, where he was able to observe the effects of—and partake himself of—hashish, the resinous by-product of cannabis (Holmstedt 1973).

Upon his return to France, Moreau investigated the therapeutic possibilities of this substance. He likely is the character known as "Dr. X" who provided hashish in the form of an electuary called *dawamesk* to such literary illuminati as Théophile Gautier, Charles Baudelaire, Alexandre Dumas and Honoré de Balzac of Le Club des Hachichins at the Hôtel Pimodan in Paris.

Moreau was among the first to apply herbal pharmacology systematically to the treatment of mental illness, using the dissociative hallucinogen *Datura stramonium* L. Solonaceae (Moreau 1841). Moreau espoused a theory that such compounds mirrored effects of insanity, and from them, physicians might gain insight into psychopathological conditions and even their amelioration. He then applied this concept to cannabis. His 1845 book, *Du Hachisch et de l'Alientation Mentale: Études Psychologiques* (Moreau 1845) is a classic in the field. Unfortunately, it is a document that few have actually viewed themselves. It had a limited press run and was never reprinted until a 1980 facsimile edition was issued by Ressources of Paris and Geneva. On the infrequent occasions that original copies appear on the rare book market, prices in the thousands of dollars are obtained.

Handbook of Cannabis Therapeutics
© 2006 by The Haworth Press, Inc. All rights reserved.
doi:10.1300/5741_03

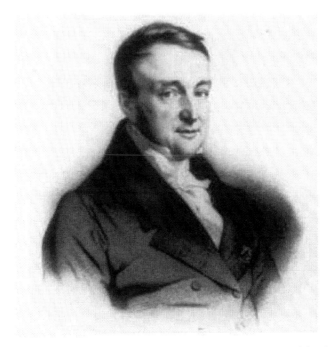

FIGURE 2.1. Portrait of Moreau in 1845, by N. E. Maurin, Library of the Academy of Medicine, Paris, France.

The book was not translated into English until 1973, as *Hashish and Mental Illness* (Moreau 1973), but this volume, too, is out of print. In an early passage, Moreau observes (p. 211):

> One of the effects of hashish that struck me most forcefully and which generally gets the most attention is that manic excitement always accompanied by a feeling of gaiety and joy inconceivable to those who have never experienced it. I saw in it a mean of effectively combatting the fixed ideas of depressives, disrupting the chain of their ideas, of unfocusing their attention on such and such a subject.

In his early efforts to apply this knowledge of cannabis to patients, Moreau observed mixed results, and he began to question its utility. However, he persisted in his efforts. Subsequently, some years later, Moreau reported an in-depth case study of a man with intractable lypemania, a type of obsessive melancholia (Moreau de Tours 1857), and its apparent resolution with cannabis therapy. Spontaneous cure might be surmised, but subsequent evidence supports a rational basis for its efficacy with the work of Muller-Vahl on obsessive-compulsive disorder (Muller-Vahl et al. 1998, 1999).

Close examination reveals that this article, presented here in English for the for the first time, was apparently written by one *"Homo, interne provisoire,"* but obviously under the close direction and supervision of Moreau at the Hospice de Bicètre. It presents an important insight into nineteenth-century medicine, psychopharmacology and cannabis usage.

According to Bo Holmstedt (Efron 1967) (p. 7), one of Moreau's favorite pronouncements was, "Insanity is the dream of the man who is awake." Moreau died in 1884 at age eighty.

In the intervening century, many have judged as a failure Moreau's efforts to therapeutically apply cannabis. This view is not universal, however. Professor E. Perrot of the Faculté de Pharmacie de Paris stated in 1926 (Rouhier 1975), "The Indian hemp, to take but one example, quite cheated the hopes of Moreau de Tours, but it would be imprudent to affirm that it will not be better utilized by the psychiatry of tomorrow!" [translation EBR] (p. IX). This sentiment is a useful one to consider in the modern age, as the search for better pharmacotherapeutic agents continues.

REFERENCES

Efron, Daniel H. 1967. *Ethnopharmacologic search for psychoactive drugs. Proceedings of a symposium held in San Francisco, California, January 28-30, 1967.* Washington, DC: U.S. Public Health Service.

Holmstedt, Bo. 1973. Introduction to Moreau de Tours. In H. Peters and G. G. Nahas (eds.), *Hashish and Mental Ilness.* New York: Raven Press.

Moreau de Tours, Jacques-Joseph. 1857. Lypemanie ave stupeur; tendance a la demence.-Traitement par l'extract (principe resineux) de cannabis indica.-Guerison. *Gazette des Hopitaux Civils et Militaires* 30:391.

Moreau, Jacques-Joseph. 1841. Traitement des hallucinations par le datura stramonium. *Gazette Medicale de Paris* (October).

Moreau, Jacques-Joseph. 1845. *Du hachisch et de l'aliénation mentale: Études psychologiques.* Paris: Fortin Masson.

Moreau, Jacques-Joseph. 1973. *Hashish and mental illness.* New York: Raven Press.

Muller-Vahl, K. R., H. Kolbe, U. Schneider, and H. M. Emrich. 1998. Cannabinoids: Possible role in patho-physiology and therapy of Gilles de la Tourette syndrome. *Acta Psychiatr Scand* 98 (6):502-506.

Muller-Vahl, K. R., U. Schneider, H. Kolbe, and H. M. Emrich. 1999. Treatment of Tourette's syndrome with delta-9-tetrahydrocannabinol [letter]. *Am J Psychiatry* 156 (3):495.

Rouhier, Alexandre. 1975. *La plante qui fait les yeux émerveillés: Le peyotl.* Nouv. éd. revue et augm. ed. [s.l.]: G. Trédaniel.

Chapter 3

Cognoscenti of Cannabis II:
Simeon Seth on Cannabis

David Deakle

Only a few original texts concerning a physician's actual practice of medicine survive from the eleventh and twelfth centuries of the Byzantine Empire. Of these, Simeon Seth's *Lexicon on the Properties of Foods (Syntagma de alimentorum facultatibus)* is perhaps the most important for understanding how dietetics were applied in Byzantine and Arabic culture.

Although his date of birth is uncertain, Simeon Seth was likely born in 1003 in Constantinople, though his family was probably from the environs of Syrian Antioch. His name appears in the English literature under a number of forms: Symeon, Symeone, Sethi, Sethy, Seth, etc. In the century prior to Seth's birth, Antioch had been reclaimed by the Byzantine Empire from the Arabs (AD 969). Seth benefited from a fluent knowledge of both the Arabic and Greek languages, and he became fascinated with the medical books of both therapeutic traditions. His translation skills, however, were not limited to medical topics. Seth was also responsible for the translation from Arabic into Greek of a popular Indian fable. At the request of Alexis I Comnenus (d. 1118). Seth translated this tale of two jackals, Calila and Dimna (in Greek, Stephanites and Ichnelates), as a moral work directed at courtly courtesans as to how people should behave.

At the age of twenty-five, Seth found favor with the imperial court, and became the medical officer in the court of three Byzantine emperors: Constantine VIII (d.1028), Romain III (1028-1034), and Michael VII Ducas (1071-1078). Seth was given the title master of the Palace at Antioch, and was physician to the emperor. In addition to his work as a physician to the court, at the age of thirty-five, Seth retired to the convent at Mount Olympus to devote himself solely to the study of science and religious life.

Handbook of Cannabis Therapeutics
© 2006 by The Haworth Press, Inc. All rights reserved.
doi:10.1300/5741_04

Seth's interests included not only medicine and religion but also the larger medieval disciplines of Aristotelean physics and natural science. He wrote *Conspectus Rerum Naturalium,* a work on natural science with reflections on heaven and earth, matter and form, place and time, soul and spirit, and the five senses. The Byzantine men of science and medicine built their theories upon the previous advances by Nicandrus, Dioscorides and Galen, but they gradually added "remedies from the east, from Arabia and Persia, to those obtained from their native flora and fauna" (Vogel 1967, p. 293). While others such as Theophanies Nonnus, Michael Psellos and John Actuarius addressed the important relation of food and health, the most important treatment of the medical properties of food and herbs was Simeon Seth's *Syntagma.* Seth was the first to mention, and to translate into Greek, the information about a number of natural substances and medications employed in the oriental world.

After a brilliant career serving the imperial court under three emperors, researching natural science and medicine, and exploring the religious life, the master of the Palace at Antioch, Simeon Seth, died at the age of seventy-eight in the year 1081 at the monastery on Mount Olympus.

Seth's *Syntagma de Alimentorum Facultatibus* is a catalog of various foods and herbs and their properties or effects. In 1868 Bernhard Langkavel produced a critical edition of Seth's *Syntagma* using a number of Greek manuscripts (Langkavel 1868).

Seth's treatment of the plants is arranged alphabetically. Under "K" (kappa in Greek) Seth treats cannabis *(Kanabos)* in a short paragraph. In Langkavel's edition there are two textual variants noted in Seth's treatment of cannabis. The first concerns the title. In manuscript K the heading reads "cannabis seeds" *(kannabourosperma).* The other variant (also in manuscript K) concerns the Greek word *touton,* which is changed from the accusative to the genitive *toutou.* This variant occurs in a phrase that is problematic and difficult to translate or understand. Perhaps the variant is an attempt to clarify the difficult meaning of the phrase, as will be noted.

Seth's treatment of cannabis has a certain medical significance. The first possibility concerns the harm of cannabis. This is found in the opening sentence when he says, "The seed of cannabis when eaten has about equal [resembling] harm as coriander." There are also several references to the psychoactive effects of cannabis and also its usage among the Arabs. Particularly, Seth notes that when "eaten without moderation . . . it produces wandering of mind [delirium]." Does the use of the phrase *without moderation* imply that cannabis was used also *with* moderation and that such usage did not produce delirium? The last phrase having possible medical significance is, "The dried leaves being drunk . . . produce a hospitable [strange?] drunkenness and lack of perception [lack of sensation/or unconsciousness] for the eater."

A translation of the Greek text of the Langkavel edition follows. The words in brackets [ ] indicate an alternative translation of a word or phrase, or a supplied word; the words in double brackets [[ ]] indicate a difficult or obscure meaning:

> The seed of cannabis when eaten has about equal [resembling] harm as coriander. For being eaten without moderation, as that [coriander?], it produces wandering of mind [delirium]. The dried leaves being drunk as/like whole meal or rather as a drink [[the same whole meal being dried]], produces a hospitable [strange] drunkenness and lack of perception [lack of sensation/or unconsciousness?] for the eater. Among the Arabs this is crushed [chewed?] in place of [instead of/for] wine and they are intoxicated; but the offspring [product of the plant] dries/drains just as camphor [literally: but it dries/drains/ parches the product just as camphor].

Some further explanation of the bracketed and double-bracketed phrases is required. In the second line the word *coriander* is not used; however, the remote demonstrative "that" *(ekeinos)* most probably refers back to coriander in the previous sentence.

In lines four and five the double-bracketed "the same whole meal being dried" does not make sense. Seth has just described the dried leaves as a drink, but then he refers to the same whole meal being dried. There is a possibility that this phrase pertains to a preparation of hashish. Vogel (1967, p. 293) indicates that Seth refers to hashish. As noted, this difficult phrase is where one manuscript has changed *touton* (accusative) to *toutou* (genitive). It should be acknowledged that the 1542 Latin translation by Leonhart Fuchs is also problematic at this same point (Fuchs 1999).

Another bracket is used in line four with the word *hospitable*. While this might mean "strange," the primary meaning of *xeven* concerns hospitableness and this is confirmed in the Fuchs' Latin translation where *hospitalem* is used.

In the sixth line "lack of perception" could also be translated "lack of sensation" or even "unconsciousness." The Greek word is literally *anaisthasian,* from which the modern term *anaesthesia* is derived. However, "lack of perception" is probably the intended meaning, given the eleventh-century context.

In line sevem "crushed" could mean "chewed," and at the end of the same line the Greek *anti* is here translated as "in place of" wine, but it may well mean "for" or "instead of" wine; the use of "for wine" is what the Latin translation by Fuchs indicates with the use of *pro uino*.

The end of line seven and all of line eight demonstrate a number of grammatical problems. The first relates to the subject-verb agreement. In the Greek text, *ekmethuousi* is an active verb, third-person plural. The meaning here is that they, the Arabs, are drunk or intoxicated by the use of cannabis. The Latin text of Fuchs changes the number to a third person singular *inebriat,* which would mean that it, the cannabis concoction, intoxicates and thus Fuchs maintains or preserves the active voice of the verb. The second grammatical problem is found in the final phrase of the paragraph. Literally the phrase reads, "but it dries/drains/parches the product just as camphor." The problem here concerns the antecedent of "it." The Greek verb *xerainei* is third-person singular. If the antecedent is the "Arabs" (meaning, they dry the plant product as they dry camphor), there is a number disagreement between the subject (Arabs) and the third-person singular verb. There is the possibility that Seth meant "the plant product is dried like camphor," but the verb is active, not passive voice. Another possibility is that the antecedent of "it" is that difficult earlier phrase "the whole meal being dried." Here Fuchs' Latin translation provides no real help for the Latin *desiccat* is also third-person singular and active voice. It should be noted that the Greek *gonan* denotes "offspring," "race" or "plant product" and probably refers to the seeds. This is confirmed by Fuchs' translation in which he employs the Latin *semen genitale,* "the offspring seed."

Given that Fuchs' Latin translation was not mentioned in Langkavel's edition, and that it may well reflect an attempt to correct some of the grammatical difficulties of Seth's Greek text, a translation of Fuchs' passage concerning Simeon Seth may be helpful. The following is a rough translation of the pertinent passage from Leonhart Fuchs, *De Historia Stirpium Commentarii Insignes,* 1542 (Fuchs 1999, vol 2, p. 392). The word in brackets [ ] indicates a supplied or implied word, and the two phrases in double brackets [[ ]] remain difficult to translate or have some obscure meaning.

> The cannabis seed, having been eaten, brings the same harm as Coriander: if it is eaten without moderation, it produces delirium as the same [i.e., Coriander]. Indeed the dried leaf, when drunk, as meal, or rather [[as dried meal for a drink]] produces a hospitable drunkenness and lack of sensation by the eater. For it is crushed or kneaded among the Arabs for wine, and it inebriates. [[It dries the offspring seed like Camphor.]]

While containing only one brief paragraph on cannabis or cannabis seeds, the *Syntagma* of Simeon Seth is yet important. Clearly this Byzantine physician and man of science reflected his knowledge of the use of cannabis in the eleventh century and included it among the many herbs used in his day. Seth indicated that the plant could be abused when taken without moderation or in excess, but he also supported the relatively negligible harm of the plant, noting it to be akin to that of coriander. He was also aware of the psychoactive properties of the herb, which may produce delirium, lack of perception or a hospitable drunkenness. While some phrases are either grammatically problematic or obscure, the tone and gist of Seth's blurb on cannabis remains clear: cannabis was known and employed as an herb in the medieval world.

BIBLIOGRAPHY

Brunet, M.-E. 1939. *Siméon Seth, Médecin de l'Empereur Michel Doucas: Sa Vie-Son Cuvre*. Bordeaux: Imprimerie–librairie Delmas.

Fuchs, L. 1999. *De Historia Stirpium Commentarii Insignes, 1542*. In F.G. Meyer, E.E. Trueblood and J.L. Heller (eds.), *The Great Herbal of Leonhart Fuchs*, 2 volumes. Stanford, CA: Stanford University Press.

Kazhdan, A.P., and A.W. Epstein. 1985. *Change in Byzantine Culture in the Eleventh and Twelfth Centuries*. Berkeley: University of California Press.

Langkavel, B. (ed.). 1868. *Simeonis Sethi, Syntagma de Alimentorum Facultatibus*. Leipzig: B.G. Teubner.

Runciman, S. 1933. *Byzantine Civilisation*. London: Edward Arnold.

Sjöberg, L.-O. 1962. *Stephanites und Ichnelates*. Stockholm: Almqvist & Wiksell.

Vogel, K. 1967. Byzantine Science. In J.M. Hussey (ed.), *The Cambridge Medieval History IV: The Byzantine Empire, Part II: Government, Church and Civilization* (pp. 264-305). Cambridge: Cambridge University.

Chapter 4

The Medical Use of Cannabis
Among the Greeks and Romans

James L. Butrica

INTRODUCTION

This chapter is intended to update our knowledge of the medical use of
cannabis in the Classical world, a topic on which the only serious discussion is Brunner (1973, largely repeated in Brunner 1977). While no previously unknown texts have been discovered in the meantime, the availability
of the Thesaurus Linguae Graecae (a searchable database of ancient Greek
literature developed by Dr. Brunner and others) now permits a more thorough investigation of the ancient sources than ever before; the result has
been not only to reveal some additional treatments not known to Brunner
but also to suggest a new understanding of some of the data.

Cannabis went by a variety of names. In the first century CE, Dioscorides
(1907-1914, *Materia Medica* 3.148) mentions *kannabion* (a diminutive form,
"little cannabis," "dear cannabis"), *skhoenostrophion* ("rope-twister"), and *aste-
rion* ("little star"). An ancient scholarly note in line 181 of Aristophanes's com-
edy *The Acharnians* says that *sphendamnos* was another name for cannabis
because its fibres were used to make slings *(sphendonai)*. Finally, the lexicon of Hesychius, compiled probably in the fifth century CE, adds *phalis* as
another equivalent *(phi, p.108)*; it is unclear whether there is any connection
with the fact that *phalis* is also attested in Pausanias as the title of a priestess
of Hera at Argos. Dioscorides notes as well that cannabis was sometimes
called "domesticated" or "tame" cannabis *(hêmeros)* to distinguish it from
another medicinal plant now identified as hemp mallow *(Althaea kan-
nabina);* this was called, in Greek, either *hydrastina* or "wild" cannabis
(agria) and, in Latin, "terminal" *(terminalis;* this use of *terminalis* is not attested in any Latin source or recognized by any Latin dictionary, probably
because we know it only from the Greek writer Dioscorides; it perhaps re-

Handbook of Cannabis Therapeutics
doi:10.1300/5741_05

23

flects a tendency of the plant to grow along paths and hedges and other borders *[termini],* as noted in the *Herbarium* of ps.-Apuleius, 106). Although wild cannabis will not be discussed in this chapter, a few of the several ancient references to its medical use are included in Appendix I on the grounds that some ancient medical writers, especially Pliny the Elder (1967), make otherwise unsupported claims about the medical use of tame cannabis that closely resemble well-attested uses of wild cannabis.

In general, cannabis was a completely uncontroversial element of everyday life for both the Greeks and the Romans, used to make mats, shoes, cloth, and especially ropes. The Romans especially favored hemp for the rope in hunting nets; among the Greeks, on the other hand, it was more often used to make the nautical ropes called *kaloi,* used for furling or rolling up the sails and hence known, in English, as "reefing ropes."

Medically, it was used to treat horses as well as humans; the evidence for its veterinary use is summarized in Appendix II. In the treatment of humans, it was part of the physician's armamentarium, though no more so than a host of other plants. Several parts of the plant could be used. Pliny mentions using the uncooked root on burns, but he may have been thinking of wild cannabis here. Another source has cannabis ash used in a poultice, but does not say which part of the plant was burned to produce it. Fresh leaves were used to dress horses' sores, dried ones against nosebleed. But it is the seeds whose use is attested most often, both "green" and mature, distinguished in Greek as *karpos* ("fruit") and *sperma* ("seed").

ABSENCE OF MENTION

Before beginning the survey proper, it is equally important to note where cannabis does *not* appear in our ancient medical texts.

First of all, though the medical use of cannabis is recorded in the encyclopedia of Pliny the Elder (written in the middle of the first century CE), it is absent from the medical writings of another contemporary encyclopedist, A. Cornelius Celsus (first half of the first century CE), and it seems to be mentioned elsewhere in Latin only in late authors who for the most part translated directly from Greek, such as Marcellus Empiricus (fifth century CE) and pseudo-Theodorus (sixth century CE?). Hence, there is nothing to show conclusively that cannabis was used medically by the Romans, though given the scarcity of evidence I would be reluctant to say that no Roman was ever treated with it. It is conceivable, for example, that when a late Roman authority like Marcellus cites an otherwise unattested use of cannabis, it comes from Roman folk medicine.

Second, the medical use of cannabis is absent from the works of such gynecologists as Soranus (second century CE), though this does not necessarily prove that it was never used in treating women. In fact, though one of the principal uses of cannabis seed is one that seems to us to be logically applicable only to males, Aëtius (sixth century CE) says that it could be used on women as well. Perhaps the most we can say is that it seems not to have been used for any condition specific to women.

Third, medical cannabis is absent from the writings of Hippocrates (fifth century BCE) and his followers, known collectively as the Hippocratic Corpus, though we need not infer that he rejected its use: despite its eventual ubiquity in the classical world, cannabis was evidently unknown to the Greeks before the fifth century BCE, and so Hippocrates's silence may well represent ignorance, not conscious rejection, though absolute certainty is of course impossible.

THE EMERGENCE OF CANNABIS

Cannabis first appears in Greek literature in the celebrated passage where the historian Herodotus, an approximate contemporary of Hippocrates, describes how the ancient Scythians used to toss cannabis seeds onto red-hot rocks and inhale the vapors that were released (4.73-75). Since Herodotus is not concerned with the medical use of the plant, there is, strictly speaking, no reason to discuss the passage at length here; but Brunner (1973, pp. 345-347) discusses it, and the archaeological discoveries alluded to there in note 45 require some rethinking of what Herodotus described, especially since modern retellings of Herodotus's account continue to abound in inaccuracies and fanciful inventions: Emboden (1972, p. 223), for example, has the Scythians using rocks from funeral pyres, and claims that Herodotus describes them dancing and singing in response.

It should be remembered that cannabis seeds were used by the Scythians not recreationally but as a part of their death ritual: instead of a wake, they put the corpse of the deceased into a wagon, and for forty days took it on visits to the homes of friends and kin, where it was served at table along with the other guests. It was at the end of this period of mourning that men resorted to the hemp baths as a form of cleansing (the head being washed first with soap), while the women pursued a different treatment (they smeared a paste of cypress, cedar, and frankincense on their bodies and allowed it stand for a day; when removed, it left their skin fragrant, clean, and shiny).

The nature of the ritual is relevant to the interpretation of the words with which Herodotus describes how the Scythians reacted to the vapor from the seeds, *agamenoi ôruontai,* which are often translated as "[they] howl with delight" or the like. The onomatopoetic verb *ôruontai* certainly describes howling and is used, for example, to describe the sound of wolves (*LSJ* [H.G. Liddell, R. Scott, H.S. Jones, *A Greek-English Lexikon* (Oxford 1968)] *s.v.* "*howl,* prop. of wolves and dogs"); the most recent translation of Herodotus (by R. Waterfield [Oxford 1998]) is therefore certainly wrong to use "shriek." As to the participle *agamenoi,* which describes the state of mind in which the Scythians do their howling, this is invariably translated as "with delight," "with pleasure," or the like; but *LSJ, s.v. ôrumomai,* offers only this passage when illustrating the sense "to howl with joy," and in fact it notes that elsewhere in Herodotus it means "to howl in mourning." The latter is closer to what one might expect in a ritual connected with death, and in fact the basic meaning of the verb *agamai* is "to be amazed" or "astounded," perhaps expressing here a state of stupefaction. The currently favoured translation may reflect a modern expectation that those who inhale such vapors ought to have a "reefer madness" experience and become hysterical, but hilarity conflicts with the fundamentally solemn nature of the experience.

The archaeological discoveries affect the interpretation of the "tents" involved. Herodotus notes that "they lean three poles against one another, cover the poles with felted woolen blankets, making sure that they fit together as tightly as possible, and then put red-hot stones from the fire on to a dish which has been placed in the middle of the pole-and-blanket structure" (4.73); subsequently "the Scythians take cannabis seeds, crawl in under the felt blankets, and throw the seeds on to the glowing stones" (trans. Waterfield). Tombs excavated in Russia have yielded not only an example of the brazier on which the stones were placed but two sets of those "tent-poles" as well. Perhaps the most accessible account is Artamonov (1965, p. 239). There is an illustration of objects recovered from one of the tombs, namely a pot containing hemp seeds, a "censer" that would have held the hot rocks onto which the seeds were thrown, and six "sticks" that "formed the frame of an 18-inch-high tent in which the hemp smoke was collected." Because of their height, however, these poles could never have formed a viable sauna or spirit lodge, which the Scythians are sometimes thought to have used, and Waterfield's translation is consistent with this, rendering the verb *hypoduô* as "crawl," as the Scythians would have to do in order to insert their heads into such a structure at ground level.

Since Herodotus's account shows that the Greeks were already familiar with vapor baths (he states at 4.75 that the seeds release a vapor which no Greek vapor bath could surpass), it should not be surprising that some of them may have adopted the Scythian habit of using hemp seed there; that much at least can be inferred from the fact that Hesychius's lexicon (*kappa* 673) records a verb *kannabisthênai* ("to get cannabissed," in effect), defined as "to grow sweaty and hot from the effect of cannabis." It is striking, however, that this definition makes no reference to the cannabis "seizing the head" (the standard euphemism for intoxication), though this just might be subsumed under "to grow hot," since we will see that cannabis seed (eaten, however, rather than inhaled in vapor form) was thought to have a "warming" effect on the body.

Apart from Herodotus, the evidence for Greek familiarity with cannabis in the late fifth and early fourth centuries BCE is ambiguous, consisting of somewhat later scholarly notes that identify certain objects mentioned in comedies of Aristophanes as made from hemp (see the scholia [ancient scholarly notes] to Aristophanes, *Acharnians* 181, *Knights* 129 and 954, *Wasps* 394, and *Plutus* 268); these interpretations, however, may be nothing more than ahistorical assumptions by scholars who lived in a world where hemp products were ubiquitous.

But by about the middle of the fourth century BCE we have evidence for a new use of cannabis seeds: their consumption as a food. Fr. 13 of the comic poet Ephippus constitutes a list of *tragêmata* or "snacks" consumed while drinking at a symposium (the ancient equivalent of the modern Greek *mezedhes*), including *kannabides*. This is a plural form, though probably not (as always assumed) of *kánnabis,* accented on the first syllable and supposedly designating cannabis seed here (though the seed is elsewhere called *karpos* or *sperma*), but of *kannabís,* accented on the last syllable and designating a confection of cannabis seeds and honey. Lexica of ancient Greek do not recognize the existence of *kannabís* = "cannabis seed cake," but the other foods in Ephippus's list are prepared rather than raw, and *kannabís* in this sense would have the same relationship to *kannabos* (an alternative form of *kannabís*) that *sesamís,* meaning "sesame seed cake," has to *sésamos,* meaning "sesame seed."

We will encounter this recreational consumption of the seeds again in the physician Galen, who confirms that they were enjoyed for their psychoactive effect.

We cannot tell when the medical use of cannabis began; since, as far as we understand, the Greeks were eating the seeds before they were using them medicinally, it was perhaps inspired by observations regarding the physiological effects of that consumption. Whenever it began, it was evidently well established by the time of our earliest references to it, which come in the first century CE.

Probably the earliest surviving account of the medical use of cannabis is the entry in the *Materia Medica* of the Greek physician Dioscorides, published around 65 CE, followed closely by the one in the *Historia*

Naturalis of Pliny the Elder, finished in 77 CE and dedicated to the emperor Titus. Despite the likelihood that Dioscorides deserves priority, I shall begin with Pliny; he is the only classical Roman writer to discuss the medical use of cannabis, and he lists more medical uses than anyone else, though he is sometimes in conflict with other authorities.

Pliny's *Historia Naturalis* has two substantial entries for hemp, one concerned principally with its use in making rope (Pliny the Elder 1967, 19.273-274), the other on its medical use (20.259):

> Cannabis in siluis primum nata est, nigrior foliis et asperior. Semen eius extinguere genituram uirorum dicitur. Sucus ex eo uermiculos aurium et quodcumque intrauerit eicit, sed cum dolore capitis, tantaque uis ei est, ut aquae infusus coagulare eam dicatur; et ideo iumentorum aluo succurrit potus in aqua. Radix articulos contractos emollit in aqua cocta, item podagras et similes impetus; ambustis cruda inlinitur, sed saepius mutatur priusquam arescat.

> Cannabis, rather dark and rough in respect to its leaves, first grew in the forests. Its seed is said to extinguish men's semen. A liquid from this casts out ear-worms and whatever animal has entered, but with a headache, and its force is so strong that it is said to coagulate water when poured into it; and so it is good for farm-animals' bellies when drunk in water. Cooked in water, the root softens contracted joints, likewise gouts and similar attacks; uncooked it is spread on burns, but is changed rather often before it dries out.

As can be seen from passage A in Appendix I, Pliny's description of the original plant as dark and rough of leaf resembles Dioscorides's description of wild cannabis as having darker and rougher leaves than tame. Perhaps this reflects a belief that tame cannabis had been bred from wild cannabis (Herodotus already distinguishes between cultivated and wild varieties of the plant known to the Scythians); or perhaps—and not for the last time—Pliny confused the two plants or carelessly ignored the distinction.

Whether or not this is the earliest surviving account of Greco-Roman medical cannabis, it is certainly our single fullest catalogue of medical uses, though Pliny is explicit about the nature of only four of the five treatments that he records:

1. *The use of the seeds:* Pliny does not say how the seeds were used, nor is he explicit about why. His comment that they "extinguish the semen" recalls modern claims about reductions in sperm levels in frequent users (cf. Brunner 1973, pp. 349, 351 [with n. 33], and 353);

but if the same phenomenon is indeed involved in both cases, one wonders just how the ancients were able to make such an observation. Brunner (1973, p. 349) interprets this and similar ancient comments as references to impotence; it is more likely, however, that they reflect a belief that the seeds have a "drying" quality (as that was understood in ancient physiology), and a passage in Aëtius will show us what appears to have been the main medical purpose of the seeds, which was precisely to "dry up" leaking semen.

2. *Its use in treating the ears:* Pliny refers to a *sucus* made from the seed that was used to clear vermin out of the ears. Unfortunately, *sucus* is a term of wide application that in a context such as this could designate either a natural juice like sap or a prepared potion. Logically, however, Pliny ought to be referring to the same thing as the *khylos* named in our Greek sources (discussed later) as a treatment for the ears, but no Greek writer has this *khylos* being used against "ear-worms." These vermin were perhaps first mentioned by the satirist Lucilius (second century BCE), but they seem to have been a particular problem in the early Empire, since Pliny records three other remedies for them (Pliny the Elder 1967, 20.256, 23.85, 28.65). Instead, Dioscorides and Galen say that the *khylos* was used for treating pains and inflammations associated with the ears. This is the first—and certainly not the last—time that we must question whether we can take Pliny at his word and assume that he has tapped into a medical tradition not attested in our other sources, or whether he was mistaken because he had difficulty in understanding a Greek source, used defective texts of Greek medical writers, or was simply confused. In fact, there is a second example of this same dilemma here, since headaches, which Pliny ascribes to the use of this *sucus* in the ears, are elsewhere associated with eating the seeds.

3. Sucus *as a remedy for the "bellies" of farm animals:* If Pliny means that it was used to prevent or control diarrhea (a Latin word meaning "therefore" connects this reference to the ability to coagulate water), this is another use known to him alone. If, on the other hand, he is alluding to the seed-based remedy for tapeworms attested in the treatment of both humans and horses (see below), this remedy does not involve the preparation of a *khylos,* only a combination of chopped seeds and water filtered to remove the grit.

4. *The use of the cooked root on joints and against gout:* No other medical authority mentions any medical use for the cannabis root; on the other hand, two passages in Dioscorides (passages A and B in Appendix I) refer to a poultice made from the boiled root of wild cannabis

supposedly effective against inflammations and chalk stones *(Materia Medica)* or against chalk stones and twisted sinews *(Euporista)*.
5. *The use of the raw root on burns:* No other medical authority mentions any use for the uncooked root of cannabis, but we have recipes (including passage C in Appendix I) for preparations supposedly effective against such eruptions on the head as melicerides (encysted tumors) that use the "dry" root of wild cannabis.

Pliny is a source that should be used with the greatest caution; while he provides information that other sources do not, some of his "facts" could be argued to result from confusing different uses of cannabis, or from confusing the medical uses of cannabis and of wild cannabis.

Dioscorides's *Materia Medica* is a complete guide to ancient medicines, describing in its botanical section both the appearance and the medical uses of the plants discussed; its entry for cannabis includes more or less the same two points with which Pliny began (Dioscorides 1907-1914, *Materia Medica* 3.149.1):

κάνναβις· φυτὸν εὔχρηστον τῷ βίῳ πρὸς τὰς τῶν εὐτονωτ σχοινίων πλοκάς. φύλλα δὲ φέρει παραπλήσια τῇ μελίᾳ, δυσώδη, κα μακρούς, κενούς, καρπὸν στρογγύλον, ἐσθιόμενον, ὃς πλείων βρ σβέννυσι γονήν· χλωρὸς δὲ χυλισθεὶς ἁρμόζει πρὸς τὰς τῶν ἀ ἀλγηδόνας ἐνσταζόμενος.

Cannabis: A plant useful for life on account of the twisting of well-strung ropes. It bears foul-smelling leaves resembling the ash, large hollow stems, a round fruit which is eaten, and when consumed in quantity extinguishes the semen; if infused when green, it is suitable for instilling against ear-aches.

Dioscorides perhaps described the leaves more clearly in another work when he wrote of the leaves of the eupatorion that they "are set at a distance and strongly split into 5 or more parts, looking much like those of the cinquefoil or cannabis" (Dioscorides 1907-1914, *Materia medica* 4.41; much the same information is provided by Pliny the Elder 1967, 25.65 and Oribasius 1933, *Collectiones medicae* 11.*epsilon*.20).

Though he too seems not to be explicit about the medical use of the seeds, Dioscorides records the valuable information, absent from Pliny's account, that they affected the body as a result of being eaten and that they had to be consumed in substantial quantities to produce the drying effect.

With regard to the treatment for earaches, Dioscorides specifies that the seeds were prepared while still green and immature. The participle *khylistheis,* translated above as "infused," shows that they were subjected to the process called *khylismos,* which resulted in a *khylos,* a juice combining substances from both the seeds and the liquid in which they were infused; such a *khylos* made from green cannabis seed is mentioned in another work of Dioscorides (Dioscorides 1907-1914, *Euporista* 1.54) as one of several preparations effective against "pains and inflammations around the ears" if instilled while warm.

Brunner (1973, pp. 350 and 353) understands the liquid used in the ears as "seed-juice," but pressing the seeds would surely yield oil rather than "juice." According to *LSJ, khylizô* means to extract juice from a plant through either infusion or decoction, but an examination of Dioscorides's actual usage reveals that the process involved only infusion, not decoction. It was evidently common enough to be mentioned well over 100 times in the *Materia Medica* alone, and it was normally applied to plants (there is an entire section on how to *khylizein* dry botanical material), though there is also one formula for asses' dung infused in wine as a remedy against scorpion bites. The plant might be worked whole, root and all, or only one part might be used (roots, stalks, grasses, leaves, and seeds are all attested explicitly), or some combination of two or more of these. Whatever was being processed was first prepared, almost always by chopping, though there are a few references to preparing roots by bruising. To this a liquid would then be added. One recipe suggests water or wine, another rain water or old wine; other liquids mentioned include warm water, *passum* (a very sweet wine made from raisins), oxymel (a combination of vinegar and honey), and honey-wine or mead (mentioned three times, twice as *melikraton,* once as *hydromel*). A period of steeping presumably followed in all cases, though it is mentioned explicitly only a few times, and only two recipes specify the length (five days in both cases; two others say "sufficient days"). This steeping did not involve the application of heat; a few formulas in the *Materia Medica* specify a period of boiling, but it always follows the steeping (hence the inappropriateness of "decoction" as a translation of *khylos*). After steeping (and sometimes boiling), the plant material would be strained (a strainer is mentioned once) or squeezed in a press (again mentioned only once, but its use was presumably standard) to extract the liquid, which constituted the *khylos*. While the creation of this liquid was obviously the goal with cannabis seed and with some of the other formulas, in other cases the goal was instead to transform the plant material itself, which would subsequently be dried, sometimes in sun, sometimes in shade, before use, while the *khylos* would apparently be discarded (if not already boiled away). Thus the preparation that was warmed and instilled into the ear against inflammations and pains would have been produced by chopping green cannabis seeds, soaking them for a period in water or some mildly alcoholic liquid such as wine, and finally pressing out the fluid. If this is indeed the same as the *sucus* mentioned by Pliny as having the ability to "coagulate" water, then uncertainties about the liquid used to produce it make it difficult to comment on the speculation offered at Brunner (1973, p. 353).

The medical use of cannabis continues to be well attested in the second century CE in the writings of the Greek physician Galen. His work *De Simplicium Medicamentorum Temperamentis et Facultatibus* (On the temperaments and properties of simple medications) offers an evaluation of the utility of the seeds which again begins with the very same two points made by Pliny and Dioscorides (Galen 1821, XII.8):

Καννάβεως ὁ καρπὸς ἄφυσός τε καὶ ξηραντικὸς εἰς τοσοῦτόν ἐστιν ὡς, εἰ πλείων βρωθείη, ξηραίνειν τὴν γονήν. ἔνιοι δὲ χλωρὸν αὐτὸν χυλίζοντες εἰς ὤτων ἀλγήματα χρῶνται τὰ κατ᾿ ἔμφραξιν, ὡς ἐμοὶ δοκεῖ, γινόμενα.

The fruit of cannabis is both nonflatulent and drying to such an extent that, if consumed in quantity, it dries up the semen. Some make an infusion of it while green and use this against those earaches, I believe, that occur through blockage.

In terms of treatment, the novelty here is the acknowledgment that the infusion works specifically against earaches caused by blockage; though (unlike Dioscorides) he does not remark that it was used warm, could Galen have realized that the *khylos* was effective simply because, like any other warm liquid, it could dislodge ear wax? Another novelty here is our first reference to the antiflatulent quality of the seeds; a later writer notes that this property is so strong that, if cannabis seeds have been eaten, there is no flatulence even after eating foods that cause it (Oribasius 1933, *Synopsis* 4.21, "the fruit of cannabis is non-flatulent even after flatulent foods"). Brunner (1973, p. 350) has the ambiguous translation "eliminates intestinal gas": "prevents" would be more precise.

Galen's account also puts the use of cannabis seeds within the context of ancient medical theory. Health was dependent not only upon the proper balance of the four humors (black bile, yellow bile, blood, and phlegm) but also upon the proper balance of the four qualities of warm, cold, dry, and moist; indeed, it could be influenced through the consumption of or abstention from those foods and medications that inherently possess these qualities or enhance them in the body. Hence we can see for the first time a connection between the drying up of semen through high level consumption of the seeds and a supposed "drying" quality inherent in the seed (see also Hesychius' lexicon [*kappa* 764], which defines cannabis as a Scythian *thumiama* [i.e., incense] that has the ability to "dry out" everyone in the vicinity).

Since many ancient medications were, as we now say, "natural source" and were in fact everyday foods as well, Galen also wrote about the eating of mature cannabis seed in another work called *De Alimentorum Facultatibus* (*On the Properties of Foods,* Galen 1821, VI.549):

Περὶ καννάβεως σπέρματος.
Οὐχ ὥσπερ αὐτὸ τὸ φυτὸν τῆς καννάβεως ἔοικε πως τῷ ἄγνῳ, καὶ τὸ σπέρμα τῷ σπέρματι παραπλήσιόν πώς ἐστι τὴν δύναμιν, ἀλλ' ἀποκεχώρηκε πάμπολυ, δύσπεπτόν τε καὶ κακοστόμαχον ὃν καὶ κεφαλαλγὲς καὶ κακόχυμον. ὅμως δ' οὖν καὶ τοῦτό τινες ἐσθίουσι φρύγοντες ἅμα τοῖς ἄλλοις τραγήμασιν. ὀνομάζω δὲ δηλονότι τραγήματα τὰ παρὰ τὸ δεῖπνον ἐσθιόμενα τῆς ἐπὶ τῷ πίνειν ἡδονῆς ἕνεκα. θερμαίνει δ' ἱκανῶς καὶ διὰ τοῦτο καὶ κεφαλῆς ἅπτεται βραχεῖ πλεῖον ληφθέν, ἀτμὸν ἀναπέμπων ἐπ' αὐτὴν θερμόν θ' ἅμα καὶ φαρμακώδη.

On the seed of cannabis:

While the cannabis-plant itself resembles to a degree the agnus plant, the seed is not at all like its seed in its power but completely different, being both hard to digest and tough on the stomach and headache-inducing and bad-tasting. All the same, however, some people eat it, munching on it together with other snacks. By "snacks" I mean the things eaten at dinner on account of the pleasure associated with drinking. It warms sufficiently, and for that reason it also intoxicates quickly when eaten in quantity by sending toward the head a vapor that is both warm and medicinal.

The word translated "vapor" here *(atmos)* is another form of the one used by Herodotus to describe what was released when the Scythians threw cannabis seed onto the hot rocks *(atmis)*. The word translated "medicinal" here is rendered by Brunner 1973, p. 350 as "toxic," but *pharmakôdês* simply means "of the nature of a *pharmakon*" *(LSJ s.v.)*, while *pharmakon* itself designates a "*drug,* whether healing or noxious" *(LSJ s.v.)*; since "drug-like" could be misleading in the context of treatment with cannabis, I have chosen "medicinal."

Again the influence of contemporary theory is evident in the reference to the "warming" quality of cannabis, naturally associated with its "drying" quality; this probably alludes not to a "warm" feeling felt by the user (Brunner 1973, p. 351) but to the ability of the seed to maintain the body's warmth, the prerequisite of life. But this passage also constitutes our best evidence for the recreational use of cannabis through consumption of the seeds (denied at Brunner 1973, p. 355), which we last saw mentioned in Ephippus in the fourth century BCE: surely it was for the intoxicating effect, and not for the unpleasant taste or for the stomachaches or headaches, that they were eaten. Galen confirms this intoxicating effect a little later in the same work (Galen 1821, VI.550) when he writes that the seed of agnus-castus doesn't "touch the head" as cannabis seed does.

One "paramedical" use worth mentioning is as a mosquito repellent (cf. Brunner 1973, p. 349). An ancient work on farming claims that "with cannabis spread below, mosquitoes will do no injustice to the one in the bed" (Anon. 1895, 13.11.9), while elsewhere it promises that "if you put a blooming sprig of fresh cannabis by you when going to bed, mosquitoes won't touch you" (13.11.4). Whether or not these actually work, they might reflect an observation by ancient hemp farmers that insects by and large tend to avoid the plant.

A work falsely attributed to Galen called *De Remediis Parabilibus (On ready remedies)* offers cannabis leaves in a treatment against nosebleeds (Galen 1821, XIV.548): "Dry some cannabis leaves, grind them and put them into the *rhothôn*" (the suggested alternative is to set fire to a piece of linen, dip it in "sharp vinegar," and insert it into the nostril!). Unfortunately, *rhothôn* does not occur elsewhere and is not found in any Greek dictionary I have consulted, but one assumes that it designates the nostrils.

Cannabis seed appears twice in remedies for tapeworms. One that is also attested for horses (see Appendix II) turns up in *On ready remedies (Opera Omnia* XIV.515):

Καννάβεως σπέρμα ξηρὸν κόψας καὶ σήσας, ὕδατι μίξας καὶ χυλῶδες ποιήσας καὶ ῥάκει καθαρῷ ἀποπιάσας δὸς πιεῖν.

Chop and sift dry cannabis seed, mix with water and make *khylos*-like, and press through a clean rag and administer.

As *sperma* shows, this involves mature seed rather than the green seed used to make the *khylos* for earaches; it is not clear, however, what the author meant by "*khylos*-like" (a brief period of steeping before filtering?). Archigenes (fr. 17) offers the second recipe, involving a drink prepared from a number of seeds, including cannabis.

Greek medicine as a form of scholarly inquiry effectively ended with Galen, and later writers, for the most part, simply rehash and recycle what we have already found.

In the fourth century, Oribasius repeats in one passage (Oribasius 1933, *Ad Eunapium* 2.1) what Galen says in *On the temperaments and properties of simple medications* about the seed drying up the semen; in another (Oribasius 1933, *Collectiones Medicae* 1.32) he abbreviates Galen's comments in "On the properties of foods" about their indigestible quality and their warming effect. In the sixth century, Aëtius writes as follows (Aëtius 1935, *Iatrica* 1.178):

Καννάβεως ὁ καρπὸς δύσπεπτός τέ ἐστι καὶ κεφαλαλγὴς καὶ κακόχυμος· εἰ δὲ καὶ φρυχθείη καὶ οὕτως ἅπτεται τῆς κεφαλῆς τῷ θερμαίνειν ἱκανῶς, ἀτμὸν ἀναπέμπων ἐπ' αὐτὴν θερμόν τε ἅμα καὶ φαρμακώδη· τῷ δὲ ξηρὰν ἔχειν τὴν κρᾶσιν καὶ ἄφυσον εἶναι ξηραίνει τὴν γονήν.

The fruit of cannabis is hard to digest, headache-inducing, and bad-tasting; even if it is roasted it intoxicates by warming the head sufficiently, sending up a warm medicinal vapor toward it; by having a dry and non-flatulent temperament it dries the semen.

This is more or less what Galen wrote in *On the properties of foods,* but perhaps a little confused; the explicit connection made here between the nonflatulent property of the seed and its ability to dry may be based upon a misunderstanding of Galen and his use of "both . . . and." (Galen probably meant that the seed was, on one hand, nonflatulent and, on the other, drying to such an extent that it dried up the semen, not that both the nonflatulent and drying properties dried up the semen.) Finally, in the seventh century, Paulus of Aegina (Paulus Aegineta 1921-1924, *Epitome Medica* 7.3.10) repeats more or less word for word the comments from Galen's work *On the temperaments and properties of simple medications.* Late Roman writers such as Marcellus Empiricus and pseudo-Theodorus closely reflect what we have already seen in Greek writers, though they sometimes add an outlandish novelty or two (cf. Brunner 1973, p. 354).

Outside these specific accounts, cannabis seed regularly appears in lists of foods with various qualities: nonflatulent foods (Oribasius 1933, *Collectiones medicae* 3.22.1, 15.1:10.9, *Synopsis ad Eustathium filium* 4.21.2, *Ad Eunapium* 1.38.1; Aëtius 1935, *Iatrica* 2.258), foods with a drying effect (Oribasius 1933, *Collectiones Medicae* 14.23.1, 15.1:10.9, *Synopsis ad Eustathium filium* 2.13.1; Aëtius 1935, *Iatrica* 2.209), foods with a warming effect (Oribasius 1933, *Collectiones medicae* 3.31.2, *Synopsis ad Eustathium filium* 4.31.2), and foods that harm the head (perhaps because of the headaches said to be associated with eating it; [Anon. 1841] *De alimentis* 31, under the designation *kannabokokka*; Oribasius 1933, *Collectiones Medicae* 3.21.3, *Synopsis ad Eustathium filium* 4.20.1). Some writers also record it as a powerful thinning agent, in other words, as having the ability to thin the body's humors (Oribasius 1933, *Collectiones medicae* 3.2.4 = *Synopsis ad Eustathium filium* 4.1.3 = *Ad Eunapium* 1.18.3, "among agents that thin powerfully enough to be medicinal is the seed of rue and of cannabis"; Aëtius 1935, *Iatrica* 2.240 gives a substantially identical text). Under the compound name *kannabosperma* ("cannabiseed," as it were), it also appears once in a list of foods that produce "sticky" humors (Anon. 1840 *De cibis* 18), specifically in a sublist of foods that also produce "cool" humors.

The imitative quality of later Greek medical writing has one advantage for us: that later writers can sometimes preserve knowledge that has otherwise been lost. In the case of cannabis seed, though we have seen numerous references to the ability of the seed to suppress semen when consumed in quantity, we have seen none that has related this explicitly to a medical use. Fortunately, a passage of Aëtius on the treatment of "gonorrheas" or involuntary discharges of sperm shows us the medical use that exploited that drying effect (Aëtius 1935, *Iatrica* 11.33):

Γονόρροια μὲν οὖν τῶν σπερματικῶν ἀγγείων ἐστὶ πάθος, οὐ τοῦ αἰδοίου. ὀδύνην μὲν οὐκ εἴωθε λίαν ἐργάζεσθαι τὸ πάθος, ἀειδίαν δὲ οὐ τὴν τυχοῦσαν καὶ συγχυσμὸν παρέχει, ἀδιαλείπτως ἐκκρινομένου τοῦ σπέρματος ἀπροαιρέτως. Ἀποτελεῖται δὲ ἐνίοτε καὶ ἐκ ῥευματισμοῦ τῶν σπερματικῶν ἀγγείων, ἔστι δὲ ὅτε καὶ σατυριάσεως προηγησαμένης ἐπιγίγνεται ἡ γονόρροια. Συμβαίνει δὲ τὸ πάθος τοῖς προηβῶσι μᾶλλον, τοῖς περὶ τὸ τεσσαρεσκαιδέκατον ἔτος· ἤδη δὲ καὶ ταῖς ἄλλαις ἡλικίαις. Ἔστι δὲ τὸ ἐκκρινόμενον σπέρμα ὑδαρὲς λεπτὸν δίχα προθυμίας τῆς περὶ τὴν συνουσίαν, τὰ πλεῖστα μὲν ἀναισθήτως, ἔστι δὲ ὅτε καὶ μετά τινος ἡδονῆς· καταφθείρεται δὲ αὐτοῖς ἠρέμα τὸ σύμπαν σῶμα ἰσχαινόμενον, ἰδίως δὲ τὰ κατὰ τὴν ὀσφύν. Παρέπεται δὲ καὶ ἀτονία πολλή, οὐ διὰ τὸ πλῆθος τοῦ ἐκκρινομένου, ἀλλὰ διὰ τὴν κυριότητα τῶν τόπων. Οὐ μόνον δὲ ἀνδράσιν, ἀλλὰ καὶ γυναιξὶ τοῦτο συμβαίνει, καὶ ἔστιν ἐπὶ τῶν γυναικῶν δυσαπάλλακτον. Θεραπεία δὲ καὶ τούτων κοινὴ ἡ ἐπὶ παντὸς ῥευματισμοῦ παραλαμβανομένη. Πρῶτον μὲν οὖν ἐπὶ ἡσυχίας καὶ ὀλιγοσιτίας καὶ ὑδροποσίας τηρεῖν· εἶτα δὲ καὶ σκέπειν τὴν ὀσφὺν καὶ τὸ ἐφήβαιον ἐρίοις βεβρεγμένοις οἴνῳ καὶ ῥοδίνῳ ἢ οἰνανθίνῳ ἢ μηλίνῳ· οὐκ ἄθετοι δὲ οὐδὲ σπόγγοι, ὀξυκράτῳ δεδευμένοι· ταῖς δὲ ἑξῆς καὶ καταπλάσμασι τοῖς διὰ φοινίκων, μήλων, ἀκακίας, ὑποκιστίδος, οἰνάνθης, ῥοὸς ἐρυθροῦ, καὶ τῶν ὁμοίων, ἐγκαθίσμασί τε χρῆσθαι στυπτικοῖς, ἀφεψήμασι σχίνου, βάτου, μυρσίνης καὶ τῶν παραπλησίων, ἑψομένων ἐν οἴνῳ αὐστηρῷ ἢ ἀκράτῳ ἢ κεκραμένῳ. Τροφαῖς δὲ χρῆσθαι δυσφθάρτοις τε καὶ δυσμεταβλήτοις καὶ ἀναξηραντικαῖς, διδόναι τε αὐτοῖς σὺν τῷ ποτῷ καὶ ταῖς τροφαῖς τοῦ ἄγνου τὸ σπέρμα καὶ τὸ τῆς καννάβεως, καὶ μᾶλλον πεφρυγμένα, καὶ τοῦ πηγάνου τὸ σπέρμα καὶ τὰ φύλλα, καὶ τῆς θριδακίνης τὸ σπέρμα καὶ τοὺς καυλούς, καὶ τῆς νυμφαίας τὴν ῥίζαν. Πίνειν δὲ κατὰ ἑκάστην ἡμέραν ἀντὶ τοῦ κοινοῦ ὕδατος ὕδωρ ἐν ᾧ σίδηρος πλειστάκις ἐναπεσβέσθη. Ἔδωκαν δέ τινες τοῖς γονορροικοῖς πίνειν ἁλικακκάβου ῥίζης τὸν φλοιὸν μετὰ ὕδατος, καὶ οὐκ ἂν εἴη ἀνοίκειον ἀποπειρᾶσθαί ποτε καὶ τούτου.

So a gonorrhea is a condition of the spermatic ducts, not of the penis. The condition generally does not cause much pain, but it does offer an unusual deformity and effusion, as the seed is incessantly being discharged involuntarily. Sometimes a gonorrhea is brought about by a discharge of the spermatic ducts, sometimes it is an aftereffect of a preceding satyriasis. The condition happens most to the young, around the age of fourteen, though at other ages as well. The seed is discharged in a watery and thin condition, unconnected with any desire for sex, mostly without being noticed, though sometimes with a certain pleasurable sensation. The entire body, but especially the areas around the loin, is gradually wasted and withered by it. Significant weakness follows, not because of the quantity of the discharge but because of the sovereignty of these areas. This happens not only to men but to women as well, and in the case of women it is difficult to cure. The general treatment of these conditions is the one for every kind of discharge. First of all, then, keep the patient rested, eating little and drinking only water; then also cover the loin and pubes with wool moistened with wine and attar of rose or grape-bloom or quince (sponges dipped in diluted sour wine are not to be rejected); in the days that follow use poultices from dates, quinces, acacia, hypocist, grape-bloom, red sumach and the like, and astringent sitz-baths, decoctions of mastich, bramble, myrtle and similar things, boiled in dry wine, either unmixed or mixed. Use foods that are hard to digest and assimilate and are drying, and give to them together with the drink and food the seed of agnus-castus and of cannabis, preferably roasted, and the seed and leaves of rue, as well as the seed and stalks of wild lettuce and the root of the water-lily. Every day, instead of ordinary water, some give water in which steel has been quenched often, some the bark from the root of the winter-cherry.

Despite the comment that this "affliction" can occur in women as well (perhaps Aëtius was thinking of vaginal secretions, though they are obviously—to us, at least—not discharges of semen), it is clear that Aëtius is discussing principally wet dreams and nocturnal emissions in teenage boys. This phenomenon evidently caused great concern to ancient physicians; the passage quoted is not even the whole of Aëtius's discussion of its treatment, but one can see that it involves plenty of rest, a restricted intake of food, and abstention from beverages other than water (obviously the physicians who administered water from the blacksmith's that had been used for quenching hot steel were engaging unconsciously in a sort of homoeopathic magic). But the logic of Aëtius' treatment is inescapable: these discharges represent leakage from the spermatic ducts, and so the drying quality of cannabis seed can be invoked to dry up those leaks.

A passage in Oribasius (Oribasius 1933, *Ad Eunapium* 4.107.2) has the fruit of wild cannabis used in this treatment, but he is very probably mistaken; his language reflects exactly what other authorities say about the effect of cannabis seed ("if drunk in quantity it dries up the semen"), and no other medical authority except the *Herbarium* of ps.-Apuleius refers to any use at all for the seed of wild cannabis. That Oribasius writes of the fruit being "drunk" rather than eaten is also likely to be an error, unless he was simply thinking about the seeds being taken together with a beverage.

This survey of the medical use of cannabis has yielded several weakly attested uses: a preparation of dry seed against tapeworms, the dried, ground leaves against nosebleed. But it has also shown that there were two principal uses, attested again and again in our major medical authorities: an infusion of the green seeds used against earaches, and consumption of the seeds in treating nocturnal emissions. For a variety of reasons, it is difficult to evaluate the effectiveness of these treatments, most obviously because of the impossibility of experimenting with the precise strains that were used in antiquity, less obviously because we cannot always be certain about the method of preparation (for example, no one tells us whether the *khylos* used in the ears was prepared with water, with wine, or even with oxymel). It may well be, however, that the lack of a technology to permit smoking cannabis meant that the ancients were denied the opportunity to make the most effective use of the plant's psychoactive and analgesic properties.

Finally, one section of a genuine work of Galen, *De Victu Attenuante (On the thinning regimen,* Galen 1923, 29), hints at some controversy over the medical use of cannabis seed. Galen is making the point that some foods exercise such a powerful effect on the body that they are little short of the properties of true medicines. His first example is the seed of the rue, followed by the seed of the agnus-castus (which we've seen associated elsewhere with the medical use of cannabis), followed by cannabis seed, which he says is not only medicinal but also headache inducing, so that "one would properly use them [i.e., the seeds of these three plants] for only one purpose, when one chooses to purify the blood through the urine." Since no other source connects cannabis seed with purification of the blood (or with the urine), it is not clear what Galen had in mind here. What does seem certain is that his words reflect a perception that there was such a thing as an *improper* use for the seed. It seems unlikely that Galen was thinking of the poorly attested use of cannabis seeds against tapeworms or even of the much better attested use of a *khylos* from them against earaches. In the absence of any other attested medical use of cannabis, this leaves the drying up of semen as his most likely target; since we know that Galen was aware that eating the seeds was not only unpleasant but could lead to intoxication as well, it is perhaps not unreasonable to suspect that the controversy underlying his words was precisely over the prescribing of cannabis seeds for the treatment of nocturnal emissions in teenage boys, inspired by observations of undesirable side effects from administering the large quantities of seed that were required to produce the "drying" effect. It is worth noting that, when Aëtius goes on to offer a specific recipe for an antidote to nocturnal emissions, it contains the seed of agnus-castus but not of the more intoxicating cannabis (see Galen, quoted previously, for agnus-castus as a non intoxicating alternative to cannabis).

APPENDIX I: PASSAGES DISCUSSING WILD CANNABIS POSSIBLY MISUNDERSTOOD AS DISCUSSING DOMESTICATED CANNABIS

A. *Dioscorides,* Materia Medica *3.149 (cf. Oribasius,* Collectiones Medicae *11.kappa.3)*

ή δὲ ἀγρία κάνναβις ῥαβδία φέρει ὅμοια τοῖς τῆς πτελέας, μελάντερα δὲ καὶ μικρότερα, τὸ ὕψος πήχεως· τὰ φύλλα ὅμοια τῇ ἡμέρῳ, τραχύτερα δὲ καὶ μελάντερα, ἄνθη ὑπέρυθρα, λυχνίδι ἐμφερῆ, σπέρμα δὲ καὶ ῥίζα ὅμοια τῇ ἀλθαίᾳ. δύναται δὲ ἡ ῥίζα καταπλασθεῖσα ἑφθὴ φλεγμονὰς παρηγορεῖν καὶ πώρους διαχεῖν· καὶ ὁ ἀπ' αὐτῆς δὲ φλοιὸς εὔθετεῖ εἰς πλοκὴν σχοινίων.

Wild cannabis bears shoots similar to those of the elm, but darker and smaller, the height of a forearm; the leaves are like the domesticated variety, but rougher and darker, the flowers reddish, similar to the toad-flax, the seed and root like the wild mallow. The root when boiled and used as a plaster can ease inflammations and disperse chalk-stones; and the inner bark from it serves for making ropes.

B. *Dioscorides,* Euporista *1.229*

πώρους δὲ τοὺς ἐπὶ ποδαγρικῶν καὶ συστροφὰς τῶν νεύρων λύει ...

κάνναβις ἀγρία καταπλασθεῖσα ...

Cures for chalk-stones in the gouty and for twistings of the sinews include ... a plaster of wild cannabis.

C. *Oribasius,* Synopsis ad Eustathium Filium *3.29.1 (cf. Aëtius 1935,* Iatrica *15.7):*

Ἀδαμαντίου πρὸς μελικηρίδας καὶ τὰ ὅμοια

Κηροῦ β', τερεβινθίνης β', λεπίδος χαλκοῦ β', νίτρου α', θείου ἀπύρου α', καννάβεως ἀγρίας ῥίζης ξηρᾶς λε' (εἰ δὲ μή, ἀριστολοχίας στρογγύλης τὸ αὐτό), κόπρου περιστερᾶς λε', ἐλαίου παλαιοῦ α'. ἐναφέψει τῷ ἐλαίῳ τὰς ῥίζας.

Adamantius' [remedy] against melicerides and the like:

Two measures of wax, 2 of terebinth, 2 of bronze chips, 1 of nitre, 1 of native sulphur, 35 of dry root of wild cannabis (otherwise the same amount of round aristolochia), 35 of pigeon-droppings, 1 of old oil. Boil down the roots in the oil.

APPENDIX II: CANNABIS IN VETERINARY MEDICINE

According to a collection of horse remedies known as the Berlin *Hippiatrica* (Anon. 1924, 96.26), the chopped leaves can be used to dress a wound: first some vinegar and pitch are brought to a full rolling boil, then wax, mustard, wheat-chaff, and roasted pine-resin are added, and the resulting mixture (presumably cooled) is applied liberally, then chopped cannabis leaves and grass trimmings are put on top before the wound is bound. This treatment evidently does not rely upon any chemical properties of cannabis leaves but simply uses them (no doubt as a waste product from cultivation for rope making) as a clean and readily available dressing.

Another collection, the Cambridge *Hippiatrica*, offers a recipe for the treatment of tapeworms which is identical to the one just cited from pseudo-Galen *On ready remedies* (Anon. 1924, 70.10).

Finally, a formula found in both the Cambridge *Hippiatrica* (Anon. 1924, 17.3) and in the *Geoponica* (Anon. 1895, *Geoponica* 16.15) specifies the use of the ash of cannabis (though we are not told whether this is from burning the stems or the leaves or even the root) combined with honey and "old urine" as a salve for wounds of the lower back (for the "back-biting" of horses and the use of cannabis to control it, cf. Brunner 1973, p. 354, with n. 40).

REFERENCES

Aëtius. 1935. *Iatrica*, ed. A. Olivieri. *Corpus Medicorum Graecorum* 8.1. Leipzig.

Anon. 1840. *De cibis*, in *Anecdota Medica Graeca*, ed. F. Z. Eremins. Leiden.

Anon. 1841. *De alimentis*, ed. J. L. Ideler. *Physici et Medici Graeci Minores* 2. Berlin.

Anon. 1895. *Geoponica*, ed. H. Beckh. Leipzig.

Anon. 1924. *Hippiatrica*, ed. E. Oder and K. Hoppe. Leipzig.

Artamonov, M. I. 1965. Frozen tombs of the Scythians. *Scientific American* 213: 233-242.

Brunner, T. 1973. Evidence of marijuana use in ancient Greece and Rome? The literary evidence. *Bulletin of the History of Medicine* 47(4): 344-355.

Brunner, T. 1977. Marijuana in ancient Greece and Rome? The literary evidence. *Journal of Psychedelic Drugs* 9(3): 221-225.

Dioscorides. 1907-1914. *Euporista* and *Materia Medica*, ed. M. Wellman. Berlin.

Emboden, W. A. Jr. 1972. Ritual use of *Cannabis sativa* L.: A historical-ethnographic survey. In P. T. Furst (ed.), *Flesh of the gods: The ritual use of hallucinogens* (pp. 214-236). New York: Praeger.

Galen. 1821. *Claudii Galeni Opera Omnia*, ed. C. G. Kühn. Leipzig.

Galen. 1923. *De Victu Attenuante*, ed. K. Kalbfleisch. *Corpus Medicorum Graecorum* 5.4.2. Leipzig.

Oribasius. 1933. *Collectiones Medicae, Synopsis ad Eustathium Filium*, and *Libri ad Eunapium*, ed. J. Raeder. *Corpus Medicorum Graecorum* 6.1.1, 6.1.2, 6.2.1, 6.2.2. Leipzig.

Paulus Aegineta. 1921-1924. *Epitomae medicae libri septem*, ed. J. L. Heiberg. *Corpus Medicorum Graecorum* 9.1, 9.2. Leipzig.

Pliny the Elder. 1967. *Historia Maturalis*, ed. I. Ian and C. Mayhoff. Stuttgart.

UPDATE

Ethan B. Russo

The ancient and medieval texts remain a treasure trove of investigational work for modern medical detectives. A newly discovered thirteenth-century vellum manuscript in the Ashmolean Museum at Oxford University contains a beautiful color rendition of cannabis and may be based on a third-century text of Pseudo-Apuleius. A new translation is planned. The phytopharmaceuticals lessons of the past are ignored at peril to our optimal realization of health in the future (Riddle 1999).

REFERENCE

Riddle, J. M. 1999. Historical data as an aid in pharmaceutical prospecting and drug safety determination. *Journal of Alternative and Complementary Medicine* 5 (2): 195-201.

Chapter 5

A Homelie Herbe: Medicinal Cannabis in Early England

Vivienne Crawford

INTRODUCTION

Although medical herbalism has an ancient and venerable history, its use in Britain since the seventeenth century has increasingly been the subject of contention. This is not a function of the perceived efficacy of plant medicine. Rather, the authorisation or prohibition of particular therapeutic practices reflects the fluctuating distribution of power by means of which the civic body, as represented by the government and the professions it recognises and licences, asserts its right to regulate the individual body of the citizen. Legal control has been particularly overt in the case of psychoactive plants such as cannabis, which possess the politically and morally charged property of changing the way we see the world.

Prohibited for common use in Britain since the 1920s, and banned even for prescription by doctors since the 1970s, cannabis is currently the subject of experimentation purporting to prove to the satisfaction of science that the plant is a cornucopia of therapeutic constituents. As in the United States of America, orthodox pharmaceutical and medical bodies have been canvassing the government to authorise clinical trials and grant licences for cannabis-based medicines. Transformed almost overnight from outlaw to commercial opportunity, cannabis is the subject of urgent investigation on the part of commercial scientists, as companies on both sides of the Atlantic scramble to patent profitable analogues. I suggest that a rational consideration of its venerable history in England, coupled with the evidence of its therapeutic properties (newly confirmed in the language of biochemistry), leads to the inescapable conclusion that the prohibition of medicinal cannabis in England is an historical anomaly that should be rectified as soon as

Handbook of Cannabis Therapeutics
© 2006 by The Haworth Press, Inc. All rights reserved.
doi:10.1300/5741_06

possible. Indeed, the British government is moving in this direction: in October 2001 cannabis was reclassified in recognition of the fact that, by any measure, it is much less dangerous than such substances as street heroin. GW Pharmaceuticals' cannabis-based medicines are in the final stages of U.K. testing. Yet there is no official will to restore cannabis to its former position in the repertory of common herbs available to qualified practitioners, let alone to legalise the growing of the plant for home consumption. Cannabis is still perceived as an alien drug and, despite reports in the popular press about its use as self-medication for pain control, or to ease the effects of neuromuscular dysfunction, one that is primarily associated with an antisocial hedonism.

Evans (1996) state that cannabis is believed to have reached Europe via Napoleonic Egypt. However, an authoritative nineteenth-century history of drugs (Flückiger and Hanbury 1879) details the way in which it became prominent in contemporary British medicine following the in vivo research carried out by O'Shaughnessy in Calcutta during the 1830s. Grinspoon (1997) adds that between 1840 and 1900 more than one hundred papers were published on its therapeutic effects.

Whilst this may be accepted as the inauguration of modern usage, hemp had in fact been a staple of indigenous European medicine for more than a millennium. In addition, like its cousin the nettle, cannabis was a source of fibre for rope and cloth. Its seeds provided food and, when crushed, yielded oil rich in essential fatty acids to nourish both people and their beasts.

Why then was it seen in the Victorian period as a new plant? Even the reputable Grieves' (1971) *Herbal* speaks of cannabis as if it reached England only in the midnineteenth century. I believe the answer is that during this period the strain of cannabis most commonly employed in Britain for both medicinal and psychotropic purposes was the variety known as *Cannabis indica* or Indian hemp, imported from the Indian subcontinent in the form of compressed resin, whereas previously, medicinal use had been made of the leaves, seeds and roots of cannabis plants grown in a northern climate.

There is no absolute consensus as to whether cannabis is a closely related genus of plants, including *Cannabis sativa, C. indica,* and *C. ruderalis,* or a single polymorphic species with variant ecotypes, each carrying different proportions of cannabinoid constituents depending on environmental circumstances (Flückiger and Hanbury 1879; Staryk 1983; Schultes and Hofmann 1992; Evans 1996). Whichever is truer, the fact that the Anglo-Saxons do not record any mind-altering effects for their homegrown hemp seems to suggest that tenth-century English-grown cannabis lacked the concentration of sunlight-induced terpenophenolic metabolites (e.g., Δ-8 and Δ-9 tetrahydrocannabinol, etc.) responsible for changes in consciousness, and consistently present in plants grown in the light and heat of Asia. Either the potentially psychotropic effects of the plant were unknown, or, if occasionally observed, were not regarded as controllable in a therapeutic context, and hence not recorded in reference texts.

CANNABIS HISTORY IN ENGLAND

Anglo-Saxon and Classical authors simply differentiated *C. sativa* (cultivated) from *C. sylvestris* or *agria* (wild). It has been suggested that the latter is *Eupatorium cannabinum*, but in the *Durham Glossary of the Names of Worts* (Cockayne 1856,Vol. 1 p. 329), *Cannabis agria*'s synonym is "holi rope," in my view an epithet applying more properly to cannabis. Reversing the usual route of plant migration, by means of which wild-growing Mediterranean herbs were introduced for cultivation into colder parts of Europe, *C. sativa* came to Greece and Italy from the northeast. Excavation of Western Altaic burial mounds has confirmed the Scythian custom of inhaling the fumes of cannabis seeds, heated in pots or on stones in an enclosed space, described by Herodotus circa 500 BCE (1978, *Histories,* bk. IV, p. 295): "it begins to smoke, giving off a vapour unsurpassed by any vapour-bath one could find in Greece. The Scythians enjoy it so much that they howl with pleasure."

Hemp has been found in Germanic burials dating back to 500 BCE (Schultes 1973). This raises the possibility that Saxon folk custom, rather than herbal lore inherited from the texts of Galen and Dioscorides, established its use in England, although subsequent monastic praxis embraced both. *Cannabis sativa* was cultivated in England during the Anglo-Saxon period (fifth through eleventh centuries CE) to make rope, but it was also noted that "manured" hemp, used for coughs and jaundice, differed in its properties from "bastard" (wild-growing) hemp, the latter being medicinal "against nodes and wennes and other hard tumours" (Schultes and Hoffmann 1992, p. 97). The *Herbarium* (eleventh century, see De Vriend 1984, CXVI, p.148) recommends "haenep" (glossed in Latin as *Cannabis sativa*) specifically for sore breasts: "gecnucude mid rysle, lege to pam breostan, heo toferep paet geswel; gyf paer hwylc gegaderung bip heo pa afeormap." (I translate this as "Rub [the herb] with fat, lay it to the breast, it will disperse the swelling; if there is a gathering of diseased matter it will purge it.")

Hemp enjoyed an enhanced respect under the Tudor monarchs, as with the onset of imperial longings, the navy's demand for rope increased. It was vigorously cultivated in England, and even planted at Jamestown, Virginia, in 1611 (Grinspoon and Bakalar 1997). Male and female plants were distinguished by the terms "carl" and "fimble" hemp, respectively, and the characteristics of summer and winter hemp assiduously noted. Parkinson's *Theatrum Botanicum* (1640) includes notes on its cultivation. The "drowning" of the carl hemp was an important part of its processing in preparation for use as fibre, and required skill, for too prolonged an immersion would cause the hemp to rot. It is interesting to note that the nineteenth-century reprint of Thomas Tusser's *Five Hundred Points of Good Husbandrie* (1810, originally published in 1557) contains an editorial comment to the effect that the neglect of the valuable hemp plant is one of the misfortunes arising from a dependence on foreign trade. The categorisation of nonpsychoactive cannabis as an indigenous or naturalised British plant, serving as a useful source of fibre, clearly remained untroubled for centuries.

But this is only one aspect of the history of cannabis use in what is now termed "early modern" England. The English Renaissance herbals clearly indicate that, as for the Anglo-Saxons, hemp was a source of therapeutic constituents as well. It is clear that the Tudor herbalists, who by 1588 depended on extra-European sources for only 15 percent of their drugs (Bellamy and Pfister 1992), were qualified by familiarity, as well as by their assimilation of Classical sources, to assess the virtues of cannabis as a medicinal herb.

"Water of hempe" was recommended in *The Vertuous Boke of Distillacioun* for headache and "for all hete wheresoe'er it be" (trans. Braunschweig, H.). John Parkinson, in *Theatrum Botanicum* (1640), and Nicholas Culpeper (1652) subsequently confirmed this indication for the aromatic water. Richard Banckes (1977) also demonstrates an awareness of the anti-pyretic property of cannabis in 1561: "its virtue is, if a man have the fever, fret well his pulse therwith, and he shall be whole."

William Turner (1551) offers his readers Latin, English, French and Dutch names for medicinal hemp, indicating widespread use in Northern Europe. He follows the Classical authors in recommending it for earache and warning that it may impede fertility, and compares Dioscorides's discussion of hemp with that of Pliny, emphasising that it "maketh soft the joints that are shrunk together" (p. 112).

Turner (1551) also echoes Simeon Sethy: the seed "if taken out of measure, taketh men's wits from them, as coriander doth" (p. 112). This does not sound like personal testimony, yet it is clear that if the English Renaissance herbalists were sufficiently in thrall to the Classical lore-masters to preserve and repeat their conclusions, they were also capable of discussing those findings and comparing them with contemporary knowledge based on the authority of experience.

What is remarkable about Turner, for instance, is his critical use of eclectic sources: he is punctilious in his attempt to differentiate between what he has read and what he has understood through his own perceptions. In the Dodoens *Herbal* translated into English by Henry Lyte (Dodoens and Lyte,

1619), Lyte warns against the ingestion of the raw seeds in what may be the voice of experience, despite being based on Galen: the seeds are "contrarie to the stomach and engendreth grosse and naughtie humors in all the bodie" (Schultes and Hoffmann 1992, p. 95). The mode of hemp preparation utilising dairy products such as butter (e.g., Culpeper 1652) is not copied from Classical sources but is a specifically Northern European practice. I conclude therefore that if Dioscorides, Galen et al. provided the literary basis of Tudor and Stuart writing about cannabis, their work was supplemented by a contemporary empirical awareness.

However, cannabis does not seem to have been recorded in English Renaissance herbals as an inebriant any more than it was documented as such by the Anglo-Saxons. This is all the more curious since Prosper Alpinus (1591) had reported on its use as an intoxicant in Egypt, and given the extraordinary cosmopolitanism of the English at that time, and the fervour with which strange plants were investigated by the early Elizabethans, it is implausible to suppose that hashish was altogether unknown. Burton's (1621) resplendent *Anatomy of Melancholy* perhaps offers a clue to this puzzle: speaking of herbs which take away grief, he mentions "another called Bang, like in effect to Opium, which puts [men] for a time into a kind of Extasis, and makes them gently to laugh" (p. 593). It is clear from the context and word choice that Burton is repeating here information gleaned from a Hispanic text: significantly, he shows no awareness that the aromatic, resinous *bhang* is in any way related to the familiar English hemp.

The generation of herbalists who followed the Renaissance practitioners in England also approached cannabis with confidence and curiosity, discovering new applications or attempting to ascertain its mechanism of action. Culpeper (1652) listed *Cannabis sativa* in his famous *Herbal*. With a wry aside on the disciplinary use of hempen rope (it is "good for something else than to make halters only" (p. 183), he applauded the healing virtues of the plant, e.g., "The emulsion of the seed is good for the jaundice, if there be ague accompanying it, for it opens obstructions of the gall, and causes digestion of choler." He recommended cannabis for fluxes, colic and rheumatic pain, adding that the fresh root, "mixed with a little oil and butter, is good for burns," and the seed, seethed in milk till it releases its oils, for hot and dry coughs (Culpeper 1652, p. 183). The use of cannabis as a drying, warming plant that "openeth the passage of the gall" is anticipated in Gerard (1633, p. 709).

Culpeper was not the first to note the significance of the hempen knot. William Bullein had earlier (1562) claimed a sociotherapeutic action for cannabis, wittily asserting that "neckwede" is specific against necrosis of the body politic. Under the heading "Many good medicines made of hepe" [sic], he notes:

if there by any yonkers troubled with idelnesse and loytryng, hauyng neither learnying, nor willyng handes to labour, or that haue studied Phisicke so longe that he can giue his Masters purse a Purgacioun, and Countinghouse, a strong vomit . . . if there be any swashbuckler, common theef, ruffen or murtherer paste grace, the next remedie is this lace or corde . . . this is a purger, not of Melancholy, but a finall banisher of al them that be not fitt to liue In a common wealth. (Fol. xxviii)

Bullein's (1562) *Booke of Simples* (Fol. xxviii-ix of the *Bulwarke of Defence*) contains an exuberant listing of all the trades cannabis can serve:

without Hempe, sayle clothes, shroudes, staies, tacles, yarde lines, warps & cables can not be made, no Plowe or Carte can be without ropes, halters, trace etc. The Fisher and Fouler muste haue Hempe, to make their nettes. And no Archer can wante [i.e., be without] his bowe string: and the Malt man for his sackes. With it the bell is rong, to seruice in the church . . .

He adds that cannabis is hot and dry, medicinally useful, *inter alia,* for conditions of cold contraction (applied as a hot poultice, the leaves and seeds "doe help against the contrarion, or shrinking of the sinewes"), and, stamped together with *Artemisia absinthum,* "to asswage swelling."

Hemp seed assumes a more sinister aspect when it appears in a narcotic mixture of herbs to be steeped in wine, strained through a cloth woven by a whore, and taken as part of a seventeenth-century ritual for questioning the dead (Deacon 1968). Further work needs to be done on herbal formulae for magical purposes, in order to determine whether the chemical components of the various plants created a desirable synergistic effect. It may be, for example, cannabis in some way modifies the effect of *Hyoscyamus niger.*

However that may be, it is certain that by 1700, cannabis had been a stalwart of English medicine for approximately a thousand years. An unproblematic component of our *Materia Medica,* it continued to be used throughout the eighteenth and nineteenth centuries. Salmon (1710, p. 510) described indications for "the emulsion of the seed" primarily in terms of its usefulness in various forms of haemorrhage and intestinal flux. He recommends a cataplasm of the root of manured (i.e., cultivated) hemp, mixed with "Barley Flower" for sciatica and pains in the hip joint. A Sheffield doctor (Short 1751) eulogised cannabis as specific for chronic uterine obstruction ("not only Months, but some Yeares"), and reports a case in which "when it could not break the Uterine or Vaginal vessels, the Woman threw up blood from the Lungs, but had [her period] naturally the next Time"

(p. 138). A uterine action for cannabis was known to the Egyptians. The Ebers Papyrus, dating to 1550 BCE, notes that hemp mingled with honey, administered intravaginally, cools and contracts the uterus (Manniche 1989).

Cannabis formed part of the antidiuretic formula in the *Medicine Britannica* (Short 1751), and he also used it for insect bites, wounds, ulcers, coughs and burns (p. 138): "An Emulsion of the Seed takes out fresh Marks of the Small Pox . . . It kills Worms in the Bowels or Ears of Man or Beast." Again, we see this English combination of the Classical herbal tradition with practical instruction: "the seed boiled in Milk till it burst, then strained, and five or six Ounces of it given several times to drink, has cured the Jaundice in many."

Ethan Russo (2001, personal communication) has made a study of equivalent European sources including Marcandier's *Traité du Chanvre,* translated into English as *A Treatise on Hemp* (1764), which though expansive in echoing its classical and renaissance medical indications, failed to demonstrate an awareness of the inebriating properties of cannabis. Once more, the English seem not to have associated their familiar domestic herb with the intoxicant enjoyed in Egypt and the East.

THE MODERN ERA

Like all plant medicines, cannabis was less prominent following the Enlightenment, until O'Shaughnessy's work in 1839 revived its popularity. Cannabis regained its status as a popular medicine in England, but this time, the condensed aromatic cannabinoids found in the blocks of imported Indian resin enabled a new emphasis to be placed on its analgesic function. Even the eminently respectable Queen Victoria used hemp sent from her new dominion for menstrual cramps (British Medical Association [BMA] 1997), and Victorian doctors treated patients for a range of illnesses, including epilepsy and nervous disorders, with extracts of *Cannabis indica*.

How did a plant which early-twentieth-century orthodox medicine enthusiastically summarised as an antipyretic, analgesic, antidiuretic, antiasthmatic, hypnotic, antianorectic, antiemetic, and anticonvulsive muscle relaxant (BMA 1997; Grinspoon 1997) come, fifty years later, to be classified as being "of no therapeutic benefit," unavailable for use, inaccessible to research, and categorized as Schedule 1 of the Misuse of Drugs Act 1971?

That question must be answered with reference to the attempts of American and European governments to control domestic consumer behaviour and influence the economies of other countries by enacting laws that distinguish acceptable drugs from those deemed pernicious. The picaresque history of cannabis legislation, recently the subject of much scholarly scrutiny, cannot be outlined here, but the historical weight of traditional usage must surely be reevaluated in the near future, and cannabis once again be restored to recognition as an herb proper to English bodies.

REFERENCES

Alpinus, Prosper. 1591. *De Medicina Aegyptiorum*. Venice.

Banckes, R. 1977. *A little herball : London, (1561?), English experience, its record in early printed books published in facsimile; no. 843*. Amsterdam. Norwood, NJ: Theatrum Orbis Terrarum; W. J. Johnson.

Bellamy, D. and A. Pfister. 1992. *World Medicine*. Oxford: Blackwell.

Braunschweig, H., and L. Andrew. 1530. *The vertuose boke of the distyllacyon of all maner of waters of the herbes in this present volume expressed, with the fygures of the stillatoryes, tr. by L. Andrew*. London: P. Treveris.

British Medical Association. 1997. *Therapeutic Uses of Cannabis*. Amsterdam: Harwood Academic publishers.

Bullein, W. 1562. *Bullein's Bulwarke of Defece* [sic] *Againste All Sicknes, Sornes, and Woundes, That Dooe Daily Assaulte Mankinde*. Facsimile edition 1971, Amsterdam: Theatrum Orbis Terrarum.

Burton, R. 1621 (reprint 1907). *The Anatomy of Melancholy*. London: Chatto & Windus.

Cockayne, O. 1856. *Leechdoms, Wortcunning and Starcraft of Early England*. Volumes I-III. London: Longman, Green, Longman.

Culpeper, N. 1652. *The British Herbal and Family Physician*. London: W. Nicholson & Sons. Reprint 1994.

Deacon, R. 1968. *John Dee: Scientist, Geographer, Astrologer and Secret Agent to Elizabeth I*. London: Frederick Muller.

De Vriend, H.J. 1984. *The Old English Herbarium and Medicina de Quadripedibus*. Oxford: Early English Text Society.

Dodoens, R., and H. Lyte. 1619. *A niewe herball, or historie of plantes. First set foorth in the Doutche tongue, and now tr. out of Fr. by H. Lyte. Corrected*. London: E. Griffin.

Evans, W.C. 1998. *Trease and Evans' Pharmacognosy*. 14th edition, London: W.B. Saunders.

Flückiger, F. and D. Hanbury. 1879. *Pharmacographia: A History of Drugs*. London: Macmillan.

Gerard, J. 1633. *The Herbal*. New York: Dover. Reprint 1975.

Grieve, M. 1971. *A Modern Herbal*. New York: Dover Publications.

Grinspoon, L. 1997. The Future of Medical Marijuana. *Forschende Komplementarmedizin* 6(3):40-43.

Herodotus. 1978. *The Histories*. Baltimore: Penguin Classics.

Manniche, L. 1989. *An Ancient Egyptian Herbal*. London: British Museum Press.

Marcandier, M. 1764. *A Treatise on Hemp*. London: T. Becket and P.A. de Hendt.

Mechoulam, R. 1986. The Pharmacohistory of *Cannabis sativa*. In R. Mechoulam (ed.), *Cannabinoids as Therapeutic Agents* (pp. 1-19). Boca Raton: CRC Press.

O'Shaughnessy, W.B. 1838-1840. On the preparations of the Indian hemp, or gunjah *(Cannabis indica);* Their effects on the animal system in health, and their utility in the treatment of tetanus and other convulsive diseases. *Transactions of the Medical and Physical Society of Bengal:*71-102, 421-461.

Parkinson, J., T. Bonham, and M. de L'Obel. 1640. *Theatrum botanicum: The theater of plants; or, An herball of a large extent ... distributed into sundry classes or tribes, for the more easie knowledge of the many herbes of one nature and property, with the chiefe notes of Dr. Lobel, Dr. Bonham, and others inserted therein.* London: Tho. Cotes.

Russo, E. 2001. Cannabis in Renaissance Europe. Private correspondence.

Salmon, W. 1710. *Botanologia: The English Herbal or, History of Plants.* London: I. Dawkes.

Schultes, R.E. 1973. Man and marijuana. *Natural History* 82:59-63, 80, 82.

Schultes, R. and A. Hoffmann. 1992. *Plants of the Gods.* Rochester, VT: Healing Arts Press.

Short, T. 1751. *Medicina Britannica.* London: Franklin and Hall.

Staryk, F. 1983. *Poisonous Plants.* London: Hamlyn.

Turner, W. 1551. *A New Herball, Part I.* Facsimile edition 1995, Chapman, G. and M. Tweddle (eds.), UK: Cambridge University Press.

Tusser, Thomas. 1810. *1599. Five hundred pointes of good husbandrie, Somers tracts, 2nd ed. vol.3.* London.

UPDATE

Ethan B. Russo

This lively entry has led to other source documents on cannabis from England. Additional entries worthy of consultation by the interested reader include those listed below.

BIBLIOGRAPHY

Mills, J.H. 2000. *Madness, Cannabis and Colonialism: The "Native Only" Lunatic Asylums of British India, 1857-1900.* New York: St. Martin's Press.

Mills, J.H. 2003. *Cannabis Britannica: Empire, Trade, and Prohibition 1800-1928.* Oxford: Oxford University Press.

Russo, E.B. 2004. History of Cannabis As Medicine. In G.W. Guy, B.A. Whittle, and P. Robson (eds.), *Medicinal Uses of Cannabis and Cannabinoids* (pp. 1-16). London: Pharmaceutical Press.

Chapter 6

Future of Cannabis and Cannabinoids in Therapeutics

Ethan B. Russo

INTRODUCTION

As is evident from preceding information in this book, an increasingly bright future seems to be on the horizon for cannabis therapeutics, whether herbally based or designed to utilize its various components. The pros and cons of cannabis proper, whether smoked, ingested orally, or vaporized, have been previously addressed. A wide variety of delivery systems is possible in the future. The present selection will detail additional preparations, particularly synthetic cannabinoids, and discuss how they and cannabis-based pharmaceuticals may be applied in future clinical therapeutics.

Nabilone

Nabilone is a synthetic cannabinoid, pharmacologically similar to THC, but with higher potency, a lesser likelihood to produce euphoria, and displaying a lower "abuse potential" (British Medical Association [BMA] 1997). It is manufactured by Eli Lilly Company as Cesamet and is available in the United Kingdom, Australia, Canada, and some European nations (Grotenhermen 2001), where it is primarily utilized as an antinausea agent in chemotherapy. Occasional reports have claimed benefit on spasticity in multiple sclerosis and dyskinesias. Lethal reactions have occurred in chronic canine usage (Mechoulam and Feigenbaum 1987).

Analgesic effects of nabilone in neuropathic pain patients have been noted (Notcutt, Price, and Chapman 1997), but prominent adverse effects included drowsiness and dysphoria. Some patients stated a clear preference for smoked cannabis in terms of side effects and analgesic efficacy.

Nabilone's cost was estimated to be ten times higher than herbal cannabis at black market rates and, all things considered, this agent would seem to have more disadvantages in the long term.

Levonantradol

Levonantradol is another synthetic cannabinoid from Pfizer. Analgesic benefits of up to six hours were noted in postoperative pain patients in a prior trial (Jain et al. 1981), but without clear dose-response effects. Adverse effects are prominent with this agent, including somnolence in 50 to 100 percent and dysphoria in 30 to 50 percent (BMA 1997), termed "unacceptable" by that authority.

Ajulemic Acid (CT3)

Ajulemic acid is a synthetic cannabinoid derived from the more stable THC-11-oic acid that does not bind to CB_1 receptors and lacks psychoactive effects. It is currently in commercial development. It has shown strong analgesic and anti-inflammatory properties in animal models of arthritis without COX-1 inhibition side effects such as ulcer production, and is advanced clinical trials (Burstein 2001, 2000). It shares antineoplastic effects with THC on a variety of cell lines (Recht et al. 2001), but is half as potent in this regard, although longer acting. Ajulemic acid has recently been demonstrated to bind to the peroxisome proliferator-activated receptor gamma, part of the nuclear receptor superfamily involved in inflammatory processes (Liu et al. 2003), and also to suppress human monocyte interleukin-1β production in vitro (Zurier et al. 2003). Ajulemic acid portends to be a valuable addition to the pantheon of cannabinoid pharmaceuticals employed for analgesic and anti-inflammatory properties.

Dexanabinol (HU-211)

Dexanabinol is a synthetic cannabinoid agent developed at Hebrew University from Δ^8-THC, but it is a nonpsychoactive enantiomer of the fabulously potent HU-210 (Pop 2000). It has demonstrated numerous interesting properties including antioxidant and anti-inflammatory effects, as well as suppression of TNF-α (tumor necrosis factor) production. Additionally, it reduced brain damage associated with soman (Sarin)-induced seizures in rats (Filbert et al. 1999), caused reduction of experimental autoimmune encephalomyelitis responses (Achiron et al. 2000) suggesting application in multiple sclerosis, and reduced damage in experimental focal ischemia

(Lavie et al. 2001). Human trials have demonstrated mixed results. In one such Phase II study of sixty-seven closed-head-injury patients, dexanabinol reduced intracranial pressure and perfusion significantly with a good adverse effect profile (Knoller et al. 2002), with some degree of improvement in clinical outcome scales after three and six months.

Dexanabinol is currently in Phase III clinical trials, and further analysis will demonstrate its relative place in the cannabinoid pharmacopoeia. As currently formulated, parenteral injection of dexanabinol is required, and it may not possess the multimodality efficacy of cannabis-based medicine extracts.

HU-308

Another agent emerging from the research of Raphael Mechoulam's laboratories in Israel is HU-308, a synthetic and specific CB_2 agonist lacking cannabinoid behavioral effects in laboratory animals (Hanus et al. 1999). Observed activities of this agent include inhibition of forskolin-stimulated cyclic AMP production, blood pressure reduction, inhibition of defecation, and production of peripheral analgesia with anti-inflammatory effects. Further testing may demonstrate an important therapeutic role for this agent.

SR141716 (Rimonabant)

Heretofore, our discussion has centered on cannabinoid agonists or analogs. However, given the profile of cannabinoid stimulation with its decremental effects on short-term memory acquisition and stimulation of hunger, it was expected that efforts would be mounted to clinically harness antagonistic cannabinoid effects. SR141716, dubbed Rimonabant, is a potent CB_1-antagonist or inverse agonist used extensively in laboratory studies. It has demonstrated antiobesity effects in mice (Ravinet Trillou et al. 2003), and is currently in human clinical trials. Preliminary results (Le Fur et al. 2001) demonstrate reduction of hunger and food intake in obese male subjects in the short term, and weight reduction in the long term, with a reportedly benign adverse effect profile. Certainly, caveats are necessary, and one might expect the emergence of depression and hyperalgesic states in patients taking this agent, such as migraine and fibromyalgia. Additionally, hypervigilance will be necessary in administering such a drug to women of child-bearing age, as SR141716 has profound effects on neonatal feeding and growth (Fride 2002b).

NEW INDICATIONS FOR CANNABINOID
PHARMACEUTICALS

Emerging concepts have demonstrated the key role that endocannabinoids play in regulation of pain (Pertwee 2001a), hormonal regulation and fertility (Bari et al. 2002), hunger (Fride 2002a) and gastrointestinal function (Pertwee 2001b), and even regulation of memory (Hampson and Deadwyler 2000), and proper extinction of aversive events (Marsicano et al. 2002).

Some of these concepts have recently been reviewed (Baker et al. 2003). In particular, the authors distinguish that cannabis and endocannabinoids may demonstrate an impairment threshold if too elevated, a range of normal function below which a deficit threshold is breached. This seems to be a simple and universal concept: for every neurotransmitter or neuromodulatory agent, there may be too much or too little, with corresponding clinical pathophysiological sequelae. With respect to endocannabinoids, this concept has been insufficiently explored. Previously, this author has postulated the likelihood of clinical endogenous cannabinoid deficiency diseases (CECDD) (Russo 2001a,b), including migraine, fibromyalgia, idiopathic bowel syndrome (IBS, "spastic colon") and possibly even psychiatric conditions, such as obsessive-compulsive disorder. In light of newer information, one may posit the addition of many other disease conditions that are seemingly unresponsive to pharmacotherapy with other agents that do not influence the endocannabinoid system: causalgia and allodynia as in brachial plexus neuropathy and phantom limb pain, post-traumatic stress disorder (PTSD), bipolar disorder (Grinspoon and Bakalar 1998), dysmenorrhea (Russo 2002), hyperemesis gravidarum (Russo 2002; Curry 2002), unexplained fetal wastage, glaucoma (Jarvinen, Pate, and Laine 2002), and many others.

In the area of pain, it may be the case that we need to renew a therapeutic maneuver of the nineteenth century (reviewed in Russo 2002), and supported in Cichewicz and Welch 2002) by combining cannabinoids and opioids, particularly postoperatively or in cases of major trauma, thereby producing analgesic synergy, reducing dosages, and adverse effect profiles with respect to opiate-induced nausea, constipation, and dysphoria.

Recently, a new indication for cannabinoid manipulation has been claimed: that of improved night vision. Based on simultaneous ethnobotanical claims of fishermen that cannabis stimulated their ability to see in the dark (West 1991; Merzouki and Molero Mesa 1999) in Jamaica and Morocco, respectively, a two-pronged pilot study was launched (Russo et al. 2003). In a double-blind controlled-dosage escalation study with THC as Marinol, improvement in scotopic sensitivity was noted in one subject, while in a subsequent field study with smoked *kif* (*Cannabis sativa/ Nicotiana rustica* mixture) in three subjects, improvement in both dark adaptation and scotopic sensitivity thresholds were noted with the SST-1 Scotopic Sensitivity Tester (Peters, Locke, and Birch 2000). Given the relative paucity of CB_1 receptors in the striate cortex (Glass, Dragunow, and Faull 1997) and their particular density in rod spherules (Straiker et al. 1999), this phenomenon seems to be of retinal rather than cortical origin. This is further supported by anecdotal claims that cannabis improves vision in retinitis pigmentosa (RP) (Arnold 1998). Based on these findings, more formal studies of RP with fully objective measures such as electroretinography seem warranted. Given the neuroprotective and antioxidant effects of cannabis and cannabinoids, extension of therapy to senile macular degeneration appears most promising.

CANNABINOIDS AND NEUROPROTECTION

In light of recent demonstration of the ability of THC and CBD to prevent cell death from glutamate toxicity (Hampson et al. 1998), a whole host of new therapeutic applications gain more than theoretical support beyond the current studies of stroke and closed head injury discussed in relation to dexanabinol. Therapeutic claims for cannabis in amyotrophic lateral sclerosis (ALS) have been advanced in a single case study (Carter and Rosen 2001), and it may prove to be that neurodegeneration may be diminished or arrested in this disorder, Huntington disease (Glass 2001), Parkinson disease (Sieradzan et al. 2001), Alzheimer disease (Volicer et al. 1997), and others. Neuroprotection is a valuable effect, as well, in treatment of seizure disorders (Cunha et al. 1980; Carlini and Cunha 1981; Wallace, Martin, and DeLorenzo 2002). The role of cannabis therapeutics in HIV encephalopathy and slow virus (prion) diseases (bovine spongiform encephalopathy [BSE] or "mad cow disease," Creutzfeldt-Jakob disease, etc.) deserves exploration based on these preliminary findings.

Emerging concepts in psychiatry support that depression is not merely attributable to deficiencies of serotonin, norepinephrine, or dopamine (Delgado and Moreno 1999) but rather may represent a disorder of neuroplasticity, suggesting the desirability to employ neuroprotective agents. An extensive history of such use over the last 4,000 years (Russo 2001b), coupled with this new information, lends credence to the hypothesis. With their unique pharmacological profiles, CBMEs deserve an effort in clinical trials.

SPASMODIC DISORDERS

The current information supporting muscle relaxant benefits of cannabis and cannabinoids in multiple sclerosis and spinal cord injury is extremely compelling. Mining the data of the past (O'Shaughnessy 1838-1840; Christison 1851; Reynolds 1868, 1890), one may wonder anew about the role of cannabinoid therapeutics in disorders such as tetanus, hiccups (Gilson and Busalacchi 1998), stiff man syndrome, the various periodic paralyses, and dystonic disorders such as torticollis, dystonia musculorum deformans, stuttering, and writer's cramp.

FORBIDDEN TERRITORIES

Obstetrics and Gynecology

This topic has been recently reviewed at length (Russo 2002a; Russo, Dreher, and Mathre 2003). Cannabis has been employed for millennia for a variety of related ills. Drugs are rightly eschewed when possible in pregnancy, but cases arise frequently wherein such treatment is necessary, even to save the life of mother and child. Close scrutiny of the literature supports the relative safety of cannabis in such applications, and particularly in episodic use, it is highly likely that the cost-benefit ratio in serious disorders is quite acceptable. Controlled studies of dysmenorrhea, hyperemesis gravidarum, and other disorders with cannabis extracts and medicines should be advanced.

Cannabinoid Medicines in Pediatrics

It is clear that cannabis and cannabinoids hold promise in for many intractable and desperate pediatric conditions, although this concept may be anathema to some.

Although it is frequently the butt of jokes, no one who has not been the parent of an affected infant can truly conceive of the stress and disturbance engendered by infantile colic. A developmental disorder appearing most often between two weeks and three months of life, this poorly understood syndrome produces nightly bouts of inconsolable crying and apparent abdominal cramping pain. Myriad remedies aimed at every imaginable neurotransmitter system of brain and gut tend to fail to stem its ravages. Perhaps infantile colic is another developmental clinical endogenous cannabinoid deficiency disorder. With its antispasmodic, analgesic, antianxiety, and soporific attributes, a THC:CBD cannabis extract holds promise where other agents have disappointed and, if so, countless new parents may be thankful.

Another possible pediatric indication for cannabis-based medicines is cystic fibrosis. In a recent study (Fride 2002a), an extremely compelling and well-conceived rationale for cannabis treatment was outlined that could vastly improve the clinical condition and well-being of affected children. Similar benefits might accrue to other serious failure-to-thrive states.

Cannabis medicines have already demonstrated remarkable success in allaying nausea and vomiting in children undergoing cancer chemotherapy (Abrahamov and Mechoulam 1995). Unfortunately, this study has been largely ignored, rather than being duplicated and extended. Any possible moral objection to such treatment holds no weight when the alternative is severe suffering and even death of a child. The recent report of cannabidiol (CBD) inhibition of glioma cell growth by promotion of apoptosis independent of cannabinoid and vanilloid receptor activity (Vaccani, Massi, and Parolaro 2003), should convince all but the most hardened detractors.

A less lethal but yet still compelling potential indication is childhood asthma. The advent of new delivery devices for cannabis medicines discussed in this volume, combining bronchodilation with modulation of leukotrienes and other mediators of inflammation, offer unique benefits to this disorder.

Finally, the area of child psychiatry deserves additional consideration. A recent book, *Jeffrey's Journey: A Determined Mother's Battle for Medical Marijuana for Her Son* (Jeffries and Jeffries 2003), documents the case study of a young man who failed every conceivable psychopharmacological agent to control his anger and other psychopathology. Only oral cannabis worked, preventing his imminent institutionalization, and allowing a return to a semblance of normal life.

This author, in his practice of child and adult neurology, has heard dozens of unsolicited testimonials to the benefits of cannabis in attention-deficit hyperactivity disorder (ADHD), supporting available anecdotal accounts (Grinspoon and Bakalar 1997). Although the idea of using cannabis-based medicines for this indication may seem surprising to most experts, controlled trials of cannabis medicines for children with ADHD seem clearly indicated, particularly in view of the controversies and side effects of existing psychotropic medications. Extension of the concept to other difficult disorders of obscure pathophysiology such as autistic spectrum and Asperger disorders may be warranted. If and when cannabis establishes its efficacy in pediatric diseases, it shall have achieved a fair measure of redemption from the derision it has elicited during the past century.

REFERENCES

Abrahamov, A., and R. Mechoulam. 1995. An efficient new cannabinoid antiemetic in pediatric oncology. *Life Sci* 56 (23-24):2097-2102.

Achiron, A., S. Miron, V. Lavie, R. Margalit, and A. Biegon. 2000. Dexanabinol (HU-211) effect on experimental autoimmune encephalomyelitis: Implications for the treatment of acute relapses of multiple sclerosis. *J Neuroimmunol* 102 (1):26-31.

Arnold, S. 1998. Seeing is believing. *Nurs Stand* 12 (22):17.

Baker, D., G. Pryce, G. Giovannoni, and A. J. Thompson. 2003. The therapeutic potential of cannabis. *Lancet Neurol* 2(May):291-298.

Bari, M., N. Battista, A. Cartoni, G. D'Arcangelo, and M. Maccarrone. 2002. Endocannabinoid degradation and human fertility. *J Cannabis Therapeutics* 2 (3-4):37-49.

British Medical Association. 1997. *Therapeutic uses of cannabis.* Amsterdam: Harwood Academic Publishers.

Bursetin, S. H. 2000. Ajulemic Acid (CT3): A potent analog of the acid metabolites of THC. *Curr Pharm Res* 6 (13):1339-1345.

Bursetin, S. H. 2001. The therapeutic potential of ajulemic acid (CT3). In F. Grotenhermen and E. Russo (eds.), *Cannabis and cannabinoids: Pharmacology, toxicology and therapeutic potential* (pp. 381-385). Binghamton, NY: The Haworth Press.

Carlini, E. A., and J. M. Cunha. 1981. Hypnotic and antiepileptic effects of cannabidiol. *J Clin Pharmacol* 21 (8-9 Suppl):417S-427S.

Carter, G. T., and B. S. Rosen. 2001. Marijuana in the management of amyotrophic lateral sclerosis. *Am J Hosp Palliat Care* 18 (4):264-270.

Christison, A. 1851. On the natural history, action, and uses of Indian hemp. *Monthly J Medical Science of Edinburgh, Scotland* 13:26-45, 117-121.

Cichewicz, D. L., and S. P. Welch. 2002. The effects of oral administration of delta-9-THC on morphine tolerance and physical dependence. Paper read at Symposium on the Cannabinoids, July 13, at Asilomar Conference Center, Pacific Grove, CA.

Cunha, J. M., E. A. Carlini, A. E. Pereira, O. L. Ramos, C. Pimentel, R. Gagliardi, W. L. Sanvito, N. Lander, and R. Mechoulam. 1980. Chronic administration of cannabidiol to healthy volunteers and epileptic patients. *Pharmacol* 21(3):175-185.

Curry, W.-N. L. 2002. Hyperemesis gravidarum and clinical cannabis: To eat or not to eat? *J Cannabis Therapeutics* 2 (3-4):63-83.

Delgado, P., and F. Moreno. 1999. Antidepressants and the brain. *Int Clin Psychopharmacol* 14 Suppl 1:S9-S16.

Filbert, M. G., J. S. Forster, C. D. Smith, and G. P. Ballough. 1999. Neuroprotective effects of HU-211 on brain damage resulting from soman-induced seizures. *Ann N Y Acad Sci* 890:505-514.

Fride, E. 2002a. Cannabinoids and cystic fibrosis: A novel approach. *J Cannabis Therapeutics* 2 (1):59-71.

Fride, E. 2002b. Cannabinoids and feeding: The role of the endogenous cannabinoid system as a trigger for newborn suckling. *J Cannabis Therapeutics* 2 (3-4): 51-62.

Gilson, I., and M. Busalacchi. 1998. Marijuana for intractable hiccups. *Lancet* 351 (9098):267.

Glass, M. 2001. The role of cannabinoids in neurodegenerative diseases. *Prog Neuropsychopharmacol Biol Psychiatry* 25 (4):743-765.

Glass, M., M. Dragunow, and R. L. Faull. 1997. Cannabinoid receptors in the human brain: A detailed anatomical and quantitative autoradiographic study in the fetal, neonatal and adult human brain. *Neurosci* 77 (2):299-318.

Grinspoon, L., and J. B. Bakalar. 1997. *Marihuana, the forbidden medicine,* Revised and expanded edition. New Haven: Yale University Press.

Grinspoon, L., and J. B. Bakalar. 1998. The use of cannabis as a mood stabilizer in bipolar disorder: Anecdotal evidence and the need for clinical research. *J Psychoactive Drugs* 30 (2):171-177.

Grotenhermen, F. 2001. Definitions and explanations. In F. Grotenhermen and E. Russo (eds.), *Cannabis and cannabinoids: Pharmacology, toxicology and therapeutic potential* (pp. xxvii-xxxi). Binghamton, NY: The Haworth Press.

Hampson, A. J., M. Grimaldi, J. Axelrod, and D. Wink. 1998. Cannabidiol and (-)Delta9-tetrahydrocannabinol are neuroprotective antioxidants. *Proc Natl Acad Sci USA* 95 (14):8268-8273.

Hampson, R. E., and S. A. Deadwyler. 2000. Cannabinoids reveal the necessity of hippocampal neural encoding for short-term memory in rats. *J Neurosci* 20 (23): 8932-8942.

Hanus, L., A. Breuer, S. Tchilibon, S. Shiloah, D. Goldenberg, M. Horowitz, R. G. Pertwee, R. A. Ross, R. Mechoulam, and E. Fride. 1999. HU-308: A specific agonist for CB(2), a peripheral cannabinoid receptor. *Proc Natl Acad Sci USA* 96 (25):14228-14233.

Jain, A. K., J. R. Ryan, F. G. McMahon, and G. Smith. 1981. Evaluation of intramuscular levonantradol and placebo in acute postoperative pain. *J Clin Pharmacol* 21 (8-9 Suppl):320S-326S.

Jarvinen, T., D. Pate, and K. Laine. 2002. Cannabinoids in the treatment of glaucoma. *Pharmacol Ther* 95 (2):203.

Jeffries, D., and L. Jeffries. 2003. *Jeffrey's journey: A determined mother's battle for medical marijuana for her son.* Rocklin, CA: LP Chronicles.

Knoller, N., L. Levi, I. Shoshan, E. Reichenthal, N. Razon, Z. H. Rappaport, and A. Biegon. 2002. Dexanabinol (HU-211) in the treatment of severe closed head injury: A randomized, placebo-controlled, phase II clinical trial. *Crit Care Med* 30 (3):548-554.

Lavie, G., A. Teichner, E. Shohami, H. Ovadia, and R. R. Leker. 2001. Long term cerebroprotective effects of dexanabinol in a model of focal cerebral ischemia. *Brain Res* 901 (1-2):195-201.

Le Fur, G., M. Arnone, M. Rinaldi-Carmona, F. Barth, and H. Heshmati. 2001. SR141716, a selective antagonist of CB1 receptors and obesity. Paper read at Symposium on the Cannabinoids, June 29, at El Escorial, Spain.

Liu, J., H. Li, S. H. Burstein, R. B. Zurier, and J. D. Chen. 2003. Activation and binding of peroxisome proliferator-activated receptor gamma by synthetic cannabinoid ajulemic acid. *Mol Pharmacol* 63 (5):983-992.

Marsicano, G., C. T. Wotjak, S. C. Azad, T. Bisogno, G. Rammes, M. G. Cascio, H. Hermann, J. Tang, C. Hofmann, W. Zieglgansberger, et al. 2002. The endogenous cannabinoid system controls extinction of aversive memories. *Nature* 418 (6897):530-534.

Mechoulam, R., and J. J. Feigenbaum. 1987. Toward cannabinoid drugs. In G. Ellis and G. West (eds.), *Progress in medicinal chemistry* (Vol. 24, pp. 159-207). Amsterdam: Elsevier Science.

Merzouki, A., and J. Molero Mesa. 1999. La [sic] chanvre *(Cannabis sativa* L.) dans la pharmacopée traditionelle du Rif (nord du Maroc). *Ars Pharmaceutica* 40 (4):233-240.

Notcutt, William, Mario Price, and Glen Chapman. 1997. Clinical experience with nabilone for chronic pain. *Pharmaceut Sci* 3:551-555.

O'Shaughnessy, W. B. 1838-1840. On the preparations of the Indian hemp, or gunjah *(Cannabis indica)*: Their effects on the animal system in health, and their utility in the treatment of tetanus and other convulsive diseases. *Transactions of the Medical and Physical Society of Bengal*:71-102, 421-461.

Pertwee, R. G. 2001a. Cannabinoid receptors and pain. *Prog Neurobiol* 63 (5):569-611.

Pertwee, R. G. 2001b. Cannabinoids and the gastrointestinal tract. *Gut* 48 (6):859-867.

Peters, A. Y., K. G. Locke, and D. G. Birch. 2000. Comparison of the Goldmann-Weekers dark adaptometer and LKC Technologies Scotopic Sensitivity tester-1. *Doc Ophthalmol* 101 (1):1-9.

Pop, E. 2000. Dexanabinol Pharmos. *Curr Opin Investig Drugs* 1 (4):494-503.

Ravinet Trillou, C., M. Arnone, C. Delgorge, N. Gonalons, P. Keane, J. P. Maffrand, and P. Soubrie. 2003. Anti-obesity effect of SR141716, a CB1 receptor antagonist, in diet-induced obese mice. *Am J Physiol Regul Integr Comp Physiol* 284 (2): R345-R353.

Recht, L. D., R. Salmonsen, R. Rosetti, T. Jang, G. Pipia, T. Kubiatowski, P. Karim, A. H. Ross, R. Zurier, N. S. Litofsky, and S. Burstein. 2001. Antitumor effects of ajulemic acid (CT3), a synthetic non-psychoactive cannabinoid. *Biochem Pharmacol* 62 (6):755-763.

Reynolds, J. R. 1868. On some of the therapeutical uses of Indian hemp. *Arch Med* 2:154-160.

Reynolds, J. R. 1890. Therapeutical uses and toxic effects of *Cannabis indica*. *Lancet* 1: 637-638.

Russo, E. B. 2001a. *Handbook of psychotropic herbs: A scientific analysis of herbal remedies for psychiatric conditions.* Binghamton, NY: The Haworth Press.

Russo, E. B. 2001b. Hemp for headache: An in-depth historical and scientific review of cannabis in migraine treatment. *J Cannabis Therapeutics* 1 (2):21-92.

Russo, E. B. 2002a. Cannabis treatments in obstetrics and gynecology: A historical review. *J Cannabis Therapeutics* 2 (3-4):5-35.

Russo, E. B. 2002b. Role of cannabis and cannabinoids in pain management. In R. S. Weiner (ed.), *Pain management: A practical guide for clinicians.* (pp. 357-375). Boca Raton, FL: CRC Press.

Russo, E. B., M. Dreher, and M. L. Mathre. 2003. *Women and cannabis: Medicine, science, and sociology.* Binghamton, NY: The Haworth Press.

Russo, E. B., A. Merzouki, J. Molero Mesa, and K. A. Frey. 2003. Cannabis improves night vision: A pilot study of dark adaptometry and scotopic sensitivity in kif smokers of the Rif Mountains of Northern Morocco. *J Ethnopharmacol* 93(1): 99-104.

Sieradzan, K. A., S. H. Fox, M. Hill, J. P. Dick, A. R. Crossman, and J. M. Brotchie. 2001. Cannabinoids reduce levodopa-induced dyskinesia in Parkinson's disease: A pilot study. *Neurol* 57(11):2108-2111.

Straiker, A., N. Stella, D. Piomelli, K. Mackie, H. J. Karten, and G. Maguire. 1999. Cannabinoid CB1 receptors and ligands in vertebrate retina: Localization and function of an endogenous signaling system. *Proc Natl Acad Sci USA* 96 (25):14565-14570.

Vaccani, A., P. Massi, and D. Parolaro. 2003. Inhibition of human glioma cell growth by the nonpsychoactive cannabidiol. Paper read at First European Workshop on Cannabinoid Research, April 4-5, at Madrid.

Volicer, L., M. Stelly, J. Morris, J. McLaughlin, and B. J. Volicer. 1997. Effects of dronabinol on anorexia and disturbed behavior in patients with Alzheimer's disease. *Int J Geriatr Psychiatry* 12 (9):913-919.

Wallace, M. J., B. R. Martin, and R. J. DeLorenzo. 2002. Evidence for a physiological role of endocannabinoids in the modulation of seizure threshold and severity. *Eur J Pharmacol* 452 (3):295-301.

West, M. E. 1991. Cannabis and night vision. *Nature* 351:703-704.

Zurier, R. B., R. G. Rossetti, S. H. Burstein, and B. Bidinger. 2003. Suppression of human monocyte interleukin-1beta production by ajulemic acid, a nonpsychoactive cannabinoid. *Biochem Pharmacol* 65 (4):649-655.

UPDATE

Ethan B. Russo

Nabilone (Cesamet) remains available in various countries, and is now being utilized in treatment of neuropathic pain. In a recent test of 2 mg of nabilone a day in six subjects with multiple sclerosis with spasticity-associated pain, the drug was said to have no significant effects on neuropsychological tests affecting driving skills (Kurzthaler et al. 2005).

Ajulemic acid (CT3, IP 751) remains in Phase II clinical trials as an analgesic and anti-inflammatory. A useful review is available (Zurier 2003). A possible new explanation for its activity may be apparent as an activator or peroxisome proliferator-activated receptor gamma (PPARγ) (Liu et al. 2003). A key point in development of this agent hinges on its analgesic effect without psychoactivity (Burstein et al. 2004). According to company materials (http://indevus.com/), the compound will soon enter human trials as a treatment for interstitial cystitis.

Dexanabinol has unfortunately failed to meet earlier hopes and expectations. In a press release (http://www.pharmoscorp.com/news/pr/pr122004. html), and article (Maas et al. 2006) the company announced that dexanabinol did not demonstrate improvement in the Extended Glasgow Coma Scale or other neurocognitive measures in an advanced Phase III clinical trial of severe traumatic brain injury patients.

SR141716A (Rimonabant, now dubbed Acomplia) remains in Phase III clinical trials for weight loss, metabolic syndrome, and smoking cessation. As with all antiobesity agents assayed in human medicine to date, the drug has no sustained effects after cessation of usage. Despite that, notable decrements in weight up to 10 percent have been noted after one year of treatment. The treatment group did display a doubling of anxiety over that in the placebo group (Le Fur 2004). Additional concerns may become evident in clinical usage once marketed, which is expected later in 2005. One case report has appeared of multiple sclerosis developing in a previously asymptomatic patient in a clinical trial with the drug (van Oosten et al. 2004).

The author's theoretical concept of clinical endocannabinoid deficiency (CECD) has been explored further in a subsequent article (Russo 2004).

REFERENCES

Burstein, S. H., M. Karst, U. Schneider, and R. B. Zurier. 2004. Ajulemic acid: A novel cannabinoid produces analgesia without a "high." *Life Sci* 75 (12):1513-1522.

Kurzthaler, I., T. Bodner, G. Kemmler, T. Entner, J. Wissel, T. Berger, and W. W. Fleischhacker. 2005. The effect of nabilone on neuropsychological functions related to driving ability: an extended case series. *Human Psychopharmacology* 20(4):291-293.

Le Fur, G. 2004. Clinical results with Rimonabant in obesity. Paper read at Conference on the Cannabinoids, June 25, at Paestum, Italy.

Liu, J., H. Li, S. H. Burstein, R. B. Zurier, and J. D. Chen. 2003. Activation and binding of peroxisome proliferator-activated receptor gamma by synthetic cannabinoid ajulemic acid. *Mol Pharmacol* 63 (5):983-992.

Maas, A. I., G. Murray, H. Henney, 3rd, N. Kassem, V. Legrand, M. Mangelus, J. P. Muizelaar, N. Stocchetti, and N. Knoller. 2006. Efficacy and safety of dexanabinol in severe traumatic brain injury: results of a phase III randomised, placebo-controlled, clinical trial. *Lancet Neurol* 5 (1):38-45.

Russo, E.B. 2004. Clinical endocannabinoid deficiency (CECD): Can this concept explain therapeutic benefits of cannabis in migraine, fibromyalgia, irritable bowel syndrome and other treatment-resistant conditions? *Neuroendocrinol Lett* 25 (1-2):31-39.

van Oosten, B. W., J. Killestein, E. M. Mathus-Vliegen, and C. H. Polman. 2004. Multiple sclerosis following treatment with a cannabinoid receptor-1 antagonist. *Mult Scler* 10 (3):330-331.

Zurier, R. B. 2003. Prospects for cannabinoids as anti-inflammatory agents. *J Cell Biochem* 88 (3):462-466.

PART II:
PHARMACOLOGY
AND PHARMACOKINETICS

Chapter 7

Clinical Pharmacokinetics
of Cannabinoids

Franjo Grotenhermen

INTRODUCTION

Among the reasons for the decline of the medical use of cannabis in the first half of the twentieth century were the pharmacokinetic properties of THC in oral preparations (tinctures, fatty extracts). With oral use, cannabis effects commence in a delayed and erratic manner, making it difficult to titrate the required dose. Overdosing and underdosing of medicinal cannabis preparations of unknown THC content were the inevitable consequences often described by physicians of the nineteenth century (See 1890).

A basic understanding of the pharmacokinetic properties of cannabinoids is necessary to comprehend many issues in context with their medical use, e.g., interactions between cannabinoids and metabolic interactions of cannabinoids with other drugs, differences in onset of action and differences in systemic bioavailability between the oral, sublingual, and rectal route of administration and inhalation.

Other questions of general interest, among them the possible effects of prenatal marijuana exposure and exposure to the nursing baby, possible health and legal consequences of passive smoking, forensic questions of drug detection, and several other topics, are easier to understand with some insight into absorption, tissue distribution and metabolism of THC.

The focus of this chapter is Δ^9-THC (tetrahydrocannabinol). The pharmacokinetics of some other natural and synthetic cannabinoids are also presented briefly.

Handbook of Cannabis Therapeutics
© 2006 by The Haworth Press, Inc. All rights reserved.
doi:10.1300/5741_08

Cannabinoids of the Δ^9-THC Type

Sixty-six phytocannabinoids have been detected, mainly belonging to one of ten subclasses or types (ElSohly 2002), consisting of the cannabigerol type (CBG), cannabichromene type (CBC), cannabidiol type (CBD), Δ^9-THC type, Δ^8-THC type, cannabicyclol type (CBL), cannabielsoin type (CBE), cannabinol type (CBN), cannabinodiol type (CBDL), or to the cannabitriol type (CBTL). It is unclear whether some types are artifacts, resulting from oxidation of the respective parent compounds: CBN from Δ^9-THC, CBL from CBC, and CBE from CBD, or through migration of the double bond in Δ^9-THC to the more thermodynamically stable position in Δ^8-THC (ElSohly 2002).

The cannabinoid acids of Δ^9-THC, cannabidiol (CBD), cannabichromene (CBC), and cannabigerol (CBG) are the quantitatively most important cannabinoids present in the plant (see Figures 7.1 and 7.2). Cannabinol (CBN), emerging from THC by oxidation, is also often found, particularly in older cannabis samples. Their relative concentrations vary, and plants have been described that mainly contain one of these cannabinoid types.

Nine cannabinoids belong to the Δ^9-THC type with side chains of 1, 3, 4, and 5 carbons (see Table 7.1). The most abundant compounds are cannabinoids with a C_5 side chain (see Figure 7.3). Large quantities of propyl homologues (C_3 side chain) have been found in some samples from the Indian subcontinent (Turner et al. 1980) and from Africa (Pitts et al. 1992), whereas the methyl (C_1 side chain) and butyl homologues (C_4 side chain) are always present in very low concentrations (Vree et al. 1972; Harvey 1976). The cannabinoid composition is determined by genetic and environmental factors. In one study, Zambian seedstock plants presented with total tetrahydrocannabivarin (THCV, C_3 side chain) levels greater than tetrahydrocannabinol (C_5 side chain), but the ratio was progressively reversed in succeeding generations of plants grown in the United Kingdom (Pitts et al. 1992). In humans, Δ^9-THCV is about one-fourth as pharmacologically active as Δ^9-THC (Hollister 1974).

The cannabinoid acids of Δ^9-THC (Δ^9-THCA) are devoid of psychotropic effects (Dewey 1986) and must be decarboxylated to the respective phenols to produce cannabis-like effects. The phenols are also responsible for most of the medicinal effects. More than 90 percent of the THC in cannabis plants grown in Europe is present as THC acids, while cannabis grown in hot climates of Africa and Asia contain considerable amounts of phenolic THC. The ratio of Δ^9-THC acids to phenolic Δ^9-THC in leaves and flowers of *Cannabis sativa* has been reported to range from 2:1 in Africa (Pitts et al. 1992) to greater than 20:1 in Switzerland (Brenneisen 1984). In

A.

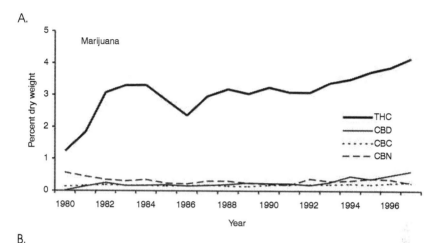

B.

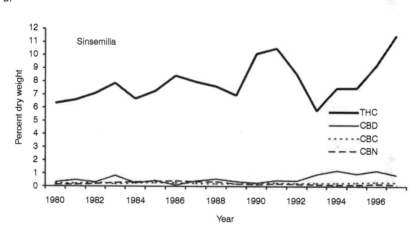

FIGURE 7.1. Average concentrations of the four cannabinoids THC, CBD, CBG, and CBN in confiscated marijuana and sinsemilla between 1980 and 1997 in the United States. (*Source:* Drawn according to data of ElSohly et al. 2000.)

plants grown in the United Kingdom from Moroccan, Sri Lankan, and Zambian seedstock, the THCA:THC ratio was 17:1, compared with 2:1 in plants from the original areas (Pitts et al. 1992). In several samples of cannabis resin (hashish) the THCA:THC ratio was reported to range between 6.1:1 and 0.5:1, the latter in hashish from India (Baker et al. 1981).

THC decarboxylation in cannabis occurs naturally over time, upon heating (Agurell and Leander 1971; Brenneisen 1984) or under alkaline conditions. Slow decarboxylation of Δ^9-THC occurs at room temperature. Five

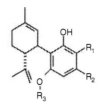

R_1 = H or COOH

R_2 = C_3 or C_5 side chain

R_3 = H or CH_3

Cannabigerol type

R_1 = H or COOH

R_2 = C_3 or C_5 side chain

Cannabichromene type

R_1 = H or COOH

R_2 = C_1, C_3, C_4, or C_5 side chain

R_3 = H or CH_3

Cannabidiol type

R_1 = H or C_3

R_2 = H or COOH

R_3 = C_1, C_3, C_4, or C_5 side chain

Cannabinol type

FIGURE 7.2. Some natural cannabinoids.

TABLE 7.1. Cannabinoids of the Δ^9-*trans*-tetrahydrocannabinol type.

Cannabinoid	Abbreviation	R_1	R_2	R_3
Δ^9-*trans*-tetrahydrocannabinolic acid A	Δ^9-THCA	COOH	C_5H_{11}	H
Δ^9-*trans*-tetrahydrocannabinolic acid B	Δ^9-THCA	H	C_5H_{11}	COOH
Δ^9-*trans*-tetrahydrocannabinol	Δ^9-THC	H	C_5H_{11}	H
Δ^9-*trans*-tetrahydrocannabinolic acid-C_4		COOH or H	C_4H_9	H or COOH
Δ^9-*trans*-tetrahydrocannabinol-C_4	Δ^9-THC-C_4	H	C_4H_9	H
Δ^9-*trans*-tetrahydrocannabivarinic acid		COOH	C_3H_7	H
Δ^9-*trans*-tetrahydrocannabivarin	Δ^9-THCV	H	C_3H_7	H
Δ^9-*trans*-tetrahydrocannabiorcolic acid		COOH or H	CH_3	H or COOH
Δ^9-*trans*-tetrahydrocannabiorcol	Δ^9-THC-C_1	H	CH_3	H

Source: Turner et al. 1980.

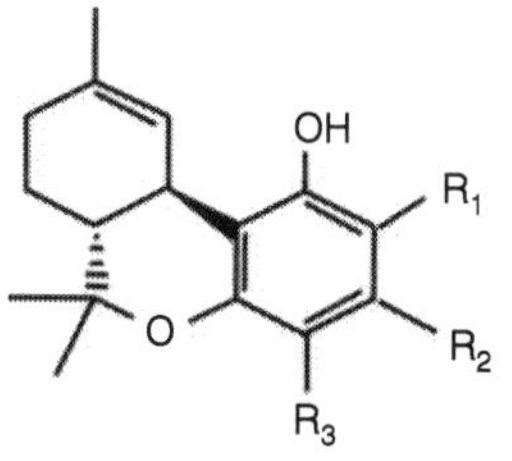

FIGURE 7.3. Cannabinoids of the Δ^9-THC type. The most widespread canna-binoids are the phenolic Δ^9-THC with 21 carbon atoms and a C_5 side chain ($R_2 = C_5H_{11}$) and its two corresponding carboxylic acids A and B (see Table 7.1).

minutes of heating to 200-210°C have been reported to be optimal for this conversion (Brenneisen 1984), but a few seconds in the blaze of a cannabis cigarette are sufficient as well. Cannabis products with a high content of phenolic THC (e.g., hashish) may be very potent without heating, but usu-ally the potency and medicinal efficacy of cannabis products is significantly increased with smoking the dried plant matter, or by cooking and baking the material.

Natural Δ^9-THC has two chiral centers at C-6a and C-10a in the *trans* configuration. Usually the acronym *THC* is applied for this naturally occur-ring ($-$)-*trans*-isomer of Δ^9-THC.

Physicochemical Properties and Degradation of Δ^9-THC

($-$)-Δ^9-*Trans*-tetrahydrocannabinol is defined as (6aR,10aR)-6a,7,8, 10a-tetrahydro-6,6,9-trimethyl-3-pentyl-6*H*-dibenzo[*b*,*d*]pyran-1-ol with the chemical short formula $C_{21}H_{30}O_2$ and a molecular weight of 314.47 Da. According to the German pharmaceutical monograph, dronabinol contains at least 95 percent of Δ^9-THC, a maximum of 2 percent Δ^8-THC and a maxi-mum of 3 percent other substances, mostly cannabinol and cannabidiol (Kommission Deutscher Arzneimittel-Codex 2001). Dronabinol as Mar-inol is available by prescription for medicinal use in several countries, in-cluding the United States, Canada, and some European countries.

At room temperature, Δ^9-THC is a light yellow, resinous sticky oil. Δ^9-THC and many of its metabolites are highly lipophilic and essentially water insoluble (Garrett and Hunt 1974). Solubility was found to be 2.8 mg/L in water at 23°C (Garrett and Hunt 1974). Calculations of the n-octanol/water partition coefficient (K_{ow}) of Δ^9-THC at neutral pH vary between 6,000 using shake-flask methodology (Mechoulam 1981) and 9.44 million by reverse-phase high-pressure liquid chromatographic estimation (Thomas et al. 1990). The wide range for aqueous solubility and K_{ow} may be attributed to the difficulty of uniformly dissolving this essentially water-insoluble substance and accurately measuring small amounts of it. The spectrophotometric pKa is 10.6 (Garrett and Hunt 1974).

Δ^9-THC is thermolabile and photolabile. Storage leads to a decrease in cumulative THC content through oxidation of THC to CBN (Agurell and Leander 1971; Fairbairn et al. 1976). Within forty-seven weeks, the THC content of dried cannabis leaves and flowers decreased by 7 percent with dark and dry storage at 5°C, and by 13 percent at 20°C (Fairbairn et al. 1976). With additional light exposure, the loss increased threefold to 36 percent. Degradation in hashish occurs much more quickly (Agurell and Leander 1971) since the cannabinoids are no longer protected against oxidation by glandular trichomes. The manufacturer recommends that dronabinol be stored tightly closed, protected from light, and in preferably completely filled containers (N. N. Monographs 2001). Stability of THC and two metabolites (11-OH-THC, THC-COOH) in blood and plasma was high for the first month of storage at -10°C, 4°C, and room temperature (Johnson et al. 1984). Concentrations of THC stored at room temperature had decreased significantly at two months but was unaltered at 4°C and -10°C for up to four months.

Δ^9-THC rapidly degrades in acid solutions. The kinetics seems to be first order and specific hydrogen-ion catalyzed (Garrett and Hunt 1974), so that significant degradation of THC was assumed to occur in the normal stomach with a $t_{1/2}$ of 1 hr at pH 1.0 (Garrett and Hunt 1974). Thus, a long exposure of THC in the stomach may considerably decrease the potency of oral cannabis preparations, e.g., when taken together with meals that are difficult to digest.

PHARMACOKINETICS OF Δ^9-THC

Most available information on the pharmacokinetics of cannabinoids pertains to Δ^9-THC (Figure 7.4). Other cannabinoids, among them the phytocannabinoids cannabidiol (Samara et al. 1988) and cannabinol (Johansson et al. 1987) and the synthetic derivative dexanabinol (HU-211) (Brewster et al. 1997), show similar kinetic profiles as the major psychotropic constituent of cannabis. Kinetics of cannabinoids are basically much the same for female and male humans (Wall et al. 1983).

Cannabis products are commonly either inhaled by smoking a cannabis cigarette, taken orally as dronabinol capsules (Marinol), or in baked foods or liquids (see Figure 7.4), doses ranging in the order of 2.5 to 40 mg THC.

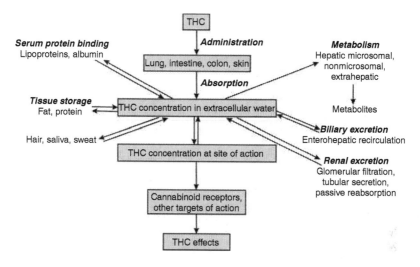

FIGURE 7.4. Pharmacokinetic properties of Δ^9-THC. (*Source:* Modified according to Brenneisen 2002.)

Various other routes of administration and delivery forms have been tested for therapeutic purposes. The rectal route with suppositories has been applied in some patients (Brenneisen et al. 1996), while dermal (Stinchcomb et al. 2001) and sublingual (Guy and Flint 2000) applications are under investigation. Other methods include eye drops to decrease intraocular pressure (Merritt et al. 1981), as well as aerosols and inhalation with vaporizers to avoid the harm associated with smoking (Williams et al. 1976; Lichtman et al. 2000). In February 2002, Unimed Pharmaceuticals, the marketer of Marinol capsules, announced its intention to develop a metered dose inhaler (MDI) of dronabinol (Grotenherman 2002c).

ABSORPTION

Absorption and metabolism of THC varies according to route of administration. The course of plasma concentration following inhalation is similar to that with intravenous administration with a high peak plasma concentration developing within minutes, which then drops quickly (Wall et al. 1983; Ohlsson, Lindgren, et al. 1980). Oral ingestion results in delayed absorption with a flat plasma course achieving its maximum usually after one to two hours (Ohlsson, Lindgren, et al. 1980; Wall et al. 1983; Frytak et al. 1984) (see Table 7.2).

TABLE 7.2. Systemic bioavailability of Δ⁹-THC following inhalation, oral, and rectal administration.

Route	Subjects	Systemic bioavailability (%) Average	Range	Formulation	References
Oral	11 frequent or infrequent users	6 ± 3	4-12	THC in chocolate cookie	Ohlsson, Lindgren, et al. 1980
	6 men, 6 women	10-20		THC in sesame oil	Wall et al. 1983
	7 men, 10 women	7 ± 3	2-14	THC in sesame oil	Sporkert et al. 2001
Inhalation	9 heavy users	23 ± 6	6-56	Marijuana cigarette	Lindgren et al. 1981
	9 light users	10 ± 7	2-22	Marijuana cigarette	Lindgren et al. 1981
	5 heavy users	27 ± 10	16-39	Marijuana cigarette	Ohlsson et al. 1982
	4 light users	14 ± 1	13-14	Marijuana cigarette	Ohlsson et al. 1982
	11 frequent or infrequent users	18 ± 6	8-24	THC in cigarette	Ohlsson, Lindgren, et al. 1980
Rectal	2 patients with spasticity	190-220% of oral bioavailability		THC-hemisuccinate	Brenneisen et al. 1996

Inhalation

Rapid absorption of THC occurs with smoking. THC is detectable in plasma only seconds after the first puff of a cannabis cigarette (Huestis et al. 1992a), with peak plasma concentrations occurring three to ten minutes after onset of smoking (Hollister et al. 1981; Lindgren et al. 1981; Ohlsson et al. 1980; Chiang and Barnett 1984; Perez-Reyes et al. 1982; Huestis et al. 1992a) (see Figure 7.5).

Systemic bioavailability in several studies ranged between 2 and 56 percent after smoking a marijuana cigarette, generally between about 10 and 35 percent, with regular users more efficient (see Table 7.2). Bioavailability varies according to depth of inhalation, puff, and breath-holding duration. About 30 percent of THC in a cannabis cigarette is assumed to be destroyed by pyrolysis. With normal smoking behavior, additional THC is lost in the butt, by side-stream smoke, and by incomplete absorption in the lungs.

A systemic bioavailability of 23 ± 16 percent (Lindgren et al. 1981) and 27 ± 10 percent for heavy users (Ohlsson et al. 1982), versus 10 ± 7 percent and 14 ± 1 percent for occasional users of the drug, was reported. In a study with a smoking machine, patterns of cannabis smoking were simulated with regard to puff duration and volume (Davis et al. 1984), resulting in a figure of 16 to 19 percent of THC retention in the mainstream smoke. If the whole cigarette was smoked in one puff, the percentage of THC in the mainstream increased to 69 percent. Smoking a pipe that produces little side stream

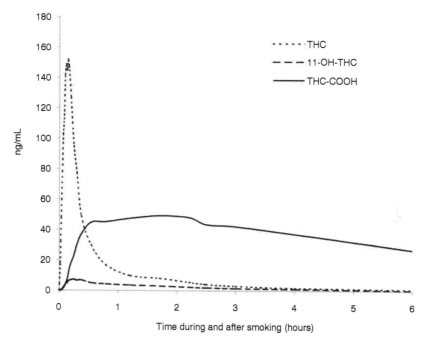

FIGURE 7.5. Mean plasma levels of THC, 11-OH-THC, and THC-COOH of six subjects during and after smoking a cannabis cigarette containing about 34 mg THC. (*Source:* Drawn from a table of Huestis et al. 1992a.)

smoke may also result in high effectiveness with 45 percent of THC transferred via the mainstream smoke in one smoker tested (Agurell and Leander 1971).

Passive smoking has been shown to result in measurable THC plasma concentrations (Cone and Johnson 1986; Perez-Reyes et al. 1983) and subsequent detection of THC metabolites in the urine (Magerl et al. 1987; Cone et al. 1987; Perez-Reyes et al. 1983). Passive exposure of five drug-free volunteers for one hour to 16 marijuana cigarettes in a small unventilated room on six consecutive days resulted in maximal plasma concentrations of 18.8 ng/mL in one participant and several urine positives with the EMIT cannabinoid assay using a cutoff of 20 ng/mL (Cone and Johnson 1986). However, passive inhalation experiments under conditions likely to reflect realistic exposure consistently resulted in values less than 10 ng/mL of cannabinoids in urine (Mule et al. 1988).

Oral Administration

With oral cannabis use, absorption is slow and erratic, resulting in maximal plasma concentrations usually after 60 to 120 minutes (Ohlsson, Lindgren, et al. 1980; Wall et al. 1983; Timpone et al. 1997) (see Figure 7.6). In several studies maximal plasma levels were observed as late as four hours (Law et al. 1984), and even six hours in some cases (Ohlsson, Lindgren, et al. 1980; Frytak et al. 1984). Several subjects showed more than one plasma peak (Ohlsson, Lindgren, et al. 1980; Hollister et al. 1981). Three daily doses of 15 mg of oral THC did not result in significantly higher THC plasma levels than a single dose (Frytak et al. 1984).

Δ^9-THC is expected to be degraded by the acid of the stomach and in the gut (Garrett and Hunt 1974). At low pH, isomerization to Δ^8-THC and protonation of the oxygen in the pyran ring may occur with cleavage to substituted CBDs (Garrett and Hunt 1974). It has been suggested that a somewhat higher bioavailability is obtained in an oil formulation

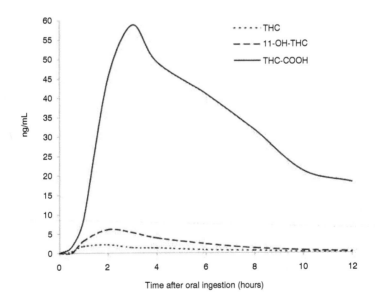

FIGURE 7.6. Mean plasma levels of THC, 11-OH-THC, and THC-COOH of six cancer patients after ingestion of one oral dose of 15 mg THC (estimated from single graphs for each patient of Frytak et al. 1984, with permission). The plasma courses of THC showed considerable interindividual variation (see Figure 7.9 for the courses of THC plasma concentrations of three patients). Used with permission of National Cancer Institute.

(Harvey and Brown 1991); however, absorption seems to be nearly complete in different vehicles. Ninety-five percent of total radioactivity of radiolabeled THC was absorbed from the gastrointestinal tract in an oil vehicle (Wall et al. 1983) and 90 to 95 percent if taken in a cherry syrup vehicle (Lemberger et al. 1972), but it is unclear from these data how much of this radioactivity was attributable to unchanged THC as opposed to its breakdown products.

An extensive first pass liver metabolism further reduces oral bioavailability of THC, i.e., much of the THC is initially metabolized in the liver before it reaches the sites of action. Ingestion of 20 mg THC in a chocolate cookie (Ohlsson, Lindgren, et al. 1980) and administration of 10 mg dronabinol (Sporkert et al. 2001) resulted in a systemic bioavailability of 6 ± 3 percent (range: 4 to 12 percent) or 7 ± 3 percent (range: 2 to 14 percent) with a high inter-individual variation (see Table 7.2).

Ophthalmic Administration

A study in rabbits with THC in light mineral oil determined a variable systemic bioavailability of 6 to 40 percent with ophthalmic administration (Chiang et al. 1983). Plasma concentrations peaked after one hour and remained high for several hours.

Rectal Administration

With rectal application, systemic bioavailability strongly differed depending on suppository formulations. Among formulations containing several polar esters of THC in various suppository bases, THC-hemisuccinate in Witepsol H15 showed the highest bioavailability in monkeys and was calculated to be 13.5 percent (ElSohly et al. 1991). The rectal bioavailability of this formulation in man was calculated to be about as twice as high (190 to 220 percent) as oral bioavailability in a small clinical study (Brenneisen et al. 1996).

Sublingual Administration

Clinical studies are under way using a liquid cannabis extract applied under the tongue. A phase 1 study in six healthy volunteers receiving up to 20 mg THC was reported to result in "relatively fast" effects (Guy and Flint 2000). In phase 2 studies, THC plasma concentrations of up to 14 ng/mL were noted (Notcutt et al. 2001).

Dermal Administration

A few experimental studies have investigated the skin permeation behavior of THC (Touitou et al. 1988; Touitou and Fabin 1988; Stinchcomb et al. 2001). In a study using the more stable Δ^8-THC isomer, the permeability coefficient of THC was significantly enhanced by water and by oleic acid in propylene glycol and ethanol (Touitou et al. 1988). Significant THC concentrations in the blood of rats treated with formulations containing 26.5 mg/g THC were measured. Recent studies designed to develop transdermal delivery of cannabinoids found a mean effective permeability coefficient for Δ^9-THC in propylene glycol of 6.3×10^{-6} cm/h (Stinchcomb et al. 2001).

DISTRIBUTION

Tissue distribution of THC and its metabolites are assumed to be governed only by their physicochemical properties, with no specific transport processes or barriers affecting the concentration of the drug in the tissues (Leuschner et al. 1986).

About 90 percent of THC in the blood is distributed to the plasma, another 10 percent to red blood cells (Widman et al. 1974); 95-99 percent of plasma THC is bound to plasma proteins, mainly to lipoproteins (Widman et al. 1974; Hunt and Jones 1980; Wahlqvist et al. 1970; Fehr and Kalant 1974) and less to albumen. Only 5 percent or less of THC is free for pharmacological activity. The metabolite 11-OH-THC appears to be even more strongly bound than the parent molecule (Harvey 1984). Protein binding of THC metabolites was lower in early phases, with values of 88 to 93 percent after 21 and 70 min of intravenous THC application, compared to 92 to 99 percent after 240 to 1,500 min (Hunt and Jones 1980).

The course of plasma concentrations of cannabinoids has been described to correspond to an open two (Wall et al. 1983; Lemberger et al. 1971), three (Barnett et al. 1982; Timpone et al. 1997; Brewster et al. 1997) or four (Hunt and Jones 1980) compartment model. Even five and six compartment concepts have been found in computer models to best fit the THC plasma course in animals (Leuschner et al. 1986). Following an absorption phase, a distribution phase is distinguished from a plasma elimination phase (two compartment model), that may be distinguished from one or more intermediate phases.

The apparent (initial) volume of distribution of THC is small for a lipophilic drug, equivalent to the plasma volume of about 2.5 to 3 L, reflecting high protein binding that complicates initial disposition. It was reported to be 2.55 ± 1.93 L in drug-free users (Hunt and Jones 1980) and 6.38 ± 4.1 in chronic users (Hunt and Jones 1980). The steady-state volume of distribution has been estimated to be more than 100 times larger, in the range of about 10 L/kg (Lemberger et al. 1971; Hunt and Jones 1980; Wall et al. 1983). These early data have been questioned because of possible inaccuracy of the quantification methods used. With the use of radiolabeled THC, some metabolites might have been considered to be THC. Based on pharmacokinetic data of two studies (Hollister et al. 1981; Lindgren et al. 1981) that applied gas chromatography/mass spectrometry (GC/MS) for analysis of THC concentration an average volume of distribution of 236 L or 3.4 L/kg (assuming a 70 kg body weight) has been calculated (Sticht and Käferstein 1998). Even smaller steady-state volumes of distribution of about 1 L/kg have been reported with GC/MS (Kelly and Jones 1992). This volume is still about 20 times the plasma volume since the majority of the lipophilic drug is in the tissues.

Distribution to Tissues and Redistribution

The lipophility of THC with high binding to tissue, and in particular to fat, causes a change of distribution pattern over time (Ryrfeldt et al. 1973). THC distribution may be divided into several phases representing several pharmacokinetic compartments (Leuschner et al. 1986) or different composites of tissues into which the cannabinoid is distributed (Chiang and Rapaka 1987). Hunt and Jones (1980) estimated that 70 percent of THC initially leaving the central compartment is taken up by tissues and 30 percent is converted via metabolism. THC rapidly penetrates highly vascularized tissues, among them liver, heart, fat, lung, jejunum, kidney, spleen, mammary gland, placenta, adrenal cortex, muscle, thyroid, and pituitary gland, resulting in a rapid decrease in plasma concentration (Ho et al. 1970). Low concentrations were found in the brain, testis and the fetus (Hutchings et al. 1989; Bailey et al. 1987; Ho et al. 1970). Only about 1 percent of THC administered through IV is found in the brain at the time of peak psychoactivity (Gill and Jones 1972). Penetration of the major THC metabolite 11-OH-THC into the brain seems to be faster and higher than that of the parent compound (Perez-Reyes et al. 1976). A ratio of 6:1 has been reported by Gill and Jones (1972). In humans, 11-OH-THC has a similar kinetic profile (Wall et al. 1976) and is as potent as THC in eliciting psychoactive and other effects (e.g., decrease of intraocular pressure) (Perez-Reyes et al. 1972). Thus, it can be expected that the metabolite will significantly contribute to the overall central effects of THC, especially with oral use, but also with inhalation to a lesser degree.

Subsequently intensive accumulation occurs in less vascularized tissues, and finally in body fat (Agurell et al. 1970; Johansson, Noren, et al. 1989; Kreuz and Axelrod 1973), the major long-term storage site, resulting in concentration ratios between fat and plasma of up to 10^4:1 (Harvey et al. 1982), while the concentration in the brain was reported to be only three to ten times higher than in plasma (Harvey 1984). Studies with tritium labeled THC determined maximal levels of radioactivity in kidneys and lung after 2 h, whereas after 72 h highest levels were found in spleen and body fat (Agurell et al. 1970), levels in body fat still increasing after 28 days of chronic administration (Kreuz and Axelrod 1973). In humans, up to 193 ng/g of wet tissue were found in fat tissues four weeks after smoking radio-labeled THC (Johansson, Noren, et al. 1989). The relatively low concentration in the brain is supposed to be due to the fact that the brain is well perfused, moving THC in and out of the brain quickly (Chiang and Rapaka 1987).

The exact composition of the material accumulated in fat is unknown (Harvey 1991), among the possibilities being unaltered THC and its hydroxy metabolites (Kreuz and Axelrod 1973). A substantial proportion of the deposits in fat seems to consist of fatty acid conjugates of 11-OH-THC (11-palmityloxy-THC, 11-stearyloxy-THC, 11-oleyloxy-THC, 11-linoley-loxy-THC) (Haggerty et al. 1986; Leighty et al. 1976). These conjugates have a more lipophilic character than THC itself (Leighty et al. 1976).

Distribution to Fetus and Breast Milk

In animal and man, Δ^9-THC rapidly crosses the placenta (Blackard and Tennes 1984). The course of THC levels in fetal blood fairly coincides with that in the maternal blood, though fetal plasma concentrations were found to be lower compared to the maternal level in rats (Hutchings et al. 1989), sheep (Abrams et al. 1985-1986), dogs (Martin et al. 1977), and monkeys (Bailey et al. 1987). The metabolites 11-OH-THC and THC-COOH cross the placenta much less efficiently than THC (Bailey et al. 1987; Martin et al. 1977).

Following oral intake, THC plasma concentrations in the fetus seem to be much lower, about one-tenth of the maternal plasma concentration (Hutchings et al. 1989), compared to intravenous and inhalation THC intake, with about one-third of the maternal plasma concentration (Martin et al. 1977; Abrams et al. 1985-1986), reflecting differences in metabolism. In humans, THC in cord blood was found to be one-third to one-sixth the concentrations in maternal blood (Blackard and Tennes, 1984). Thus, oral intake may be less toxic for the fetus compared to inhalation. Additionally, there seems to be a considerable variation in fetal exposure to maternal THC in dependency of placenta function. In a twin study with six dizygotic pairs (where each of the twins has an individual placenta) there were large differences between the pairs in cannabinoid concentrations in hair and meconium (Boskovic et al. 2001). Given that twins are theoretically exposed to similar maternal drug levels, these findings suggest that the placenta may have a major role in modulating the amounts of THC reaching the fetus. The ratio of concentrations in maternal and fetal plasma was maintained with multiple administrations (Martin et al. 1977; Hutchings et al. 1989), indicating that the maternal plasma THC and not the fetal tissue is the actual source for the fetal plasma THC.

THC passes into breast milk. In monkeys, 0.2 percent of the THC ingested by the mother appeared in the milk (Chao et al. 1976). Chronic administration leads to accumulation (Perez-Reyes and Wall 1982). In a human female, the THC concentration in milk was 8.4 times higher than in plasma (Perez-Reyes and Wall 1982a). Thus, the nursing infant might ingest daily THC amounts in the range of about 0.01-0.1 mg from the milk of her mother who is consuming 1 to 2 cannabis cigarettes a day, assuming an average daily ingestion of 700 mL milk.

Distribution to Saliva and Sweat

THC was detected in oral fluid (saliva) and forehead wipes (sweat) in 16 of 198 injured drivers admitted to an emergency hospital (Kintz et al. 2000). Concentrations varied between 1 and 103 ng per salivette in oral fluid and between 4 and 152 ng per pad in sweat of the forehead applying GC/MS technology. In a study by Niedbala et al. (2001) with ten volunteers who had been administered single doses of marijuana by smoked and oral routes, THC was detectable in oral fluid for an average of 34 h with a high interindividual variability (range: 1-72 hours), and THC-COOH for 13 h (range: 1-24 hours) by gas chromatography-tandem mass spectrometry (GC-MS-MS) with a 0.5 ng/mL cutoff concentration.

Results of roadside studies using screening devices (immunoassays) for saliva and sweat have provided conflicting results with regard to sensitivity. While screening methods show high sensitivity and specifity for the hydrophilic amphetamines and opiates, they are less sensitive for the lipophilic cannabinoids (Gronholm and Lillsunde 2001). High rates of false negative and false positives have been observed (Samyn and van Haeren 2000; Mura et al. 1999), while others reported good correlation of screening results with later GC/MS analysis of the blood; at least positive results in the screening could mostly be confirmed by GC/MS (Steinmeyer et al. 2001).

METABOLISM

Metabolism of THC occurs mainly in the liver by microsomal hydroxylation and oxidation catalyzed by enzymes of the cytochrome P-450 complex (Matsunaga et al. 1995; Narimatsu et al. 1992), a member of the CYP2C subfamily of isoenzymes playing the major role in humans (Watanabe et al. 1995). Because of its high lipophility, THC needs considerable structural modification to ease excretion. Metabolism of THC occurs quickly. In rats, more than 80 percent of intravenous THC was metabolized within five minutes (Alozie et al. 1980).

Metabolic rates show relevant interspecies differences that may be in part responsible for some problems of interspecies extrapolation of pharmacological and toxicological effects (Grotenhermen 2002b). Borys and Karler (1979) found three times higher metabolic rates in mice than in rats. Differences in composition of metabolic compounds may be attributed to different profiles of cytochrome P-450 isoenzymes (Harvey and Brown 1991). In humans, allylic oxidation, epoxidation, alphatic oxidation, decarboxylation and conjugation have been described (Chiang and Rapaka 1987) (see Figures 7.7 and 7.8).

Besides the liver, other tissues are able to metabolize cannabinoids, but to a much lesser degree, among them the heart and the lung (Nakazawa and Costa 1971; Widman et al. 1975; Harvey and Paton 1976). Nearly 100 metabolites have been identified for THC (Harvey and Brown 1991). Biotransformation of THC produces mono-, di-, and trihydroxy metabolites (Wall et al. 1972; Lemberger et al. 1970; 1971). Further oxidation results in a series of carboxylic acids and their hydroxy derivatives (Wall and Perez Reyes 1981).

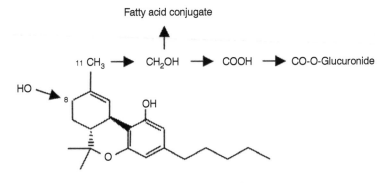

FIGURE 7.7. Main metabolic pathways of THC.

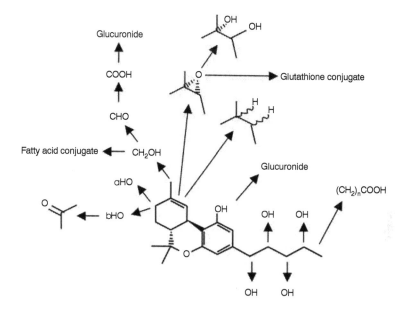

FIGURE 7.8. Summary of metabolic pathways of THC. (*Source:* Modified according to Harvey 1991.)

Major metabolites are monohydroxylated compounds, but the pattern of hydroxylation varies considerably between species (Harvey and Brown 1991). In man (Widman et al. 1978; Halldin, Andersson, et al. 1982; Wall 1971) and many other species, among them mouse, rat, guinea pig, rabbit, and gerbil (Harvey and Paton 1976; Harvey and Brown 1991), C-11 is the major site attacked (see Figure 7.7). Hydroxylation results in 11-hydroxy-THC (11-OH-THC), and further oxidation in 11-nor-9-carboxy-THC (THC-COOH). THC-COOH may be glucuronated to 11-nor-9-carboxy-THC beta-glucuronide. Long-chain fatty acid conjugates of 11-OH-THC are proposed to be a form in which THC may be stored within tissues (Leighty 1973). The C-8 position is also attacked in humans but to a much lesser degree than C-11 (Widman et al. 1978; Halldin, Carlson, et al. 1982).

Average plasma clearance rates have been reported to be 197 ± 50 mL/min for females and 248 ± 62 mL/min for males (Wall et al. 1983) while others reported higher clearance rates of 760-1190 mL/min (Ohlsson et al. 1982) or 605 ± 149 mL/min for naive THC users and 977 ± 304 mL/min for chronic users (Hunt and Jones 1980) (Table 7.3). The higher values are similar to the volume of hepatic blood flow, indicating that it is the limiting step

TABLE 7.3. Pharmacokinetic data for Δ^9-THC.

	Subjects	Dosage (mg)	AUC (ng/ml) × min	C_{max} (ng/ml)	$t_{1/2\beta}$ (h)	V_D (L)	Cl_r (ml/min)	References
Intravenous	4 non-users	0.5			57 ± 4	658 ± 174		Lemberger et al. 1971
	5 regular users	0.5			27 ± 1	597 ± 76		Lemberger et al. 1971
	6 males (drug free)	2			19.6 ± 4.1	626 ± 296	605 ± 149	Hunt and Jones 1980
	6 males (chronic)	2			18.7 ± 4.2	742 ± 331	977 ± 304	Hunt and Jones 1980
	6 males	4		70 ± 30	36	734 ± 444	248 ± 62	Wall et al. 1983
	6 females	2.2		85 ± 26	29	523 ± 217	197 ± 50	Wall et al. 1983
	11 males	5	4330 ± 620	161-316				Hollister et al. 1981; Ohlsson, Lindgren, et al. 1980
	9 heavy users	5	4300 ± 1670	288 ± 119				Lindgren et al. 1981
	9 light users	5	6040 ± 2.21	302 ± 95				Lindgren et al. 1981
	5 heavy users	5	5180 ± 830		> 20		980 ± 150	Ohlsson et al. 1982
	4 light users	5	5460 ± 1180		> 20		950 ± 200	Ohlsson et al. 1982
	4 heavy users	5	9908 ± 3785	438 ± 36	1.9 ± 0.3	75 ± 16	777 ± 690	Kelly and Jones 1992
	4 light users	5	7094 ± 2248	386 ± 29	1.6 ± 0.5	74 ± 35	771 ± 287	Kelly and Jones 1992
Oral	6 males	20		14.5 ± 9.7	25			Wall et al. 1983
	6 females	15		9.4 ± 4.5	25			Wall et al. 1983
	11 males	20	1020 ± 320	4.4-11				Hollister et al. 1981; Ohlsson, Lindgren, et al. 1980
	3 males	3 × 15		4-6				Frytak et al. 1984
	3 males, 3 females	15		3-5				Frytak et al. 1984
	20 AIDS patients	2 × 2.5		2.01 (0.58-12.48)				Timpone et al. 1997

	Subjects	Dosage (mg)	AUC (ng/ml) × min	C_{max} (ng/ml)	$t_{1/2\beta}$ (h)	V_D (L)	Cl_T (ml/min)	References
	7 men, 10 women	10	610 ± 310	4.7 ± 3.0				Sporkert et al. 2001
Inhalation	11 males	19	1960 ± 650	33-118				Hollister et al. 1981; Ohlsson, Lindgren, et al. 1980
	9 heavy users	19	2160 ± 1030	98 ± 44				Lindgren et al. 1981
	9 light users	19	1420 ± 740	67 ± 38				Lindgren et al. 1981
	5 heavy users	10	2450 ± 530					Ohlsson et al. 1982
	4 light users	10	1420 ± 340					Ohlsson et al. 1982
	6 males	15.8		84 (50-129)				Huestis et al. 1992a
	6 males	33.8		162 (76-267)				Huestis et al. 1992a

AUC = Area under the curve; C_{max} = Maximum plasma concentration; $t_{1/2\beta}$ = plasma elimination half-life; Cl_T = total clearance; V_D = volume of distribution.

of the metabolic rate. These high clearance rates explain the high degree of first-pass metabolism, the low systemic bioavailability of THC after oral use, and the much higher concentration of 11-OH-THC after oral administration compared to inhalation.

Only slight differences in pharmacokinetic parameters were observed after single and repeat dosing, indicating that the tolerance after chronic THC administration is not or only slightly due to altered metabolism or excretion after repeated dosing (Hunt and Jones 1980). Neither enzyme induction nor enzyme inhibition appear to have much effect on metabolic clearance of THC.

COURSE OF PLASMA CONCENTRATION OF THC AND METABOLITES

Intravenous infusion of 5 mg THC over 2 min caused average plasma levels within 2 min after the end of infusion of 438 ng/mL in frequent and of 386 ng/mL in infrequent users, that fell rapidly to an average of 25 and 20 ng/mL at 90 min (Kelly and Jones 1992).

The course of plasma THC levels after inhalation resembles that after IV administration (Perez-Reyes et al. 1982; Huestis et al. 1992a). Smoking a single cannabis cigarette containing 16 to 34 mg THC caused average peak levels of 84.3 ng/mL (range: 50.0 to 129.0) for the lower dose and 162.2 ng/mL (range: 76.0 to 267.0) for the higher dose, than rapidly decreased to low levels of about 1 to 4 ng/mL within 3 to 4 hours (Huestis et al. 1992a) (see Figure 7.5).

The maximal THC plasma level after smoking a marijuana cigarette (3.55 percent THC) was reported to exceed the maximal THC-COOH level by threefold and 11-OH-THC by twentyfold (Huestis et al. 1992a). However, THC/11-OH-THC ratios declined and reached a ratio of about 2:1 after 2 to 3 hours (Huestis et al. 1992a). Peak concentrations for THC were observed 8 minutes (range: 6 to 10) after onset of smoking. After onset of smoking, 11-OH-THC peaked 15 minutes (range: 9 to 23) and THC-COOH peaked 81 min (range: 32 to 133) (Huestis et al. 1992a).

After oral application the THC plasma concentration shows a flat course with peaks ranging from 4.4 to 11 ng/mL following 20 mg THC (Ohlsson, Lindgren, et al. 1980), from 2.7 to 6.3 ng/mL with 15 mg THC (Frytak et al. 1984) and from 0.58 to 12.48 ng/mL with 2.5 mg THC (Timpone et al. 1997). The plasma course of THC and 11-OH-THC is much more variable than after smoking (see Figure 7.9). Much higher amounts of 11-OH-THC are formed as with inhalative or intravenous application (Wall et al. 1983; Frytak et al. 1984; Brenneisen et al. 1996). In a study by Wall et al. (1983) the ratio of THC and 11-OH-THC plasma levels in men and women was about 2:1 to 1:1. In several clinical studies (Frytak et al. 1984; Timpone et al. 1997) 11-OH-THC levels even exceeded the THC levels in patients. In a clinical study with 2.5 mg dronabinol daily medium maximal THC levels were 2.01 ng/mL compared to 4.61 ng/mL 11-OH-THC (Timpone et al. 1997).

ELIMINATION

Elimination from Plasma

About six hours after intravenous dosing of THC a pseudoequilibrium is reached between plasma and tissues (Chiang and Rapaka 1987). Concentration in plasma usually has dropped below 2 ng/mL at this time and then decreases more slowly with increasing time from use (Perez-Reyes et al; 1982b; Huestis et al. 1992a). Residual THC plasma levels may persist in frequent cannabis users for several days after last use and may cause difficulties in predicting time of inhalation from THC plasma levels (Huestis et al. 1992b).

After smoking a low-dose cannabis cigarette (1.75 percent THC, about 16 mg) the detection limit of 0.5 ng/mL THC in plasma was reached after

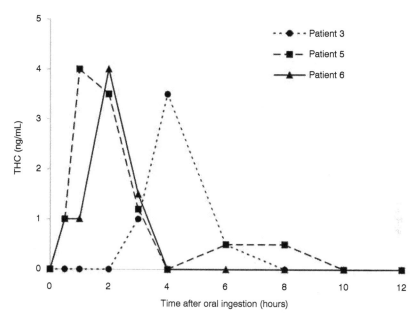

FIGURE 7.9. Mean plasma levels of THC, 11-OH-THC, and THC-COOH of three of the six cancer patients of Figure 7.6 after ingestion of one oral dose of 15 mg THC. (*Source:* Estimated from graphs of Figure 2 of Frytak et al. 1984.)

7.2 h (range: 3 to 12 h) and following a high dose cigarette (3.55 percent THC, about 34 mg) a plasma concentration of 0.5 ng/mL THC was reached within 12.5 h (range: 6 to 27 h). Metabolites disappear more slowly. THC-COOH was detectable for 3.5 days (range: 2 to 7 d) after the low dose and for 6.3 days (range 3 to 7 days) after smoking the high dose cigarette (Huestis et al. 1992a). After a single oral dose of 20 mg overall Δ^9-THC metabolites reached the detection limit of 0.4 ng/mL in plasma after five days (Law et al. 1984).

The major reason for the slow elimination of THC from the plasma is the slow rediffusion of THC from body fat and other tissues into the blood (Leuschner et al. 1986).

The true elimination half-life of THC from the plasma is difficult to calculate, as the concentration equilibrium ratio plasma/fatty tissue is only slowly reached, resulting in very low plasma levels that are difficult to analyze. In a study by Wall et al. (1983) the terminal phase $t_{1/2\beta}$ ranged from 25 to 36 h for THC, from 12 to 36 h for 11-OH-THC and from 25 to 55 h for THC-COOH after oral or intravenous dosing in man and women. The plasma concentration was followed for 72 h in this study, not long enough to determine the half life accurately. Similar elimination half lives for THC in the range of 20 to 30 h covering similar periods have been reported by others (Lemberger et al. 1971; Hunt and Jones 1980; Ohlsson et al. 1982).

Longer half-lives of THC plasma elimination have been determined after higher doses and longer periods of measurement in animals (Harvey et al. 1982) and humans (Johansson, Halldin, et al. 1989). In a study by Johansson, Halldin, et al. (1989), regular users of cannabis were asked to smoke 56 mg radiolabeled THC during two days and then abstain from all cannabis use. A terminal half-life of 4.3 ± 1.6 days has been determined in 5 subjects whose plasma levels were followed for 2 weeks. In 2 subjects followed for 4 weeks terminal half-lives of 9.6 and 12.6 d were noted. However, it is unclear whether THC could be reliably distinguished from its metabolites in this study, thus overestimating the length of the half live (Kelly and Jones 1992). Studies using sensitive GC/MC that follow THC plasma concentrations for long periods are needed to determine the elimination half-life of THC from plasma. Kelly and Jones (1992) measured a terminal half-life for THC of only 117 min for frequent and 93 min for infrequent users, applying GC/MS technology.

The elimination half-life for THC metabolites from plasma is longer than the elimination half life of the parent molecule. In a study by Hunt and Jones (1980), the terminal half-life of THC for chronic users was 18.7 ± 4.2 h and of the overall metabolites 52.9 ± 3.7 h. In the study by Kelly and Jones (1992), the plasma elimination half-life for THC-COOH was 5.2 ± 0.8 days for frequent and 6.2 ± 6.7 days for infrequent cannabis users.

Studies in humans have found no difference in elimination kinetics between heavy and light users (Ohlsson et al. 1982; Hunt and Jones 1980). Differences between regular and casual users in an earlier study (Lemberger et al. 1971) may be attributed to insufficiencies of the detection method (Cone and Huestis 1993). No relevant differences between men and women have been noted (Wall and Perez-Reyes 1981).

Excretion with Urine and Feces

THC is excreted within days and weeks, mainly as metabolites, about 20 to 35 percent in urine and 65 to 80 percent in feces, less than 5 percent of an oral dose as unchanged drug in the feces (Wall et al. 1983; Hunt and Jones 1980). After three days, overall excretion rates were about 65 percent following oral and about 45 percent with intravenous administration (Wall et al. 1983) (see Table 7.4). Excretion rates for urine were similar with both

TABLE 7.4. Mean cumulative cannabinoid excretion, according to Wall et al. (1983).

Subjects	Urine (%) 24 h	Urine (%) 72 h	Feces (%) 24 h	Feces (%) 72 h	Total (%) 72 h	% of Total in Urine 72 h
Women intravenous	11 ± 2	16 ± 3	9 ± 11	26 ± 19	42	38.1
Men intravenous	10 ± 5	15 ± 4	14 ± 11	35 ± 11	50	30.0
Women oral	12.5 ± 3.0	15.9 ± 3.6	9 ± 11	48 ± 6	63.9	24.9
Men oral	10.3 ± 2.1	13.4 ± 2.0	24 ± 42	53 ± 18	66.4	20.2

routes of application, but excretion rates in feces were substantially higher after oral use.

After smoking cannabis, the urine started to test positive for THC-COOH by GC/MS after an average time of four hours (range: two to eight h) (Niedbala et al. 2001). A single dose of THC may result in detectable metabolites in urine for up to twelve days (Law et al. 1984), usually for three to five days (Schwartz et al. 1985). In one study, the average time to the first negative result in urine screening for THC metabolites (enzyme immunoassay with a cutoff calibration of 20 ng/mL) was 8.5 days (range: 3 to 18 d) for infrequent users and 19.1 days (range: 3 to 46 d) for regular users (Ellis et al. 1985). Since urine excretion of metabolites does not monotonously decrease, urine screenings may fluctuate between positive and negative results for several days (see Figure 7.10). The average time until the latest positive result was 12.9 d (3 to 29 d) for light users and 31.5 d (4 to 77 d) for heavy users (Ellis et al. 1985). Similar results with detection times of up to 1 to 2 months for regular cannabis users and even longer in single cases were reported by others (Daldrup et al. 1988).

An average urinary excretion half-life for THC-COOH of about 30 h was observed with a 7-day monitoring period and of 44 to 60 h with a 14-day period (Huestis and Cone 1998). Other groups calculated similar average values of 1.9 and 2 days for frequent and infrequent cannabis users with a 12-day monitoring period (Kelly and Jones 1992) and of about 3 days (range: 0.9 to 9.8 days) when THC-COOH was measured for 25 days (Johansson and Halldin 1989).

Mainly acids are excreted with the urine of which 18 have been identified (Halldin, Andersson, et al. 1982; Halldin, Carlsson, et al. 1982), the main metabolite being the acid glucuronide of THC-COOH (Williams and Moffat 1980). Free THC-COOH is not excreted in the urine in significant concentration (Law et al. 1984). It was proposed that unconjugated THC-COOH cannot be detected in urine of infrequent users (Alburges and

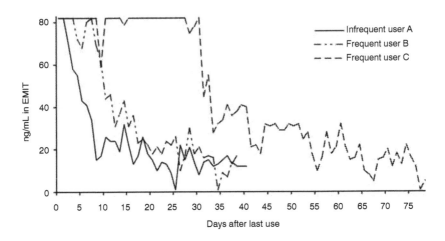

FIGURE 7.10. Course of urine concentration of THC-COOH in one infrequent and two frequent users who abstained from cannabis use at day 0, measured with enzyme immunoassay (EMIT). (*Source:* Drawn according to data of Ellis et al. 1985.)

Peat 1986), while others found free THC-COOH concentrations of 1 ± 1.5 ng/mL one day after intravenous administration of THC in casual cannabis smokers (Kelly and Jones 1992). In regular users, free THC-COOH is usually found and was present in concentrations of 2.8 ± 2.7 ng/mL one day after intravenous administration of THC (Kelly and Jones 1992). The detection of 8β,11-dihydroxy-THC above levels of 15 to 20 ng/mL was proposed to be indicative of use within the previous four to six hour (McBurney et al. 1986).

Several authors reported that the concentrations of THC and 11-OH-THC in urine were insignificant (Garrett and Hunt 1974; Wall and Perez-Reyes 1981), but a recent study found significant concentrations of these neutral cannabinoids using an enzymatic hydrolysis step in the extraction protocol, with THC concentrations peaking at 21.5 ng/mL (range: 3.2 to 53.3) after 2 h of smoking 27 mg THC in cannabis cigarettes, 11-OH-THC peaking at 77.3 ± 29.7 ng/mL after 3 h, and THC-COOH peaking at 179.4 ± 146.9 ng/mL after 4 h (Manno et al. 2001) (see Figure 7.11).

Renal clearance is not constant and has been reported to decrease from a maximum of 20 mL/min at approximately 100 min to 1 mL/min after 4 days of THC administration (Hunt and Jones 1980). The high lipophilicity of

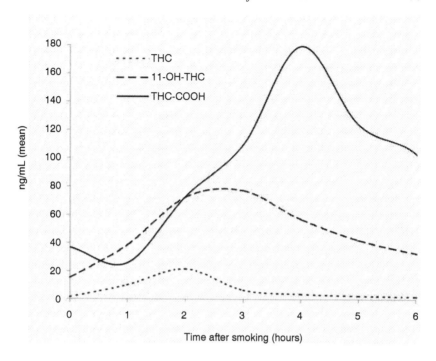

FIGURE 7.11. Mean urine concentrations of unchanged THC and its major metabolites after smoking a cannabis cigarette containing about 27 mg THC by eight subjects with self-reported history of light marijuana use (one to three cigarettes per week or less). One subject later admitted regular use and presented with high baseline concentrations of 11-OH-THC and THC-COOH. (*Source:* Drawn from a table of Manno et al. 2001.)

THC resulting in complete tubular reabsorption explains the lack of significant renal excretion of the unchanged drug (Garrett and Hunt 1974).

The marked enterohepatic recirculation of metabolites and the high protein binding explains the dominance of fecal excretion. The metabolites in the feces are only present in the nonconjugated form (Wall et al. 1983). Acids metabolites, among them THC-COOH, and neutral metabolites, in particular 11-OH-THC, have been found (Mikes et al. 1971; Wall et al. 1983). Differences in metabolite composition have been reported in dependency of route of administration for excretion in both urine and feces. More unaltered THC, less of the hydroxy metabolite, and more THC-COOH is excreted in feces after oral compared to intravenous dosing (Wall et al. 1983).

TIME EFFECT RELATIONSHIP

The peak psychotropic effects ("high") after intravenous and inhalative THC application were noted after 20 to 30 min and decreased to low levels after 3 h, and to baseline after 4 h (Hollister et al. 1981; Lindgren et al. 1981; Chiang and Barnett 1984) (see Figure 7.12). Maximum increase of heart rate was noted within a few minutes (1 to 5 min), decreasing to baseline after 3 h (Lindgren et al. 1981). Conjunctival injection was noted within a few minutes and subsided in some participants by 3 h after smoking (Ohlsson, Lindgren, et al. 1980). Duration of maximal effects is dose dependent and was found to be 45 min after 9 mg THC (Harder and Rietbrock 1997) and more than 60 min with higher doses (Robbe 1994).

Following inhalation, THC plasma concentrations have already dropped significantly before maximal psychotropic effects are achieved (Chiang and Barnett 1984; Ohlsson, Lindgren, et al. 1980). A plot of THC plasma levels versus THC effects shows a counterclockwise hysteresis (Chiang and Barnett 1984). During the first 15 minutes the intensity of psychic effects is still rising while plasma levels are falling (Ohlsson,

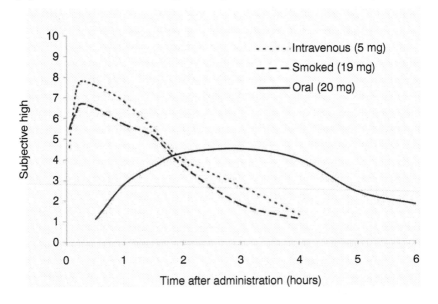

FIGURE 7.12. Time course of subjective effects following three modes of administration. A rating of the degree of "high" was made by subjects on a 0 to 10 scale. (*Source:* Estimated from figures of Hollister et al. 1981 and Ohlsson, Lindgren, et al. 1980.)

Lindgren, et al. 1980). It has been proposed that the first hour represents the distribution phase (Sticht and Käferstein 1998) and that after 1 h the central compartment has reached equilibrium with effect compartment (Chiang and Barnett 1984). Hence, about 1 to 4 h after smoking there is a good correlation between plasma level and effects (Chiang and Barnett 1984). There was also a good correlation between THC plasma level and other effects in this phase, with heart rate (Cocchetto et al. 1981) and with psychomotor impairment (Barnett et al. 1985). Overall correlations between log plasma concentrations and ratings of "high" were reported to be moderately positive (r = 0.53) (Ohlsson, Lindgren, et al. 1980), with better correlations at lower THC levels.

After oral use (20 mg THC in a cookie), reddening of the conjunctivae occurred within 30 to 60 min and was maximal from 60 to 180 min, gradually lessening thereafter (Ohlsson, Lindgren, et al. 1980). As with inhalation, the pulse rate often returned to baseline or below even while the participants felt "high" (Ohlsson, Lindgren, et al. 1980). Psychotropic effects after oral use set in after 30 to 90 minutes (Wall et al. 1983; Hollister et al. 1981), were maximal between 2 to 4 h, and declined to low levels after 6 h (Hollister et al. 1981). Maximal psychotropic effects usually were delayed for 1 to 3 h when the plasma levels started to fall (Hollister et al. 1981) (see Figure 7.13). Correlations between log plasma concentrations and ratings of "high" were reported to be slightly lower compared to inhalation (r = 0.42) (Ohlsson, Lindgren, et al. 1980).

Pharmacokinetic Pharmacodynamic Modeling

With both inhalation and oral use the association between THC levels in the plasma and subsequent psychotropic effects describes a hysteresis over time (see Figure 7.13). Intensity of THC effects depends on concentration in the effect compartment. THC quickly crosses the blood brain barrier (Nyoni et al. 1996). The short delay in psychotropic THC effects compared to plasma levels is attributed to the time needed to penetrate the barrier and bind the cannabinoid receptors. While plasma levels are already falling, the brain concentrations are still rising (Ohlsson, Widman, et al. 1980; Nyoni et al. 1996). In monkeys, an IV dose of radiolabelled THC resulted in peak radioactivity levels in the brain after 15 to 60 minutes in accordance with the time of maximal effect after intravenous and inhalative administration in man (McIsaac et al. 1971). The equilibrium half-life with the effect compartment was calculated to be 29 minutes after smoking a cannabis cigarette (Harder and Rietbrock 1997). Chiang and Barnett (1984) have proposed a kinetic and dynamic model based on an open two compartment model (see

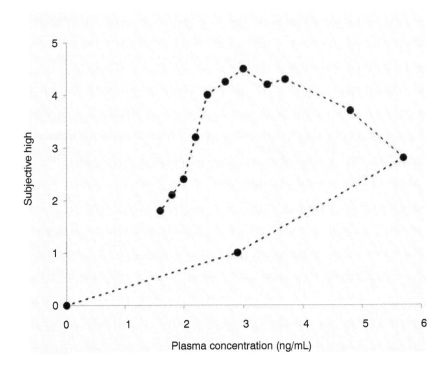

FIGURE 7.13. Phase plots of subjective high/plasma THC levels after oral ingestion of 15 mg THC in a chocolate cookie from 0 to 360 minutes (estimated from figures by Hollister et al. 1981 with some extrapolated data). Every thick point in the figure marks 30 minutes of the whole time. The maximum THC plasma concentration (5.7 ng/mL) was reached after 60 minutes, while the maximum subjective high (on a 0 to 10 scale, see Figure 7.12) was noted 2 to 4 hours after intake of the cannabinoid.

Figure 7.14). Similar kinetic models have been proposed by others (Harder and Rietbrock 1997).

According to the Hill equation there is an association between the intensity of the high effects *(E)* and the amount of THC in the effect compartment.

$$E = \frac{(k_{e0} \times A_e lk_{e1} \times V_1)^{\gamma}}{(k_{e0} \times A_e lk_{e1} \times V_1)^{\gamma} + C_{ss}(50)}$$

The steady-state plasma concentration at the 50 percent of maximum high effect $C_{ss}(50)$ was ascertained to be 25-29 (ng/mL) by using cannabis ciga-

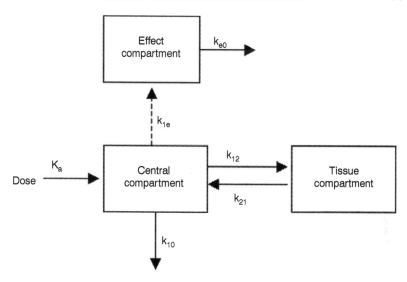

FIGURE 7.14. Kinetic and dynamic model for THC (modified according to Chiang and Barnett 1984). K_a, k_{12}, k_{21}, and k_{10} describe THC kinetics in the empiric two-compartment model. The rate constants k_{1e} and k_{e0} characterize the effect compartment.

rettes of three different potencies (Chiang and Barnett 1984). The elimination rate constant from the effect compartment (k_{e0}) ranged from 0.03 to 0.04 per min, the sigmoid parameter γ (the degree of sigmoidicity of the effect/amount relationship) was 1.5 to 2.0. The transfer rate constant k_{21} from the tissue compartment was much smaller (0.0078 to -0.012 per min) than the elimination rate constant. Thus, the time course of effect must precede the time course of the THC amount in the tissue compartment. The rate constant k_{10} is probably consisting of a mixture of constants for metabolism and distribution between the central and deep tissue compartments (Chiang and Barnett 1984).

Predicting Time of Administration

Several models have been applied to predict time of cannabis use from blood concentrations. Recent cannabis use and possible significant impairment was assumed with THC plasma levels of more than 2 to 3 ng/mL (McBurney et al. 1986) or more than 10 ng/mL (Law and Moffat 1985).

Hanson et al. (1983) were the first to propose the ratio of metabolites to parent molecule for time estimation of last use. Law et al. (1984) stated that a ratio of overall metabolites and THC of less than 20 was indicative of recent use, although the ratio could be greater than 30 in regular users due to accumulation of THC-COOH. Other authors assumed that a THC-COOH/THC ratio less than 1 was indicative for use within the past 30 min, a ratio of 2:1 within one h, a ratio of 3:1 within two, of 4:1 within three and a ratio of 7:1 within 24 h (Garriott et al. 1986).

Huestis et al. (1992b) proposed two mathematical models, derived from linear regression analysis of plasma THC concentration and elapsed time after cannabis use (Model I, $r = 0.949$), and from linear regression analysis of plasma THC-COOH:THC ratios versus elapsed time after use (Model II, $r = 0.919$):

Model I: Log (time in h) = -0.698 log [THC] + 0.687

Model II: Log (time in h) = $(0.576 \times$ [THC-COOH]/[THC]$) - 0.176$

Medium deviation from the correct time of use was about 1 to 2 h two to four hours after use and about 2.5 to 4 h four to eight hours after use (Huestis et al. 1992b). Model I was more accurate following inhalation in infrequent and frequent users, but less reliable with oral use of cannabis, while Model II was more accurate for infrequent inhalation and oral ingestion but tended to overestimate time of usage in frequent users.

Daldrup (1996) proposed a CIF (cannabis influence factor) consisting of a ratio of THC together with 11-OH-THC and THC-COOH weighted with constants.

$$CIF = \frac{\dfrac{[THC]}{314.5} + \dfrac{[11\text{-}OH\text{-}THC]}{330.5}}{\dfrac{[THC\text{-}COOH] \times 0.01}{344.5}}$$

Individuals with a CIF greater than 10 were classified as being severely impaired with regard to driving abilities. This author applied Daldrup's equation to data of a paper by Huestis et al. (1992a). A CIF of greater than 10 was usually reached 2.5 to 4 h after smoking a marijuana cigarette with great interindividual variability (Grotenhermen 2001).

PHARMACOKINETICS OF OTHER CANNABINOIDS

The pharmacokinetics of other cannabinoids resembles the kinetics of THC with regard to plasma course, terminal half-lives and other parameters. These will be reviewed briefly for the natural cannabinoids CBD and CBN, for nabilone, a synthetic 9-ketocannabinoid and psychotropic derivative of cannabinol available on prescription in several countries, and for dexa-nabinol, a nonpsychotropic analog of Δ^8-THC under clinical investigation.

Cannabidiol (CBD)

Average systemic bioavailability of inhaled CBD in a group of cannabis users was 31 percent (range: 11 to 45 percent) (Ohlsson et al. 1984). The plasma pattern was similar to that of THC with high levels of about 100 ng/mL within minutes after smoking, and a fast decrease to a concentration of about 10 ng/mL after one hour. After oral administration of 40 mg CBD, the plasma course over 6 h was in the same range as the course after 20 mg THC (Agurell et al. 1981). Daily oral doses of 10 mg/kg CBD per day for 6 weeks in patients with Huntington's disease resulted in mean weekly plasma levels of 5.9 to 11.2 ng/mL (Consroe et al. 1991). The distribution volume was about 30 L/kg, greater than for THC (Ohlsson et al. 1984). In rats receiving intravenous THC and CBD (1 mg/kg body weight each), brain concentrations of unchanged CBD were higher than that of THC 5 minutes after administration (Alozie et al. 1980).

The plasma clearance ranged from 960 to 1560 mL/min (Ohlsson et al. 1984). An average terminal half-life of 24 h (range: 18 to 33 h) was deter-mined after intravenous injection of 20 mg during an observation period of 72 h (Ohlsson et al. 1984).

Thirty-three metabolites were identified in the urine of a patient treated with CBD and further four metabolites were partially characterized (Harvey and Mechoulam 1990). The metabolic pattern is similar to THC (Wall et al. 1976). The widely used dibenzopyran system for the numbering of cannabinoids cannot be applied to CBD. Metabolites of CBD have to be numbered according to the monoterpene system which can cause some confusion, since the main attacked carbon is numbered C-7 instead of C-11 (see Figure 7.15), resulting in the hydroxy metabolite 7-OH-THC. Several cyclicized cannabinoids were identified as well, among them Δ^9-THC, Δ^8-THC, and cannabinol (Harvey and Mechoulam 1990). The excretion rate of metabolites in humans in urine (16 percent in 72 h) is similar to that of THC (Wall et al. 1976). Unlike THC, unchanged CBD is excreted in large percentages in the feces (Wall et al. 1976).

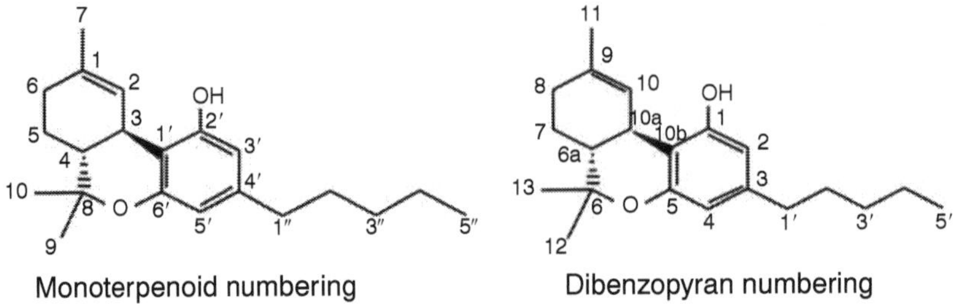

Monoterpenoid numbering   Dibenzopyran numbering

FIGURE 7.15. Numbering of cannabinoids. Chemical structure of THC, according to the monoterpenoid system (Δ^1-THC) and dibenzopyran system (Δ^9-THC).

Cannabinol (CBN)

Average systemic bioavailability after smoking 19 mg CBN was 26 percent (range: 8 to 65 percent), similar or somewhat higher than the values for THC (Johansson et al. 1987). The plasma course following oral ingestion (Agurell et al. 1981), inhalation (Ohlsson et al. 1985; Johansson et al. 1987), and intravenous administration (Ohlsson et al. 1985; Johansson et al. 1987) was similar to that of CBD. The volume of distribution was determined to 23 L/kg (Johansson et al. 1987). The apparent terminal half-lives for CBN were 17 h and 29 h after intravenous administration and smoking, respectively (Johansson et al. 1987). Metabolic patterns in humans were similar to THC with a main attack at C-11 (Wall et al. 1976). Excretion was slower with about 8 percent eliminated with urine and 35 percent excreted in feces within 72 h (Wall et al. 1976).

Nabilone

The absorption of oral nabilone (Figure 7.16) (as a polyvinylpyrrolidone coprecipitate) is nearly complete (Lemberger et al. 1982) with plasma levels peaking at 1 to 4 h. Nabilone was reported to disappear from plasma relatively fast, with a half life of about 2 h (Rubin et al. 1977; Lemberger et al. 1982), while total radioactivity disappeared slowly with a half-life of 30 h (Lemberger et al. 1982). Circulating metabolites in plasma include isomeric carbinols with long half-lives formed by reduction of the ketone at C-9 (Rubin et al. 1977; Sullivan et al. 1978; Sullivan et al. 1987). About 91 percent of nabilone was excreted within 7 days, 23 percent in urine, and 67 percent in the feces (Lemberger et al. 1982).

Dexanabinol (HU-211)

The pharmacokinetics of the synthetic nonpsychotropic cannabinoid dexanabinol (HU-211) (Figure 7.17) was evaluated with doses of 48 mg, 100 mg, and 200 mg as short IV infusions in healthy volunteers. The plasma course best corresponded to a three-compartment model with a terminal elimination half-life of approximately 9 h (Brewster et al. 1997). The plasma clearance of the drug (about 1,700 mL/min) and the volume of distribution (about 15 L/kg) were somewhat higher than seen with THC.

METABOLIC INTERACTIONS

Interactions of cannabinoids with other drugs may depend on activity on similar effector systems or metabolic interactions (Pryor et al. 1976). Since cannabinoids are strongly bound to proteins, interactions with other protein-bound drugs may also occur. However, the latter effect has never been reported.

Metabolic Interactions Between Cannabinoids

Metabolic interaction between cannabinoids has been observed, but only cannabidiol seems to have a significant effect on THC by inhibiting hepatic

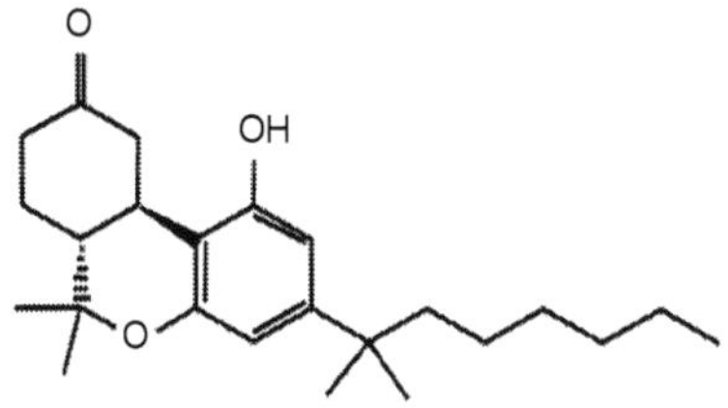

FIGURE 7.16. Nabilone.

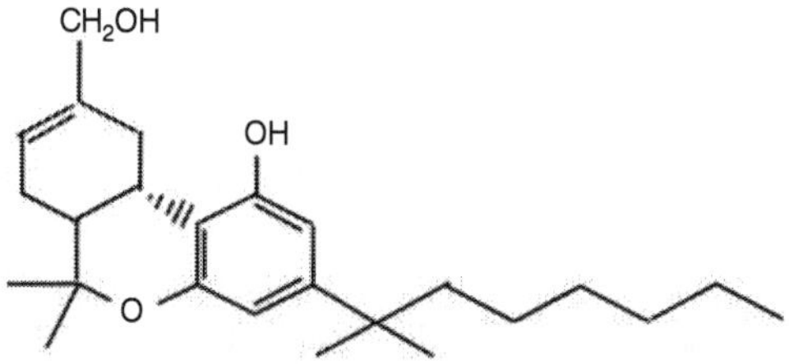

FIGURE 7.17. Dexanabinol (HU-211).

microsomal THC metabolism through inactivation of the cytochrome P-450 oxidative system (Watanabe et al. 1987; Bornheim and Grillo 1998; Jaeger et al. 1996; Yamamoto et al. 1995). Preincubation of human liver microsomes with cannabidiol selectively decreased the formation of tetra-hydrocannabinol metabolites catalyzed by cytochrome P450-3A but had no effect on P450-2C9-catalyzed metabolites (Jaeger et al. 1996).

Treatment of mice with high doses of CBD (120 mg/kg) resulted in changes of metabolism of 12 mg/kg THC and modest elevation of THC blood levels (Bornheim et al. 1995). The plasma area under the curve (AUC) of THC was increased by 50 percent as a function of decreased clearance, while brain levels of THC increased by nearly 3-fold and brain AUC by 7- to 15-fold (Bornheim et al. 1995). The inhibition of cytochrome P-450 isoenzymes by CBD has been proposed to be a reason for recreational use of cannabis together with other drugs that need cytochrome P-450 for metabolism (cocaine, phencyclidine) (Reid and Bornheim 2001); however, THC and THC metabolites (Bornheim et al. 1994; Watanabe et al. 1986), other cannabinoid receptor agonists (Costa et al. 1996) and even CBD (Bornheim et al. 1994) seem to increase the activity of cytochrome P450 with repeated administration through enzyme induction.

In humans, *pretreatment* with 40 mg oral CBD resulted in a delayed, longer, and only slightly reinforced action of 20 mg oral THC (Hollister and Gillespie 1975), while *simultaneous* administration of CBD and THC resulted in a significant block of several THC effects, among them anxiety and other subjective alterations caused by THC (Zuardi et al. 1982), and tachycardia (Karniol et al. 1974), if CBD and THC were given in a ratio of 1:1 or higher, presumably due to antagonistic interaction of CBD at the cannabinoid-1 receptor (Petitet et al. 1998). There were no or only minimal effects of CBD on plasma levels of THC in man (Agurell et al. 1981; Hunt et al. 1981), and there may be a minimal effect on the formation and excretion of metabolites (Hunt et al. 1981).

Metabolic Interactions with Other Drugs

Metabolic interactions of THC with other drugs may occur if these drugs are metabolized by the same isoenzymes of the cytochrome P-450 complex.

A Swiss study found lower plasma levels of the antipsychotic drugs clozapine and olanzapine in smokers of tobacco and cannabis, which was attributed to induction of CYP1A2 of the cytochrome P-450 complex by some smoke constituents (Zullino et al. 2002). Two patients treated with these antipsychotics who stopped smoking experienced adverse drug effects due to increased plasma levels of the drugs, which made dose adjustment necessary (Zullino et al. 2002).

Authors of a case report of a young man who presented with myocardial infarction after taking Viagra (sildenafil citrate, that is metabolized predominantly by the cytochrome P450-3A4 enzyme) in combination with cannabis supposed that the harmfulness of this combination was mainly due to the inhibition of the cytochrome P450-3A4 isoenzyme by cannabinoids (McLeod et al. 2002). However, it seems more likely that the combination of the cardiovascular effects of both drugs were the main reason (see Mittleman et al. 2001), since a relevant inhibition of this enzyme by natural cannabinoids would have only been expected with high doses of CBD.

In a clinical study with AIDS patients, there was only a minor influence of cannabis smoking and oral dronabinol on pharmacokinetic parameters of antiretroviral medication used in HIV infection and metabolized by cytochrome P-450 enzymes, and the use of cannabinoids was regarded as unlikely to impact antiretroviral efficacy (Kosel et al. 2002).

Most interactions of cannabinoids with other drugs are not based on metabolic interactions but on their activity on similar effector systems (Grotenhermen 2002a).

CONCLUSION

With regard to the absorption of cannabinoids, efforts are made to compensate the special disadvantages of oral use and inhalation. Sublingual administration of cannabis-based medicines is used in current clinical studies to accelerate the onset of action, which is slow and erratic with dronabinol capsules or cannabis confections. The use of vaporizers and the development of inhalers are intended to avoid the harm caused by combustion products inhaled with the smoke of herbal material. Further promising alternatives to the most common routes of administration of today are rectal and transdermal administration, increasing either bioavailability or duration of action.

With regard to distribution and redistribution, cannabinoids cause several problems in forensic science. It is difficult or impossible to assess the actual degree of impairment of drivers from cannabinoid levels in body fluids or to estimate the time of the last consumption. In contrast to the hydrophilic alcohol, cannabinoids are lipophilic and there is only weak correlation between THC levels in the effect compartment (central nervous system) and THC levels in blood or other body fluids. Therefore, it seems reasonable to assess actual impairment with other means, e.g., reactions of the eye pupils to light. Amplitude, contraction speed, and dilation speed of the pupils following a defined light stimulus show a dose dependent behavior with maximal effects in the first hour after smoking cannabis and a gradual decline thereafter (Kelly et al. 1993).

Questions of interest with regard to metabolism include different patterns of metabolism in dependency of administration route, and interactions between natural cannabinoids and with other drugs. Since cannabinoids are metabolized by enzymes of the cytochrome P-450 complex, both decreased (through inhibition by CBD) and increased (through enzyme induction by all cannabinoids) activity of these enzymes may occur. This complex metabolic interaction may be further complicated by other forms of interaction (e.g., interactions at the receptor site). Thus, CBD may reinforce the activity of THC by reducing its metabolic rate and antagonize its activity at the CB_1 receptor site, which may explain contradictory results in studies investigating the interaction of the two phytocannabinoids. In general, it can be expected that metabolic interactions of cannabis products (that usually contain only low amounts of CBD) with other drugs are based more on enzyme induction than on inhibition, but this topic needs further investigation.

The increased formation of 11-OH-THC with oral use compared to inhalation is often made responsible for stronger psychotropic effects of oral cannabinoids. But it seems that this metabolite has a similar pharmacological profile as THC in man and binds to the CB_1 receptor, making it unclear how this metabolic difference may cause differences in effects. There seems to be no relevant difference between single THC and whole plant cannabis taken both orally and inhaled with regard to psychotropic and other subjective effects (Wachtel et al. 2002), supporting the view that the differences in scheduling cannabis and THC (dronabinol) in the narcotics acts of many countries are based more on political than on pharmacological grounds.

REFERENCES

Abrams, R.M., C.E. Cook, K.H. Davis, K. Niederreither, M.J. Jaeger, and H.H. Szeto. 1985-1986. Plasma delta-9-tetrahydrocannabinol in pregnant sheep and fetus after inhalation of smoke from a marijuana cigarette. *Alcohol Drug Res* 6(5):361-369.

Agurell, S., S. Carlsson, J.E. Lindgren, A. Ohlsson, H. Gillespie, and L. Hollister. 1981. Interactions of delta 1-tetrahydrocannabinol with cannabinol and cannabidiol following oral administration in man. Assay of cannabinol and cannabidiol by mass fragmentography. *Experientia* 37(10):1090-1092.

Agurell, S., and K. Leander. 1971. Stability, transfer and absorption of cannabinoid constituents of cannabis (hashish) during smoking. *Acta Pharm Suec* 8(4):391-402.

Agurell, S., I.M. Nilsson, A. Ohlsson, and F. Sandberg. 1970. On the metabolism of tritium-labelled, Δ1-tetrahydrocannabinol in the rabbit. *Biochem Pharmacol* 19(4):1333-1339.

Alburges, M.E., and M.A. Peat. 1986. Profiles of delta 9-tetrahydrocannabinol metabolites in urine of marijuana users: preliminary observations by high performance liquid chromatography-radioimmunoassay. *J Forensic Sci* 31(2):695-706.

Alozie, S.O., B.R. Martin, L.S. Harris, and W.L. Dewey. 1980. 3H-delta 9-tetrahydrocannabinol, 3H-cannabinol and 3H-cannabidiol: Penetration and regional distribution in rat brain. *Pharmacol Biochem Behav* 12(2):217-221.

Bailey, J.R., H.C. Cunny, M.G. Paule, and W. Slikker Jr. 1987. Fetal disposition of delta 9-tetrahydrocannabinol (THC) during late pregnancy in the rhesus monkey. *Toxicol Appl Pharmacol* 90(2):315-321.

Baker, P.B., B.J. Taylor, and T.A. Gough. 1981. The tetrahydrocannabinol and tetrahydrocannabinolic acid content of cannabis products. *J Pharm Pharmacol* 33(6): 369-372.

Barnett, G., C.W. Chiang, M. Perez-Reyes, and S.M. Owens. 1982. Kinetic study of smoking marijuana. *J Pharmacokinet Biopharm* 10(5):495-506.

Barnett, G., V. Licko, and T. Thompson. 1985. Behavioral pharmacokinetics of marijuana. *Psychopharmacology* 85(1):51-56.

Blackard, C., and K. Tennes. 1984. Human placental transfer of cannabinoids. *N Engl J Med* 311(12):797.

Bornheim, L.M., E.T. Everhart, J. Li, and M.A. Correia. 1994. Induction and genetic regulation of mouse hepatic cytochrome P450 by cannabidiol. *Biochem Pharmacol* 48(1):161-171.

Bornheim, L.M., and M.P. Grillo. 1998. Characterization of cytochrome P450 3A inactivation by cannabidiol: Possible involvement of cannabidiol-hydroxyquinone as a P450 inactivator. *Chem Res Toxicol* 11(10):1209-1216.

Bornheim, L.M., K.Y. Kim, J. Li, B.Y. Perotti, and L.Z. Benet. 1995. Effect of cannabidiol pretreatment on the kinetics of tetrahydrocannabinol metabolites in mouse brain. *Drug Metab Dispos* 23(8):825-831.

Borys, H.K., and R. Karler. 1979. Cannabidiol and delta 9-tetrahydrocannabinol metabolism. In vitro comparison of mouse and rat liver crude microsome preparations. *Biochem Pharmacol* 28(9):1553-1559.

Boskovic, R., J. Klein, C. Woodland, T. Karaskov, and G. Koren. 2001. The role of the placenta in variability of fetal exposure to cocaine and cannabinoids: A twin study. *Can J Physiol Pharmacol* 79(11):942-945.

Brenneisen, R. 1984. Psychotrope Drogen. II. Bestimmung der Cannabinoide in *Cannabis sativa* L. und in Cannabisprodukten mittels Hochdruckflüssigkeitschromatographie (HPLC). *Pharmaceutica Acta Helvetiae* 59(9-10):247-259.

Brenneisen, R. 2002. Pharmacokinetics. In F. Grotenhermen and E. Russo (eds.), *Cannabis and cannabinoids. Pharmacology, toxicology, and therapeutic potential* (pp. 67-72). Binghamton, NY: The Haworth Press, Inc.

Brenneisen, R., A. Egli, M.A. Elsohly, V. Henn, and Y. Spiess. 1996. The effect of orally and rectally administered delta 9-tetrahydrocannabinol on spasticity: A pilot study with 2 patients. *Int J Clin Pharmacol Ther* 34(10):446-452.

Brewster, M.E., E. Pop, R.L. Foltz, S. Reuschel, W. Griffith, S. Amselem, and A. Biegon. 1997. Clinical pharmacokinetics of escalating i.v. doses of dexanabinol (HU-211), a neuroprotectant agent, in normal volunteers. *Int J Clin Pharmacol Ther* 35(9):361-365.

Chao, F.C., D.E. Green, I.S. Forrest, J.N. Kaplan, A. Winship-Ball, and M. Braude. 1976. The passage of 14C-delta-9-tetrahydrocannabinol into the milk of lactating squirrel monkeys. *Res Commun Chem Pathol Pharmacol* 15(2):303-317.

Chiang, C.W., and G. Barnett. 1984. Marijuana effect and delta-9-tetrahydrocannabinol plasma level. *Clin Pharmacol Ther* 36(2):234-238.

Chiang, C.W., G. Barnett, and D. Brine. 1983. Systemic absorption of delta 9-tetrahydrocannabinol after ophthalmic administration to the rabbit. *J Pharm Sci* 72(2): 136-138.

Chiang, C.N., and R.S. Rapaka. 1987. Pharmacokinetics and disposition of cannabinoids. *NIDA Res Monogr* 79:173-188.

Cocchetto, D.M., S.M. Owens, M. Perez-Reyes, S. DiGuiseppi, and L.L. Miller. 1981. Relationship between plasma delta-9-tetrahydrocannabinol concentration and pharmacologic effects in man. *Psychopharmacology* 75(2):158-164.

Cone, E.J., and M.A. Huestis. 1993. Relating blood concentrations of tetrahydrocannabinol and metabolites to pharmacologic effects and time of marijuana usage. *Ther Drug Monit* 15(6):527-532.

Cone E.J., and R.E. Johnson. 1986. Contact highs and urinary cannabinoid excretion after passive exposure to marijuana smoke. *Clin Pharmacol Ther* 40(3):247-256.

Cone, E.J., R.E. Johnson, W.D. Darwin, D. Yousefnejad, L.D. Mell, B.D. Paul, and J. Mitchell. 1987. Passive inhalation of marijuana smoke: Urinalysis and room air levels of delta-9-tetrahydrocannabinol. *J Anal Toxicol* 11(3):89-96.

Consroe, P., J. Laguna, J. Allender, S. Snider, L. Stern, R. Sandyk, K. Kennedy, and K. Schram. 1991. Controlled clinical trial of cannabidiol in Huntington's disease. *Pharmacol Biochem Behav* 40(3):701-708.

Costa, B., D. Parolaro, and M. Colleoni. 1996. Chronic cannabinoid, CP-55,940, administration alters biotransformation in the rat. *Eur J Pharmacol* 313(1-2):17-24.

Daldrup, Th. 1996. *Cannabis im Straßenverkehr. Final report commissioned by the Ministry of Economy, Technology and Traffic of North Rhine-Westphalia.* Düsseldorf: University of Düsseldorf.

Daldrup, Th., T. Thompson, and G. Reidenbach. 1988. Cannabiskonsum-Nachweisbarkeitsdauer, zeitlicher Verlauf, forensische Bedeutung. In W. Arnold, W.E. Poser, and M.R. Möller (eds.), *Suchtkrankheiten, Diagnose, Therapie und analytischer Nachweis* (pp. 39-51). Berlin, Heidelberg: Springer-Verlag.

Davis, K.H., J.A. McDaniell, L.W. Cadwell, and P.L. Moody. 1984. Some smoking characteristics of marijuana cigarettes. In S. Agurell, W.L. Dewey, and R.E.

Willette (eds.), *The cannabinoids: Chemical, pharmacologic and therapeutic aspects* (pp. 245-261). New York: Academic Press.

Dewey, W.L. 1986. Cannabinoid pharmacology. *Pharmacol Rev* 38(2):151-178.

Ellis, G.M. Jr., M.A. Mann, B.A. Judson, N.T. Schramm, and A. Tashchian. 1985. Excretion patterns of cannabinoid metabolites after last use in a group of chronic users. *Clin Pharmacol Ther* 38(5):572-578.

ElSohly, M.A. 2002. Chemical constituents of cannabis. In F. Grotenhermen and E. Russo (eds.), *Cannabis and cannabinoids: Pharmacology, toxicology, and therapeutic potential* (pp. 27-36). Binghamton, NY: The Haworth Press, Inc.

ElSohly, M.A., S.A. Ross, Z. Mehmedic, R. Arafat, B. Yi, and B.F. Banahan. 2000. Potency trends of Δ^9-THC and other cannabinoids in confiscated marijuana from 1980-1997. *J Forensic Sci* 45(1):24-30.

ElSohly, M.A., D.F. Stanford, E.C. Harland, A.H. Hikal, L.A. Walker, T.L. Little Jr., J.N. Rider, and A.B. Jones. 1991. Rectal bioavailability of delta-9-tetrahydrocannabinol from the hemisuccinate ester in monkeys. *J Pharm Sci* 80(10):942-945.

Fairbairn, J.W., J.A. Liebmann, and M.G. Rowan. 1976. The stability of cannabis and its preparations on storage. *J Pharm Pharmacol* 28(1):1-7.

Fehr, K.O., and H. Kalant. 1974. Fate of 14C-delta1-THC in rat plasma after intravenous injection and smoking. *Eur J Pharmacol* 25(1):1-8.

Frytak, S., C.G. Moertel, and J. Rubin. 1984. Metabolic studies of delta-9-tetrahydrocannabinol in cancer patients. *Cancer Treat Rep* 68(12):1427-1431.

Garrett, E.R., and C.A. Hunt. 1974, Physiochemical properties, solubility, and protein binding of Δ^9-tetrahydrocannabinol. *J Pharm Sci* 63(7):1056-1064.

Garriott, J.C., V.J. Di Maio, and R.G. Rodriguez. 1986. Detection of cannabinoids in homicide victims and motor vehicle fatalities. *J Forensic Sci* 31(4):1274-1282.

Gill, E.W., and G. Jones. 1972. Brain levels of Δ1-tetrahydrocannabinol and its metabolites in mice–correlation with behaviour, and the effect of the metabolic inhibitors SKF 525A and piperonyl butoxide. *Biochem Pharmacol* 21(16):2237-2248.

Gronholm, M., and P. Lillsunde. 2001. A comparison between on-site immunoassay drug-testing devices and laboratory results. *Forensic Sci Int* 121(1-2):37-46.

Grotenhermen, F. 2001. Grenzwertmodelle zur Bestimmung der Fahrtüchtigkeit und Messverfahren. In F. Grotenhermen and M. Karus (eds.), *Cannabiskonsum, Straßenverker und Arbeitswelt [Cannabis use, driving and workplace]* (pp. 313-344). Heidelberg: Springer-Verlag.

Grotenhermen, F. 2002a. Practical hints. In F. Grotenhermen and E. Russo (eds.), *Cannabis and cannabinoids. Pharmacology, toxicology, and therapeutic potential* (pp. 345-353). Binghamton, NY: The Haworth Press, Inc.

Grotenhermen, F. 2002b. Review of unwanted actions of Cannabis and THC. In F. Grotenhermen and E. Russo (eds.), *Cannabis and cannabinoids. Pharmacology, toxicology, and therapeutic potential* (pp. 233-247). Binghamton, NY: The Haworth Press, Inc.

Grotenherman, F. 2002c. IAMC Bulletin, March 3. http://www.cannabis-med.org/english/nav/home-bulletin.htm.

Guy, G.W., and M.E. Flint. 2000. A phase one study of sublingual Cannabis based medicinal extracts. *2000 Symposium on the Cannabinoids,* Burlington, VT: International Cannabinoid Research Society, p. 115.

Haggerty, G.C., R. Deskin, P.J. Kurtz, A.F. Fentiman, and E.G., Leighty. 1986. The pharmacological activity of the fatty acid conjugate 11-palmitoyloxy-delta 9-tetrahydrocannabinol. *Toxicol Appl Pharmacol* 84(3):599-606.

Halldin, M.M., L.K. Andersson, M. Widman, and L.E. Hollister. 1982. Further urinary metabolites of delta 1-tetrahydrocannabinol in man. *Arzneimittelforschung* 32(9):1135-1138.

Halldin, M.M., S. Carlsson, S.L. Kanter, M. Widman, and S. Agurell. 1982. Urinary metabolites of delta 1-tetrahydrocannabinol in man. *Arzneimittelforschung* 32(7): 764-768.

Hanson, V., M. Buonarati, R. Baselt, N. Wade, C. Yep, A. Biasotti, V. Reeve, A. Wong, and M. Orbanowsky. 1983. Comparison of ^{3}H- and ^{125}I-Radioimmunoassay and gas chromatography/mass spectrometry for the determination of Δ^9-tetrahydrocannabinol and cannabinoids in blood and serum. *J Anal Toxicol* 7(2):96-102.

Harder, S., and S. Rietbrock. 1997. Concentration-effect relationship of delta-9-tetrahydrocannabiol and prediction of psychotropic effects after smoking marijuana. *Int J Clin Pharmacol Ther* 35(4):155-159.

Harvey, D.J. 1976. Characterization of the butyl homologues of delta1-tetrahydrocannabinol, cannabinol and cannabidiol in samples of cannabis by combined gas chromatography and mass spectrometry. *J Pharm Pharmacol* 28(4):280-285.

Harvey, D.J. 1984. Chemistry, metabolism and pharmacokinetics of the cannabinoids. In G. Nahas (ed.), *Marihuana in Science and Medicine* (pp. 37-107). New York: Raven Press.

Harvey, D.J. 1991. Metabolism and pharmacokinetics of the cannabinoids. In R.R. Watson (ed.), *Biochemistry and Physiology of Substance Abuse* (pp. 279-295), Volume III. Boca Raton, FL: CRC Press.

Harvey, D.J., and N.K. Brown. 1991. Comparative in vitro metabolism of the cannabinoids. *Pharmacol Biochem Behav* 40(3):533-540.

Harvey, D.J., J.T. Leuschner, and W.D. Paton. 1982. Gas chromatographic and mass spectrometric studies on the metabolism and pharmacokinetics of delta 1-tetrahydrocannabinol in the rabbit. *J Chromatogr* 239:243-250.

Harvey, D.J., and R. Mechoulam. 1990. Metabolites of cannabidiol identified in human urine. *Xenobiotica* 20(3):303-320.

Harvey, D.J., and W.D.M. Paton. 1976. Examination of the metabolites of Δ1-tetrahydrocannabinol in mouse, liver, heart and lung by combined gas chromatography and mass spectrometry. In G.G. Nahas (ed.), *Marihuana: Chemistry, Biochemistry and Cellular Effects* (pp. 93-109). New York: Springer-Verlag.

Ho, B.T., G.E. Fritchie, P.M. Kralik, L.F. Englert, W.M. McIsaac, and J. Idanpaan-Heikkila. 1970. Distribution of tritiated-1 delta 9-tetrahydrocannabinol in rat tissues after inhalation. *J Pharm Pharmacol* 22(7):538-539.

Hollister, L.E. 1974. Structure-activity relationships in man of cannabis constituents, and homologs and metabolites of delta9-tetrahydrocannabinol. *Pharmacology* 11(1):3-11.

Hollister, L.E., and H. Gillespie. 1975. Interactions in man of delta-9-tetrahydrocannabinol. II. Cannabinol and cannabidiol. *Clin Pharmacol Ther* 18(1):80-83.

Hollister, L.E., H.K. Gillespie, A. Ohlsson, J.E. Lindgren, A. Wahlen, and S. Agurell. 1981. Do plasma concentrations of delta 9-tetrahydrocannabinol reflect the degree of intoxication? *J Clin Pharmacol* 21(8-9 Suppl):171S-177S.

Huestis, M.A., and E.J. Cone. 1998. Urinary excretion half-life of 11-nor-9-carboxy-Δ^9-tetrahydrocannabinol in humans. *Ther Drug Monit* 20(5):570-576.

Huestis, M.A., J.E. Henningfield, and E.J. Cone. 1992a. Blood cannabinoids. I. Absorption of THC and formation of 11-OH-THC and THCCOOH during and after smoking marijuana. *J Anal Toxicol* 16(5):276-282.

Huestis, M.A., J.E. Henningfield, E.J. Cone. 1992b. Blood cannabinoids. II. Models for the prediction of time of marijuana exposure from plasma concentrations of delta 9-tetrahydrocannabinol (THC) and 11-nor-9-carboxy-delta 9-tetrahydrocannabinol (THCCOOH). *J Anal Toxicol* 16(5):283-290.

Hunt, C.A. and R.T. Jones. 1980. Tolerance and disposition of tetrahydrocannabinol in man. *J Pharmacol Exp Ther* 215(1):35-44.

Hunt, C.A., R.T. Jones, R.I. Herning, and J. Bachman. 1981. Evidence that cannabidiol does not significantly alter the pharmacokinetics of tetrahydrocannabinol in man. *J Pharmacokinet Biopharm* 9(3):245-260.

Hutchings, D.E., B.R. Martin, Z. Gamagaris, N. Miller, and T. Fico. 1989. Plasma concentrations of delta-9-tetrahydrocannabinol in dams and fetuses following acute or multiple prenatal dosing in rats. *Life Sci* 44(11):697-701.

Jaeger, W., L.Z. Benet, and L.M. Bornheim. 1996. Inhibition of cyclosporine and tetrahydrocannabinol metabolism by cannabidiol in mouse and human microsomes. *Xenobiotica* 26(3):275-284.

Johansson, E., and M.M. Halldin. 1989. Urinary excretion half-life of delta 1-tetrahydrocannabinol-7-oic acid in heavy marijuana users after smoking. *J Anal Toxicol* 13(4):218-223.

Johansson, E., M.M. Halldin, S. Agurell, L.E. Hollister, and H.K. Gillespie. 1989. Terminal elimination plasma half-life of delta 1-tetrahydrocannabinol (delta 1-THC) in heavy users of marijuana. *Eur J Clin Pharmacol* 37(3):273-277.

Johansson, E., K. Noren, J. Sjovall, and M.M. Halldin. 1989. Determination of delta 1-tetrahydrocannabinol in human fat biopsies from marihuana users by gas chromatography-mass spectrometry. *Biomed Chromatogr* 3(1):35-38.

Johansson, E., A. Ohlsson, J.E. Lindgren, S. Agurell, H. Gillespie, and L.E. Hollister. 1987. Single-dose kinetics of deuterium-labelled cannabinol in man after intravenous administration and smoking. *Biomed Environ Mass Spectrom* 14(9):495-499.

Johnson, J.R., T.A. Jennison, M.A. Peat, and R.L. Foltz. 1984. Stability of delta 9-tetrahydrocannabinol (THC), 11-hydroxy-THC, and 11-nor-9-carboxy-THC in blood and plasma. *J Anal Toxicol* 8(5):202-204.

Karniol, I.G., I. Shirakawa, N. Kasinski, A. Pfeferman, and E.A. Carlini. 1974. Cannabidiol interferes with the effects of delta 9-tetrahydrocannabinol in man. *Eur J Pharmacol* 28(1):172-177.

Kelly, T.H., R.W. Foltin, C.S. Emurian, and M.W. Fischman. 1993. Performance-based testing for drugs of abuse: Dose and time profiles of marijuana, amphetamine, alcohol, and diazepam. *J Anal Toxicol* 17(5):264-272.

Kelly, P., and R.T. Jones. 1992. Metabolism of tetrahydrocannabinol in frequent and infrequent marijuana users. *J Anal Toxicol* 16(4):228-235.

Kintz, P., V. Cirimele, and B. Ludes. 2000. Detection of cannabis in oral fluid (saliva) and forehead wipes (sweat) from impaired drivers. *J Anal Toxicol* 24(7): 557-561.

Kommission Deutscher Arzneimittel-Codex. 2001. Monograph: Dronabinol. In *Deutscher* Arzneimittel-Codex (DAC), Loose-Leaf Collection of 2001, edited by Bundesvereinigung Deutscher Apothekerverbände. Eschborn, Germany: Govi-Verlag Pharmazeutischer Verlag/Stuttgart, Germany: Deutscher Apotheker-Verlag.

Kosel, B.W., F.T. Aweeka, N.L. Benowitz, S.B. Shade, J.F. Hilton, P.S. Lizak, and D.I. Abrams. 2002. The effects of cannabinoids on the pharmacokinetics of indinavir and nelfinavir. *AIDS* 16(4):543-550.

Kreuz, D.S., and J. Axelrod. 1973. Delta-9-tetrahydrocannabinol: localization in body fat. *Science* 179 (71):391-393.

Law, B., P.A. Mason, A.C. Moffat, R.I. Gleadle, and L.J. King. 1984. Forensic aspects of the metabolism and excretion of cannabinoids following oral ingestion of cannabis resin. *J Pharm Pharmacol* 36(5):289-294.

Law, B., and A.C. Moffat. 1985. In D.J. Harvey (ed.), *Marijuana '84* (pp. 197-204). Proceedings of the Oxford Symposium on Cannabis. Oxford: IRL Press Limited.

Leighty, E.G., 1973. Metabolism and distribution of cannabinoids in rats after different methods of administration. *Biochem Pharmacol* 22(13):1613-1621.

Leighty, E.G., A.F. Fentiman Jr., and R.L. Foltz. 1976. Long-retained metabolites of Δ^9- and Δ^8-tetrahydrocannabinols identified as novel fatty acid conjugates. *Res Commun Chem Pathol Pharmacol* 14(1):13-28.

Lemberger, L., A. Rubin, R. Wolen, K. DeSante, H. Rowe, R. Forney, and P. Pence. 1982. Pharmacokinetics, metabolism and drug-abuse potential of nabilone. *Cancer Treat Rev* 9(Suppl B):17-23.

Lemberger, L., S.D. Silberstein, J. Axelrod, and I.J. Kopin. 1970. Marihuana: Studies on the disposition and metabolism of delta-9-tetrahydrocannabinol in man. *Science* 170(964):1320-1322.

Lemberger, L., N.R. Tamarkin, J. Axelrod, and I.J. Kopin. 1971. Delta-9-tetrahydrocannabinol: metabolism and disposition in long-term marihuana smokers. *Science* 173(991):72-74.

Lemberger, L., J.L. Weiss, A.M. Watanabe, I.M. Galanter, R.J. Wyatt, and P.V. Cardon. 1972. Delta-9-tetrahydrocannabinol. Temporal correlation of the psychologic effects and blood levels after various routes of administration. *N Engl J Med* 286(13):685-688.

Leuschner, J.T., D.J. Harvey, R.E. Bullingham, and W.D. Paton. 1986. Pharmacokinetics of delta 9-tetrahydrocannabinol in rabbits following single or multiple intravenous doses. *Drug Metab Dispos* 4(2):230-238.

Lichtman, A.H., J. Peart, J.L. Poklis, D.T. Bridgen, R.K. Razdan, D.M. Wilson, A. Poklis, Y. Meng, P.R. Byron, B.R. Martin. 2000. Pharmacological evaluation of aerosolized cannabinoids in mice. *Eur J Pharmacol* 399(2-3):141-149.

Lindgren, J.E., A. Ohlsson, S. Agurell, L. Hollister, H. Gillespie. 1981. Clinical effects and plasma levels of delta 9-tetrahydrocannabinol (delta 9-THC) in heavy and light users of cannabis. *Psychopharmacology* 74(3):208-212.

Magerl, H., C. Wiegand, E. Schulz. 1987. Cannabinoid-Aufnahme durch Passivrauchen. *Arch Kriminol* 179(1-2):31-37.

Manno, J.E., B.R. Manno, P.M. Kemp, D.D. Alford, I.K. Abukhalaf, M.E. McWilliams, F.N. Hagaman, and M.J. Fitzgerald. 2001. Temporal indication of marijuana use can be estimated from plasma and urine concentrations of Δ9-tetrahydrocannabinol, 11-hydroxy-Δ 9-tetrahydrocannabinol, and 11-nor-Δ 9-tetrahydrocannabinol-9-carboxylic acid. *J Anal Toxicol* 25(7):538-549.

Martin, B.R., W.L. Dewey, L.S. Harris, and J.S. Beckner. 1977. 3H-delta 9-tetrahydrocannabinol distribution in pregnant dogs and their fetuses. *Res Commun Chem Pathol Pharmacol* 17: 457-470.

Matsunaga, T., Y. Iwawaki, K. Watanabe, I. Yamamoto, T. Kageyama, and H. Yoshimura. 1995. Metabolism of delta 9-tetrahydrocannabinol by cytochrome P450 isozymes purified from hepatic microsomes of monkeys. *Life Sci* 56(23-24): 2089-2095.

McBurney, L.J., B.A. Bobbie, and L.A. Sepp. 1986. GC/MS and EMIT analyses for delta 9-tetrahydrocannabinol metabolites in plasma and urine of human subjects. *J Anal Toxicol* 10(2):56-64.

McIsaac, W., G. Fritchie, J. Idanpaan-Heikkila, B. Ho, and L. Englert. 1971. Distribution of marihuana in monkey brain and concomitant behavioural effects. *Nature* 230(5296):593-594.

McLeod, A.L., C.J. McKenna, and D.B. Northridge. 2002. Myocardial infarction following the combined recreational use of Viagra and cannabis. *Clin Cardiol* 25(3): 133-134.

Mechoulam, R. 1981. Chemistry of cannabis. *Handbook Exp Pharmacol* 53:119-134.

Merritt, J.C., J.L. Olsen, J.R. Armstrong, and S.M. McKinnon. 1981. Topical delta 9-tetrahydrocannabinol in hypertensive glaucomas. *J Pharm Pharmacol* 33(1): 40-41.

Mikes, F., A. Hofmann, and P.G. Waser. 1971. Identification of (−)-delta 9-6a,10a-trans-tetrahydrocannabinol and two of its metabolites in rats by use of combination gaschromatography-mass spectrometry and mass fragmentography. *Biochem Pharmacol* 20(9): 2469-2476.

Mittleman, M.A., R.A. Lewis, M. Maclure, J.B. Sherwood, and J.E. Muller. 2001. Triggering myocardial infarction by marijuana. *Circulation* 103(23):2805-2809.

Mule, S.J., P. Lomax, and S.J. Gross. 1988. Active and realistic passive marijuana exposure tested by three immunoassays and GC/MS in urine. *J Anal Toxicol* 12(3): 113-116.

Mura, P., P. Kintz, Y. Papet, G. Ruesch, and A. Piriou. 1999. Evaluation de six tests rapides pour le depistage du cannabis dans la sueur, la salive et les urines. *Acta Clin Belg* Suppl 1:35-38.

N. N. Monographs. 2001. Dronabinol capsules 2.5 / 5 or 10 mg (NRF 22.7.); oily dronabinol drops 2.5 percent (NRF 22.8). In *Deutscher Arzneimittel-Codex (DAC), Loose-Leaf Collection of 2001,* edited by Bundesvereinigung Deutscher Apothekerverbände. Eschborn, Germany: Govi-Verlag Pharmazeutischer Verlag/ Stuttgart, Germany: Deutscher Apotheker-Verlag.

Nakazawa, K., and E. Costa. 1971. Metabolism of delta-9-tetrahydrocannabinol by lung and liver homogenates of rats treated with methylcholanthrene. *Nature* 234(5323): 48-49.

Narimatsu, S., K. Watanabe, T. Matsunaga, I. Yamamoto, S. Imaoka, Y. Funae, and H. Yoshimura. 1992. Cytochrome P-450 isozymes involved in the oxidative metabolism of delta 9-tetrahydrocannabinol by liver microsomes of adult female rats. *Drug Metab Dispos* 20(1):79-83.

Niedbala, R.S., K.W. Kardos, D.F. Fritch, S. Kardos, T. Fries, J. Waga, J. Robb, and E.J. Cone. 2001. Detection of marijuana use by oral fluid and urine analysis following single-dose administration of smoked and oral marijuana. *J Anal Toxicol* 25(5):289-303.

Notcutt, W., M. Price, R. Miller, S. Newport, C. Sansom, and S. Simmonds. 2001. Medicinal cannabis extracts in chronic pain: (5) cognitive function and blood cannabinoid levels. 2001 Congress on Cannabis and the Cannabinoids, Cologne, Germany: International Association for Cannabis as Medicine, p. 28.

Nyoni, E.C., B.R. Sitaram, and D.A. Taylor. 1996. Determination of delta 9-tetrahydrocannabinol levels in brain tissue using high-performance liquid chromatography with electrochemical detection. *J Chromatogr B Biomed Appl* 679 (1-2): 79-84.

Ohlsson, A., E. Johansson, J.E. Lindgren, S. Agurell, H. Gillespie, and L.E. Hollister. 1985. Kinetics of cannabinol in man. In D.J. Harvey (ed.), *Marihuana '85*. Oxford: IRL Press.

Ohlsson, A., J.E. Lindgren, S. Andersson, S. Agurell, H. Gillespie, and L.E. Hollister. 1984. Single dose kinetics of cannabidiol in man. In S. Agurell, W.L. Dewey, and R. Willette (eds.), *The cannabinoids: Chemical, pharmacologic, and therapeutic aspects* (pp. 219-225). New York: Academic Press.

Ohlsson, A., J.E. Lindgren, A. Wahlen, S. Agurell, L.E. Hollister, and H.K. Gillespie. 1980. Plasma delta-9 tetrahydrocannabinol concentrations and clinical effects after oral and intravenous administration and smoking. *Clin Pharmacol Ther* 28(3): 409-416.

Ohlsson, A., J.E. Lindgren, A. Wahlen, S. Agurell, L.E. Hollister, and H.K. Gilles-pie. 1982. Single dose kinetics of deuterium labelled Δ1-tetrahydrocannabinol in heavy and light cannabis users. *Biomed Mass Spectrom* 9(1):6-10.

Ohlsson, A., M. Widman, S. Carlsson, T. Ryman, and C. Strid. 1980. Plasma and brain levels of delta 6-THC and seven monooxygenated metabolites correlated to the cataleptic effect in the mouse. *Acta Pharmacol Toxicol (Copenh)* 47(4):308-317.

Perez-Reyes, M., S. Di Guiseppi, K.H. Davis, V.H. Schindler, and C.E. Cook. 1982. Comparison of effects of marihuana cigarettes to three different potencies. *Clin Pharmacol Ther* 31(5):617-24.

Perez-Reyes, M., S. Di Guiseppi, A.P. Mason, and K.H. Davis. 1983. Passive inhala-tion of marihuana smoke and urinary excretion of cannabinoids. *Clin Pharmacol Ther* 34(1):36-41.

Perez-Reyes, M., J. Simmons, D. Brine, G.L. Kimmel, K.H. Davis, and M.E. Wall. 1976. Rate of penetration of Δ⁹-tetrahydrocannabinol and 11-hydroxy-Δ⁹-tetra-hydrocannabinol to the brain of mice. In G.G. Nahas (ed.), *Marihuana: Chemis-try, Biochemistry, and Cellular Effects* (pp. 179-187). New York: Springer.

Perez-Reyes, M., M. Timmons, M. Lipton, K. Davis, and M. Wall. 1972. Intrave-nous injection in man of delta-9-tetrahydrocannabinol and 11-OH-delta-9-tetra-hydrocannabinol. *Science* 177(49):633-635.

Perez-Reyes, M., and M.E. Wall. 1982. Presence of delta 9-tetrahydrocannabinol in human milk. *N Engl J Med* 307:819-820.

Petitet, F., B. Jeantaud, M. Reibaud, A. Imperato, and M.C. Dubroeucq. 1998. Com-plex pharmacology of natural cannabinoids: evidence for partial agonist activity of Δ 9-tetrahydrocannabinol and antagonist activity of cannabidiol on rat brain cannabinoid receptors. *Life Sci* 63(1): PL1-PL6.

Pitts, J.E., J.D. Neal, and T.A. Gough. 1992. Some features of Cannabis plants grown in the United Kingdom from, seeds of known origin. *J Pharm Pharmacol* 44(12): 947-951.

Pryor, G.T., S. Husain, and C. Mitoma. 1976. Acute and subacute interactions be-tween delta-9-tetrahydrocannabinol and other drugs in the rat. *Ann N Y Acad Sci* 281: 171-189.

Reid, M.J., and L.M. Bornheim. 2001. Cannabinoid-induced alterations in brain disposition of drugs of abuse. *Biochem Pharmacol* 61(11):1357-1367.

Robbe, H.W.J. 1994. *Influence of marijuana on driving.* Maastricht: Institut for Hu-man Psychopharmacology, University of Limburg.

Rubin, A., L. Lemberger, P. Warrick, R.E. Crabtree, H. Sullivan, H. Rowe, and B.D. Obermeyer. 1977. Physiologic disposition of nabilone, a cannabinol derivative, in man. *Clin Pharmacol Ther* 22(1):85-91.

Ryrfeldt, A., C.H. Ramsay, I.M. Nilsson, M. Widman, and S. Agurell. 1973. Whole-body autoradiography of Δ1-tetrahydrocannabinol and Δ1(6)-tetrahydrocan-nabinol in mouse. Pharmacokinetic aspects of Δ1-tetrahydrocannabinol and its metabolites. *Acta Pharm Suec* 10(1): 13-28.

Samara, E., M. Bialer, and R. Mechoulam. 1988. Pharmacokinetics of cannabidiol in dogs. *Drug Metab Dispos* 16(3):469-472.

Samyn, N., and C. van Haeren. 2000. On-site testing of saliva and sweat with Drugwipe and determination of concentrations of drugs of abuse in saliva, plasma and urine of suspected users. *Int J Legal Med* 113(3):150-154.

Schwartz, R.H., G.F. Hayden, and M. Riddile. 1985. Laboratory detection of marijuana use. Experience with a photometric immunoassay to measure urinary cannabinoids. *Am J Dis Child* 139(11):1093-1096.

See, G. 1890. Anwendung der Cannabis indica in der Behandlung der Neurosen und gastrischen Dyspepsieen. *Dtsch Med Wschr* 60(31-34):679-682, 727-730, 748-754, 771-774.

Sporkert, F., F. Pragst, C.J. Ploner, A. Tschirch, and A.M. Stadelmann. 2001. Pharmacokinetic investigation of delta-9-tetrahydrocannabinol and its metabolites after single administration of 10 mg Marinol in attendance of a psychiatric study with 17 volunteers. *Poster at the 39th Annual International Meeting, The International Association of Forensic Toxicologists,* Prague, Czech Republic, August 26-30, 62.

Steinmeyer, S., H. Ohr, H.J. Maurer, and M.R. Moeller. 2001. Practical aspects of roadside tests for administrative traffic offences in Germany. *Forensic Sci Int* 121(1-2):33-36.

Sticht, G., and H. Käferstein. 1998. Grundbegriffe, Toxikokinetik und Toxikodynamik. In G. Berghaus, H.P. Krüger (eds.), *Cannabis im Straßenverkehr* (p. 1-11). Stuttgart: Gustav Fischer.

Stinchcomb, A., P. Challapalli, K. Harris, and J. Browe. 2001. Optimization of in vitro experimental conditions for measuring the percutaneous absorption of Δ9-THC, cannabidiol, and WIN55,212-2. 2001 Symposium on the Cannabinoids. Burlington Vermont: International Cannabinoid Research Society.

Sullivan, H.R., G.K. Hanasono, W.M. Miller, and P.G. Wood. 1987. Species specificity in the metabolism of nabilone. Relationship between toxicity and metabolic routes. *Xenobiotica* 17(4):459-468.

Sullivan, H.R., D.L. Kau, and P.G. Wood. 1978. Pharmacokinetics of nabilone, a psychotropically active 9-ketocannabinoid, in the dog. Utilization of quantitative selected ion monitoring and deuterium labeling. *Biomed Mass Spectrom* 5(4): 296-301.

Thomas, B.F., D.R. Compton, and B.R. Martin. 1990. Characterization of the lipophilicity of natural and synthetic analogs of delta 9-tetrahydrocannabinol and its relationship to pharmacological potency. *J Pharmacol Exp Ther* 255(2): 624-630.

Timpone, J.G., D.J. Wright, N. Li, M.J. Egorin, M.E. Enama, J. Mayers, G. Galetto, and the DATRI 004 Study Group. 1997. The safety and pharmacokinetics of single-agent and combination therapy with megestrol acetate and dronabinol for the treatment of HIV wasting syndrome. *AIDS Res Hum Retroviruses* 13(4):305-315.

Touitou, E., and B. Fabin. 1988. Altered skin permeation of a highly lipophilic molecule: Tetrahydrocannabinol. *Int J Pharm* 43:17-22.

Touitou, E., B. Fabin, S. Dany, and S. Almog. 1988. Transdermal delivery of tetrahydrocannabinol. *Int J Pharm* 43: 9-15.

Turner, C., M.A. ElSohly, and E. Boeren. 1980. Constituent of *Cannabis sativa* L. XVII. A review of the natural constituents. *Journal of Natural Products* 43(2): 169-234.

Vree, T.B., D.D. Breimer, C.A. van Ginneken, and J.M. van Rossum. 1972. Identification in hashish of tetrahydrocannabinol, cannabidiol and cannabinol analogues with a methyl side-chain. *J Pharm Pharmacol* 24(1):7-12.

Wachtel, S.R., M.A. ElSohly, S.A. Ross, J. Ambre, and H. De Wit. 2002. Comparison of the subjective effects of delta(9)-tetrahydrocannabinol and marijuana in humans. *Psychopharmacology* 161(4):331-339.

Wahlqvist, M., I.M. Nilsson, F. Sandberg, and S. Agurell. 1970. Binding of delta-1-tetrahydrocannabinol to human plasma proteins. *Biochem Pharmacol* 19(9): 2579-2584.

Wall, M.E. 1971. The in vivo and in vitro metabolism of tetrahydrocannabinol. *Ann N Y Acad Sci* 191:23-29.

Wall, M.E., D.R. Brine, and M. Perez-Reyes. 1976. Metabolism of cannabinoids in man. In M.C. Braude, S. Szara (eds.), *Pharmacology of marihuana* (pp. 93-113). New York: Raven Press.

Wall, M.E., D.R. Brine, C.G. Pitt, and M. Perez-Reyes. 1972. Identification of Δ9-tetrahydrocannabinol and metabolites in man. *J Am Chem Soc* 94(24): 8579-8581.

Wall, M.E., and M. Perez-Reyes. 1981. The metabolism of delta 9-tetrahydrocannabinol and related cannabinoids in man. *J Clin Pharmacol* 21(8-9 Suppl): 178S-189S.

Wall, M.E., B.M. Sadler, D. Brine, H. Taylor, and M. Perez-Reyes. 1983. Metabolism, disposition, and kinetics of delta-9-tetrahydrocannabinol, in men and women. *Clin Pharmacol Ther* 34(3):352-363.

Watanabe, K., M. Arai, S. Narimatsu, I. Yamamoto, and H. Yoshimura. 1986. Effect of repeated administration of 11-hydroxy-delta 8-tetrahydrocannabinol, an active metabolite of delta 8-tetrahydrocannabinol, on the hepatic microsomal drug-metabolizing enzyme system of mice. *Biochem Pharmacol* 35(11):1861-1865.

Watanabe, K., M. Arai, S. Narimatsu, I. Yamamoto, and H. Yoshimura. 1987. Self-catalyzed inactivation of cytochrome P-450 during microsomal metabolism of cannabidiol. *Biochem Pharmacol* 36(20):3371-3377.

Watanabe, K., T. Matsunaga, I. Yamamoto, Y. Funae, and H. Yoshimura. 1995. Involvement of CYP2C in the metabolism of cannabinoids by human hepatic microsomes from an old woman. *Biol Pharm Bull* 18(8):1138-1141.

Widman, M., S. Agurell, M. Ehrnebo, and G. Jones. 1974. Binding of (+)- and (−)-Δ 1-tetrahydrocannabinols and (−)-7-hydroxy-Δ 1-tetrahydrocannabinol to blood cells and plasma proteins in man. *J Pharm Pharmacol* 26(11):914-916.

Widman, M., M. Halldin, and B. Martin. 1978. In vitro metabolism of tetrahydrocannabinol by rhesus monkey liver and human liver. *Adv Biosci* 22-23:101-103.

Widman, M., M. Nordqvist, C.T. Dollery, and R.H. Briant. 1975. Metabolism of delta1-tetrahydrocannabinol by the isolated perfused dog lung. Comparison with in vitro liver metabolism. *J Pharm Pharmacol* 27(11):842-848.

Williams, S.J., J.P. Hartley, and J.D. Graham. 1976. Bronchodilator effect of delta1-tetrahydrocannabinol administered by aerosol of asthmatic patients. *Thorax* 31(6): 720-723.

Williams, P.L., and A.C. Moffat. 1980. Identification in human urine of delta 9-tetrahydrocannabinol-11-oic acid glucuronide: A tetrahydrocannabinol metabolite. *J Pharm Pharmacol* 32(7):445-448.

Yamamoto, I., K. Watanabe, S. Narimatsu, and H. Yoshimura. 1995. Recent advances in the metabolism of cannabinoids. *Int J Biochem Cell Biol* 27(8): 741-746.

Zuardi, A.W., I. Shirakawa, E. Finkelfarb, and I.G. Karniol. 1982. Action of cannabidiol on the anxiety and other effects produced by delta 9-THC in normal subjects. *Psychopharmacology* 76(3):245-250.

Zullino, D.F., D. Delessert, C.B. Eap, M. Preisig, and P. Baumann. 2002. Tobacco and cannabis smoking cessation can lead to intoxication with clozapine or olanzapine. *Int Clin Psychopharmacol* 17(+3):141-143.

Chapter 8

Clinical Pharmacodynamics of Cannabinoids

Franjo Grotenhermen

INTRODUCTION

Unlike the opiates and many other medicinally used plant constituents, the cannabinoids were not identified before the twentieth century, which occasionally resulted in dosing problems of oral medicinal extracts which had been in use in the nineteenth century in Europe and North America. In the 1930s and 1940s, the chemical structure of the first phytocannabinoids had been successfully characterized (Loewe 1950), and the first synthetic derivatives of THC (parahexyl, DMHP) were successfully tested in clinical studies for epilepsy (Davis and Ramsey 1949), depression (Stockings 1947) and dependency to alcohol and opiates (Thompson and Proctor 1953). However, it was not until 1964 that Δ^9-tetrahydrocannabinol (Δ^9-THC, dronabinol), mainly responsible for the pharmacological effects of the cannabis plant (Dewey 1986; Hollister 1986), was stereochemically defined, and synthesized (Gaoni and Mechoulam 1964). Another scientific breakthrough in cannabinoid research was the detection of a system of specific cannabinoid receptors in mammals and their endogenous ligands within the past fifteen years. Both detections resulted in a considerable boost in research activities (see Figure 8.1).

Cannabinoids were originally thought to be present only in the cannabis plant (*Cannabis sativa* L.), but recently some cannabinoid-type bibenzyls have also been found in liverwort *(Radula perrottetii* and *Radula marginata)* (Toyota et al. 2002), the chemical structure of perrottetinenic acid in liverwort being similar to that of Δ^9-THC in cannabis.

About 65 cannabinoids have been detected in the cannabis plant, mainly belonging to 1 of 10 subclasses or types (ElSohly 2002), of which the cannabigerol type (CBG), the cannabichromene type (CBC), the cannabidiol type

Handbook of Cannabis Therapeutics
© 2006 by The Haworth Press, Inc. All rights reserved.
doi:10.1300/5741_09

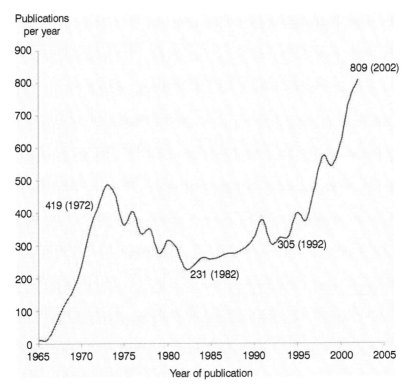

FIGURE 8.1. Dynamic of cannabinoid publications. Annual number of publications found in PubMed (http://www.ncbi.nlm.nih.gov/PubMed/) by using the keywords "cannabis, cannabinoids, THC, marijuana" between 1965 and 2002.

(CBD), the Δ^9-THC type (with nine cannabinoids), and the cannabinol type (CBN) are the most relevant in quantity. Cannabinoid distribution varies between different cannabis strains and usually only three or four cannabinoids are found in one plant in relevant concentrations. Other cannabis compounds of possible pharmacological interest are terpenes (about 120) which are responsible for the specific smell of the plant, flavonoids (21), and nitrogenous compounds (27) including two spermidine-type alkaloids.

Δ^9-THC, the main cannabinoid in cannabis of the drug type with concentrations in a range between 2 and 30 percent in the flowering tops and upper leaves of the female plant, given alone produced similar effects as whole plant-drug cannabis (marijuana) in healthy volunteers (Hart et al. 2002; Wachtel et al. 2002) and patients (Abrams et al. 2001). In one study, pure THC and whole cannabis were either smoked or taken orally in a double-blind, cross-over design with five experimental conditions: a low and a high dose of

THC only, a low and a high dose of whole-plant cannabis, and placebo (Wachtel et al. 2002). In both the oral study and the smoking study, THC-only and whole-plant cannabis produced similar subjective effects, with only minor differences. The THC main effects, including medicinal properties, may be modulated by other cannabinoids, mainly CBD, and other cannabis constituents (McPartland and Russo 2001).

In addition to these phytocannabinoids, synthetic agonists and antagonists at the cannabinoid receptor and other modulators of the endogenous cannabinoid system are under investigation for therapeutic purposes.

MECHANISM OF ACTION

The mechanism of action of cannabinoids is best investigated for Δ^9-THC (THC, dronabinol; see Figure 8.2 for chemical structure) and other cannabinoid receptor agonists, while the mode of action of other cannabinoids of therapeutic interest, among them CBD, as well as the carboxy metabolite of THC (11-nor-9-carboxy-Δ^9-THC) and its analogues (e.g., ajulemic acid, CT-3) is less well established. Previous reviws on cannabis include two by Grotenhermen (2002a,c).

Mechanism of Action of Δ^9-THC

The majority of THC effects are mediated through agonistic actions at cannabinoid receptors. Some non-CB-mediated effects of THC and synthetic derivatives have also been described, e.g., some effects on the immune system (Bueb et al. 2001), some neuroprotective effects (Hampson 2002), and antiemetic effects. The antiemetic effects of THC are supposed to be mediated in part by CB_1 receptors (Parker et al. 2003) and in part by

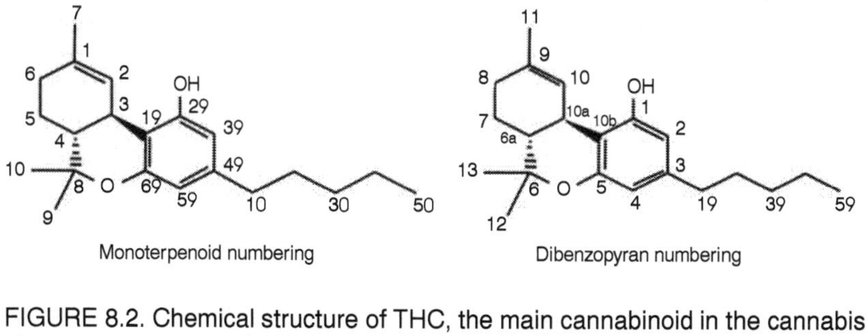

FIGURE 8.2. Chemical structure of THC, the main cannabinoid in the cannabis plant, according to the monoterpenoid system (Δ^1-THC) and dibenzopyran system (Δ^9-THC).

non-CB mechanisms, the rationale for the clinical use of THC as an anti-emetic in children receiving cancer chemotherapy (Abrahamov and Mechoulam 1995). Due to the lower CB_1 receptor density in the brain of children compared with adults, they tolerated relatively high doses of Δ^8-THC in a clinical study, without significant CB_1 receptor mediated adverse effects (Abrahamov and Mechoulam 1995). In a study with cells stably transfected with the human 5-HT$_{3A}$ receptor, several (endo)cannabinoids (THC, WIN55, 212-2, anandamide, etc.) directly inhibited currents induced by 5-hydroxytryptamine (Barann et al. 2002). Since 5-HT$_3$ antagonists are potent antiemetic drugs, this may be one mechanism by which cannabinoids act as antiemetics.

It is possible that several effects previously thought to be nonreceptor mediated are mediated by cannabinoid receptor subtypes that have not yet been identified.

Mechanism of Action of Cannabidiol

The mode of action of cannabidiol (see Figure 8.3 for chemical structure) is not fully understood and several mechanisms have been proposed: (1) CBD acts as antagonist at the central CB_1 receptor and is able to inhibit several CB_1-mediated THC effects (Zuardi et al. 1982). In a study by Petitet et al. (1998), CBD considerably reduced the receptor activation by the potent classical CB_1 receptor agonist CP55940. (2) CBD stimulates the vanilloid receptor type 1 (VR_1) with a maximum effect similar in efficacy to that of capsaicin (Bisogno et al. 2001). (3) CBD inhibits the uptake and hydrolysis of the endocannabinoid anandamide, thus increasing its concentration (Bisogno et al. 2001; Mechoulam and Hanus 2002). (4) Finally, CBD may also increase the plasma THC level (Bornheim et al. 1995) by inhibiting hepatic microsomal THC metabolism through inactivation of the cytochrome P-450 oxidative system (Bornheim and Grillo 1998; Jaeger et al. 1996). However, there was no or minimal effect of CBD on plasma levels of THC in man (Agurell et al. 1981; Hunt et al. 1981).

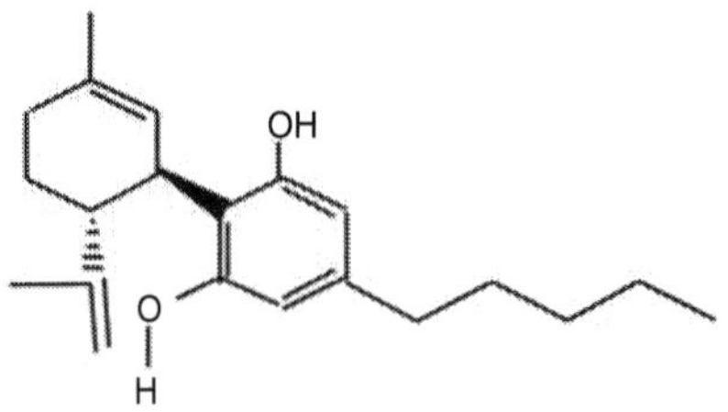

FIGURE 8.3. Cannabinoid.

In a study that analyzed the mode of action of the anti-inflammatory and antihyperalgesic effects of CBD, simultaneous administration of a VR_1 receptor antagonist fully reversed the antihyperalgesic effects (Costa et al. 2003). A CB_2 receptor antagonist was partly effective and a CB_1 receptor antagonist had no effect. The anti-inflammatory efficacy of CBD was unrelated to cyclooxygenase (COX) activity, but inhibited the endothelial isoform of nitric oxide synthase (eNOS). In a rat model of arthritis, low doses of CBD decreased prostaglandin E_2, nitric oxide and lipid peroxide level, mediators that are all known to be involved in the development and maintenance of arthritis (Costa et al. 2003).

CANNABINOID RECEPTORS

To date two cannabinoid receptors have been identified, the CB_1 (cloned in 1990), and the CB_2 receptor (cloned in 1993) (Pertwee 1997), exhibiting 48 percent amino acid sequence identity. Besides their difference in amino acid sequence, they differ in signaling mechanisms, tissue distribution, and sensitivity to certain agonists and antagonists that show marked selectivity for one or the other receptor type (Howlett 2002). Both receptor types are coupled through inhibiting G proteins (G_i proteins), negatively to adenylate cyclase, and positively to mitogen-activated protein kinase. Activation of G_i proteins causes inhibition of adenylate cyclase, thus inhibiting the conversion of ATP to cyclic AMP (cAMP). CB_1 receptors are also coupled to certain kinds of calcium channels and potassium channels (Pertwee 2002). They may also mobilize arachidonic acid and close $5\text{-}HT_3$ receptor ion channels (Pertwee 2002). Under certain conditions, they may also activate adenylate cyclase through stimulating G proteins (G_s proteins) (Glass and Felder 1997).

CB_1 receptors are mainly found on neurons in the brain, spinal cord and peripheral nervous system, but are also present in certain peripheral organs and tissues, among them endocrine glands, leukocytes, spleen, heart and parts of the reproductive, urinary and gastrointestinal tracts (Pertwee 1997). In the central nervous system the CB_1 receptor is the most abundant G-protein-coupled receptor. One of its functions is inhibition of neurotransmitter release. Their endogenous agonists probably serve as retrograde synaptic messengers. CB_1 receptors are highly expressed in the basal ganglia, cerebellum, hippocampus and dorsal primary afferent spinal cord regions, which reflect the importance of the cannabinoid system in motor control, memory processing and pain modulation, while their expression in the brainstem is low (Howlett 2002), which may account for the lack of cannabis- related acute fatalities, e.g., due to depression of respiration.

CB_2 receptors occur principally in immune cells, among them leukocytes, spleen and tonsils (Pertwee 2002). In contrast to CB_1 receptors they are not coupled to ion channels. Immune cells also express both CB_1 receptors but there is markedly more mRNA for CB_2 than CB_1 receptors in the immune system. Levels of CB_1 and CB_2 mRNA in human leukocytes have been shown to vary with cell type (B cells > natural killer cells > monocytes > polymorphonuclear neutrophils, T4 and T8 cells) (Galiègue et al. 1995). One of the functions of CB receptors in the immune system is modulation of cytokine release.

Activation of the CB_1 receptor produces marijuana-like effects on psyche and circulation, while activation of the CB_2 receptor does not. Hence, selective CB_2 receptor agonists have become an increasingly investigated target for therapeutic uses of cannabinoids, among them analgesic, anti-inflammatory and antineoplastic actions (Recht et al. 2001; Sanchez et al. 2001).

There is increasing evidence for the existence of additional cannabinoid receptor subtypes in the brain and periphery (Breivogel et al. 2001; Di Marzo, Breivogel, et al. 2000; Fride et al. 2003; Pertwee, 1999a; Wiley and Martin 2002). These receptors are more likely to be functionally related to the known cannabinoid receptors than have a similar structure as there is no evidence for additional cannabinoid receptors in the human genome (Baker et al. 2001).

ENDOCANNABINOIDS

The identification of cannabinoid receptors was followed by the detection of endogenous ligands for these receptors, endogenous cannabinoids or endocannabinoids, a family of eicosanoids (Devane et al. 1992; Giuffrida et al. 2001; Sugiura et al. 1995). To date five endocannabinoids have been identified. These are *N*-arachidonylethanolamide (anandamide) (Devane et al. 1992), 2-arachidonylglycerol (2-AG) (Mechoulam et al. 1995; Sugiura et al. 1995), 2-arachidonylglyceryl ether (noladin ether) (Hanus et al. 2001), *O*-arachidonyl-ethanolamine (virodhamine) (Porter et al. 2002) and *N*-arachidonyl-dopamine (NADA) (Huang et al. 2002).

Cannabinoid receptors and their endogenous ligands together constitute the "endogenous cannabinoid system," or the "endocannabinoid system" which is teleologically millions of years old and has been found in mammals and many other species (De Petrocellis et al. 1999).

Endocannabinoids serve as neurotransmitters or neuromodulators (Howlett 2002). Anandamide and NADA do not only bind to cannabinoid receptors but also stimulate vanilloid receptors (VR_1) (Al-Hayani et al. 2001; Huang et al. 2002), nonselective ion channels associated with hyperalgesia. Thus, the historical designation of anandamide as an endocannabinoid seems to be only one part of the physiological reality, and cannabinoid receptors seem to amount only to some of the "anandamide receptors." Some non-CB effects may be mediated by vanilloid receptors, e.g., inhibition of cell proliferation of rat C6 glioma cells by endocannabinoids was reported to involve combined activation of both vanilloid receptors and to a lesser extent cannabinoid receptors (Jacobsson et al. 2001).

The first two discovered endocannabinoids, anandamide (Figure 8.4) and 2-AG (Figure 8.5), are the best to be studied. They are produced "on demand" by cleavage of membrane lipid precursors and released from cells in a stimulus-dependent manner (Giuffrida et al. 2001). The production of anandamide and 2-AG involves phospholipases D and C. After release, they are rapidly deactivated by uptake into cells and metabolized. Metabolism of anandamide and 2-AG occurs by enzymatic hydrolysis by the fatty acid amide hydrolase (FAAH) (Di Marzo 1998; Giuffrida et al. 2001). FAAH degrades anandamide to arachidonic acid and ethanolamide. In mice, lack of FAAH resulted in supersensitivity to anandamide and enhanced endogenous cannabinoid signalling (Cravatt et al. 2001). Other metabolic processes include hydrolysis of 2-AG by monoglyceride lipase (Dinh et al. 2002), acylation of noladin ether (Fezza et al. 2002), oxidation of anandamide and 2-AG and methylation of the aromatic moiety of NADA.

In all cases cellular uptake must preceed metabolism since metabolism occurs only in the cells. Endocannabinoid uptake by cells seems to happen by "enhanced diffusion" through the cell membrane (Fowler and Jacobsson

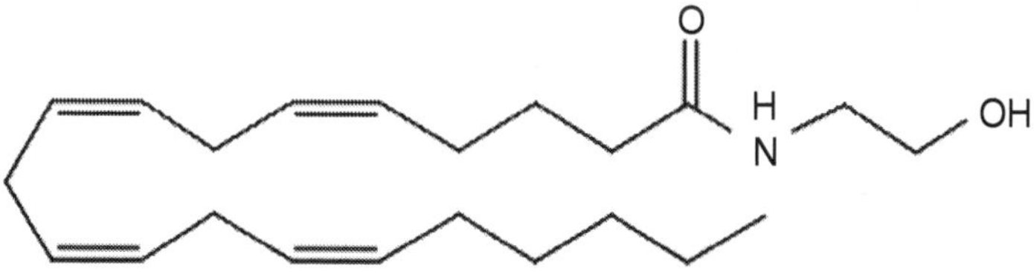

FIGURE 8.4. Arachidonylethanolamide (anandamide).

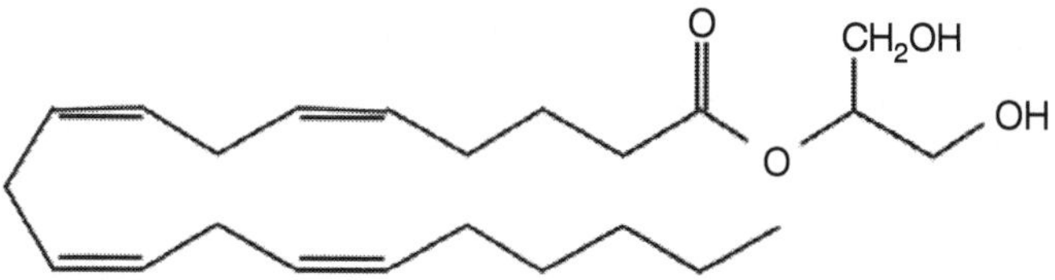

FIGURE 8.5. 2-Arachidonylglycerol (2-AG).

2002; Huang et al. 2002; Porter et al. 2002), even though an active carrier system has not been detected so far. Simple passive diffusion following a concentration gradient into the cells, where they are quickly metabolized by FAAH, is regarded as unlikely, since several substances have been developed that are thought to inhibit anandamide cellular uptake without inhibiting FAAH, among them Arvanil (Di Marzo et al. 2002) and VDM11 (Baker et al. 2001), and noladine ether and NADA are rapidly taken up into cells despite they are rather stable or refractory to enzymatic hydrolysis (Fezza et al. 2002; Huang et al. 2002). However, the discussion on the existence of a transport system is not finished, and one group demonstrated that arvanil and other substances regarded as anandamide transporters (olvanil, AM404) were actually inhibitors of FAAH (Glaser et al. 2003). Intracellular uptake of endocannabinoids is a temperature-dependent and rapid process with a half time of a few minutes, compared to hours in the case of exogenous plant cannabinoids.

Affinity to the Cannabinoid Receptor

Cannabinoids show differing affinities for CB_1 and CB_2 receptors. Synthetic cannabinoids have been developed that act as highly selective agonists or antagonists at one of these receptor types (Abadji et al. 1994; Pertwee 1999b; Pertwee 2002). Δ^9-THC has approximately equal affinity for the CB_1 and CB_2 receptor, while anandamide has marginal selectivity for CB_1 receptors (Pertwee 1999b). However, the efficacy of THC and anandamide is less at CB_2 than at CB_1 receptors. In contrast to the anandamide, 2-AG and noladine ether, which act as agonists at both CB receptor types, virodhamine acts as an antagonist at the CB_1 receptor and as a full agonist at the CB_2 receptor (Porter et al. 2002).

Tonic Activity of the Endocannabinoid System

When administered by themselves, cannabinoid receptor antagonists may behave as inverse agonists in several bioassay systems, i.e., not only block the effects of exogenous cannabinoids but produce effects that are opposite in direction from those produced by cannabinoid receptor agonists, e.g., cause hyperalgesia (Jaggar et al. 1998), suggesting that the endogenous cannabinoid system is tonically active. Tonic activity may be due to a constant release of endocannabinoids or from a portion of cannabinoid receptors that exist in a constitutively active state (Pertwee 2002).

Tonic activity of the endogenous cannabinoid system has been demonstrated in several conditions. Endocannabinoids have been shown to be tonically active in the dorsal horn neurons of the spinal cord, thus, attenuating acute nociceptive transmission at the level of the spinal cord (Chapman 1999). Endocannabinoid levels have been demonstrated to be increased in a pain circuit of the brain (periaqueductal gray) following painful stimuli (Walker et al. 1999). Tonic control of spasticity by the endocannabinoid system has been observed in chronic relapsing experimental autoimmune encephalomyelitis (CREAE) in mice, an animal model of multiple sclerosis (Baker et al. 2001). An increase of cannabinoid receptors following nerve damage was demonstrated in a rat model of chronic neuropathic pain (Siegling et al. 2001) and in a mouse model of intestinal inflammation (Izzo et al. 2001). This may increase the potency of cannabinoid agonists used for the treatment of these conditions. Tonic activity has also been demonstrated with regard to appetite control (Di Marzo, Berrendero, et al. 2000) and with regard to vomiting in emetic circuits of the brain (Darmani 2001). Elevated endocannabinoid levels have been detected in the cerebrospinal fluid of schizophrenic patients (Leweke et al. 1999). In other models tonic or enhanced activity could not be demonstrated, e.g., in a rat model of inflammatory hyperalgesia (Beaulieu et al. 2000).

PHARMACOLOGICAL EFFECTS OF THC

The pharmacological activity of Δ^9-THC is stereoselective, with the natural $(-)$-trans isomer (dronabinol) being 6-100 times more potent than the (+)-trans isomer, depending on the assay (Dewey 1986).

The activation of the cannabinoid system through THC and other phytocannabinoids, synthetic and endogenous cannabinoids causes numerous actions that have been extensively reviewed (see Exhibit 8.1) (Adams and Martin 1996; Dewey 1986; Grotenhermen and Russo 2002; Hall et al. 1994; Hollister 1986; House of Lords 1998; Joy et al. 1999; Kalant et al. 1999). Additional nonreceptor mediated effects have come into focus as well (Hampson 2002). Some effects of cannabinoid receptor agonists show a biphasic behavior in dependency of dose, e.g., low doses of anandamide stimulated phagocytosis and stimulated behavioral activities in mice while high doses decreased activities and caused inhibitory effects on immune functions (Sulcova et al. 1998).

TOXICITY

The median lethal dose (LD_{50}) of oral THC in rats was 800-1900 mg/kg depending on sex and strain (Thompson et al. 1973). There were no cases of

**EXHIBIT 8.1. Effects of THC
The Following Dose-Dependent Effects were
Observed in Clinical Studies, in vivo, or in vitro**

Psyche and perception. Fatigue, euphoria, enhanced well-being, dysphoria, anxiety, reduction of anxiety, depersonalization, increased sensory perception, heightened sexual experience, hallucinations, alteration of time perception, aggravation of psychotic states, sleep.

Cognition and psychomotor performance. Fragmented thinking, enhanced creativity, disturbed memory, unsteady gait, ataxia, slurred speech, weakness, deterioration or amelioration of motor coordination.

Nervous system. Analgesia, muscle relaxation, appetite stimulation, vomiting, anti-emetic effects, neuroprotection in ischemia and hypoxia.

Body temperature. Decrease of body temperature.

Cardiovascular system. Tachycardia, enhanced heart activity, increased output, increase in oxygen demand, vasodilation, orthostatic hypotension, hypertension (in horizontal position), inhibition of platelet aggregation.

Eye. Injected (reddened) conjunctivae, reduced tear flow, decrease of intraocular pressure.

Respiratory system. Bronchodilation, hyposalivation and dry mouth.

Gastrointestinal tract. Reduced bowel movements and delayed gastric emptying.

Hormonal system. Influence on LH, FSH, testosterone, prolactin, somatotropin, TSH, glucose metabolism, reduced sperm count and sperm motility, disturbed menstrual cycle and suppressed ovulation.

Immune system. Impairment of cell-mediated and humoral immunity, immune stimulation, anti-inflammatory and antiallergic effects.

Fetal development. Malformations, growth retardation, impairment to fetal and postnatal cerebral development, impairment of cognitive functions.

Genetic material and cancer. Antineoplastic activity, inhibition of synthesis of DNA, RNA and proteins.

death due to toxicity following the maximum oral THC dose in dogs (up to 3000 mg/kg THC) and monkeys (up to 9000 mg/kg THC) (Thompson et al. 1973). Acute fatal cases in humans have not been substantiated. However, myocardial infarction may be triggered by THC due to effects on circulation (Bachs and Morland 2001; Mittleman et al. 2001). However, this is unlikely to occur in healthy subjects, but possibly in persons with coronary heart disease for whom orthostatic hypotension or a moderately increased heart rate may pose a risk.

Adverse effects of medical cannabis use are within the range of effects tolerated for other medications (House of Lords 1998; Joy et al. 1999). It is controversial whether heavy regular consumption may impair cognition (Pope et al. 2001; Pope 2002; Solowij et al. 2002), but this impairment seems to be minimal if it exists (Lyketsos et al. 1999; Pope et al. 2001). Early users who started their use before the age of 17 presented with poorer cognitive performance, especially verbal IQ compared to users who started later or nonusers (Pope et al. 2003). Possible reasons for this difference may be (1) innate differences between groups in cognitive ability, antedating first cannabis use; (2) a neurotoxic effect of cannabis on the developing brain; or (3) poorer learning of conventional cognitive skills by young cannabis users who have eschewed school and university (Pope et al. 2003).

Long-term medical use of cannabis for more than 15 years has been reported to be well-tolerated without significant physical or cognitive impairment (Russo et al. 2002). There is conflicting evidence that infants exposed to THC in utero suffer developmental and cognitive impairment (Fried et al. 1998). Marijuana can induce a schizophrenic psychosis in vulnerable persons (Hall et al. 1994; Solowij and Grenyer 2002) and there is increasing evidence that there is a distinct cannabis psychosis (Nunez and Gurpegui 2002).

The harmful effects of combustion products produced by smoking cannabis have to be distinguished from effects by cannabis or single cannabinoids (Joy et al. 1999).

PSYCHE, COGNITION AND BEHAVIOR

In many species the behavioral actions of low doses of THC are characterized by an unique mixture of depressant and stimulant effects in the CNS (Dewey 1986).

In humans, THC or cannabis consumption is usually described as a pleasant and relaxing experience. Use in a social context may result in laughter and talkativeness. Occasionally there are unpleasant feelings such as anxiety that may escalate to panic. A sense of enhanced well-being may alternate with dysphoric phases. THC improves taste responsiveness and enhances the sensory appeal of foods (Mattes et al. 1994). It may induce sleep (Freemon 1972; Lissoni et al. 1986).

Acute THC intoxication impairs learning and memory (Hampson and Deadwyler 1999; Heyser et al. 1993; Slikker et al. 1992), and may adversely affect psychomotor and cognitive performance (Solowij and Grenyer 2002), reducing the ability to drive a car and to operate machinery. Reduced reaction time also affects the response of the pupil of the eye. A brief light flash shows decreased amplitude of constriction and a decelerated velocity of constriction and dilation (Kelly et al. 1993).

The most conspicuous psychological effects of THC in humans have been divided into four groups: affective (euphoria and easy laughter), sensory (increased perception of external stimuli and of the person's own body), somatic (feeling of the body floating or sinking in the bed), and cognitive (distortion of time perception, memory lapses, difficulty in concentration) (Perez-Reyes 1999).

These effects only appear if an individually variable threshold of dose is exceeded. During a study on the efficacy of dronabinol (THC) in 24 patients with Tourette syndrome who received up to 10 mg THC daily for 6 weeks, no detrimental effects were seen on neuropsychological performance (learning, recall of word lists, visual memory, divided attention) (Müller-Vahl, Prevedel, et al. 2003).

CENTRAL NERVOUS SYSTEM AND NEUROCHEMISTRY

Most THC effects (analgesia, appetite enhancement, muscle relaxation, hormonal actions, etc.) are mediated by central cannabinoid receptors, their distribution reflecting many of the medicinal benefits and side effects (Hampson and Deadwyler 1999; Pertwee 2002; Sañudo-Peña et al. 1999).

Cannabinoids interact with a multitude of neurotransmitters and neuro-modulators (Dewey 1986; Pertwee 1992), among them acetylcholine, dopamine, α-aminobutyric acid (GABA), histamine, serotonin, glutamate, norepinephrine, prostaglandins and opioid peptides (see Table 8.1). A number of pharmacological effects can be explained (at least in part) on the basis of such interactions. For example, tachycardia and hyposalivation with dry mouth (Domino 1999; Mattes et al. 1994) are mediated by effects of THC on release and turnover of acetylcholine (Domino 1999). In a rat model, cannabinoid agonists inhibited activation of $5\text{-}HT_3$ receptors, explaining antiemetic properties of cannabinoids to be based on interactions with serotonin (Fan 1995). Therapeutic effects in movement and spastic disorders could be ascribed in part to interactions with GABAergic, glutamergic

TABLE 8.1. Neurotransmitter functions under cannabinoid control.

Neurotransmitter	Associated disorder
Excitatory amino acids	
Glutamate	Epilepsy, nerve-cell death in ischemia and hypoxia (stroke, head trauma, nerve gas toxicity)
Inhibitory amino acids	
GABA	Spinal cord motor disorders, epilepsy, anxiety
Glycine	Startle syndromes
Monoamines	
Noradrenaline	Autonomic homeostasis, hormones, depression
Serotonin	Depression, anxiety, migraine, vomiting
Dopamine	Parkinson's disease, schizophrenia, vomiting, pituitary hormones, drug addiction
Acetylcholine	Neuromuscular disorders, autonomic homeostasis (heart rate, blood pressure), dementia, parkinsonism, epilepsy, sleep-wake cycle
Neuropeptides	Pain, movement, neural development, anxiety

Source: Modified according to Baker et al. 2001.

and dopaminergic transmitters systems (Müller-Vahl et al. 2002; Musty and Consroe 2002).

Cannabinoids influence the activity of most neurotransmitters in a complex manner, which sometimes may result in contradictory effects with suppression or induction/intensification of convulsion, emesis, pain and tremor depending on subject and condition. Cannabis and dronabinol are used against nausea and vomiting caused by antineoplastic drugs but rarely may cause vomiting. They are used as analgesics but sometimes may increase pain, etc. These observations are probably based on the control of these effects by several neuronal circuits influenced by cannabinoids. Influence on neurotransmitters may depend on brain region. Thus, dopamine activity may be reduced by cannabinoids in brain areas responsible for motor control (Giuffrida et al. 2001) but enhanced in the reward system (Gardner 2002). Interactions of cannabinoids with other neurotransmitter systems may cause unexpected effects. While studies in animals have demonstrated that opioid receptor antagonists precipitated a cannabinoid-like withdrawal syndrome in cannabinoid-dependent rats (Lichtman et al. 2001) and blocked other effects related to behavioral effects of CB_1 agonists (Braida et al. 2001; Tanda et al. 1997), in humans opioid receptor antagonists did not block the subjective effects of THC in one study (Wachtel and de Wit 2000) and even increased the subjective effects THC in another study (Haney et al. 2003).

One important physiological role of endocannabinoids seems to be neuroprotection (Mechoulam 2002). Ischemia and hypoxia in the CNS induce abnormal glutamate hyperactivity and other processes that cause neuronal damage. These processes also play a role in chronic neurodegenerative diseases such as Parkinson's and Alzheimer's disease and multiple sclerosis. Neuroprotective mediators are also released in ischemia and hypoxia, including anandamide and 2-AG. When these two cannabinoids were administered after traumatic brain injury in animals, they reduced brain damage (Mechoulam 2002). Neuroprotective cannabinoid mechanisms observed in animal studies include reduction of glutamate toxicity by inhibition of excessive glutamate production, inhibition of calcium influx into cells, antioxidant properties which reduce damage caused by oxygen radicals and modulation of vascular tone (Grundy 2002; Hampson 2002; Mechoulam 2002). THC was neuroprotective in rats given the toxic agent ouabain. THC-treated animals showed reduced volume of edema by 22 percent in the acute phase and 36 percent less nerve damage after 7 days (van der Stelt et al. 2001). Whether these effects may be of therapeutic benefit in acute or chronic diseases has to be elucidated. Clinical studies under way investigating the therapeutic potential of a non-psychotropic derivative of THC in acute conditions (head trauma, stroke and nerve gas intoxication) showed initial positive results (Knoller et al. 2002).

CIRCULATORY SYSTEM

THC can induce tachycardia (Perez-Reyes 1999) and increase cardiac output with increased cardiac labor and oxygen demand (Tashkin et al. 1977). It can also produce peripheral vasodilation, orthostatic hypotension (Benowitz and Jones 1975; Hollister 1986) and reduced platelet aggregation (Formukong et al. 1989). There was no change of mean global cerebral blood flow after smoking cannabis but increases and decreases in several regions (O'Leary et al. 2002).

In young healthy subjects the heart is under control of the vagus which mediates bradycardia. Tachycardia by THC may easily be explained by vagal inhibition (inhibited release of acetylcholine) through presynaptic

CB_1 receptors (Szabo et al. 2001), which can be attenuated by beta-blockers (Perez-Reyes 1999) and blocked by the selective CB_1 antagonist SR141716A (Huestis et al. 2001). Regular use can lead to bradycardia (Benowitz and Jones 1975). The endogenous cannabinoid system seems to play a major role in the control of blood pressure. Hypotension is mediated by central inhibition of the sympathetic nervous system, obviously by activation of CB_1 receptors since this effect can also be prevented by a CB_1 antagonist (Lake et al. 1997). Endocannabinoids are produced by the vascular endothelium, circulating macrophages and platelets (Wagner et al. 1998). Vascular resistance in the coronaries and the brain is lowered primarily by direct activation of vascular cannabinoid CB_1 receptors (Wagner et al. 2001).

SOME OTHER ORGAN SYSTEMS AND EFFECTS

Antibacterial and Antiviral Actions

Antibacterial actions have been demonstrated for CBD, CBG and THC (Van Klingeren and Ten Ham 1976). Incubation with THC reduced the infectious potency of herpes simplex viruses (Lancz et al. 2002).

Appetite and Eating

The endogenous cannabinoid system plays a critical role in milk ingestion of newborn mice (Fride et al. 2003). Blockade of the CB_1 receptor results in death of newborns in this setting (Fride and Shohami 2002). Anandamide induces overeating in rats through a CB_1-receptor-mediated mechanism (Williams and Kirkham 1999). Endocannabinoids in the hypothalamus are part of the brain's complex system for controlling appetite which is regulated by leptin (Di Marzo et al. 2001). Leptin is the primary signal through which the hypothalamus senses nutritional state and modulates food intake and energy balance. Leptin reduces food intake by upregulating appetite-reducing neuropeptides, such as alpha-melanocyte-stimulating hormone, and downregulating appetite-stimulating factors, primarily neuropeptide Y. In animal research reduced levels of leptin were associated with elevated levels of endocannabinoids in the hypothalamus, and application of leptin reduced endocannabinoid levels (Di Marzo et al. 2001). Cannabinoid-induced eating is ascribed to an increase of the incentive value of food (Williams and Kirkham 2002).

Bones

Preliminary observations show that endocannabinoids seem to stimulate bone formation (Mechoulam et al. 2003). Reverse transcription polymerase chain reaction of differentiating osteoblastic precursor cells demonstrated progressive increase in mRNA levels of CB_2 but not of CB_1. In addition, normal mice treated systematically with 2-AG showed a dose dependent increase in trabecular bone formation (Mechoulam et al. 2003). The peptide leptin is known to negatively regulate both osteoblastic and endocannabinoid activity (Di Marzo et al. 2001).

Digestive Tract

Cannabinoid agonists inhibit gastrointestinal motility and gastric emptying in rats (Shook and Burks 1989). In a study with humans, THC caused a significant delay in gastric emptying (McCallum et al. 1999). In addition, CB agonists inhibited pentagastrin-induced gastric acid secretion in the rat (Coruzzi et al. 1999), mediated by suppression of vagal drive to the stomach through activation of CB_1 receptors (Adami et al. 2002).

Eye

The evidence of cannabinoid receptors at different sites (anterior eye, retina, corneal epithelium) suggests that cannabinoids influence different physiological functions in the human eye (Pate 2002). Vasodilation in the eye is observed as conjunctival reddening after THC exposure (Dewey 1986). THC and some other cannabinoids decrease intraocular pressure (Colasanti 1990; Pate 2002). CB_1 receptors in the eye are involved in this effect while CB_2 receptor agonists do not reduce intraocular pressure (Laine et al. 2003).

Genetic and Cell Metabolism

THC can inhibit DNA, RNA and protein synthesis, and can influence the cell cycle. However, very high doses are required to produce this effect in vitro (Tahir et al. 1992). Cannabinoid agonists inhibited human breast cancer cell proliferation in vitro (De Petrocellis et al. 1998; Melck et al. 2000), and, directly applied at the tumor site, showed antineoplastic activity against malignant gliomas in rats (Galve-Roperh et al. 2000).

Hormonal System and Fertility

THC interacts with the hypothalamic-pituitary adrenal axis influencing numerous hormonal processes (Murphy 2002). Minor changes in human hormone levels due to acute cannabis or THC ingestion usually remain in the normal range (Hollister 1986). Tolerance develops to these effects, however, and even regular cannabis users demonstrate normal hormone levels.

Immune System

Animal and cell experiments have demonstrated that THC exerts complex effects on cellular and humoral immunity (Cabral 2002; Melamede 2002). It is not clear whether and to what extent these effects are of clinical relevance in humans with respect to beneficial inflammation (Evans et al. 1987; Sofia et al. 1973), allergies (Jan et al. 2003), autoimmune processes (Melamede 2002) and undesirable effects (decreased resistance toward pathogens and carcinogens) (Cabral 2002). THC was shown to modulate the immune response of T lymphocytes (Yuan et al. 2002). It suppressed the proliferation of T cells and changed the balance of T helper 1 (Th1) and T helper 2 (Th2) cytokines. It decreased the proinflammatory Th1 reaction (e.g., the production of interferon-gamma) and increased the Th2 reaction. This may explain why THC is effective against inflammation with a strong Th1 reaction, e.g., in multiple sclerosis, Crohn's disease and arthritis. The regulation of the activation and balance of human Th1/Th2 cells seems to be mediated by a CB_2 receptor-dependent pathway (Yuan et al. 2002).

Sperm

After several weeks of daily smoking eight to ten cannabis cigarettes, a slight decrease in sperm count was observed in humans, without impairment of their function (Hembree et al. 1978). In animal studies high doses of cannabinoids inhibited the acrosome reaction (Chang et al. 1993).

PHARMACOLOGICAL ACTIVITY OF THC METABOLITES

11-Hydroxy-Δ^9-THC

The most important psychotropic metabolite of Δ^9-THC is 11-OH-Δ^9-tetrahydrocannabinol (11-OH-THC) (Figure 8.6), with a similar spectrum of actions and similar kinetic profiles as the parent molecule (Lemberger et al. 1972; Perez-Reyes et al. 1972). After intravenous administration in humans, 11-OH-THC was equipotent to THC in causing psychic effects and reduction in intraocular pressure (Perez-Reyes et al. 1972). In some pharmacological animal tests, 11-OH-THC was three to seven times more potent than THC (Karler and Turkanis 1987).

11-Nor-9-Carboxy-Δ⁹-THC

The most important nonpsychotropic metabolite of Δ^9-THC is 11-nor-9-carboxy-THC (THC-COOH) (Figure 8.7). It possesses anti-inflammatory and analgesic properties by mechanisms similar to nonsteroidal anti- inflammatory drugs (Burstein et al. 1989; Burstein 1999; Doyle et al. 1990). THC-COOH antagonizes some effects of the parent drug through an unknown mechanism, e.g., the cataleptic effect in mice (Burstein et al. 1987). Ajulemic acid (CT-3), a synthetic derivative of THC-COOH, shows a similar pharmacological profile as the natural substance. Recently, a possible mechanism of action was proposed for this derivative (Liu et al. 2003). Ajulemic acid bounds directly and specifically to the peroxisome proliferator-activated receptor gamma (PPAR gamma), a pharmacologically important member of the nuclear receptor superfamily. In addition, it was shown that ajulemic acid inhibited interleukin-8 promoter activity in a PPAR gamma-dependent manner, suggesting a link between the anti-inflammatory action of the cannabinoid acid and the activation of PPAR gamma.

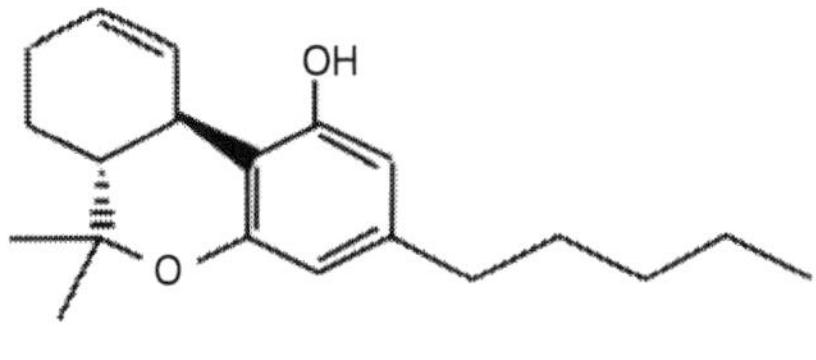

FIGURE 8.6. 11-OH-THC (11-hydroxy-Δ⁹-THC).

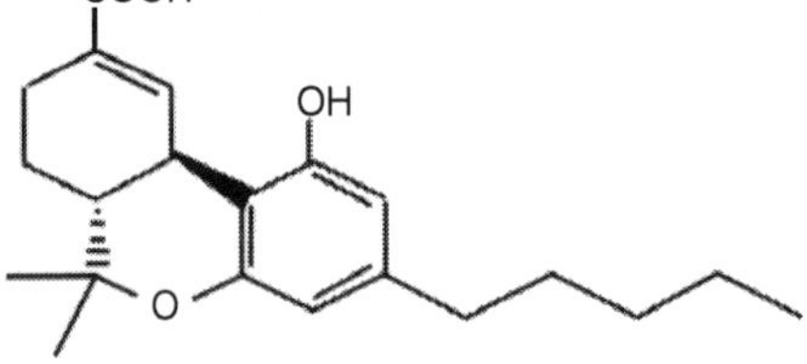

FIGURE 8.7. THC-COOH (11-nor-9-carboxy-Δ⁹-THC).

PHARMACOLOGICAL EFFECTS
OF OTHER CANNABINOIDS

Phytocannabinoids

Cannabidiol (CBD) is a nonpsychotropic cannabinoid, for which sedating (Zuardi et al. 2002), antiepileptic (Karler and Turkanis 1981), antidystonic (Consroe et al. 1986), antiemetic (Parker et al. 2002) and antiinflammatory (Malfait et al. 2000) effects have been observed. It reduced intraocular pressure (Colasanti et al. 1984), was neuroprotective (Hampson 2002) and antagonized the psychotropic and several other effects of THC (Zuardi et al. 1982). Anxiolytic and antipsychotic properties might prove useful in psychiatry (Zuardi et al. 1982; Zuardi et al. 2002).

The nonpsychotropic cannabinoids cannabigerol (CBG) and cannabichromene (CBC) showed sedative effects. CBG has been observed to decrease intraocular pressure (Colasanti 1990), showed antitumor activity against human cancer cells (Baek et al. 1998) and has antibiotic properties.

Endocannabinoids

Anandamide (arachidonylethanolamide), an endocannabinoid, produces pharmacological effects similar to those of THC. However, there are apparently some significant differences to THC. Under certain circumstances, anandamide acts as a partial agonist at the CB_1 receptor (Fride et al. 1995), and very low doses of anandamide antagonized the actions of THC. It is assumed that low doses of anandamide activated stimulating G_s protein pathways and not inhibiting G_i proteins, or caused an allosteric modulation of the cannabinoid receptor (Fride et al. 1995).

Classical Synthetic Cannabinoids

Among the classical synthetic cannabinoids that retain the phytocannabinoid ring structures and their oxygen atoms are nabilone (Figure 8.8), HU-210 and HU-211 (Figure 8.9). Nabilone is available by prescription in several countries with a similar pharmacological profile as THC (Archer et al. 1986). HU-210, an analogue of Δ^8-THC with a dimethylheptyl side chain, is between 80 and 800 times more active than THC (Little et al. 1989; Ottani and Giuliani 2001), while its enantiomer (mirror image) HU-211 is completely devoid of psychoactivity (Titishov et al. 1989). The latter, also called dexanabinol, is an NMDA antagonist with neuroprotective properties in hypoxia and ischemia (Mechoulam and Shohami 2002). It is under

clinical investigation for the treatment of brain injuries and stroke (Mechoulam and Shohami 2002). CT-3 or ajulemic acid (Figure 8.10), a derivative
of the Δ^8-THC metabolite THC-COOH, is under clinical investigation for
the treatment of inflammation and pain (Burstein 2002; Perez-Reyes et al.
1976).

Nonclassical Synthetic Cannabinoids

Levonantradol, from Pfizer, under clinical investigation for the treatment
of pain (Jain et al. 1981) and the side effects of chemotherapy (Citron et al.

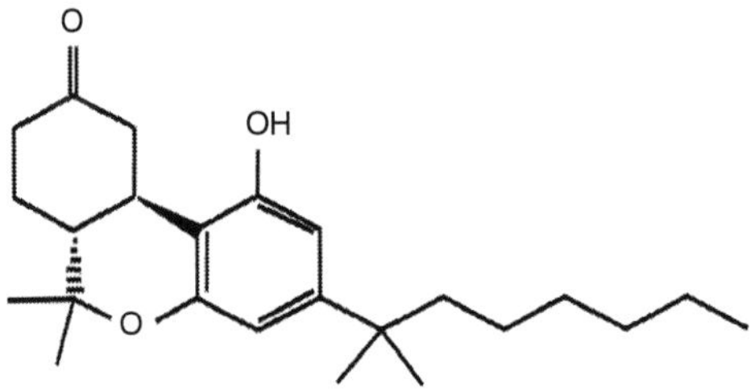

FIGURE 8.8. Nabilone.

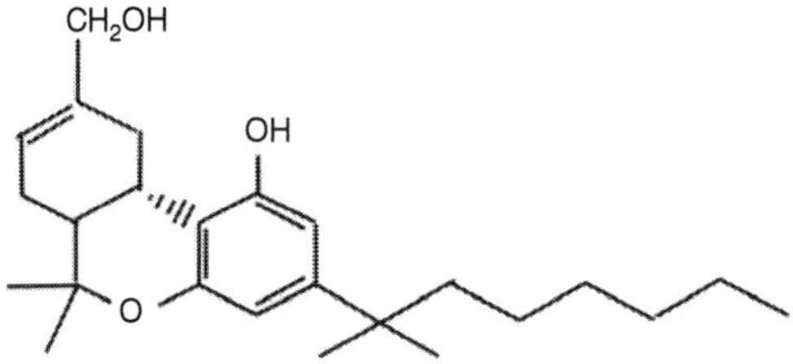

FIGURE 8.9. Dexanabinol (HU-211).

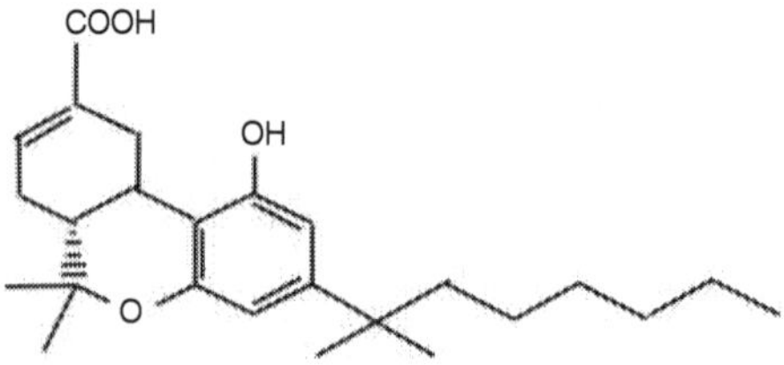

FIGURE 8.10. CT-3 (ajulemic acid).

1985) and radiotherapy (Lucraft and Palmer 1982), is a nonclassical cannabinoid with a more radical deviation of the typical structure. Other nonclassical cannabinoids are the aminoalkylindol WIN-55,212-2, which has a 6.75-fold selective affinity toward the CB_2 receptor (Showalter et al. 1996) and the bicyclic cannabinoid analogue CP-55,940, a widely used agonist for the testing of cannabinoid receptor affinity, with potency 4 to 25 times greater than THC, depending on assay (Melvin et al. 1993).

Anandamide Analogues

Several anandamide congeners have been synthesized (Abadji et al. 1994), among them (R)-(+)-α-methanandamide that possesses both a fourfold higher affinity for the CB_1 receptor and a greater catabolic resistance than anandamide. Fatty-acid-based compounds have been synthesized that mimic the structure of anandamide, but act as inhibitors of the catabolic amidase enzyme, the "fatty acid amide hydrolase" (FAAH) (Di Marzo 1998).

AM-404 is a synthetic fatty amide that acts as a selective inhibitor of anandamide transport, thus preventing cellular reuptake of anandamide (Beltramo et al. 1997) and increasing circulating anandamide levels (Giuffrida et al. 2001).

Therapeutic Potential of Antagonists

SR141716A (Figure 8.11) has been shown to improve memory in rodents (Terranova et al. 1996) and cause hyperalgesia (Jaggar et al. 1998).

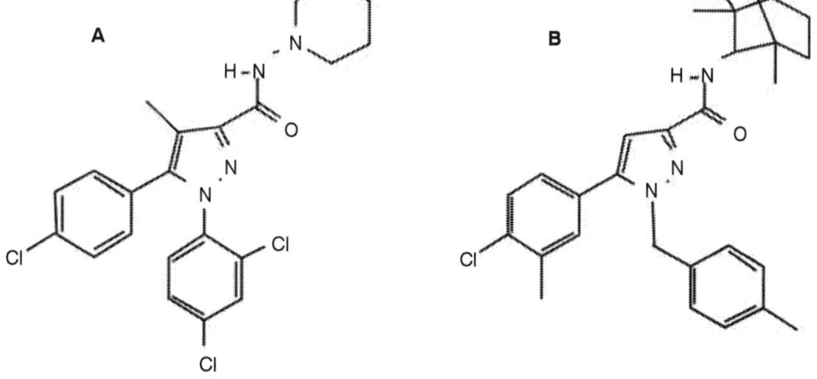

FIGURE 8.11. Cannabinoid receptor antagonists, SR141716A (A), a selective CB_1 receptor antagonist, and SR144528 (B), a selective CB_2 receptor antagonist.

This antagonist was also able to block the psychological and physiological effects of THC in humans in a dose-dependent manner (Huestis et al. 2001). A possible therapeutic potential was proposed for obesity (Huestis et al. 2001), schizophrenia (Huestis et al. 2001), in conditions with lowered blood pressure, e.g., liver cirrhosis (Wagner et al. 2001), Parkinson's disease (Di Marzo, Hill, et al. 2000), Huntington's disease (Müller-Vahl et al. 1999), alcohol dependency (Vacca et al. 2002; Racz et al. 2003) and to improve memory in Alzheimer's disease (Huestis et al. 2001).

TOLERANCE AND DEPENDENCY

Tolerance

Tolerance develops to most of the THC effects (Romero et al. 1997), among them the cardiovascular, psychological and skin hypothermic effects (Jones et al. 1976; Stefanis 1978), analgesia (Bass and Martin 2000), immunosuppression (Luthra et al. 1980), corticosteroid release (Miczek and Dixit 1980), and disruption of the hypothalamo-hypophyseal axis (Smith et al. 1983), causing alterations in endocannabinoid formation and contents in the brain (Di Marzo, Berrendero, et al. 2000). In a 30-day study, volunteers received daily doses of 210 mg oral THC and developed tolerance to cognitive and psychomotor impairment and to the psychological high by the end of the study (Jones and Benowitz 1976). After a few days an increased heart rate was replaced by a normal or a slowed heart rate. Tolerance develops also to orthostatic hypotension (Benowitz and Jones 1975).

Tolerance can mainly be attributed to pharmacodynamic changes, presumably based on receptor downregulation and/or receptor desensitisation (Di Marzo, Berrendero, et al. 2000; Rubino, Vigano, Massi, et al. 2000). Rate and duration of tolerance varies with different effects. Rats receiving THC over a period of five days exhibited a decreased specific binding ranging from 20 to 60 percent in different receptor sites of the brain compared to controls (Romero et al. 1997). However, in another study no significant alteration in receptor binding was observed after chronic administration of THC resulting in a 27-fold behavioral tolerance (Abood et al. 1993). Chronic administration of anandamide as well resulted in behavioral tolerance without receptor down-regulation (Rubino, Vigano, Costa, et al. 2000), and it was proposed that desensitization of the CB_1 receptor might account for this observation (Rubino, Vigano, Costa, et al. 2000). Tolerance has been observed to occur together with modified biotransformation activities with regard to mitochondrial oxygen consumption, monooxygenase activities, and the content of liver microsomal cytochrome P-450 (Costa et al. 1996).

However, only a small proportion of tolerance can be attributed to changes in metabolism (Hunt and Jones 1980).

Withdrawal and Dependency

After abrupt cessation of chronic dosing with high doses of THC, withdrawal has been observed in humans (Georgotas and Zeidenberg 1979; Jones et al. 1976). Subjects complained of inner unrest, irritability, and insomnia and presented "hot flashes," sweating, rhinorrhea, loose stools, hiccups, and anorexia. Withdrawal symptoms in humans are usually mild and the risk for physical and psychic dependency is low compared to opiates, tobacco, alcohol and benzodiazepines (Anthony et al. 1994; Kleiber et al. 1997; Roques 1998). A review of several indicators of the abuse potential of oral dronabinol in a therapeutic context found little evidence of such a problem (Calhoun et al. 1998).

THERAPEUTIC USES

Cannabis preparations have been employed in the treatment of numerous diseases, with marked differences in the available supporting data (British Medical Association 1997; Grotenhermen and Russo 2002; House of Lords 1998; Joy et al. 1999). Besides phytocannabinoids, several synthetic cannabinoid derivatives are under clinical investigation that are devoid of psychotropic effects, and modulators of the endocannabinoid system (re-uptake inhibitors, antagonists at the CB receptor, etc.) will presumably follow.

Clinical studies with single cannabinoids, or, less often with whole plant preparations (smoked marijuana, encapsulated cannabis extract), have often been inspired by positive anecdotal experiences of patients employing crude cannabis products (usually without legal sanction). The antiemetic (Dansak 1997) and the appetite-enhancing effects (Plasse et al. 1991), muscle relaxation (Clifford 1983), analgesia (Noyes and Baram 1974) and therapeutic use in Tourette's syndrome (Müller-Vahl et al. 1997) were all discovered or rediscovered in this manner.

Incidental observations have also revealed therapeutically useful effects. This occurred in a study of Volicer et al. (1997) in patients with Alzheimer's disease wherein the primary issue was an examination of the appetite-stimulating effects of Δ^9-THC. Not only appetite and body weight increased, but disturbed behavior among the patients also decreased following the intake of the drug. The discovery of decreased intraocular pressure with THC administration in the beginning of the 1970s was also serendipitous (Hepler and Frank 1971), when several research groups screened for effects of marijuana on the human body.

HIERARCHY OF THERAPEUTIC EFFECTS

Possible indications for cannabis preparations have been extensively reviewed (British Medical Association 1997; Grinspoon and Bakalar 1993; Grotenhermen and Russo 2002; Gotenhermen 2002b; House of Lords 1998; Joy et al. 1999; Mathre 1997; Mechoulam 1986). To do justice to the scientific evidence with regard to different indications, a hierarchy of therapeutic effects can be devised, with established, relatively well-confirmed, less confirmed and effects at a basic research stage. However, the history of research into the therapeutic benefits of cannabis and cannabinoids has demonstrated that the scientific evidence for a specific indication does not necessarily reflect the actual therapeutic potential for a given disease, but sometimes obstacles to clinical research.

Established Effects

Marinol (dronabinol, Δ^9-THC) is approved for medical use in refractory nausea and vomiting caused by antineoplastic drugs used for the treatment of cancer (Abrahamov and Mechoulam 1995; Dansak 1997; Lane et al. 1991; Sallan et al. 1980) and for appetite loss in anorexia and cachexia of HIV/AIDS patients (Beal et al. 1995, 1997; Plasse et al. 1991). These effects can be regarded as established effects for THC and cannabis. THC is also effective in cancer cachexia (Jatoi et al. 2002) and nausea induced by syrup of ipecac (Soderpalm et al. 2001). Cesamet (nabilone) is approved for nausea and vomiting associated with cancer chemotherapy.

Relatively Well-Confirmed Effects

Spasticity due to spinal cord injury (Brenneisen et al. 1996; Maurer et al. 1990; Petro 1980), multiple sclerosis (MS) (Brenneisen et al. 1996; Killestein et al. 2002; Martyn et al. 1995; Meinck et al. 1989; Petro 1980; Petro and Ellenberger 1981; Ungerleider et al. 1987) and other reasons (Lorenz 2002), chronic painful conditions, especially neurogenic pain (Elsner et al. 2001; Holdcroft et al. 1997; Maurer et al. 1990; Notcutt et al. 2001a,b; Noyes, Brunk, Avery, and Canter 1975; Noyes, Brunk, Baram, and Canter 1975; Petro 1980; Wade et al. 2003), movement disorders (including Tourette's syndrome, dystonia and levodopa-induced dyskinesia) (Clifford 1983; Fox et al. 2002; Hemming and Yellowlees 1993; Müller-Vahl et al.

1999, 2002; Müller-Vahl et al. 2003a,b; Sandyk and Awerbuch 1998; Sieradzan et al. 2001), asthma (Hartley et al. 1978; Tashkin et al. 1974; Williams et al. 1976) and glaucoma (Crawford and Merritt 1979; Hepler and Frank 1971; Hepler and Petrus 1976; Merritt et al. 1980; Merritt et al. 1981) can be regarded as relatively well-confirmed effects with small placebo-controlled trials demonstrating benefits. However, results were sometimes conflicting. In contrast to other studies, Clermont-Gnamien et al. (2002) did not find any therapeutic effect of oral dronabinol titrated to the maximum dose of 25 mg/day (mean dose: 15 ± 6 mg), during an average of 55 days in seven patients with chronic refractory neuropathic pain. Killestein et al. (2002) were unable to find any benefits of THC and capsulated cannabis extract in MS patients with severe spasticity but doses applied (2×2.5 mg or 2×5 mg THC) were probably too low to get the desired therapeutic effects.

Less Confirmed Effects

There are several indications in which mainly case reports suggest benefits. These are allergies (Schnelle et al. 1999), inflammation (Joy et al. 1999), epilepsy (Gordon and Devinsky 2001), intractable hiccups (Gilson and Busalacchi 1998), depression (Beal et al. 1995), bipolar disorders (Grinspoon and Bakalar 1998), anxiety disorders (Joy et al. 1999), dependency to opiates and alcohol (Mikuriya 1970; Schnelle et al. 1999), withdrawal symptoms (Mikuriya 1970) and disturbed behavior in Alzheimer's disease (Volicer et al. 1997).

BASIC RESEARCH STAGE

Basic research shows promising possible future therapeutic uses, among them neuroprotection in hypoxia and ischemia due to traumatic head injury, nerve gas damage and stroke (Hampson 2002; Mechoulam and Shohami 2002). Some immunological mechanisms of THC hint to possible benefits in autoimmune diseases, such as multiple sclerosis, arthritis, and Crohn's disease (Melamede 2002). In a murine model of multiple sclerosis, cannabinoids significantly improved the neurological deficits in a long-lasting way. On a histological level they reduced microglial activation and decreased the number of CD4+ infiltrating T cells in the spinal cord (Arevalo-Martin et al. 2003). Another group found that amelioration of clinical disease in the same MS model was associated with down-regulation of myelin epitope-specific Th1 effector functions (delayed-type hypersensitivity and IFN-gamma production) and the inhibition of the proinflammatory cytokines, TNF-alpha, interleukin 1-beta, and interleukin-6 (Croxford and

Miller 2003). Several phytocannabinoids possess an anti-allergic potential. THC and cannabinol attenuated the increase of the interleukins IL-2, IL-4, IL-5, and IL-13 in reaction to sensitization with ovalbumin in mice. In addition, the elevation of serum IgE and the mucus overproduction induced by ovalbumin was markedly attenuated by the two cannabinoids (Jan et al. 2003).

Antineoplastic activity of THC came into the focus of research after a long-term animal study, designed to investigate THC's potential carcinogenicity, resulted in better survival of rats dosed with THC than controls due to lower incidence for several types of cancer (Chan et al. 1996). Frequency of testicular interstitial cell, pancreas and pituitary gland adenomas in male rats and mammary gland fibroadenoma and uterus stromal polyp in female rats was reduced in a dose-related manner. Later studies showed that cannabinoids exerted antineoplastic activity in malignant gliomas (Jacobsson et al. 2001; Sanchez et al. 2001) and malignant skin tumors (Casanova et al. 2003). CB_1 and CB_2 receptor agonists were both effective. Cannabinoids seem to be able to control the cell survival/death decision (Guzman et al. 2001). Thus cannabinoids may induce proliferation, growth arrest or apoptosis in a number of cells depending on dose (Guzman et al. 2001). Cannabinoids were also shown to inhibit angiogenesis of malignant gliomas by at least two mechanisms, direct inhibition of vascular endothelial cell migration and survival as well as the decrease of the expression of proangiogenic factors (Blazquez et al. 2003). A first human Phase I-II trial to investigate the tolerability and efficacy of intracranially applied THC (dronabinol) in glioblastoma multiforme is underway in Spain.

Other fields of research are disorders of circulation and blood pressure (Ralevic and Kendall 2001; Wagner et al. 2001). In rats, daily application of a CB_1 agonist after experimental infarction prevented signs of heart failure, endothelial dysfunction and hypotension; however, the cannabinoid also increased left-ventricular end-diastolic pressure, which may be negative in the long run (Wagner et al. 2003).

Several effects observed in animal studies provide the basis for further research, among them effects against diarrhea in mice (Izzo et al. 2000), inhibition of bronchospasm provoked by chemical irritants in rats (Calignano et al. 2000) and stabilization of respiration in sleep-related breathing disorders (e.g., apnea) (Carley et al. 2002).

Some effects that are usually regarded as side effects may be also of advantage in certain pathological situations, among them the disturbance of short-term memory. Patients suffering from posttraumatic stress disorders want to forget and there are anecdotal reports on their benefits from cannabis (Gieringer 2001). Animal research has demonstrated that CB_1-deficient mice showed strongly impaired short-term and long-term extinction of aversive memories (Marsicano et al. 2002), which may explain some of the anxiety-reducing effects in post-traumatic stress disorder and similar conditions (Sah 2002).

DRUG INTERACTIONS

Interactions with other drugs may depend on activity on similar effector systems or metabolic interactions (Pryor et al. 1976). Since cannabinoids are strongly bound to proteins, interactions with other protein bound drugs may also occur. They might also interact with drugs that, such as THC, are metabolized by enzymes of the cytochrome P-450 complex. However, there was only a minor influence of cannabis smoking and oral dronabinol on pharmacokinetic parameters of antiretroviral medication used in HIV infection and metabolized by cytochrome P-450 enzymes, and the use of cannabinoids was regarded as unlikely to impair antiretroviral efficacy (Kosel et al. 2002). Tobacco and cannabis smoking cessation was reported to result in elevated blood levels of antipsychotic medication (clozapine or olanzapine), due to cessation of induction of cytochrome $P450_{1A2}$ (CYP1A2) by smoke constituents (Zullino et al. 2002).

Other medicines may enhance or attenuate certain actions of THC or certain actions of these medicines may be enhanced or attenuated by THC (Hollister 1999; Sutin and Nahas 1999). Moreover, it is possible that certain effects are enhanced and others reduced, as is the case with phenothiazines applied against side effects of cancer chemotherapy. In a study by Lane et al. (1991), a combination of prochlorperazine and dronabinol was more effective in reducing unwanted effects of the antineoplastic medication than the phenothiazine alone and the incidence of cannabinoid-induced adverse effects was decreased when dronabinol was combined with prochlorperazine, which also has antipsychotic properties. Cannabis, caffeine and tobacco reduced the blood pressure reactivity protection of ascorbic acid, probably through their dopaminergic effects (Brody and Preut 2002).

Of greatest clinical relevance is reinforcement of the sedating effects of other psychotropic substances (alcohol, benzodiazepines), and the interaction with substances that act on heart and circulation (amphetamines, adrenaline, atropine, beta-blockers, diuretics, tricyclic antidepressants, etc.) (Hollister 1999; Sutin and Nahas 1999).

A number of additive effects may be desirable, such as the enhancement of muscle relaxants, bronchodilators and antiglaucoma medication (Pate 2002), of analgesia by opiates (Welch and Eads 1999; Cichewicz and McCarthy 2003), the antiemetic effect of phenothiazines (Lane et al. 1991), and the antiepileptic action of benzodiazepines (Koe et al. 1985).

THC may antagonize the antipsychotic actions of neuroleptics (Sutin and Nahas 1999) and may improve their clinical responsiveness in motor disorders (Moss et al. 1989). A combination with other drugs may be desirable not only to reduce side effects of the single drugs but also to prevent the development of tolerance. In animal studies, tolerance to morphine was reduced by simultaneous administration of THC (Cichewicz and Welch 2003). Chronic treatment with high doses of oral morphine produced a threefold tolerance of pain-reducing effects. Tolerance to morphine was prevented in groups receiving a daily cotreatment with low doses of THC (Cichewicz and Welch 2003).

Since the endocannabinoid system is linked with hormonal control there may be interactions in this area. The progesterone receptor inhibitor mifepristone, which is approved for the termination of early pregnancy, and the glucocorticoid synthesis inhibitor metyrapone was recently shown to potentiate the sedating effects of high THC doses in mice (Pryce et al. 2003).

The cyclooxygenase inhibitors indomethacin, acetylsalicylic acid, and other non-steroidal anti-inflammatory drugs antagonize THC effects. Indomethacin significantly reduced subjective "high" (Perez-Reyes et al. 1991), tachycardia (Perez-Reyes et al. 1991), decrease of contractile performance in heart muscle (Bonz et al. 2003) and decrease of intraocular pressure following topical THC (eye drops) (Green et al. 2001), reflecting the involvement of cyclooxygenase activity in several THC effects.

CONCLUSIONS

The discovery, within the past 15 years, of a system of specific cannabinoid receptors in humans and their endogenous ligands has strongly stimulated research with about 800 articles published in Medline listed journals in 2002, compared to about 250 twenty years ago. It becomes apparent that the endocannabinoid system is playing a major role in signal transduction in neuronal cells, and arachidonylethanolamide (anandamide) seems to be a central inhibitory compound in the central nervous system (Mechoulam et al. 1998).

Mechanisms of action of cannabinoids are complex, not only involving activation of and interaction at the cannabinoid receptor, but also activation of vanilloid receptors (Jacobsson et al. 2001), influence of endocannabinoid concentration (Bisogno et al. 2001), antioxidant activity (Hampson 2002), metabolic interaction with other compounds, and several others. There is still much to learn about the physiological role of the natural ligands to the CB receptors and about long-term effects of cannabis use. However, due to the millennia-long use of cannabis for recreational, religious and medicinal purposes, which in recent decades was accompanied by scientific investigation in several disciplines, we do not expect to encounter with the medicinal use of cannabinoids the same unpleasant surprises that occasionally occur with newly designed synthetic drugs.

Many people who suffer from severe illnesses have discovered cannabis as a beneficial remedy, and public opinion surveys in Europe and North America show that increasing numbers of citizens reject criminal prosecution of patients who benefit from the drug. The psychotropic and circulatory effects of CB_1 receptor agonists and the stigma of cannabis as a recreational and addicting drug are still major obstacles to the legal therapeutic utilization of the whole range of potentially beneficial effects. Properly designed and executed clinical studies are necessary to verify anecdotal experiences and the results from smaller uncontrolled studies, and to overcome uncertainties and skepticism.

Aside from phytocannabinoids and cannabis preparations, cannabinoid analogues that do not bind to the CB_1 receptor are attractive compounds for clinical research, among them dexanabinol and CT-3. Additional ideas for the separation of the desired therapeutic effects from the psychotropic action comprise the concurrent administration of THC and CBD, the design of CB_1 receptor agonists that do not cross the blood-brain barrier, and the development of compounds that influence endocannabinoid levels by inhibition of their membrane transport (transport inhibitors) or hydrolysis (FAAH inhibitors). For example, blockers of anandamide hydrolysis were able to reduce anxiety in animal tests (Kathuria et al. 2003). These benzodiazepine-like properties were accompanied by augmented brain levels of anandamide and were prevented by CB_1 receptor blockade. It is remarkable that FAAH inhibitors may already be in clinical use as proposed by Fowler (2003). The nonsteroidal anti-inflammatory agent fluriprofen inhibits the metabolism of FAAH and intrathecally administrated fluriprofen reduced inflammatory pain by a mechanism that was blocked by a CB_1 receptor antagonist (Fowler 2003).

The future will show which drugs that target the endogenous cannabinoid system will follow dronabinol and nabilone into the pharmacy and which indications will prove successful in clinical trials.

REFERENCES

Abadji, V., S. Lin, T. Gihan, G. Griffen, L.A. Stevenson, G.R. Pertwee, and A. Makriyannis. 1994. (R)-methanandamide: A chiral novel anandamide possessing higher potency and metabolic stability. *J Med Chem* 37:1889-1893.

Abood, M.E., C. Sauss, F. Fan, C.L. Tilton, and B.R. Martin. 1993. Development of behavioral tolerance to delta 9-THC without alteration of cannabinoid receptor binding or mRNA levels in whole brain. *Pharmacol Biochem Behav* 46(3):575-579.

Abrahamov, A., and R. Mechoulam. 1995. An efficient new cannabinoid antiemetic in pediatric oncology. *Life Sci* 56(23-24):2097-2102.

Abrams, D.I., R.J. Leiser, J.F. Hilton, S.B. Shade, T.A. Elbeik, F.A. Aweeka, J.A. Aberg, L.N. Benowitz, B.M. Bredt, S.G. Deeks, et al. 2001. Short-term effects of cannabinoids in patients with HIV infection. *2001 Congress on Cannabis and the Cannabinoids*, Cologne, Germany: International Asociation for Cannabis as Medicine, p. 7.

Adami, M., P. Frati, S. Bertini, A. Kulkarni-Narla, D.R. Brown, G. de Caro, G. Coruzzi, and G. Soldani. 2002. Gastric antisecretory role and immunohisto-chemical localization of cannabinoid receptors in the rat stomach. *Br J Pharmacol* 135(7):1598-1606.

Adams, I.B., and B.R. Martin. 1996. Cannabis: Pharmacology and toxicology in animals and humans. *Addiction* 91(11):1585-1614.

Agurell, S., S. Carlsson, J.E. Lindgren, A. Ohlsson, H. Gillespie, and L. Hollister. 1981. Interactions of delta 1-tetrahydrocannabinol with cannabinol and cannabidiol following oral administration in man. Assay of cannabinol and cannabidiol by mass fragmentography. *Experientia* 37(10):1090-1092.

Al-Hayani, A., K.N. Wease, R.A. Ross, R.G. Pertwee, and S.N. Davies. 2001. The endogenous cannabinoid anandamide activates vanilloid receptors in the rat hippocampal slice. *Neuropharmacology* 41(8):1000-1005.

Anthony, J.C., L.A. Warner, and R.C. Kessler. 1994. Comparative epidemiology of dependence on tobacco, alcohol, controlled substances, and inhalants: basic findings from the National Comorbidity Survey. *Experimental and Clin Psychopharmacol* 2:244-268.

Archer, R.A., P. Stark, and L. Lemberger. 1986. Nabilone. In R. Mechoulam (ed.), *Cannabinoids as therapeutic agents* (pp. 85-103). Boca Raton: CRC Press.

Arevalo-Martin, A., J.M. Vela, E. Molina-Holgado, J. Borrell, and C. Guaza. 2003. Therapeutic action of cannabinoids in a murine model of multiple sclerosis. *J Neurosci* 23(7):2511-2516.

Bachs, L., and H. Morland. 2001. Acute cardiovascular fatalities following cannabis use. *Forensic Sci Int* 124(2-3):200-203.

Baek, S.H., Y.O. Kim, J.S. Kwag, K.E. Choi, W.Y. Jung, and D.S. Han. 1998. Boron trifluoride etherate on silica-A modified Lewis acid reagent (VII). Antitumor activity of cannabigerol against human oral epitheloid carcinoma cells. *Arch Pharm Res* 21(3):353-356.

Baker, D., G. Pryce, J.L. Croxford, P. Brown, R.G. Pertwee, A. Makriyannis, A. Khanolkar, L. Layward, F. Fezza, T. Bisogno, and V. Di Marzo. 2001. Endo-cannabinoids control spasticity in a multiple sclerosis model. *FASEB J* 15(2): 300-302.

Barann, M., G. Molderings, M. Bruss, H. Bonisch, B.W. Urban, and M. Gothert. 2002. Direct inhibition by cannabinoids of human 5-HT3A receptors: probable involvement of an allosteric modulatory site. *Br J Pharmacol* 137(5):589-596.

Bass, C.E., and B.R. Martin. 2000. Time course for the induction and maintenance of tolerance to Δ^9-tetrahydrocannabinol in mice. *Drug Alcohol Depend* 60(2): 113-119.

Beal, J.E., R. Olson, L. Laubenstein, J.O. Morales, P. Bellman, B. Yangco, L. Lefkowitz, Plasse T.F., and Shepard K.V. 1995. Dronabinol as a treatment for anorexia associated with weight loss in patients with AIDS. *J Pain Symptom Manage* 10(2):89-97.

Beal, J.E., R. Olson, L. Lefkowitz, L. Laubenstein, P. Bellman, B. Yangco, J.O. Morales, R. Murphy, W. Powderly, T.F. Plasse, et al. 1997. Long-term efficacy and safety of dronabinol for acquired immunodeficiency syndrome-associated anorexia. *J Pain Symptom Manage* 14(1):7-14.

Beaulieu, P., T. Bisogno, S. Punwar, W.P. Farquhar-Smith, G. Ambrosino, V. Di Marzo, and A.S. Rice. 2000. Role of the endogenous cannabinoid system in the formalin test of persistent pain in the rat. *Eur J Pharmacol* 396(2-3):85-92.

Beltramo, M., N. Stella, A. Calignano, S.Y. Lin, A. Makriyannis, and D. Piomelli. 1997. Functional role of high-affinity anandamide transport, as revealed by selective inhibition. *Science* 277(5329):1094-1097.

Benowitz, N.L., and R.T. Jones. 1975. Cardiovascular effects of prolonged delta-9-tetrahydrocannabinol ingestion. *Clin Pharmacol Ther* 18(3):287-297.

Bisogno, T., L. Hanus, L. De Petrocellis, S. Tchilibon, D.E. Ponde, I. Brandi, A.S. Moriello, J.B. Davis, R. Mechoulam, and V. Di Marzo. 2001. Molecular targets for cannabidiol and its synthetic analogues: effect on vanilloid VR1 receptors and on the cellular uptake and enzymatic hydrolysis of anandamide. *Br J Pharmacol* 134(4):845-852.

Blazquez, C., M.L. Casanova, A. Planas, T.G. Del Pulgar, C. Villanueva, M.J. Fernandez-Acenero, J. Aragones, J.W. Huffman, J.L. Jorcano, and M. Guzman. 2003. Inhibition of tumor angiogenesis by cannabinoids. *FASEB J* 17(3):529-531.

Bonz, A., M. Laser, S. Kullmer, S. Kniesch, J. Babin-Ebell, V. Popp, G. Ertl, and J.A. Wagner. 2003. Cannabinoids acting on CB1 receptors decrease contractile performance in human atrial muscle. *J Cardiovasc Pharmacol* 41(4):657-664.

Bornheim, L.M., and M.P. Grillo. 1998. Characterization of cytochrome P450 3A inactivation by cannabidiol: Possible involvement of cannabidiol-hydroxyquinone as a P450 inactivator. *Chem Res Toxicol* 11(10):1209-1216.

Bornheim, L.M., K.Y. Kim, J. Li, B.Y. Perotti, and L.Z. Benet. 1995. Effect of cannabidiol pretreatment on the kinetics of tetrahydrocannabinol metabolites in mouse brain. *Drug Metab Dispos* 23(8):825-831.

Braida, D., M. Pozzi, R. Cavallini, and M. Sala. 2001. Conditioned place preference induced by the cannabinoid agonist CP 55,940: Interaction with the opioid system. *Neuroscience* 104(4):923-926.

Breivogel, C.S., G. Griffin, V. Di Marzo, and B.R. Martin. 2001. Evidence for a new G protein-coupled cannabinoid receptor in mouse brain. *Mol Pharmacol* 60(1): 155-163.

Brenneisen, R., A. Egli, M.A. Elsohly, V. Henn, Y. Spiess. 1996. The effect of orally and rectally administered delta 9-tetrahydrocannabinol on spasticity: A pilot study with 2 patients. *Int J Clin Pharmacol Ther* 34(10):446-452.

British Medical Association. 1997. *Therapeutic uses of cannabis.* Amsterdam: Harwood Academic Publishers.

Brody, S., and R. Preut. 2002. Cannabis, tobacco, and caffeine use modify the blood pressure reactivity protection of ascorbic acid. *Pharmacol Biochem Behav* 72(4): 811-816.

Bueb, J.L., D.M. Lambert, and E.J. Tschirhart. 2001. Receptor-independent effects of natural cannabinoids in rat peritoneal mast cells in vitro. *Biochim Biophys Acta* 1538(2-3):252-259.

Burstein, S. 1999. The cannabinoid acids: nonpsychoactive derivatives with therapeutic potential. *Pharmacol Ther* 82(1):87-96.

Burstein, S. 2002. Therapeutic potential of ajulemic acid (CT3). In F. Grotenhermen and E. Russo (eds.), *Cannabis and cannabinoids. Pharmacology, toxicology, and therapeutic potential* (pp. 381-388). Binghamton, NY: The Haworth Press.

Burstein, S., C.A. Audette, S.A. Doyle, K. Hull, S.A. Hunter, and V. Latham. 1989. Antagonism to the actions of platelet activating factor by a nonpsychoactive cannabinoid. *J Pharmacol Exp Ther* 251(2):531-535.

Burstein, S., S.A. Hunter, V. Latham, and L. Renzulli. 1987. A major metabolite of delta 1-tetrahydrocannabinol reduces its cataleptic effect in mice. *Experientia* 43(4):402-403.

Cabral, G. 2002. Immune system. In F. Grotenhermen and E. Russo (eds.), *Cannabis and cannabinoids. Pharmacology, toxicology, and therapeutic potential* (pp. 279-288). Binghamton, NY: The Haworth Press.

Calhoun, S.R., G.P. Galloway, and D.E. Smith. 1998. Abuse potential of dronabinol (Marinol). *J Psychoactive Drugs* 30(2):187-196.

Calignano, A., I. Katona, F. Desarnaud, A. Giuffrida, G. La Rana, K. Mackie, T.F. Freund, and D. Piomelli. 2000. Bidirectional control of airway responsiveness by endogenous cannabinoids. *Nature* 408(6808):96-101.

Carley, D.W., S. Paviovic, M. Janelidze, and M. Radulovacki. 2002. Functional role for cannabinoids in respiratory stability during sleep. *Sleep* 25(4):391-398.

Casanova, M.L., C. Blazquez, J. Martinez-Palacio, C. Villanueva, M.J. Fernandez-Acenero, J.W. Huffman, J.L. Jorcano, and M. Guzman. 2003. Inhibition of skin tumor growth and angiogenesis in vivo by activation of cannabinoid receptors. *J Clin Invest* 111(1):43-50.

Chan, P.C., R.C. Sills, A.G. Braun, J.K. Haseman, and J.R. Bucher. 1996. Toxicity and carcinogenicity of delta 9-tetrahydrocannabinol in Fischer rats and B6C3F1 mice. *Fundam Appl Toxicol* 30(1):109-117.

Chang, M.C., D. Berkery, R. Schuel, S.G. Laychock, A.M. Zimmerman, S. Zimmerman, and H. Schuel. 1993. Evidence for a cannabinoid receptor in sea urchin sperm and its role in blockade of the acrosome reaction. *Mol Reprod Dev* 36(4):507-516.

Chapman, V. 1999. The cannabinoid CB1 receptor antagonist, SR141716A, selectively facilitates nociceptive responses of dorsal horn neurones in the rat. *Br J Pharmacol* 127(8):1765-1767.

Cichewicz, D.L., and E.A. McCarthy. 2003. Antinociceptive synergy between Δ9-tetrahydrocannabinol and opioids after oral administration. *J Pharmacol Exp Ther* 304(3):1010-1015.

Cichewicz, D.L., and S.P. Welch. 2003. Modulation of oral morphine antinociceptive tolerance and naloxone-precipitated withdrawal signs by oral Δ9-THC. *J Pharmacol Exp Ther* 305(3):812-817.

Citron, M.L., T.S. Herman, F. Vreeland, S.H. Krasnow, and B.E. Fossieck, Jr. 1985. Antiemetic efficacy of levonantradol compared to delta-9-tetrahydrocannabinol for chemotherapy-induced nausea and vomiting. *Cancer Treat Rep* 69:109-112.

Clermont-Gnamien, S., S. Atlani, N. Attal, F. Le Mercier, F. Guirimand, and L. Brasseur. 2002. [The therapeutic use of D9-tetrahydrocannabinol (dronabinol) in refractory neuropathic pain] [Article in French]. *Presse Med* 31(39 Pt 1): 1840-1845.

Clifford, D.B. 1983. Tetrahydrocannabinol for tremor in multiple sclerosis. *Ann Neurol* 13(6):669-671.

Colasanti, B.K. 1990. A comparison of the ocular and central effects of delta 9-tetrahydrocannabinol and cannabigerol. *J Ocul Pharmacol* 6(4):259-269.

Colasanti, B.K., R.E. Brown, and C.R. Craig. 1984. Ocular hypotension, ocular toxicity, and neurotoxicity in response to marihuana extract and cannabidiol. *Gen Pharmacol* 15(6):479-484.

Consroe, P., R. Sandyk, and S.R. Snider. 1986. Open label evaluation of cannabidiol in dystonic movement disorders. *Int J Neurosci* 30(4):277-282.

Coruzzi, G., M. Adami, G. Coppelli, P. Frati, and G. Soldani. 1999. Inhibitory effect of the cannabinoid receptor agonist WIN 55,212-2 on pentagastrin-induced gastric acid secretion in the anaesthetized rat. *Naunyn Schmiedebergs Arch Pharmacol* 360(6):715-718.

Costa, B., G. Giagnoni, S. Conti, D. Parolaro, and M. Colleoni. 2003. Cannabidiol is an oral effective therapeutic agent both in acute inflammation and in chronic FCA-induced arthritis. *First European Workshop on Cannabinoid Research*. Madrid (Spain).

Costa, B., D. Parolaro, and M. Colleoni. 1996. Chronic cannabinoid, CP-55,940, administration alters biotransformation in the rat. *Eur J Pharmacol* 313(1-2): 17-24.

Cravatt, B.F., K. Demarest, M.P. Patricelli, M.H. Bracey, D.K. Giang, B.R. Martin, and A.H. Lichtman. 2001. Supersensitivity to anandamide and enhanced endogenous cannabinoid signaling in mice lacking fatty acid amide hydrolase. *Proc Natl Acad Sci U S A* 98(16):9371-9376.

Crawford, W.J., and J.C. Merritt. 1979. Effects of tetrahydrocannabinol on arterial and intraocular hypertension. *Int J Clin Pharmacol Biopharm* 17(5):191-196.

Croxford, J.L., and S.D. Miller. 2003. Immunoregulation of a viral model of multiple sclerosis using the synthetic cannabinoid R(+)WIN55,212. *J Clin Invest* 111(8):1231-1240.

Dansak, D.A. 1997. As an antiemetic and appetite stimulant in cancer patients. In M.L. Mathre (ed.), *Cannabis in medical practice: A legal, historical and pharmacological overview of the therapeutic use of marijuana* (pp. 69-83). Jefferson, NC: McFarland and Co.

Darmani, N.A. 2001. Delta-9-tetrahydrocannabinol differentially suppresses cisplatin-induced emesis and indices of motor function via cannabinoid CB(1) receptors in the least shrew. *Pharmacol Biochem Behav* 69(1-2):239-249.

Davis, J.P., and H.H. Ramsey. 1949. Antiepileptic action of marijuana active substances. *Fed Proc* 8:284.

De Petrocellis, L., D. Melck, T. Bisogno, A. Milone, and V. Di Marzo. 1999. Finding of the endocannabinoid signalling system in Hydra, a very primitive organism: Possible role in the feeding response. *Neuroscience* 92(1):377-387.

De Petrocellis, L., D. Melck, A. Palmisano, T. Bisogno, C. Laezza, M. Bifulco, and V. Di Marzo. 1998. The endogenous cannabinoid anandamide inhibits human breast cancer cell proliferation. *Proc Natl Acad Sci USA* 95(14):8375-8380.

Devane, W.A., L. Hanus, A. Breuer, R.G. Pertwee, L.A. Stevenson, G. Griffin, D. Gibson, A. Mandelbaum, A. Etinger, and R. Mechoulam. 1992. Isolation and structure of a brain constituent that binds to the cannabinoid receptor. *Science* 258(5090):1946-1949.

Dewey, W.L. 1986. Cannabinoid pharmacology. *Pharmacol Rev* 38(2):151-178.

Di Marzo, V. 1998. "Endocannabinoids" and other fatty acid derivatives with cannabimimetic properties: biochemistry and possible physiopathological relevance. *Biochim Biophys Acta* 1392(2-3):153-175.

Di Marzo, V., F. Berrendero, T. Bisogno, S. Gonzalez, P. Cavaliere, J. Romero, M. Cebeira, J.A. Ramos, and J.J. Fernandez-Ruiz. 2000. Enhancement of anandamide formation in the limbic forebrain and reduction of endocannabinoid contents in the striatum of Δ^9–tetrahydrocannabinol-tolerant rats. *J Neurochem* 74(4):1627-1635.

Di Marzo, V., C.S. Breivogel, Q. Tao, D.T. Bridgen, R.K. Razdan, A.M. Zimmer, A. Zimmer, and B.R. Martin. 2000. Levels, metabolism, and pharmacological activity of anandamide in CB(1) cannabinoid receptor knockout mice: Evidence for non-CB(1), non-CB(2) receptor-mediated actions of anandamide in mouse brain. *J Neurochem* 75(6):2434-2444.

Di Marzo, V., S.K. Goparaju, L. Wang, J. Liu, S. Batkai, Z. Jarai, F. Fezza, G.I. Miura, R.D. Palmiter, T. Sugiura, and G. Kunos. 2001. Leptin-regulated endocannabinoids are involved in maintaining food intake. *Nature* 410(6830):822-825.

Di Marzo, V., G. Griffin, L. De Petrocellis, I. Brandi, T. Bisogno, W. Williams, M.C. Grier, S. Kulasegram, A. Mahadevan, R.K. Razdan, and B.R. Martin. 2002. A structure/activity relationship study on arvanil, an endocannabinoid and vanilloid hybrid. *J Pharmacol Exp Ther* 300(3):984-991.

Di Marzo, V., M.P. Hill, T. Bisogno, A.R. Crossman, and J.M. Brotchie. 2000. Enhanced levels of endogenous cannabinoids in the globus pallidus are associated with a reduction in movement in an animal model of Parkinson's disease. *FASEB J* 14(10):1432-1438.

Dinh, T.P., T.F. Freund, and D. Piomelli. 2002. A role for monoglyceride lipase in 2-arachidonoylglycerol inactivaion. *Chem Phys Lipids* 121(1-2):149-158.

Domino, E.F. 1999. Cannabinoids and the cholinergic system. In G. Nahas, K.M. Sutin, D.J. Harvey, and S. Agurell (eds.), *Marihuana and medicine* (pp. 223-226). Totowa, NJ: Humana Press.

Doyle, S.A., S.H. Burstein, W.L. Dewey, and S.P. Welch. 1990. Further studies on the antinociceptive effects of delta 6-THC-7-oic acid. *Agents Actions* 31(1-2):157-163.

Elsner, F., L. Radbruch, and R. Sabatowski. 2001. Tetrahydrocannabinol zur Therapie chronischer Schmerzen [Tetrahydrocannabinol for treatment of chronic pain]. *Schmerz* 15(3):200-204.

ElSohly, M.A. 2002. Chemical constituents of cannabis. In F. Grotenhermen and E. Russo (eds.), *Cannabis and cannabinoids. Pharmacology, toxicology, and therapeutic potential* (pp. 27-36). Binghamton, NY: The Haworth Press.

Evans, A.T., E.A. Formukong, and F.J. Evans. 1987. Actions of cannabis constituents on enzymes of arachidonate, metabolism: anti-inflammatory potential. *Biochem Pharmacol* 36(12):2035-2037.

Fan, P. 1995. Cannabinoid agonists inhibit the activation of 5-HT3 receptors in rat nodose ganglion neurons. *J Neurophysiol* 73(2):907-910.

Fezza, F., T. Bisogno, A. Minassi, G. Appendino, R. Mechoulam, and V. Di Marzo. 2002. Noladin ether, a putative novel endocannabinoid: Inactivation mechanisms and a sensitive method for its quantification in rat tissues. *FEBS Lett* 513(2-3):294-298.

Formukong, E.A., A.T. Evans, and F.J. Evans. 1989. The inhibitory effects of cannabinoids, the active constituents of *Cannabis sativa* L. on human and rabbit platelet aggregation. *J Pharm Pharmacol* 41(10):705-709.

Fowler, C.J., and S.O. Jacobsson. 2002. Cellular transport of anandamide, 2-arachidonoylglycerol and palmitoylethanolamide—targets for drug development? *Prostaglandins Leukot Essent Fatty Acids* 66(2-3):193-200.

Fowler, C.W. 2003. Biochemistry and pharmacology of fatty acid amide hydrolase, the enzyme responsible for the metabolism of anandamide and related N-acyl ethanolamines. *First European Workshop on Cannabinoid Research.* Madrid (Spain).

Fox, S.H., M. Kellett, A. P. Moore, A.R. Crossman, and J.M. Brotchie. 2002. Randomised, double-blind, placebo-controlled trial to assess the potential of cannabinoid receptor stimulation in the treatment of dystonia. *Mov Disord* 17(1):145-149.

Freemon, F.R. 1972. Effects of marihuana on sleeping states. *JAMA* 220(10):1364-1365.

Fride, E., J. Barg, R. Levy, D. Saya, E. Heldman, R. Mechoulam, and Z. Vogel. 1995. Low doses of anandamides inhibit pharmacological effects of delta 9-tetrahydrocannabinol. *J Pharmacol Exp Ther* 272(2):699-707.

Fride, E., A. Foox, E. Rosenberg, M. Faigenboim, V. Cohen, L. Barda, H. Blau, and R. Mechoulam. 2003. Milk intake and survival in newborn cannabinoid CB(1) receptor knockout mice: Evidence for a "CB(3)" receptor. *Eur J Pharmacol* 461(1):27-34.

Fride, E., and E. Shohami. 2002. The endocannabinoid system: Function in survival of the embryo, the newborn and the neuron. *Neuroreport* 13(15):1833-1841.

Fried, P.A., B. Watkinson, and R. Gray. 1998. Differential effects on cognitive functioning in 9- to 12-year olds prenatally exposed to cigarettes and marihuana. *Neurotoxicol Teratol* 20(3):293-306.

Galiègue, S., S. Mary, J. Marchand, D. Dussossoy, D. Carrière, P. Carayon, M. Bouaboula, D. Shire, G. Le Fur, and P. Casellas. 1995. Expression of central and peripheral cannabinoid receptors in human immune tissues and leukocyte subpopulations. *Eur J Biochem* 232:54-61.

Galve-Roperh, I., C. Sanchez, M.L. Cortes, T.G. del Pulgar, M. Izquierdo, and M. Guzman. 2000. Anti-tumoral action of cannabinoids: Involvement of sustained ceramide accumulation and extracellular signal-regulated kinase activation. *Nat Med* 6(3):313-319.

Gaoni, Y., and R. Mechoulam. 1964. Isolation, structure and partial synthesis of the active constituent of hashish. *J Am Chem Soc* 86:1646-1647.

Gardner, E.L. 2002. Addictive potential of cannabinoids: The underlying neurobiology. *Chem Phys Lipids* 121(1-2):267-290.

Georgotas, A., and P. Zeidenberg. 1979. Observations on the effects of four weeks of heavy marihuana smoking on group interaction and individual behavior. *Compr Psychiatry* 20(5):427-432.

Gieringer, D. 2002. Medical use of cannabis: Experience in California. In F. Grotenhermen and E. Russo (eds.), *Cannabis and cannabinoids. Pharmacology, toxicology, and therapeutic potential* (pp. 143-151). Binghamton, NY: The Haworth Press.

Gilson, I., and M. Busalacchi. 1998. Marijuana for intractable hiccups. *Lancet* 351 (9098):267.

Giuffrida, A., M. Beltramo, and D. Piomelli. 2001. Mechanisms of endocannabinoid inactivation: Biochemistry and pharmacology. *J Pharmacol Exp Ther* 298(1):7-14.

Glaser, S.T., N.A. Abumrad, F. Fatade, M. Kaczocha, K.M. Studholme, D.G. Deutsch. 2003. Evidence against the presence of an anandamide transporter. *Proc Natl Acad Sci USA* 100(7):4269-4274.

Glass, M., and C.C. Felder. 1997. Concurrent stimulation of cannabinoid CB1 and dopamine D2 receptors augments cAMP accumulation in striatal neurons: Evidence for a G_s linkage to the CB1 receptor. *J Neurosci* 17:5327-5333.

Gordon, E., and O. Devinsky. 2001. Alcohol and marijuana: Effects on epilepsy and use by patients with epilepsy. *Epilepsia* 42(10):1266-1272.

Green, K., E.C. Kearse, and O.L. McIntyre. 2001. Interaction between Delta-9-tetrahydrocannabinol and indomethacin. *Ophthalmic Res* 33(4):217-220.

Grinspoon, L., and J.B. Bakalar. 1993. *Marihuana, the forbidden medicine.* New Haven, CT: Yale University Press.

Grinspoon, L., and J.B. Bakalar. 1998. The use of cannabis as a mood stabilizer in bipolar disorder: Anecdotal evidence and the need for clinical research. *J Psychoactive Drugs* 30(2):171-177.

Grotenhermen, F. 2002a. Effects of cannabis and the cannabinoids. In F. Grotenhermen and E. Russo (eds.), *Cannabis and cannabinoids. Pharmacology, toxicology, and therapeutic potential* (pp. 55-66). Binghamton, NY: The Haworth Press.

Grotenhermen, F. 2002b. Review of therapeutic effects. In F. Grotenhermen and E. Russo (eds.), *Cannabis and cannabinoids. Pharmacology, toxicology, and therapeutic potential* (pp. 123-142). Binghamton, NY: The Haworth Press.

Grotenhermen, F. 2002c. Review of unwanted actions of Cannabis and THC. In F. Grotenhermen and E. Russo (eds.), *Cannabis and cannabinoids. Pharmacology, toxicology, and therapeutic potential* (pp. 233-245). Binghamton, NY: The Haworth Press.

Grotenhermen, F., and E. Russo (eds.). 2002. *Cannabis and cannabinoids: Pharmacology, toxicology, and therapeutic potential.* Binghamton, NY: The Haworth Press.

Grundy, R.I. 2002. The therapeutic potential of the cannabinoids in neuroprotection. *Expert Opin Investig Drugs* 11(10):1365-1374.

Guzman, M., C. Sanchez, and I. Galve-Roperh. 2001. Control of the cell survival/death decision by cannabinoids. *J Mol Med* 78(11):613-625.

Hall, W., N. Solowij, and J. Lemon. 1994. *The health and psychological consequences of cannabis use.* Canberra: Commonwealth Department of Human Services and Health, Monograph Series No. 25.

Hampson, A. 2002. Cannabinoids as neuroprotectants against ischemia. In F. Grotenhermen and E. Russo (eds.), *Cannabis and cannabinoids. Pharmacology, toxicology, and therapeutic potential* (pp. 101-110). Binghamton, NY: The Haworth Press.

Hampson, R.E., and S.A. Deadwyler. 1999. Cannabinoids, hippocampal function and memory. *Life Sci* 65:715-723.

Haney, M., A. Bisaga, and R.W. Foltin. 2003. Interaction between naltrexone and oral THC in heavy marijuana smokers. *Psychopharmacology (Berl)* 166(1):77-85.

Hanus, L., S. Abu-Lafi, E. Fride, A. Breuer, Z. Vogel, D.E. Shalev, I. Kustanovich, and R. Mechoulam. 2001. 2-arachidonyl glyceryl ether, an endogenous agonist of the cannabinoid CB1 receptor. *Proc Natl Acad Sci U S A* 98(7):3662-3665.

Hart, C.L., A.S. Ward, M. Haney, S.D. Comer, R.W. Foltin, and M.W. Fischman. 2002. Comparison of smoked marijuana and oral Δ9-tetrahydrocannabinol in humans. *Psychopharmacology (Berl)* 164(4):407-415.

Hartley, J.P., S.G. Nogrady, and A. Seaton. 1978. Bronchodilator effect of delta1-tetrahydrocannabinol. *Br J Clin Pharmacol* 5(6):523-525.

Hembree 3d, W.C., G.G. Nahas, P. Zeidenberg, and H.F. Huang. 1978. Changes in human spermatozoa associated with high dose marihuana smoking. *Adv Biosci* 22-23:429-439.

Hemming, M., and P.M. Yellowlees. 1993. Effective treatment of Tourette's syndrome with marijuana. *J Psychopharmacol* 7:389-391.

Hepler, R.S., and I.R. Frank. 1971. Marihuana smoking and intraocular pressure. *JAMA* 217(10):1392.

Hepler, R.S., and R.J. Petrus. 1976. Experiences with administration of marihuana to glaucoma patients. In S. Cohen and R.C. Stillman (eds.), *The therapeutic potential of marihuana* (pp. 63-75). New York: Plenum Medical Book.

Heyser, C.J., R.E. Hampson, and S.A. Deadwyler. 1993. Effects of delta-9-tetrahydrocannabinol on delayed match to sample performance in rats: Alterations in short-term memory associated with changes in task specific firing of hippocampal cells. *J Pharmacol Exp Ther* 264(1):294-307.

Holdcroft, A., M. Smith, A. Jacklin, H. Hodgson, B. Smith, M. Newton, and F. Evans. 1997. Pain relief with oral cannabinoids in familial Mediterranean fever. *Anaesthesia* 52(5):483-486.

Hollister, L.E. 1986. Health aspects of cannabis. *Pharmacological Reviews* 38:1-20.

Hollister, L.E. 1999. Interactions of marihuana and Δ^9-THC with other drugs. In G. Nahas, K.M. Sutin, D.J. Harvey, and S. Agurell (eds.), *Marihuana and medicine* (pp. 273-277). Totowa, NJ: Humana Press.

House of Lords Select Committee on Science and Technology. 1998. *Cannabis. The scientific and medical evidence.* London: The Stationery Office.

Howlett, A.C. 2002. The cannabinoid receptors. *Prostaglandins Other Lipid Mediat* 68-69:619-631.

Huang, S.M., T. Bisogno, M. Trevisani, A. Al-Hayani, L. De Petrocellis, F. Fezza, M. Tognetto, T.J. Petros, J.F. Krey, C.J. Chu, et al. 2002. An endogenous capsaicin-like substance with high potency at recombinant and native vanilloid VR1 receptors. *Proc Natl Acad Sci U S A* 99(12):8400-8405.

Huestis, M.A., D.A Gorelick, S.J. Heishman, K.L. Preston, R.A. Nelson, E.T. Moolchan, and R.A. Frank. 2001. Blockade of effects of smoked marijuana by the CB1-selective cannabinoid receptor antagonist SR141716. *Arch Gen Psychiatry* 58(4):322-328.

Hunt, C.A., R.T. Jones. 1980. Tolerance and disposition of tetrahydrocannabinol in man. *J Pharmacol Exp Ther* 215(1):35-44.

Hunt, C.A., R.T. Jones, R.I. Herning, and J. Bachman. 1981. Evidence that cannabidiol does not significantly alter the pharmacokinetics of tetrahydrocannabinol in man. *J Pharmacokinet Biopharm* 9(3):245-260.

Izzo, A.A., F. Fezza, R. Capasso, T. Bisogno, L. Pinto, T. Iuvone, G. Esposito, N. Mascolo, V. Di Marzo, and F. Capasso. 2001. Cannabinoid CB1-receptor mediated regulation of gastrointestinal motility in mice in a model of intestinal inflammation. *Br J Pharmacol* 134(3):563-570.

Izzo, A.A., L. Pinto, F. Borrelli, R. Capasso, N. Mascolo, and F. Capasso. 2000. Central and peripheral cannabinoid modulation of gastrointestinal transit in physiological states or during the diarrhoea induced by croton oil. *Br J Pharmacol* 129(8):1627-1632.

Jacobsson, S.O., T. Wallin, and C.J. Fowler. 2001. Inhibition of rat C6 glioma cell proliferation by endogenous and synthetic cannabinoids. Relative involvement of cannabinoid and vanilloid receptors. *J Pharmacol Exp Ther* 299(3):951-959.

Jaeger, W., L.Z. Benet, and L.M. Bornheim. 1996. Inhibition of cyclosporine and tetrahydrocannabinol metabolism by cannabidiol in mouse and human microsomes. *Xenobiotica* 26(3):275-284.

Jaggar, S.I., F.S. Hasnie, S. Sellaturay, and A.S. Rice. 1998. The anti-hyperalgesic actions of the cannabinoid anandamide and the putative CB2 receptor agonist palmitoylethanolamide in visceral and somatic inflammatory pain. *Pain* 76(1-2):189-199.

Jain, A.K., J.R. Ryan, F.G. McMahon, and G. Smith. 1981. Evaluation of intramuscular levonantrodol and placebo in acute postoperative pain. *Journal of Clinical Pharmacology* 21(Suppl):320S-326S.

Jan, T.R., A.K. Farraj, J.R. Harkema, and N.E. Kaminski. 2003. Attenuation of the ovalbumin-induced allergic airway response by cannabinoid treatment in A/J mice small star, filled. *Toxicol Appl Pharmacol* 188(1):24-35.

Jatoi, A., H.E. Windschitl, C.L. Loprinzi, J.A. Sloan, S.R. Dakhil, J.A. Mailliard, S. Pundaleeka, C.G. Kardinal, T.R. Fitch, J.E. Krook, et al. 2002. Dronabinol versus megestrol acetate versus combination therapy for cancer-associated anorexia: A North Central Cancer Treatment Group study. *J Clin Oncol* 20(2):567-573.

Jones, R.T., N. Benowitz, and J. Bachman. 1976. Clinical studies of cannabis tolerance and dependence. *Ann N Y Acad Sci* 282:221-239.

Joy, J.E., S.J. Watson, and J.A. Benson. 1999. *Marijuana and medicine: Assessing the science base.* Washington DC: Institute of Medicine, National Academy Press.

Kalant, H., W. Corrigal, W. Hall, and R. Smart. 1999. *The health effects of cannabis.* Toronto (Canada): Centre for Addiction and Mental Health.

Karler, R., and S.A. Turkanis. 1981. The cannabinoids as potential antiepileptics. *J Clin Pharmacol* 21(8-9 Suppl):437S-448S.

Karler, R., and S.A. Turkanis. 1987. Different cannabinoids exhibit different pharmacological and toxicological properties. *NIDA Res Monogr* 79:96-107.

Kathuria, S., S. Gaetani, D. Fegley, F. Valino, A. Duranti, A. Tontini, M. Mor, G. Tarzia, G. La Rana, A. Calignano, et al. 2003. Modulation of anxiety through blockade of anandamide hydrolysis. *Nat Med* 9(1):76-81.

Kelly, T.H., R.W. Foltin, C.S. Emurian, and M.W. Fischman. 1993. Performance-based testing for drugs of abuse: Dose and time profiles of marijuana, amphetamine, alcohol, and diazepam. *J Anal Toxicol* 17(5):264-272.

Killestein, J., E.L. Hoogervorst, M. Reif, N.F. Kalkers, A.C. Van Loenen, P.G. Staats, R.W. Gorter, B.M. Uitdehaag, and C.H. Polman. 2002. Safety, tolerability, and efficacy of orally administered cannabinoids in MS. *Neurology* 58(9):1404-1407.

Kleiber, D., R. Soellner, and P. Tossmann. 1997. *Cannabiskonsum in der Bundesrepublik* Deutschland: Entwicklungstendenzen, Konsummuster und Einflußfaktoren. Bonn: Federal Ministry of Health.

Knoller, N., L. Levi, I. Shoshan, E. Reichenthal, N. Razon, Z.H. Rappaport, and A. Biegon. 2002. Dexanabinol (HU-211) in the treatment of severe closed head injury: A randomized, placebo-controlled, phase II clinical trial. *Crit Care Med* 30(3):548-554.

Koe, B.K., G.M. Milne, A. Weissman, M.R. Johnson, and L.S. Melvin. 1985. Enhancement of brain [3H]flunitrazepam binding and analgesic activity of synthetic cannabimimetics. *Eur J Pharmacol* 109(2):201-212.

Kosel, B.W., F.T. Aweeka, N.L. Benowitz, S.B. Shade, J.F. Hilton, P.S. Lizak, and D.I. Abrams. 2002. The effects of cannabinoids on the pharmacokinetics of indinavir and nelfinavir. *AIDS* 16(4):543-550.

Laine, K., K. Jarvinen, and T. Jarvinen. 2003. Topically administered CB(2)-receptor agonist, JWH-133, does not decrease intraocular pressure (IOP) in normotensive rabbits. *Life Sci* 72(7):837-842.

Lake, K.D., D.R. Compton, K. Varga, B.R. Martin, and G. Kunos. 1997. Cannabinoid-induced hypotension and bradycardia in rats is mediated by CB1-like cannabinoid receptors. *J Pharmacol Exp Ther* 281:1030-1037.

Lane, M., C.L. Vogel, J. Ferguson, S. Krasnow, J.L. Saiers, J. Hamm, K. Salva, P.H. Wiernik, C.P. Holroyde, S. Hammill, et al. 1991. Dronabinol and prochlorperazine in combination for treatment of cancer chemotherapy-induced nausea and vomiting. *J Pain Symptom Manage* 6(6):352-359.

Lemberger, L., R.E. Crabtree, and H.M. Rowe. 1972. 11-hydroxy-Δ9-tetrahydrocannabinol: Pharmacology, disposition, and metabolism of a major metabolite of marihuana in man. *Science* 177(43):62-64.

Leweke, F.M., A. Giuffrida, U. Wurster, H.M. Emrich, and D. Piomelli. 1999. Elevated endogenous cannabinoids in schizophrenia. *Neuroreport* 10(8):1665-1669.

Lichtman, A.H., S.M. Sheikh, H.H. Loh, and B.R. Martin. 2001. Opioid and cannabinoid modulation of precipitated withdrawal in delta(9)-tetrahydrocannabinol and morphine-dependent mice. *J Pharmacol Exp Ther* 298(3):1007-1014.

Lissoni, P., M. Resentini, R. Mauri, D. Esposti, G. Esposti, D. Rossi, G. Legname, and F. Fraschini. 1986. Effects of tetrahydrocannabinol on melatonin secretion in man. *Horm Metab Res* 18(1):77-78.

Little, P.J., D.R. Compton, R. Mechoulam, and B. Martin. 1989. Stereochemical effects of 11-OH-Δ8-THC-dimethylheptyl in mice and dogs. *Pharmacol Biochem Behav* 32:661-666.

Liu, J., H. Li, S.H. Burstein, R.B. Zurier, and J.D. Chen. 2003. Activation and binding of peroxisome proliferator-activated receptor gamma by synthetic cannabinoid ajulemic acid. *Mol Pharmacol* 63(5):983-992.

Loewe, S. 1950. Cannabiswirkstoffe und Pharmakologie der Cannabinole. *Archiv für Experimentelle Pathologie und Pharmakologie* 211:175-193.

Lorenz, R. 2002. A casuistic rationale for the treatment of spastic and myocloni in a childhood neurodegenerative disease: neuronal ceroid lipofuscinosis of the type Jansky-Bielschowsky. *Neuroendocrinol Lett* 23(5-6):387-390.

Lucraft, H.H., and M.K. Palmer. 1982. Randomized clinical trial of levonantradol and chlorpromazine in the prevention of radiotherapy-indiced vomiting. *Clin Radiol* 33(6):621-622.

Luthra, Y.K., H.J. Esber, D.M. Lariviere, and H. Rosenkrantz. 1980. Assessment of tolerance to immunosuppressive activity of delta 9-tetrahydrocannabinol in rats. *J Immunopharmacol* 2(2):245-256.

Lyketsos, C.G., E. Garrett, K.Y. Liang, and J.C. Anthony. 1999. Cannabis use and cognitive decline in persons under 65 years of age. *Am J Epidemiol* 149(9):794-800.

Malfait, A.M., R. Gallily, P.F. Sumariwalla, A.S. Malik, E. Andreakos, R. Mechoulam, M. Feldmann. 2000. The nonpsychoactive cannabis constituent cannabidiol is an oral anti-arthritic therapeutic in murine collagen-induced arthritis. *Proc Natl Acad Sci USA* 97(17):9561-9566.

Martyn, C.N., L.S. Illis, and J. Thom. 1995. Nabilone in the treatment of multiple sclerosis. *Lancet* 345(8949):579.

Mathre, M.L. 1997. *Cannabis in medical practice: A legal, historical and pharmacological overview of the therapeutic use of marijuana.* Jefferson, NC: McFarland and Co.

Mattes, R.D., L.M. Shaw, and K. Engelman. 1994. Effects of cannabinoids (marijuana) on taste intensity and hedonic ratings and salivary flow of adults. *Chem Senses* 19(2):125-140.

Maurer, M., V. Henn, A. Dittrich, and A. Hofmann. 1990. Delta-9-tetrahydrocannabinol shows antispastic and analgesic effects in a single case double-blind trial. *Eur Arch Psychiatry Neurol Sci* 240(1):1-4.

McCallum, R.W., I. Soykan, K.R. Sridhar, D.A. Ricci, R.C. Lange, and M.W. Plankey. 1999. Delta-9-tetrahydrocannabinol delays the gastric emptying of solid food in humans: A double-blind, randomized study. *Aliment Pharmacol Ther* 13(1):77-80.

McPartland, J.M., and E.B. Russo. 2001. Cannabis and cannabis extracts: Greater than the sum of their parts? *J Cannabis Ther* 1(3/4):103-132.

Mechoulam, R. 1986. *Cannabinoids as therapeutic agents.* Boca Raton: CRC Press.

Mechoulam, R. 2002. Discovery of endocannabinoids and some random thoughts on their possible roles in neuroprotection and aggression. *Prostaglandins Leukot Essent Fatty Acids* 66(2-3):93-99.

Mechoulam, R., S. Ben-Shabat, L. Hanus, M. Ligumsky, N.E. Kaminski, A.R. Schatz, A. Gopher, S. Almog, B.R. Martin, and D.R. Compton. 1995. Identification of an endogenous 2-monoglyceride, present in canine gut, that binds to cannabinoid receptors. *Biochem Pharmacol* 50(1):83-90.

Mechoulam, R., and L. Hanus. 2002. Cannabidiol: An overview of some chemical and pharmacological aspects. Part I: chemical aspects. *Chem Phys Lipids* 121(1-2):35-43.

Mechoulam, R., and E. Shohami. 2002. HU-211: Cannabinoid Neuroprotective Agent. In F. Grotenhermen and E. Russo (eds.), *Cannabis and cannabinoids. Pharmacology, toxicology, and therapeutic potential* (pp. 389-400). Binghamton, NY: The Haworth Press.

Mechoulam, R., E. Shohami, E. Fride, and I. Bab. 2003. The ubiquitous role of endocannabinoids in physiological processes: examples in neuroprotection, feeding and bone formation. *First European Workshop on Cannabinoid Research.* Madrid (Spain).

Meinck, H.M., P.W. Schonle, and B. Conrad. 1989. Effect of cannabinoids on spasticity and ataxia in multiple sclerosis. *J Neurol* 236(2):120-122.

Melamede, R. 2002. Possible mechanisms in autoimmune diseases. In F. Grotenhermen and E. Russo (eds.), *Cannabis and cannabinoids. Pharmacology, toxicology, and therapeutic potential* (pp. 111-122). Binghamton, NY: The Haworth Press.

Melck, D., L. De Petrocellis, P. Orlando, T. Bisogno, C. Laezza, M. Bifulco, and V. Di Marzo. 2000. Suppression of nerve growth factor Trk receptors and prolactin receptors by endocannabinoids leads to inhibition of human breast and prostate cancer cell proliferation. *Endocrinology* 141(1):118-126.

Melvin, L.S., G.M. Milne, M.R. Johnson, B. Subramaniam, G.H. Wilken, and A.C. Howlett. 1993. Structure-activity relationships for cannabinoid receptor-binding and analgesic activity: Studies of bicyclic cannabinoid analogs. *Mol Pharmacol* 44(5):1008-1015.

Merritt, J.C., W.J. Crawford, P.C. Alexander, A.L. Anduze, and S.S. Gelbart. 1980. Effect of marihuana on intraocular and blood pressure in glaucoma. *Ophthalmology* 87(3):222-228.

Merritt, J.C., J.L. Olsen, J.R. Armstrong, and S.M. McKinnon. 1981. Topical delta 9-tetrahydrocannabinol in hypertensive glaucomas. *J Pharm Pharmacol* 33(1): 40-41.

Miczek, K.A., and B.N. Dixit. 1980. Behavioral and biochemical effects of chronic delta 9-tetrahydrocannabinol in rats. *Psychopharmacology (Berl)* 67(2):195-202.

Mikuriya, T.H. 1970. Cannabis substitution. An adjunctive therapeutic tool in the treatment of alcoholism. *Med Times* 98(4):187-191.

Mittleman, M.A., R.A. Lewis, M. Maclure, J.B. Sherwood, and J.E. Muller. 2001. Triggering myocardial infarction by marijuana. *Circulation* 103(23):2805-2809.

Moss, D.E., P.Z. Manderscheid, S.P. Montgomery, A.B. Norman, and P.R. Sanberg. 1989. Nicotine and cannabinoids as adjuncts to neuroleptics in the treatment of Tourette syndrome and other motor disorders. *Life Sci* 44(21):1521-1525.

Müller-Vahl, K.R., H. Kolbe, and R. Dengler. 1997. Gilles de la Tourette-Syndrom. Einfluß von Nikotin, Alkohol und Marihuana auf die klinische Symptomatik [Gilles de la Tourette-Syndrom. Influence of nicotine, alcohol and marijuana on clinical symptoms] [published in German]. *Nervenarzt* 68:985-989.

Müller-Vahl, K.R., H. Prevedel, K. Theloe, H. Kolbe, H.M. Emrich, and U. Schneider. 2003. Treatment of Tourette syndrome with delta-9-tetrahydrocannabinol (delta 9-THC): no influence on neuropsychological performance. *Neuropsychopharmacology* 28(2):384-388.

Müller-Vahl, K.R., U. Schneider, A. Koblenz, M. Jobges, H. Kolbe, T. Daldrup, and H.M. Emrich. 2002. Treatment of Tourette's syndrome with Δ⁹-tetrahydrocannabinol (THC): a randomized crossover trial. *Pharmacopsychiatry* 35(2):57-61.

Müller-Vahl, K.R., U. Schneider, H. Kolbe, and H.M. Emrich. 1999. Treatment of Tourette's syndrome with delta-9-tetrahydrocannabinol. *Am J Psychiatry* 156(3): 495.

Müller-Vahl, K.R., U. Schneider, H. Prevedel, K. Theloe, H. Kolbe, T. Daldrup, and H.M. Emrich. 2003. Δ9-tetrahydrocannabinol (THC) is effective in the treatment of tics in Tourette syndrome: a 6-week randomized trial. *J Clin Psychiatry* 64(4): 459-465.

Murphy, L. 2002. Hormonal system and reproduction. In F. Grotenhermen and E. Russo (eds.), *Cannabis and cannabinoids. Pharmacology, toxicology, and therapeutic potential* (pp. 289-298). Binghamton, NY: The Haworth Press.

Musty, R.E., P. Consroe. 2002. Spastic disorders. In F. Grotenhermen and E. Russo (eds.), *Cannabis and cannabinoids. Pharmacology, toxicology, and therapeutic potential* (pp. 195-204). Binghamton, NY: The Haworth Press.

Notcutt, W., M. Price, R. Miller, S. Newport, C. Sansom, and S. Simmonds. 2001a. Medicinal cannabis extracts in chronic pain: (2) comparison of two patients with back pain and sciatica. *2001 Congress on Cannabis and the Cannabinoids*, Cologne, Germany: International Association for Cannabis as Medicine, p. 25.

Notcutt, W., M. Price, R. Miller, S. Newport, C. Sansom, and S. Simmonds. 2001b. Medicinal cannabis extracts in chronic pain: (3) comparison of two patients with multiple sclerosis. *2001 Congress on Cannabis and the Cannabinoids*, Cologne, Germany: International Association for Cannabis as Medicine, p. 26.

Noyes, R., D.A. Baram. 1974. Cannabis analgesia. *Compreh Psychiatr* 15:531-535.

Noyes, R. Jr, S.F. Brunk, D.A.H. Avery, and A.C. Canter. 1975. The analgesic properties of delta-9-tetrahydrocannabinol and codeine. *Clin Pharmacol Ther* 18(1): 84-89.

Noyes, R. Jr, S.F. Brunk, D.A. Baram, and A. Canter. 1975. Analgesic effect of delta-9-tetrahydrocannabinol. *J Clin Pharmacol* 15(2-3):139-143.

Nunez, L.A., and M. Gurpegui M. 2002. Cannabis-induced psychosis: a cross-sectional comparison with acute schizophrenia. *Acta Psychiatr Scand* 105(3):173-178.

O'Leary, D.S., R.I. Block, J.A. Koeppel, M. Flaum, S.K. Schultz, N.C. Andreasen, L.B. Ponto, G.L. Watkins, R.R. Hurtig, and R.D. Hichwa. 2002. Effects of smoking marijuana on brain perfusion and cognition. *Neuropsychopharmacology* 26(6):802-816.

Ottani, A., and D. Giuliani. 2001. Hu 210: a potent tool for investigations of the cannabinoid system. *CNS Drug Rev* 7(2):131-145.

Parker, L.A., R. Mechoulam, and C. Schlievert. 2002. Cannabidiol, a non-psychoactive component of cannabis and its synthetic dimethylheptyl homolog suppress nausea in an experimental model with rats. *Neuroreport* 13(5):567-570.

Parker, L.A., R. Mechoulam, C. Schlievert, L. Abbott, M.L. Fudge, and P. Burton. 2003. Effects of cannabinoids on lithium-induced conditioned rejection reactions in a rat model of nausea. *Psychopharmacology (Berl)* 166(2):156-162.

Pate, D. 2002. Glaucoma and cannabinoids. In F. Grotenhermen and E. Russo (eds.), *Cannabis and cannabinoids. Pharmacology, toxicology, and therapeutic potential* (pp. 215-224). Binghamton, NY: The Haworth Press.

Perez-Reyes, M. 1999. The psychologic and physiologic effects of active cannabinoids. In G. Nahas, K.M. Sutin, D.J. Harvey, and S. Agurell (eds.), *Marihuana and medicine* (pp. 245-252). Totowa, NJ: Humana Press.

Perez-Reyes, M., S.H. Burstein, W.R. White, S.A. McDonald, and R.E. Hicks. 1991. Antagonism of marihuana effects by indomethacin in humans. *Life Sci* 48(6):507-515.

Perez-Reyes, M., J. Simmons, D. Brine, G.L. Kimmel, K.H. Davis, and M.E. Wall. 1976. Rate of penetration of Δ^9-tetrahydrocannabinol and 11-hydroxy-Δ^9-tetrahydrocannabinol to the brain of mice. In G.G. Nahas (eds.), *Marihuana: Chemistry, biochemistry, and cellular effects* (pp. 179-185). New York: Springer.

Perez-Reyes, M., M. Timmons, M. Lipton, K. Davis, and M. Wall. 1972. Intravenous injection in man of delta-9-tetrahydrocannabinol and 11-OH-delta-9-tetrahydrocannabinol. *Science* 177(49):633-635.

Pertwee, R. 1992. In vivo interactions between pschotropic cannabinoids and other drugs involving central and peripheral neurochemical mediators. In L. Myrphy and A. Bartke (eds.), *Marijuana/cannabinoids: Neurobiology and neurophysiology* (pp. 165-218). Boca Raton, FL: CRC Press.

Pertwee, R.G. 1997. Pharmacology of cannabinoid CB1 and CB2 receptors. *Pharmacol Ther* 74(2):129-180.

Pertwee, R.G. 1999a. Evidence for the presence of CB1 cannabinoid receptors on peripheral neurones and for the existence of neuronal non-CB1 cannabinoid receptors. *Life Sci* 65:597-605.

Pertwee, R.G. 1999b. Pharmacology of cannabinoid receptor ligands. *Curr Med Chem* 6:635-664.

Pertwee, R.G. 2002. Sites and Mechanisms of Action. In F. Grotenhermen and E. Russo (eds.), *Cannabis and cannabinoids. Pharmacology, toxicology, and therapeutic potential* (pp. 73-88). Binghamton, NY: The Haworth Press.

Petitet, F., B. Jeantaud, M. Reibaud, A. Imperato, and M.C. Dubroeucq. 1998. Complex pharmacology of natural cannabinoids: Evidence for partial agonist activity of Δ^9-tetrahydrocannabinol and antagonist activity of cannabidiol on rat brain cannabinoid receptors. *Life Sci* 63(1):PL1-PL6.

Petro, D.J. 1980. Marihuana as a therapeutic agent for muscle spasm or spasticity. *Psychosomatics* 21(1):81, 85.

Petro, D.J., and C. Ellenberger Jr. 1981. Treatment of human spasticity with delta 9-tetrahydrocannabinol. *J Clin Pharmacol* 21(8-9 Suppl):413S-416S.

Plasse, T.F., R.W. Gorter, S.H. Krasnow, M. Lane, K.V. Shepard, and R.G. Wadleigh. 1991. Recent clinical experience with dronabinol. *Pharmacol Biochem Behav* 40(3):695-700.

Pope, H.J. 2002. Cannabis, cognition, and residual confounding. *JAMA* 287(9): 1172-1174.

Pope, H.G., A.J. Gruber, J.I. Hudson, G. Cohane, M.A. Huestis, and D. Yurgelun-Todd. 2003. Early-onset cannabis use and cognitive deficits: What is the nature of the association? *Drug Alcohol Depend* 69(3):303-310.

Pope, H.G. Jr., A.J. Gruber, J.I. Hudson, M.A. Huestis, and D. Yurgelun-Todd. 2001. Neuropsychological performance in long-term cannabis users. *Arch Gen Psychiatry* 58(10):909-915.

Porter, A.C., J.M. Sauer, M.D. Knierman, G.W. Becker, M:J. Berna, J. Bao, G.G. Nomikos, P. Carter, F.P. Bymaster, A.B. Leese, and C.C. Felder. 2002. Characterization of a novel endocannabinoid, virodhamine, with antagonist activity at the CB1 receptor. *J Pharmacol Exp Ther* 301(3):1020-1024.

Pryce, G., G. Giovannoni, and D. Baker. 2003. Mifepristone or inhibition of 11 beta-hydroxylase activity potentiates the sedating effects of the cannabinoid receptor-1 agonist Delta(9)-tetrahydrocannabionol in mice. *Neurosci Lett* 341(2):164-166.

Pryor, G.T., S. Husain, and C. Mitoma. 1976. Acute and subacute interactions between delta-9-tetrahydrocannabinol and other drugs in the rat. *Ann N Y Acad Sci* 281:171-189.

Racz, I., A. Bilkei-Gorzo, Z.E. Toth, K. Michel, M. Palkovits, and A. Zimmer. 2003. A critical role for the cannabinoid CB1 receptors in alcohol dependence and stress-stimulated ethanol drinking. *J Neurosci* 23(6):2453-2458.

Ralevic, V., and D.A. Kendall. 2001. Cannabinoid inhibition of capsaicin-sensitive sensory neurotransmission in the rat mesenteric arterial bed. *Eur J Pharmacol* 418(1-2):117-125.

Recht, L.D., R. Salmonsen, R. Rosetti, T. Jang, G. Pipia, T. Kubiatowski, P. Karim, A.H. Ross, R. Zurier, N.S. Litofsky, and S. Burstein. 2001. Antitumor effects of ajulemic acid (CT3), a synthetic non-psychoactive cannabinoid. *Biochem Pharmacol* 62(6):755-763.

Romero, J., E. Garcia-Palomero, J.G. Castro, L. Garcia-Gil, J.A. Ramos, and J.J. Fernandez-Ruiz. 1997. Effects of chronic exposure to Δ^9-tetrahydrocannabinol on cannabinoid receptor binding and mRNA levels in several rat brain regions. *Brain Res Mol Brain Res* 46(1-2):100-108.

Roques, B. 1998. *Problemes posées par la dangerosité des drogues.* Rapport du professeur Bernhard Roques au Secrétaire d'Etat à la Santé. Paris.

Rubino, T., D. Vigano, B. Costa, M. Colleoni, and D. Parolaro. 2000. Loss of cannabinoid-stimulated guanosine 5'-O-(3-[(35)S]Thiotriphosphate) binding without receptor down-regulation in brain regions of anandamide-tolerant rats. *J Neurochem* 75(6):2478-2484.

Rubino, T., D. Vigano, P. Massi, and D. Parolaro. 2000. Changes in the cannabinoid receptor binding, G protein coupling, and cyclic AMP cascade in the CNS of rats tolerant to and dependent on the synthetic cannabinoid compound CP55,940. *J Neurochem* 75(5):2080-2086.

Russo, E., M.L. Mathre, A. Byrne, R. Velin, P.J. Bach, J. Sanchez-Ramos, and K.A. Kirlin. 2002. Chronic cannabis use in the compassionate investigational new drug program: An examination of benefits and adverse effects of legal medical cannabis. *J Cannabis Ther* 2(1):3-57.

Sallan, S.E., C. Cronin, M. Zelen, and N.E. Zinberg. 1980. Antiemetics in patients receiving chemotherapy for cancer: A randomized comparison of delta-9-tetra-hydrocannabinol and prochlorperazine. *N Engl J Med* 302(3):135-138.

Sanchez, C., M.L. de Ceballos, T.G. del Pulgar, D. Rueda, C. Corbacho, G. Velasco, I. Galve-Roperh, J.W. Huffman, S. Ramon y Cajal, and M. Guzman. 2001. Inhibition of glioma growth in vivo by selective activation of the CB(2) cannabinoid receptor. *Cancer Res* 2001; 61(15):5784-5789.

Sandyk, R., and G. Awerbuch. 1998. Marijuana and Tourette's syndrome. *J Clin Psychopharmacol* 8:844.

Sañudo-Peña, M.C., K. Tsou, and J.M. Walker. 1999. Motor actions of cannabinoids in the basal ganglia output nuclei. *Life Sci* 65:703-713.

Schnelle, M., F. Grotenhermen, M. Reif, and R.W. Gorter. 1999. Ergebnisse einer standardisierten Umfrage zur medizinischen Verwendung von Canna-bisprodukten im deutschen Sprachraum, [Results of a standardized survey on the medical use of cannabis products in the German-speaking area]. (Suppl 3) 28-36. *Forsch Komplementarmed* [Res Complementary Med] (Suppl 3) 28-36.

Shook, J.E., and T.F. Burks. 1989. Psychoactive cannabinoids reduce gastrointestinal propulsion and motility in rodents. *J Pharmacol Exp Ther* 249(2):444-449.

Showalter, V.M., D.R. Compton, B.R. Martin, and M.E. Abood. 1996. Evaluation of binding in a transfected cell line expressing a peripheral cannabinoid receptor (CB2): Identification of cannabinoid receptor subtype selective ligands. *J Pharmacol Exp Ther* 278(3):989-999.

Siegling, A., H.A. Hofmann, D. Denzer, F. Mauler, and J. De Vry. 2001. Cannabinoid CB(1) receptor upregulation in a rat model of chronic neuropathic pain. *Eur J Pharmacol* 415(1):R5-R7.

Sieradzan, K.A., S.H. Fox, M. Hill, J.P. Dick, A.R. Crossman, and J.M. Brotchie. 2001. Cannabinoids reduce levodopa-induced dyskinesia in Parkinson's disease: A pilot study. *Neurology* 57(11):2108-2111.

Slikker, W. Jr., M.G. Paule, S.F. Ali, A.C. Scallet, and J.R. Bailey. 1992. Behavioral, neurochemical and neurhistochemical effects of chronic marijuana smoke exposure in the nonhuman primate. In L. Myrphy and A. Bartke (eds.), *Marijuana/ Cannabinoids: Neurobiology and neurophysiology* (pp. 219-73). Boca Raton, FL: CRC Press.

Smith, C.G., R.G. Almirez, J. Berenberg, and R. H. Asch. 1983. Tolerance develops to the disruptive effects of delta 9-tetrahydrocannabinol on primate menstrual cycle. *Science* 219(4591):1453-1455.

Soderpalm, A.H., A. Schuster, and H. de Wit. 2001. Antiemetic efficacy of smoked marijuana: Subjective and behavioral effects on nausea induced by syrup of ipecac. *Pharmacol Biochem Behav* 69(3-4):343-350.

Sofia, R.D., S.D. Nalepa, J.J. Harakal, and V.B. Vassar. 1973. Anti-edema and analgesic properties of Δ^9-tetrahydrocannabinol (THC). *J Pharmacol Exp Ther* 186(3):646-655.

Solowij, N., and B.F.S. Grenyer. 2002b. Long term effects of cannabis on psyche and cognition. In F. Grotenhermen and E. Russo (eds.), *Cannabis and cannabinoids. Pharmacology, toxicology, and therapeutic potential* (pp. 299-312). Binghamton, NY: The Haworth Press.

Solowij, N., R.S. Stephens, R.A. Roffman, T. Babor, R. Kadden, M. Miller, K. Christiansen, B. McRee, and J. Vendetti. 2002. Cognitive Functioning of Long-term Heavy Cannabis Users Seeking Treatment. *JAMA* 287(9):1123-1131.

Stefanis, C. 1978. Biological aspects of cannabis use. *NIDA Res Monogr* 19:149-178.

Stockings, G.T. 1947. A new euphoriant for depressive mental states. *BMJ* 1:918-922.

Sugiura, T., S. Kondo, A. Sukagawa, S. Nakane, A. Shinoda, K. Itoh, A. Yamashita, and K. Waku. 1995. 2-Arachidonoylglycerol: A possible endogenous cannabinoid receptor ligand in brain. *Biochem Biophys Res Commun* 215(1):89-97.

Sulcova, E., R. Mechoulam, and E. Fride. 1998. Biphasic effects of anandamide. *Pharmacol Biochem Behav* 59(2):347-352.

Sutin, K.M., and G.G. Nahas. 1999. Physiological and pharmacological interations of marihuana (Δ^9-THC) with drugs and anesthetics. In G. Nahas, K.M. Sutin, D.J. Harvey, and S. Agurell (eds.), *Marihuana and medicine* (pp. 253-271). Totowa, NJ: Humana Press.

Szabo, B., U. Nordheim, and N. Niederhoffer. 2001. Effects of cannabinoids on sympathetic and parasympathetic neuroeffector transmission in the rabbit heart. *J Pharmacol Exp Ther* 297:819-826.

Tahir, S.K., J.E. Trogadis, J.K. Stevens, and A.M. Zimmerman. 1992. Cytoskeletal organization following cannabinoid treatment in undifferentiated and differentiated PC12 cells. *Biochem Cell Biol* 70(10-11):1159-1173.

Tanda, G., F.E. Pontieri, and G. Di Chiara. 1997. Cannabinoid and heroin activation of mesolimbic dopamine transmission by a common mu1 opioid receptor mechanism. *Science* 276(5321):2048-2050.

Tashkin, D.P., J.A. Levisman, A.S. Abbasi, B.J. Shapiro, and N.M. Ellis. 1977. Short-term effects of smoked marihuana on left ventricular function in man. *Chest* 72(1):20-26.

Tashkin, D.P., B.J. Shapiro, and I.M. Frank. 1974. Acute effects of smoked marijuana and oral Δ^9-tetrahydrocannabinol on specific airway conductance in asthmatic subjects. *Am Rev Respir Dis* 109(4):420-428.

Terranova, J.-P., J.-J. Storme, N. Lafon, A. Perio, Rinaldi-Carmona, G. Le Fur, and P. Soubrie. 1996. Improvement of memory in rodents by the selective CB1 cannabinoid receptor antagonist, SR 141716. *Psychopharmacology* 126:165-172.

Thompson, G.R., H. Rosenkrantz, U.H. Schaeppi, and M.C. Braude. 1973. Comparison of acute oral toxicity of cannabinoids in rats, dogs and monkeys. *Toxicol Appl Pharmacol* 25(3):363-372.

Thompson, L.J., and R.C. Proctor. 1953. The use of pyrahexyl in the treatment of alcoholic and drug withdrawal conditions. *N Carolina Med J* 14:520-523.

Titishov, N., R. Mechoulam, and A.M. Zimmerman. 1989. Stereospecific effects of (–)- and (+)-7-hydroxy-delta-6-tetrahydrocannabinol-dimethylheptyl on the immune system of mice. *Pharmacology* 39(6):337-349.

Toyota, M., T. Shimamura, H. Ishii, M. Renner, J. Braggins, and Y. Asakawa. 2002. New bibenzyl cannabinoid from the New Zealand liverwort Radula marginata. *Chem Pharm Bull (Tokyo)* 50(10):1390-1392.

Ungerleider, J.T., T. Andyrsiak, L. Fairbanks, G.W. Ellison, and L.W. Myers. 1987. Delta-9-THC in the treatment of spasticity associated with multiple sclerosis. *Adv Alcohol Subst Abuse* 7(1):39-50.

Vacca, G., S. Serra, G. Brunetti, M.A. Carai, G.L. Gessa, and G. Colombo. 2002. Boosting effect of morphine on alcohol drinking is suppressed not only by naloxone but also by the cannabinoid CB1 receptor antagonist, SR 141716. *Eur J Pharmacol* 445(1-2):55-59.

Van der Stelt, M., W.B. Veldhuis, P.R. Bar, G.A. Veldink, J.F. Vliegenthart, and K. Nicolay. 2001. Neuroprotection by delta-9-tetrahydrocannabinol, the main active compound in marijuana, against ouabain-induced in vivo excitotoxicity. *J Neurosci* 21(17):6475-6479.

Van Klingeren, B., and M. Ten Ham. 1976. Antibacterial activity of delta-9-tetrahydrocannabinol and cannabidiol. *Antonie Van Leeuwenhoek* 42(1-2):9-12.

Volicer, L., M. Stelly, J. Morris, J. McLaughlin, and B.J. Volicer. 1997. Effects of dronabinol on anorexia and disturbed behavior in patients with Alzheimer's disease. *Int J Geriatr Psychiatry* 12(9):913-919.

Wachtel, S.R., and H. de Wit. 2000. Naltrexone does not block the subjective effects of oral Δ9-tetrahydrocannabinol in humans. *Drug Alcohol Depend* 59(3):251-260.

Wachtel, S.R., M.A. ElSohly, S.A. Ross, J. Ambre, and H. De Wit. 2002. Comparison of the subjective effects of Delta(9)-tetrahydrocannabinol and marijuana in humans. *Psychopharmacology* 161(4):331-339.

Wade, D.T., P. Robson, H. House, P. Makela, and J. Aram. 2003. A preliminary controlled study to determine whether whole-plant cannabis extracts can improve intractable neurogenic symptoms. *Clin Rehabil* 17:18-26.

Wagner, J.A., K. Hu, J. Karcher, J. Bauersachs, A. Schafer, M. Laser, H. Han, and G. Ertl. 2003. CB(1) cannabinoid receptor antagonism promotes remodeling and cannabinoid treatment prevents endothelial dysfunction and hypotension in rats with myocardial infarction. *Br J Pharmacol* 138(7):1251-1258.

Wagner, J.A., Z. Jarai, S. Batkai, and G. Kunos. 2001. Hemodynamic effects of cannabinoids: coronary and cerebral vasodilation mediated by cannabinoid CB(1) receptors. *Eur J Pharmacol* 423(2-3):203-210.

Wagner, J.A., K. Varga, and G. Kunos. 1998. Cardiovascular actions of cannabinoids and their generation during shock. *J Mol Med* 76(12):824-836.

Walker, J.M., S.M. Huang, N.M. Strangman, K. Tsou, and M.C. Sanudo-Pena. 1999. Pain modulation by release of the endogenous cannabinoid anandamide. *Proc Natl Acad Sci U S A* 96(21):12198-12203.

Welch, S.P., and M. Eads. 1999. Synergistic interactions of endogenous opioids and cannabinoid systems. *Brain Res* 848(1-2):183-190.

Wiley, J.L., and B.R. Martin. 2002. Cannabinoid pharmacology: Implications for additional cannabinoid receptor subtypes. *Chem Phys Lipids* 121(1-2):57-63.

Williams, C.M., and T.C. Kirkham. 1999. Anandamide induces overeating: mediation by central cannabinoid (CB1) receptors. *Psychopharmacology* 143(3):315-317.

Williams, C.M., and T.C. Kirkham. 2002. Observational analysis of feeding induced by Delta(9)-THC and anandamide. *Physiol Behav* 76(2):241-250.

Williams, S.J., J.P. Hartley, and J.D. Graham. 1976. Bronchodilator effect of delta1-tetrahydrocannabinol administered by aerosol of asthmatic patients. *Thorax* 31(6):720-773.

Yuan, M., S.M. Kiertscher, Q. Cheng, R. Zoumalan, D.P. Tashkin, and M.D. Roth. 2002. Delta 9-Tetrahydrocannabinol regulates Th1/Th2 cytokine balance in activated human T cells. *J Neuroimmunol* 133(1-2):124-131.

Zuardi, A.W., F.S. Guimarães, V.M.C. Guimarães, and E.A. Del Bel. 2002. Cannabidiol: Possible therapeutic application. In F. Grotenhermen and E. Russo (eds.), *Cannabis and cannabinoids. Pharmacology, toxicology, and therapeutic potential* (pp. 359-370). Binghamton, NY: The Haworth Press.

Zuardi, A.W., I. Shirakawa, E. Finkelfarb, and I.G. Karniol. 1982. Action of cannabidiol on the anxiety and other effects produced by delta 9-THC in normal subjects. *Psychopharmacology* 76(3):245-250.

Zullino, D.F., D. Delessert, C.B. Eap, M. Preisig, and P. Baumann. 2002. Tobacco and cannabis smoking cessation can lead to intoxication with clozapine or olanzapine. *Int Clin Psychopharmacol* 17(3):141-143.

UPDATE

Franjo Grotenhermen

Research into the pharmacodynamics of cannabinoids is quickly advancing. Additionally, inhibitors of endocannabinoid degradation and cannabinoid receptor blockers are interesting targets of clinical investigation.

Besides Sanofi-Synthelabo, which is conducting Phase III trials with Rimonabant, several other pharmaceutical companies have patented CB receptor antagonists, among them Pfizer, Bayer, Merck, Solvay Pharmaceuticals, Hoffmann-La Roche and AstraZeneca (Lange and Kruse 2004).

Further therapeutic uses have been suggested for CB receptor antagonists, including problems in sexual behavior and sexual performance, and asthma (Lange and Kruse 2004). It was reported that the density of CB_1 receptors and the levels of anandamide and 2-AG in the dorsolateral prefrontal cortex of alcoholic suicide victims was higher than in a control group of chronic alcoholics, suggesting a hyperactivity of endocannabinoidergic signaling and a therapeutic potential for CB_1 antagonists (Vinod et al. 2005).

Recently it has been shown that two selective inhibitors of the putative endocannabinoid transporter, and hence of endocannabinoid inactivation, provide an effective therapy for Theiler murine encephalomyelitis, a virus-induced demyelinating disease and animal model of multiple sclerosis (Mestre et al. 2005). Treatment of infected mice with the transport inhibitors OMDM1 and OMDM2 enhanced anandamide levels in the spinal cord, ameliorated motor symptoms and decreased inflammatory responses. This effect resembles that of exogenous cannabinoid receptor agonists (Ni et al. 2004).

The endocannabinoid system may also serve as a novel approach to the treatment of anxiety-related disorders. Endocannabinoid signaling negatively modulates the function of the hypothalamic-pituitary-adrenal axis in a context-dependent manner (Patel et al. 2004). Upon exposure of mice to acute stress, hypothalamic 2-arachidonoyl glycerol content was reduced compared with the control value; however, after five days of stress that resulted in an attenuated corticosterone response, the hypothalamic 2-AG content was increased compared with the control value. The CB_1 receptor agonist CP55940 reduced blood corticosterone levels in stressed mice while a CB_1 receptor antagonist increased corticosterone concentrations (Patel et al. 2004). A similar effect was achieved by the administration of the putative endocannabinoid transport inhibitor AM404 or the FAAH inhibitor URB597. Another group observed reduced hippocampal 2-AG levels following chronic stress (Hill et al. 2005). Chronic stress impaired reversal learning and induced perseveratory behavior in the Morris water maze, an impairment that was reversed by exogenous cannabinoid administration, suggesting deficient endocannabinoid signaling.

Anandamide levels during pregnancy show a characteristic pattern (Habayeb et al. 2004). Mean plasma levels were 0.9 nanomole (nm) in the first trimester and 0.4 nm in the second and third trimester. During labor, anandamide plasma levels rose to 2.5 nm. Postmenopausal and luteal-phase levels were similar to those in the first trimester. It is currently unclear whether implantation of the embryo can be disrupted by THC or cannabis.

The consequences of the use of cannabis products by patients with liver cirrhosis is unclear. In experimental studies activation of the CB_2 receptor was shown to cause antifibrogenic effects (Julien et al. 2005). In liver biopsy specimens from patients with active cirrhosis of various etiologies, CB_2 receptors were expressed in non-parenchymal cells. In contrast, CB_2 receptors were not detected in normal human liver. In cultured hepatic myofibroblasts and in activated hepatic stellate cells activation of CB_2 receptors triggered potent antifibrogenic effects, namely, growth inhibition and apoptosis. On the other hand, an epidemiological study suggests that daily use of cannabis may promote the development of liver cirrhosis in persons with chronic hepatitis C, while moderate use did not increase the risk (Hezode et al. 2005).

Foci of continued interest are the neuroprotective effects of cannabinoids, among them possible therapeutic effects in Alzheimer's disease (AD). Enhanced amyloid-beta peptide deposition along with glial cell activation in senile plaques plays a major role in the pathology of AD. CB_1 positive neurons are greatly reduced in areas of microglial activation and CB_1 receptor protein expression is markedly decreased in AD brains (Ramirez et al. 2005). Amyloid-beta induced activation of microglial cells, cognitive impairment and loss of neuronal markers was prevented by cannabinoids in rats (Ramirez et al. 2005).

Case reports suggest that cannabis may have medicinal value in attention-deficit hyperactivity disorder (ADHD). Basic research with an animal model of ADHD, the spontaneously hypertensive rat (SHR), gives support to this observation (Adriani et al. 2003). A very impulsive subgroup of SHRs presented a reduced density of CB_1 cannabinoid receptors in the prefrontal cortex of the brain. The administration of WIN55,212-2 normalized the impulsive behavioral profile in this subgroup but had no effect on controls.

Experimental research also suggests that some cannabinoids may be protective in a quite different area, preventing cartilage resorption, in part, by inhibiting proteoglycan degradation and also by inhibiting cytokine production of chondrocytes induced by the free radical nitric oxide (NO) (Mbvundula et al. 2005).

Current clinical research with cannabis-based drugs has focused prominently on neuropathic pain and spasticity. Berman et al. (2004) observed a significant decrease in pain and improved sleep by two different cannabis extracts in 48 patients with neuropathic pain from brachial plexus avulsion (Berman et al. 2004). And there are several reports of pain reduction in multiple sclerosis by THC (Svendsen et al. 2004; Zajicek et al. 2003) and cannabis (Zajicek et al. 2003). One new publication described significant analgesic effects of THC and cannabis in chronic pain of different origins (multiple sclerosis, spinal cord injury, brachial plexus avulsion, stiff-man syndrome, etc.) (Notcutt et al. 2004). In contrast to these studies Attal et al. (2004) found a therapeutic effect of oral THC in only one of seven patients with chronic refractory neuropathic pain.

Large placebo-controlled trials for the investigation of the efficacy of cannabis and THC in spasticity were restricted to MS patients (Brady et al. 2004; Vaney et al. 2004; Wade et al. 2004; Zajicek 2004; Zajicek et al. 2003), and there is only one small study on cannabinoids in spasticity due to spinal cord injury conducted in the past few years (Hagenbach et al. 2005). Most studies usually found significant effects in only subjective parameters but not in objective spasticity scores (Vaney et al. 2004; Wade et al. 2004; Zajicek et al. 2003). Preliminary results of a first long-term study of THC and cannabis in MS suggest that THC may have long-term beneficial effects on the course of the disease (Zajicek 2004). Results of the short-term trial (15 weeks) with 630 eligible patients had been conflicting (Zajicek et al. 2003). Eighty percent of the original study population participated in a 12-month follow-up study. In the 15-week study, 657 patients with stable MS and muscle spasticity received a maximum daily dose of 10 to 25 mg THC as single agent or in a cannabis extract. There was no significant effect of cannabinoids on objective spasticity scores according to the Ashworth scale, but patients reported subjective improvements in pain and spasticity. In the long-term study there was a significant improvement of spasticity scores in the THC group.

REFERENCES

Adriani, W., A. Caprioli, O. Granstrem, M. Carli, and G. Laviola. 2003. The spontaneously hypertensive-rat as an animal model of ADHD: Evidence for impulsive and non-impulsive subpopulations. *Neurosci Biobehav Rev* 27 (7):639-651.

Attal, N., L. Brasseur, D. Guirimand, S. Clermond-Gnamien, S. Atlami, and D. Bouhassira. 2004. Are oral cannabinoids safe and effective in refractory neuropathic pain? *Eur J Pain* 8 (2):173-177.

Berman, J. S., C. Symonds, and R. Birch. 2004. Efficacy of two cannabis based medicinal extracts for relief of central neuropathic pain from brachial plexus avulsion: results of a randomised controlled trial. *Pain* 112 (3):299-306.

Brady, C. M., R. DasGupta, C. Dalton, O. J. Wiseman, K. J. Berkley, and C. J. Fowler. 2004. An open-label pilot study of cannabis-based extracts for bladder dysfunction in advanced multiple sclerosis. *Mult Scler* 10 (4):425-433.

Habayeb, O.M., A. H. Taylor, M. D. Evans, M. S. Cooke, D. J. Taylor, S. C. Bell, and J. C. Konje. 2004. Plasma levels of the endocannabinoid anandamide in women—A potential role in pregnancy maintenance and labor? *J Clin Endocrinol Metab* 89 (11):5482-5487.

Hezode, C., F. Roudot-Thoraval, S. Nguyen, P. Grenard, B. Julien, E. S. Zafrani, J. M. Pawlostky, D. Dhumeaux, S. Lotersztajn, and A. Mallat. 2005. Daily cannabis smoking as a risk factor for progression of fibrosis in chronic hepatitis C. *Hepatology* 42(1):63-71.

Hill, M. N., S. Patel, E. J. Carrier, D. J. Rademacher, B. K. Ormerod, C. J. Hillard, and B. B. Gorzalka. 2005. Downregulation of endocannabinoid signaling in the hippocampus following chronic unpredictable stress. *Neuropsychopharmacology* 30 (3):508-15.

Julien, B., P. Grenard, F. Teixeira-Clerc, J. T. Van Nhieu, L. Li, M. Karsak, A. Zimmer, A. Mallat, and S. Lotersztajn. 2005. Antifibrogenic role of the cannabinoid receptor CB2 in the liver. *Gastroenterology* 128 (3):742-755.

Lange, J. H., and C. G. Kruse. 2004. Recent advances in CB1 cannabinoid receptor antagonists. *Curr Opin Drug Discov Devel* 7 (4):498-506.

Mbvundula, E. C., R. A. Bunning, and K. D. Rainsford. 2005. Effects of cannabinoids on nitric oxide production by chondrocytes and proteoglycan degradation in cartilage. *Biochem Pharmacol* 69 (4):635-640.

Mestre, L., F. Correa, A. Arevalo-Martin, E. Molina-Holgado, M. Valenti, G. Ortar, V. Di Marzo, and C. J. Guaza. 2005. Pharmacological modulation of the endocannabinoid system in a viral model of multiple sclerosis. *J Neurochem* 92 (6):1327-1339.

Ni, X., E. B. Geller, M. J. Eppihimer, T. K. Eisenstein, M. W. Adler, and R. F. Tuma. 2004. Win 55212-2, a cannabinoid receptor agonist, attenuates leukocyte/endothelial interactions in an experimental autoimmune encephalomyelitis model. *Mult Scler* 10 (2):158-164.

Notcutt, W., M. Price, R. Miller, S. Newport, C. Phillips, S. Simmons, and C. Sansom. 2004. Initial experiences with medicinal extracts of cannabis for chronic pain: results from 34 'N of 1' studies. *Anaesthesia* 59 (5):440-452.

Patel, S., C. T. Roelke, D. J. Rademacher, W. E. Cullinan, and C. J. Hillard. 2004. Endocannabinoid signaling negatively modulates stress-induced activation of the hypothalamic-pituitary-adrenal axis. *Endocrinology* 145 (12):5429-5430.

Ramirez, B. G., C. Blazquez, T. Gomez del Pulgar, M. Guzman, and M. L. de Ceballos. 2005. Prevention of Alzheimer's disease pathology by cannabinoids: neuroprotection mediated by blockade of microglial activation. *J Neurosci* 25 (8):1904-1913.

Svendsen, K. B., T. S. Jensen, and F. W. Bach. 2004. Does the cannabinoid dronabinol reduce central pain in multiple sclerosis? Randomised double blind placebo controlled crossover trial. *BMJ* 329 (7460):253.

Vaney, C., M. Heinzel-Gutenbrunner, P. Jobin, F. Tschopp, B. Gattlen, U. Hagen, M. Schnelle, and M. Reif. 2004. Efficacy, safety and tolerability of an orally administered cannabis extract in the treatment of spasticity in patients with multiple sclerosis: a randomized, double-blind, placebo-controlled, crossover study. *Mult Scler* 10 (4):417-424.

Vinod, K.Y., V. Arango, S. Xie, S. A. Kassir, J. J. Mann, T. B. Cooper, and B. L. Hungund. 2005. Elevated levels of endocannabinoids and CB1 receptor-mediated G-protein signaling in the prefrontal cortex of alcoholic suicide victims. *Biol Psychiatry* 57 (5):480-486.

Wade, D.T., P. Makela, P. Robson, H. House, and C. Bateman. 2004. Do cannabis-based medicinal extracts have general or specific effects on symptoms in multiple sclerosis? A double-blind, randomized, placebo-controlled study on 160 patients. *Mult Scler* 10 (4):434-441.

Zajicek, J. 2004. The cannabinoids in MS study—Final results from 12 months follow-up. *Mult Scler* 10 (suppl 2):115.

Zajicek, J., P. Fox, H. Sanders, D. Wright, J. Vickery, A. Nunn, and A. Thompson. 2003. Cannabinoids for treatment of spasticity and other symptoms related to multiple sclerosis (CAMS study): Multicentre randomised placebo-controlled trial. *Lancet* 362 (9395):1517-1526.

Chapter 9

Cannabis and Cannabis Extracts: Greater Than the Sum of Their Parts?

John M. McPartland
Ethan B. Russo

INTRODUCTION

Cannabis is an herb; it contains hundreds of pharmaceutical compounds (Turner et al. 1980). Herbalists contend that polypharmaceutical herbs provide two advantages over single-ingredient synthetic drugs: (1) *therapeutic effects* of the primary active ingredients in herbs may be synergized by other compounds, and (2) *side effects* of the primary active ingredients may be mitigated by other compounds. Thus, cannabis has been characterized as a "synergistic shotgun," in contrast to Marinol (Δ^9-tetrahydrocannabinol, THC), a synthetic, single-ingredient "silver bullet" (McPartland and Pruitt 1999).

Mechoulam et al. (1972) suggested that other compounds present in herbal cannabis might influence THC activity. Carlini et al. (1974) determined that cannabis extracts produced effects "two or four times greater than that expected from their THC content." Similarly, Fairbairn and Pickens (1981) detected the presence of unidentified "powerful synergists" in cannabis extracts causing 330 percent greater activity in mice than THC alone.

Other compounds in herbal cannabis may ameliorate the side effects of THC. Whole cannabis causes fewer psychological side effects than synthetic THC, seen as symptoms of dysphoria, depersonalization, anxiety, panic reactions, and paranoia (Grinspoon and Bakalar 1997). This difference in side effect profiles may also be due, in part, to differences in administration: THC taken by mouth undergoes "first-pass metabolism" in the small intestine and liver, to 11-hydroxy-THC; the metabolite is more psy-

The authors thank David Pate and Vincenzo Di Marzo for presubmission reviews.

choactive than THC itself (Browne and Weissman 1981). Inhaled THC undergoes little first-pass metabolism, so less 11-hydroxy-THC is formed. Thus, "smoking cannabis is a satisfactory expedient in combating fatigue, headache and exhaustion, whereas the oral ingestion of cannabis results chiefly in a narcotic effect which may cause serious alarm" (Walton 1938, p. 49).

Respiratory side effects from inhaling cannabis smoke may be ameliorated by both cannabinoid and noncannabinoid components in cannabis. For instance, throat irritation may be diminished by anti-inflammatory agents, mutagens in the smoke may be mitigated by antimutagens, and bacterial contaminants in cannabis may be annulled by antibiotic compounds (McPartland and Pruitt 1997). The pharmaceutically active compounds in cannabis that enhance beneficial THC activity and reduce side effects are relatively unknown. The purpose of this chapter is to review the biochemistry and physiological effects of those other compounds.

MATERIALS AND METHODS

MEDLINE (1966-2000) was searched using MeSH keywords: *cannabinoids, marijuana, tetrahydrocannabinol.* AGRICOLA (1990-1999) was searched using the keywords *cannabis, hemp,* and *marijuana.* Phytochemical and ethnobotanical databases were searched via the Agricultural Research Service Web page (http://www.ars-grin.gov/~ngrlsb/). All reports were scanned for supporting bibliographic citations; antecedent sources were retrieved to the fullest possible extent. Data validity was assessed by source (peer-reviewed article versus popular press), identification methodology (analytical chemistry versus clinical history), and the frequency of independent observations.

RESULTS AND DISCUSSION

Turner et al. (1980) listed more than 420 compounds in cannabis. Sparacino et al. (1990) listed 200 additional compounds in cannabis smoke. We will highlight six cannabinoids beyond THC, a dozen-odd terpenoids, three flavonoids, and one phytosterol. Other noncannabinoids with proven pharmacological activity include poorly characterized glycoproteins, alkaloids, and compounds that remain completely unidentified (Gill et al. 1970).

CANNABINOIDS

Mechoulam and Gaoni (1967) defined cannabinoids as a group of C_{21} terpenophenolic compounds uniquely produced by cannabis. The subsequent development of synthetic cannabinoids (e.g., HU-210) has blurred this definition, as has the discovery of endogenous cannabinoids (e.g., anandamide), defined as "endocannabinoids" by Di Marzo and Fontana (1995). Thus, Pate (1999) proposed the term *phytocannabinoids* to designate the C_{21} compounds produced by cannabis. Phytocannabinoids exhibit very low mammalian toxicity, and mixtures of cannabinoids are less toxic than pure THC (Thompson et al. 1973).

Cannabidiol (CBD) is the next-best studied phytocannabinoid after THC (Table 9.1). The investigation of CBD by marijuana researchers is rather paradoxical, considering its concentrations are notably lower in drug varieties of cannabis than in fiber cultivars (Turner et al. 1980).

CBD possesses sedative properties (Carlini and Cunha, 1981), and a clinical trial showed that it reduces the anxiety and other unpleasant psychological side effects provoked by pure THC (Zuardi et al. 1982). CBD modulates the pharmacokinetics of THC by three mechanisms: (1) it has a slight affinity for cannabinoid receptors (Ki at CB1 = 4350 nM, compared to THC = 41 nM; Showalter et al. 1996), and it signals receptors as an antagonist or reverse agonist (Petitet et al. 1998); (2) CBD may modulate signal transduction by perturbing the fluidity of neuronal membranes, or by remodeling G proteins that carry intracellular signals downstream from cannabinoid receptors; and (3) CBD is a potent inhibitor of cytochrome P450-3A11 metabolism, thus it blocks the hydroxylation of THC to its 11-hydroxy metabolite (Bornheim et al. 1995). The 11-hydroxy metabolite is four times more psychoactive than unmetabolized THC (Browne and Weissman 1981) and four times more immunosuppressive (Klein et al. 1987).

CBD provides antipsychotic benefits (Zuardi et al. 1995). It increases dopamine activity, serves as a serotonin uptake inhibitor, and enhances norepinephrine activity (Banerjee et al. 1975; Poddar and Dewey 1980). CBD protects neurons from glutamate toxicity and serves as an antioxidant, more potently than ascorbate and α-tocopherol (Hampson et al. 1998). Auspiciously, CBD does *not* decrease acetylcholine (ACh) activity in the brain (Domino 1976; Cheney et al. 1981). THC, in contrast, reduces hippocampal ACh release in rats (Carta et al. 1998), and this correlates with loss of short-term memory consolidation. In the hippocampus THC also inhibits *N*-methyl-D-aspartate (NMDA) receptor activity (Misner and Sullivan 1999; Shen and Thayer 1999), and NMDA synaptic transmission is crucial for memory consolidation (Shimizu et al. 2000). CBD, unlike THC, does not dampen

TABLE 9.1. Phytocannabinoids.

Structure[a]	Concentration[b] (% dry weight)	Boiling point °C[c]	Properties
Δ-9-tetrahydrocannabinol (THC)	0.1-25	157	Euphoriant Analgesic Antiinflammatory Antioxidant Antiemetic
cannabidiol (CBD)	0.1-2.89	160-180	Anxiolytic Analgesic Antipsychotic Antiinflammatory Antioxidant Antispasmodic
cannabinol (CBN)	0.0-1.6	185	Oxidation breakdown product Sedative Antibiotic
cannabichromene (CBC)	0.0-0.65	220	Antiinflammatory Antibiotic Antifungal
cannabigerol (CBG)	0.03-1.15	MP 52	Antiinflammatory Antibiotic Antifungal

TABLE 9.1 *(continued)*

Structure[a]	Concentration[b] (% dry weight)	Boiling point °C[c]	Properties
Δ-8-tetrahydrocannabinol (Δ-8-THC)	0.0-0.1	175-178	Resembles Δ-9-THC Less psychoactive More stable Antiemetic
tetrahydrocannabivarin (THCV)	0.0-1.36	< 220	Analgesic Euphoriant

[a] Structures of constituents obtained from Bisset and Wichtl 1994; British Medical Association 1997; Buckingham 1992; Iversen 2000; Tisserand and Balacs 1995; Turner et al. 1980.

[b] Concentrations of constituents (v/w or w/w) were calculated from various sources. Cannabinoid concentrations (presented as a range, including cannabinoids and cannabinoidic acids) were primarily obtained from Small 1979; Veszki et al. 1980; Fournier et al. 1987; and Pitts et al. 1992. Terpenoid data (presented as maximum values) were calculated from Ross and ElSohly 1996; and Mediavilla and Steinemann 1997. Flavonoid data came from Paris et al. 1976; and Barrett et al. 1986.

[c] Boiling/melting points (MP) recorded at atmospheric pressure (760 mmHg) unless otherise noted; values obtained from various sources, primarily Buckingham 1992; Guenther 1948; Parry 1918; and Mechoulam (personal communication, April 2001).

the firing of hippocampal cells (Heyser et al. 1993) and does not disrupt learning (Brodkin and Moerschbaecher 1997).

Consroe (1998) presented an excellent review of CBD in neurological disorders. In some studies, it ameliorates symptoms of Huntington's disease, such as dystonia and dyskinesia. CBD mitigates other dystonic conditions, such as torticollis, in rat studies and uncontrolled human studies. CBD functions as an anticonvulsant in rats, on a par with phenytoin (Dilantin, a standard antiepileptic drug).

CBD demonstrated a synergistic benefit in the reduction of intestinal motility in mice produced by THC (Anderson et al. 1974). This may be an important component of observed benefits of cannabis in inflammatory bowel diseases.

The CBD in cannabis smoke may explain why inhaling it causes less airway irritation and inflammation than inhalation of pure THC (Tashkin et al. 1977). CBD imparts analgesia (more potently than THC), it inhibits erythema (much more than THC), it blocks cyclooxygenase (COX) activity with a greater maximum inhibition than THC, and it blocks lipoxygenase (the enzyme that produces asthma-provoking leukotrienes), again more effectively than THC (Evans 1991). Mice with inflammatory collagen- induced arthritis (a mouse model for rheumatoid arthritis) were given oral CBD (5 mg/kg per day) and showed clinical improvement, and the treatment effectively blocked progression of the arthritis (Malfait et al. 2000).

CBD reportedly has little or no effect on the immune system (reviewed by Klein et al. 1998), although the mouse arthritis study by Malfait et al. (2000) showed CBD decreases the production of tumor necrosis factor (TNF) and Interferon-gamma (IFN-γ), which are two immunomodulatory cytokines described later. CBD actually kills bacteria and fungi, with greater potency than THC (Klingeren and Ham 1976; ElSohly et al. 1982; McPartland 1984). Thus, cannabis may have less microbial contamination than other herbs, an important consideration for immunocompromised individuals (McPartland and Pruitt 1997).

Cannabinol (CBN) is the degradation product of THC (Turner et al. 1980), and is found most often in aged cannabis products (Table 9.1). CBN potentiates the effects of THC in man (Musty et al. 1976), yet it antagonizes the effects of THC in mice (Formukong et al. 1988). Studies reporting CBN's effects upon norepinephrine and dopamine also conflict—CBN may have negligible effects on these biogenic amines (Banerjee et al. 1975), enhance their release (Poddar and Dewey 1980), or decrease their release (Dalterio et al. 1985). CBN increases plasma concentrations of follicle-stimulating hormone, and enhances the production of testicular testosterone (Dalterio et al. 1985). CBN shares some characteristics with CBD; for example, it has anticonvulsant activity (Turner et al. 1980) and anti-inflammatory activity (Evans 1991).

CBN has affinity for CB_1 receptors (Ki at CB1 = 308 nM) and signals as an agonist (Showalter et al. 1996). Further down the signal transduction cascade, it stimulates the binding of GTP-γ-S (Petitet et al. 1998), but with half the efficacy of THC; when CBN is added to THC, the effects are not significantly additive. CBN has a threefold greater affinity for CB_2 receptors (Ki = 96 nM) (Showalter et al. 1996), thus it may affect cells of the immune system more than the central nervous system (Klein et al. 1998). CBN modulates thymocytes (Herring and Kaminski 1999) by attenuating the activity of the c-AMP response element-binding protein (CREB), nuclear factor κB (NF-κB), and interleukin-2 (IL-2). IL-2 is regulated by activator protein-1 (AP-1) transcription factor, a complex of c-Fos and c-Jun proteins (Foletta et al. 1998); CBN inhibits the expression of these proteins in splenocytes, via decreased activation of ERK MAP kinases (Faubert and Kaminski 2000).

Cannabichromene (CBC) is the fourth major cannabinoid, found predominantly in tropical *Cannabis* spp. strains (Table 9.1). Until the mid-1970s, CBC was frequently misidentified as CBD, because CBC and CBD have nearly the same retention times in gas chromatography. Like CBD, CBC decreases inflammation (Wirth et al. 1980) and provides analgesic effects (Davis and Hatoum 1983). CBC inhibits prostaglandin synthesis in vitro, but less potently than CBD or THC (Burstein et al. 1973). CBC exhibits strong antibacterial activity and mild antifungal activity, superior to THC and CBD in most instances (ElSohly et al. 1982). Unlike CBD, CBC has no effect on cytochrome P-450 enzymes (Kapeghian et al. 1983), nor does it function as an anticonvulsant in rats (Davis and Hatoum 1983).

The molecular affinity of CBC for cannabinoid receptors has not been measured. In mice, CBC causes hypothermia, sedation, and synergizes the depressant effects of hexobarbital (Hatoum et al. 1981). CBC also sedates dogs and decreases muscular coordination in rats, but causes no cannabimimetic activity in monkeys and people (Turner et al. 1980). In rats, the coadministration of CBC with THC potentiates THC changes in heart rate, but does not potentiate THC's hypotensive effects (O'Neil et al. 1979). Co-administration of CBC lowers the LD_{50} dose of THC in mice (Hatoum et al. 1981).

Cannabigerol (CBG) is the biosynthetic precursor of CBC, CBD, and THC, and is present only in minor amounts (Table 9.1). CBG has been called "inactive" when compared to THC, but CBG has slight affinity for CB_1 receptors, approximately the same as CBD (Devane et al. 1988). In rat brains, CBG inhibits the uptake of serotonin and norepinephrine, less effectively than CBD and THC, but CBG inhibits GABA uptake more effectively than CBD and THC (Banerjee et al. 1975). CBG acts as an analgesic (more potently than THC), it inhibits erythema (much more than THC), and it blocks lipoxygenase, again more effectively than THC (reviewed by Evans 1991).

CBG has antibacterial properties (Mechoulam and Gaoni 1965). Its activity against gram-positive bacteria, mycobacteria, and fungi is superior to that of THC, CBD, and CBC (ElSohly et al. 1982). CBG inhibits the growth of human oral epitheloid carcinoma cells (Baek et al. 1998).

Delta-8-THC (Δ^8-THC) is an isomer of delta-9-THC; it differs only by the location of the double bond in the cyclohexal C ring. The Ki of Δ^8-THC is 126 nM (Compton et al. 1993), and this loosely correlates with human studies, which show Δ^8-THC is less psychoactive than Δ^9-THC (Hollister 1974). The chemical stability of Δ^8-THC and its relative ease of synthesis compared to Δ^9-THC have made Δ^8-THC the template for the development of two important synthetic derivatives, the extremely potent psychoactive CB_1 agonist, HU-210 (Mechoulam and Ben-Shabat 1999), and the non-psychoactive antiemetic and neuroprotectant, HU-211 (dexanabinol) (Achiron et al. 2000; Biegon and Joseph 1995; Gallily et al. 1997). Δ^8-THC was employed clinically in an important study (Abrahamov and Mechoulam 1995) in which 8 children with hematological malignancies were treated with the drug over the course of 8 months at a dose of 18 mg/m^2 to treat chemo-therapy-associated nausea and vomiting. Interestingly, not only was this agent uniformly effective as an antiemetic, but it was also free of psychoactive effects in this age range (2 to 13 years).

Tetrahydrocannabivarin (THCV) is a propyl analogue of Δ^9-THC, primarily appearing in *indica* and *afghanica* varieties of cannabis, such as hashish from Nepal (Merkus 1971), dagga from South Africa (Boucher et al. 1977), and in plants cultivated from seeds from Zambia (Pitts et al. 1992) (Table 9.1). THCV is only 20 to 25 percent as psychoactive as Δ^9-THC (Hollister 1974). It has a quicker onset of action than Δ^9-THC (Gill et al. 1970) and is of briefer duration (Clarke 1998). THCV may be clinically effective in migraine treatment (Personal communication, HortaPharm, November 2000). Kubena and Barry (1972) suggested THCV synergizes the effects of THC, but did not hypothesize a mechanism. As a legal fine point, this analogue is not controlled in the Netherlands, and is not specified in the United States as a Schedule I drug, but would likely be considered illegal under the Controlled Substance Analogue Enforcement Act of 1986 (Public Law 99-570). THCV is of interest from a medical-legal standpoint in that is has been suggested as a biochemical marker of illicit cannabis use, since it is not a metabolite of Marinol (synthetic THC) (ElSohly et al. 1999).

TERPENOIDS

The unique smell of cannabis does not arise from cannabinoids, but from more than 100 terpenoid compounds (Turner et al. 1980). Terpenoids derive from repeating units of isoprene (C_5H_8), such as monoterpenoids (with C_{10} skeletons), sesquiterpenoids (C_{15}), diterpenoids (C_{20}), and triterpenoids (C_{30}). The final structure of terpenoids ranges from simple linear chains to complex polycyclic molecules, and they may include alcohol, ether, aldehyde, ketone, or ester functional groups. These compounds are easily extracted from plant material by steam distillation or vaporization. This distillate is called the *essential oil* or *volatile oil* of the plant. A range of researchers cite different yields of essential oil from different types of cannabis: Martin et al. (1961) cited yields of 0.05 to 0.11 percent essential oil from fresh green leaves and flowers of mixed male and female plants, from feral hemp growing in Canada. Nigam et al. (1965) yielded 0.1 percent essential oil from fresh whole male plants from Kashmir. Malingré et al. (1973) yielded 0.12 percent essential oil from fresh leaves of "strain X" obtained from birdseed in the Netherlands. Ross and ElSohly (1996) yielded 0.29 percent essential oil from fresh marijuana buds, reputed to be the Afghani variety "Skunk #1." Drying the plant material led to a loss of water content and net weight, concentrating the essential oil to 0.80 percent in buds that had been dried at room temperature for one week (Ross and ElSohly 1996).

Field-cultivated cannabis yields about 1.3 liter of essential oil per metric ton of freshly harvested plant material (Mediavilla and Steinemann 1997). Preventing pollination increases the yield of essential oil: 18 L/ha in sinsemilla crops versus 8 L/ha in pollinated crops (Meier and Mediavilla 1998). The composition of terpenoids varies between strains of cannabis (Mediavilla and Steinemann 1997) and varies between harvest dates (Meier and Mediavilla 1998).

Many terpenoids vaporize near the same temperature as THC, which boils at 157°C (see Tables 9.1 and 9.2). Terpenoids are lipophilic and permeate lipid membranes. Many cross the blood-brain barrier (BBB) after inhalation (Buchbauer et al. 1993; Nasel et al. 1994).

Meschler and Howlett (1999) discussed several mechanisms by which terpenoids modulate THC activity. For instance, terpenoids may bind to cannabinoid receptors. Thujone, from *Artemisia absinthium*, has a weak affinity for CB_1 receptors (Ki at CB_1 = 130,000 nM). Terpenoids might modulate the affinity of THC for its own receptor, by sequestering THC, by perturbing annular lipids surrounding the receptor, or by increasing the fluidity of neuronal membranes. Further downstream, terpenoids may alter the signal cascade by remodeling G proteins. Terpenoids may alter the pharmacokinetics of THC by changing the BBB; cannabis extracts are known to cause a significant increase in BBB permeability (Agrawal et al. 1989). Terpenoids may also act on other receptors and neurotransmitters. Some terpenoids act as serotonin uptake inhibitors (as does Prozac), enhance norepinephrine activity (as do tricyclic antidepressants), increase dopamine activity (as do monoamine oxidase inhibitors and bupropion), and augment GABA (as do baclofen and the benzodiazepines). Recently, strong seroto-

TABLE 9.2. Terpenoid essential oil components of cannabis.

Cannabis constituent structure[a]	Concentration[b] (% dry weight)	Boiling point °C[c]	Properties
β-myrcene	0.47	166-168	Analgesic Anti-inflammatory Antibiotic Antimutagenic
β-caryophyllene	0.05	119	Anti-inflammatory Cytoprotective (gastric mucosa) Antimalarial
d-limonene	0.14	177	Cannabinoid agonist? Immune potentiator Antidepressant Antimutagenic
linalool	0.002	198	Sedative Antidepressant Anxiolytic Immune potentiator
pulegone	0.001	224	Memory booster? AChE inhibitor Sedative Antipyretic
1,8-cineole (eucalyptol)	>0.001	176	AChE inhibitor Increases cerebral blood flow Stimulant Antibiotic Antiviral Anti-inflammatory Antinociceptive
α-pinene	0.04	156	Anti-inflammatory Bronchodilator Stimulant Antibiotic Antineoplastic AChE inhibitor

TABLE 9.2 *(continued)*

Cannabis constituent structure[a]	Concentration[b] (% dry weight)	Boiling point °C[c]	Properties
α-terpineol	0.02	217-218	Sedative Antibiotic AChE inhibitor Antioxidant Antimalarial
terpineol-4-ol	0.0004	209	AChE inhibitor Antibiotic
p-cymene	0.0004	177	Antibiotic Anticandidal AChE inhibitor
borneol	0.008	210	Antibiotic
Δ-3-carene	0.004	168	Anti-inflammatory

[a] Structures of constituents obtained from Bisset and Wichtl 1994; British Medical Association 1997; Buckingham 1992; Iversen 2000; Tisserand and Balacs 1995; Turner et al. 1980.

[b] Concentrations of constituents (v/w or w/w) were calculated from various sources. Cannabinoid concentrations (presented as a range, including cannabinoids and cannabinoidic acids) were primarily obtained from Small 1979; Veszki et al. 1980; Fournier et al. 1987; and Pitts et al. 1992. Terpenoid data (presented as maximum values) were calculated from Ross and ElSohly 1996; and Mediavilla and Steinemann 1997. Flavonoid data came from Paris et al. 1976; and Barrett et al., 1986.

[c] Boiling/melting points (MP) recorded at atmospheric pressure (760 mmHg) unless otherise noted; values obtained from various sources, primarily Buckingham 1992; Guenther 1948; Parry 1918; and Mechoulam (personal communication, April 2001).

nin activity at the $5\text{-}HT_{1A}$ and $5\text{-}HT_{2a}$ receptors has been demonstrated (Russo et al. 2000; Russo 2001) that may support synergistic contributions of terpenoids on cannabis-mediated pain and mood effects. Further studies are in progress to identify the most active terpenoid components responsible and whether synergism of the components is demonstrable.

The essential oil of cannabis is traditionally employed as an anti-inflammatory in the respiratory and digestive tracts without known contraindications at physiological dosages (Franchomme and Pénoël 1990). The essential oil of black pepper, *Piper nigrum,* has a composition of terpenes that is qualitatively quite similar to that of cannabis (Lawless 1995). It has often been claimed anecdotally that smoked cannabis may substitute for nicotine in attempts at smoking cessation. Aside from cannabinoid influences, current evidence supports this contention based on terpene content and its activity. A recent study has shown that inhalation of black pepper essential oil vapor significantly reduced withdrawal symptoms and anxiety in tobacco smokers (Rose and Behm 1994). Interestingly, the authors posited not a central biochemical mechanism but rather a peripheral one, assuming physical cues of bronchial sensation as operative in the origin of the benefit. The true scope of the essential oil benefits in this context may be quite a bit broader.

Pate (1994), McPartland (1997), and McPartland et al. (2000) have reviewed the pesticidal properties of cannabis attributable to its terpenoid content. The essential oil of *Eugenia dysenterica* was recently demonstrated to have significant inhibitory effects on *Cryptococcus neoformans* strains isolated from HIV patients with cryptococcal meningitis (Costa et al. 2000). Key components of that oil were common to cannabis: β-caryophyllene, α-humulene, α-terpineol, and limonene.

Additionally, monoterpenes such as those abundant in cannabis resin have been suggested to (1) inhibit cholesterol synthesis, (2) promote hepatic enzyme activity to detoxify carcinogens, (3) stimulate apoptosis in cells with damaged DNA, and (4) inhibit protein isoprenylation implicated in malignant deterioration (Jones 1999).

Myrcene, specifically β-myrcene, a noncyclic monoterpene, is the most abundant terpenoid produced by cannabis (Ross and ElSohly 1996; Mediavilla and Steinemann 1997). It also occurs in high concentrations in hops *(Humulus lupulus)* and lemongrass *(Cymbopogon citratus)*. Myrcene is a potent analgesic, acting at central sites that are antagonized by naloxone (Rao et al. 1990). Myrcene also works via a peripheral mechanism shared by CBD, CBG, and CBC—by blocking the inflammatory activity of prostaglandin E_2 (Lorenzetti et al. 1991). This activity is expressed by other terpenoids in cannabis smoke, such as carvacrol, which is more potent than THC or CBG (Burstein et al. 1975). The activity of many terpenoids may be cumulative: unfractionated cannabis essential oil exhibits greater anti-inflammatory activity than its individual constituents, suggesting synergy (Evans et al. 1987).

Myrcene also synergizes the antibiotic potency of other essential oil components, against *Staphylococcus aureus, Bacillus subtilis, Pseudomonas aeruginosa,* and a specific strain of *Escherichia coli* (Onawunmi et al. 1984). Myrcene inhibits cytochrome P450-2B1, an enzyme implicated in the metabolic activation of promutagens (De Oliveira et al. 1997). Aflatoxin B_1 is a promutagen produced by *Aspergillus flavus* and *Aspergillus parasiticus,* two fungal contaminants of moldy marijuana (reviewed by McPartland and Pruitt 1997). After aflatoxin B_1 is metabolized by P450- 2B1, it becomes extremely hepatocarcinogenic. Myrcene blocks this metabolism, as do other terpenoids in cannabis, including limonene, α-pinene, α-terpinene, and citronellal (De Oliveira et al. 1997).

β-Caryophyllene is the most common sesquiterpenoid in cannabis (Mediavilla and Steinemann 1997). It is the main component of copaiba balsam, from *Copaifera* spp. (Lawless 1995), which is a popular oral and topical anti-inflammatory agent in Brazil (Basile et al. 1988). The latter authors were able to demonstrate anti-inflammatory effects of the oleoresin in rats comparable to phenylbutazone, in reduction of granuloma formation. A decreased vascular permeability to injected histamine was also observed.

A gastric cytoprotective effect of β-caryophyllene was demonstrated in rats against challenge with absolute ethanol and hydrochloric acid (Tambe et al. 1996). This benefit was noted without influence on gastric acid or pepsin secretion. The authors suggested this agent as clinically safe, and potentially useful. Campbell et al. (1997) have demonstrated a moderate antimalarial effect against two strains of *Plasmodium falciparum* by an essential oil rich in β-caryophyllene and α-terpineol.

Limonene is a monocyclic monoterpenoid and a major constituent of citrus rinds (Tisserand and Balacs 1995). It finds extensive use as a solvent and in the perfumery and flavor industries. Because of limonene's widespread occurrence and application, its biological activity is well-known. Limonene is highly absorbed by inhalation and quickly appears in the bloodstream (Falk-Flilipsson et al. 1993). According to Ross and ElSohly (1996), limonene is the second most common terpenoid in an unidentified cultivar of cannabis.

Limonene may have a low-affinity interaction with cannabinoid receptors (Meschler and Howlett 1999). Studies of long-term inhalation of lemon fragrance (predominately limonene) have demonstrated inhibition of thymic involution in stress-induced immunosuppression in mice (Ortiz de Urbina et al. 1989).

Limonene was the primary component of the essential oil mixture employed by Komori et al. (1995) in their clinical study of immune function and depressive states in humans. The key result of this experiment was the ability to markedly reduce the dosage of, or even eliminate the need for, synthetic antidepressant drugs.

As mentioned in the myrcene section, limonene protects against aflatoxin B_1-induced cancer by inhibiting the hepatic metabolism of the promutagen to its active form. Limonene also blocks this process at two earlier steps by inhibiting the growth of *Aspergillus* fungi and inhibiting their production of aflatoxins (Greene-McDowelle et al. 1999). Limonene and other terpenoids suppress the growth of many species of fungi and bacteria, demonstrated in hundreds of published studies (reviewed by McPartland 1997).

Limonene blocks the carcinogenesis induced by benz[α]anthracene (Crowell 1999), a component of the "tar" generated by the combustion of herbal cannabis. Thus, this terpenoid may reduce the harm caused by inhaling cannabis smoke. Limonene blocks carcinogenesis by multiple mechanisms. It detoxifies carcinogens by inducing Phase II carcinogen-metabolizing enzymes (Crowell 1999). It selectively inhibits the isoprenylation of Ras proteins, thus blocking the action of mutant *ras* oncogenes (Hardcastle et al. 1999). It induces redifferentiation of cancer cells (by enhancing expression of transforming growth factor β1 and growth factor II receptors), and it induces apoptosis of cancer cells (Crowell 1999). Orally administered limonene is currently undergoing Phase II clinical trials in the treatment of breast cancer (Vigushin et al. 1998); it also protects against lung, liver, colon, pancreas, and skin cancers (Vigushin et al. 1998; Crowell 1999; Setzer et al. 1999).

Linalool is a noncyclic monoterpenoid, commonly extracted from lavender (*Lavandula* spp.), rose (*Rosa* spp.), and neroli oil (from *Citrus aurantium*). It usually constitutes 5 percent or less of cannabis essential oil (Ross and ElSohly 1996). Linalool nevertheless exhibits strong biological activity. Buchbauer et al. (1993) assayed the sedative effects of more than 40 terpenoids upon *inhalation* by mice; linalool was the most powerful, reducing mouse motility 73 percent after 1 hour of inhalation. The study demonstrated that other terpenoids found in cannabis, such as citronellol and α-terpineol, are also deeply sedating upon inhalation, even in low concentrations. Furthermore, combinations of these terpenoids (e.g., neroli oil) are synergistic in their sedative effects. These terpenoids may mitigate the anxiety provoked by pure THC. Inhalation of such terpenoids also provides antidepressant effects (Komori et al. 1995).

Reducing anxiety and depression will improve immune function via the neuroendocrine system, by damping down the hypothalamic-pituitary-adrenal (HPA) axis. Hence, inhalation of terpenoids reduces the secretion of HPA stress hormones (e.g., corticosterone), and normalizes CD4-CD8 ratios (Komori et al. 1995). By a similar mechanism, terpenoids in *Ginkgo biloba* inhibit corticosterone secretion by attenuating corticotropin-releasing factor (CRF) expression (Marcihac et al. 1998). CRF not only induces corticosterone secretion via the HPA axis, it is also associated with anxiety. Rodríguez de Fonseca et al. (1996) showed that the psychoactive cannabinoid HU-210 caused a release of CRF. Thus, the terpenoids act synergistically with nonpsychoactive CBD, which may decrease CRF by inhibiting IFN-γ (Malfait et al. 2000).

Pulegone, a monocyclic monoterpenoid, is a minor constituent of cannabis (Turner et al. 1980). Higher concentrations of pulegone are found in rosemary (*Rosmarinus officinalis*), "the herb of remembrance." Pulegone may alleviate a major side effect of THC—loss of short-term memory consolidation. THC causes acetylcholine (ACh) deficits in the hippocampus. Hippocampal ACh deficits are also seen in people with Alzheimer's disease. Alzheimer's patients can be treated with tacrine (Cognex), a drug that increases ACh activity by inhibiting acetylcholinesterase (AChE). Indeed, tacrine has blocked THC-induced memory loss behavior in rats. Pulegone exhibits the same activity as tacrine, that of AChE inhibition (Miyazawa et al. 1997). Other terpenoids in cannabis also provide AChE inhibition, including limonene, limonene oxide, α-terpinene, γ-terpinene, terpinen-4-ol, carvacrol, l- and d-carvone, 1,8-cineole, *p*-cymene, fenchone, and pulegone-1,2-epoxide (Perry et al. 1996; McPartland and Pruitt 1999). The beneficial effects of AChE inhibitors, however, are decreased in individuals carrying the E4 subtype of the apolipoprotein E gene, ApoE E4 (Poirier et al. 1995). Pulegone has also demonstrated significant sedative and antipyretic properties in a study in rats (Ortiz de Urbina et al. 1989).

1,8-Cineole, a bicyclic monoterpenoid, is a minor constituent of cannabis and the major aromatic found in *Eucalyptus* species. Studies show the inhalation of 1,8-cineole increases cerebral blood flow and enhances cortical activity (Nasel et al. 1994). Brain function is enhanced by administering terpenoids that improve cerebral blood flow, much as the ginkgolides in *Ginkgo biloba* (Russo 2000). Similarly, cerebral blood flow increases after inhaling cannabis smoke, and this increase is *not* related to plasma levels of THC (Mathew and Wilson 1993).

A stimulatory effect on rat locomotion was demonstrated employing a 1,8-cineole-rich essential oil of rosemary with a terpene profile similar to that of cannabis (Kovar et al. 1987). Blood levels correlated with the degree of stimulation observed. Antinociceptive and anti-inflammatory effects of 1,8-cineole were demonstrated at high doses in rats, using carrageenan rat paw and cotton pellet-induced granuloma models (Santos and Rao 2000). An analgesic effect of an essential oil was demonstrated in another animal study, and correlated with the 1,8-cineole concentration (Aydin et al. 1999).

1,8-Cineole demonstrated antibacterial activity against *Bacillus subtilis,* and antifungal properties against *Trichophyton mentagrophytes, Cryptococcus neoformans,* and *Candida albicans* (Hammerschmidt et al. 1993). In subsequent assays, this essential oil component was cidal against *Candida albicans* and *Escherichia coli,* and bacteriostatic against *Staphylococcus aureus* (Carson and Riley 1995). In a rat study, 1,8-cineole prevented the sexual transmission of *Herpes simplex* virus type 2 (HSV-2). HSV-2 is a frequently comorbid condition with HIV, and its prevention has been suggested as one method of lowering HIV transmission risks (Gwanzura et al. 1998).

Perry et al. (2000) demonstrated that 1,8-cineole was an inhibitor of human erythrocyte acetylcholinesterase, but that an essential oil of *Salvia lavandulaefolia* containing 1,8-cineole and other terpenoids produced a synergistic inhibition of acetylcholinesterase that suggested utility in the clinical treatment of Alzheimer's disease. A similar mechanism may operate in cannabis essential oil with the same components.

α-Pinene, a bicyclic monoterpenoid, was effective in prevention of acute inflammation in a carrageenan-induced plantar edema model (Gil et al. 1989). A pharmacokinetics study of inhaled α-pinene in humans demonstrated 60 percent uptake, and a relative bronchodilation effect (Falk et al. 1990). After 1 hour of inhalation, α-pinene produced a 13.8 percent increase in mouse motility measures (Buchbauer et al. 1993). α-Pinene has inhibited acetylcholinesterase in a variety of assays (Perry et al. 1996; McPartland and Pruitt 1999), suggesting utility in the clinical treatment of Alzheimer's disease. The antibiotic properties of α -pinene, α -terpineol, and terpinen-4-ol have been demonstrated against *Staphylococcus aureus, S. epidermidis,* and *Propionibacterium acnes* (Raman et al. 1995). α-Pinene and its isomer β-pinene were both cytotoxic in vitro against Hep-G2 (human hepatocellular carcinoma) and Sk-Mel-28 (human melanoma) tumor cell lines (Setzer et al. 1999).

α-Terpineol, terpinen-4-ol, and 4-terpineol are three closely related monoterpenoids. Inhalation of α-terpineol reduced mouse motility 45 percent (Buchbauer et al. 1993). Burits and Bucar (2000) demonstrated that 4-terpineol exhibits "respectable" radical scavenging and antioxidant properties. Terpinen-4-ol, α-terpineol, and α-pinene demonstrated dose-dependent antibiotic properties against *Staphylococcus aureus, S. epidermidis,* and *Propionibacterium acnes* (Raman et al. 1995). Similar studies have demonstrated antimicrobial activity against a wide range of pathogenic organisms, excluding *Pseudomonas* (Carson and Riley 1995). Campbell et al. (1997) have demonstrated a moderate antimalarial effect against two strains of *Plasmodium falciparum* by an essential oil with major α-terpineol and α-caryophyllene components.

Cymene, or *p*-cymene, a monoterpenoid, is active against *Bacterioides fragilis, Candida albicans,* and *Clostridium perfringens* (Carson and Riley 1995).

Borneol, a bicyclic monoterpenoid, was tested in walnut oil as an external treatment for purulent otitis media (Liu 1990), where it proved to be 98 percent effective ($P < 0.001$), to a greater degree than neomycin, and without toxicity.

Δ^3-Carene, a bicyclic monoterpenoid, was effective in prevention of acute inflammation in a carrageenan-induced plantar edema model (Gil et al. 1989).

FLAVONOIDS

Flavonoids are aromatic, polycyclic phenols. Cannabis produces about 20 of these compounds as free flavonoids and conjugated glycosides (Turner et al. 1980). Paris et al. (1976) estimated that cannabis leaves consist of 1 percent flavonoids. Some flavonoids are volatile, lipophilic, permeate membranes and apparently retain pharmacological activity in cannabis smoke (Sauer et al. 1983). Flavonoids may modulate the pharmacokinetics of THC, via a mechanism shared by CBD, the inhibition of P450-3A11 and P450-3A4 enzymes. Naringenin, a flavonoid in grapefruit juice, also inhibits these enzymes, thus blocking the metabolism of cyclosporine, caffeine, benzodiazepines, and calcium antagonists (Fuhr 1998). Two related enzymes, P450-3A4 and P450-1A1, metabolize environmental toxins from procarcinogens to their activated forms. Thus, P450-suppressing compounds serve as chemoprotective agents, shielding healthy cells from the activation of benzo[α]pyrene and aflatoxin B_1 (Offord et al. 1997), which are two procarcinogens potentially found in cannabis smoke (McPartland and Pruitt 1997).

Apigenin is a flavone found in nearly all vascular plants (Table 9.3). It exerts a wide range of biological effects, including many properties shared by terpenoids and cannabinoids. Apigenin is the primary anxiolytic agent found in chamomile, *Matricaria recutita* (reviewed in Russo 2000). It selectively binds with high affinity to central benzodiazepine receptors, which are located in α- and β-subunits of GABA$_A$ receptors (Salgueiro et al. 1997); this anxiolytic activity is not associated with the unwanted side effects caused by synthetic benzodiazepines, such as muscular relaxation, amnesia, and sedation.

Apigenin inhibits the production of tumor necrosis factor-alpha (TNF-α), a cytokine primarily expressed by monocytes and macrophages (Gerritsen et al. 1995). TNF-α induces and maintains inflammation, a

TABLE 9.3. Flavonoid and phytosterol components of cannabis.

Cannabis constituent structure[a]	Concentration[b] (% dry weight)	Boiling point °C[c]	Properties
apigenin	>0.1%	178	Anxiolytic Anti-inflammatory Estrogenic
quercetin	>0.1%	250	Antioxidant Antimutagenic Antiviral Antineoplastic
cannflavin A	0.02%	182	COX inhibitor LO inhibitor
β-sitosterol	?	134	Anti-inflammatory 5-α-reductase inhibitor

[a]Structures of constituents obtained from Bisset and Wichtl 1994; British Medical Association 1997; Buckingham 1992; Iversen 2000; Tisserand and Balacs 1995; Turner et al. 1980.

[b]Concentrations of constituents (v/w or w/w) were calculated from various sources. Cannabinoid concentrations (presented as a range, including cannabinoids and cannabinoidic acids) were primarily obtained from Small 1979; Veszki et al. 1980; Fournier et al. 1987; and Pitts et al. 1992. Terpenoid data (presented as maximum values) were calculated from Ross and ElSohly 1996; and Mediavilla and Steinemann 1997. Flavonoid data came from Paris et al. 1976; and Barrett et al. 1986.

[c]Boiling/melting points (MP) recorded at atmospheric pressure (760 mmHg) unless otherise noted; values obtained from various sources, primarily Buckingham 1992; Guenther 1948; Parry 1918; and Mechoulam (personal communication, April 2001).

pathological condition in rheumatoid arthritis and multiple sclerosis. THC decreases TNF-α, probably by a nonreceptor-mediated mechanism (Burnette-Curley and Cabral 1995), although one study suggested THC might induce TNF-α (Shivers et al. 1994). Either way, apigenin provides beneficial suppression of TNF-α, whether in concert with THC or counteracting THC.

Apigenin and other flavonoids interact with estrogen receptors, and appear to be the primary estrogenic agents in cannabis smoke (Sauer et al. 1983). Although apigenin has a high affinity for estrogen receptors (especially β-estrogen receptors), it has low estrogenic activity; apigenin actually inhibits estradiol-induced proliferation of breast cancer cells (Wang and Kurzer 1998).

Quercetin is a flavonol found in nearly all vascular plants, including cannabis (Turner et al. 1980). Quercetin is a potent antioxidant; by some measures more potent than ascorbic acid, α-tocopherol, and BHT (Gadow et al. 1997). Combinations of quercetin and other antioxidants work synergistically (Hudson and Mahgoub 1981). The antioxidant potential of quercetin and other flavonoids should be tested against CBD, another potent antioxidant (Hampson et al. 1998). Perhaps flavonoids can induce chemical reduction of CBD, effectively recycling CBD as an antioxidant. Flavonoids block free radical formation at several steps: by scavenging superoxide anions (in both enzymatic and non-enzymatic systems), by quenching intermediate peroxyl and alkoxyl radicals, and by chelating iron ions, which catalyze many Fenton reactions leading to free radical formation (Musonda and Chipman 1998).

Free radicals activate NF-κB, a transcription factor protein that induces the expression of oncogenes, inflammation, and apoptosis. Quercetin arrests the formation of NF-κB, by blocking the PKC-induced phosphorylation of an inhibitory subunit of NF-κB called IκB (Musonda and Chipman 1998), consequently quercetin hinders carcinogenesis and inflammatory diseases. NF-κB also plays a role in the activation of HIV-1 (Greenspan 1993), so quercetin may hinder the replication of that virus. In a similar fashion, silymarin (a flavonoid produced by milk thistle, *Silybum marianum*) impedes NF-κB-induced replication of the hepatitis C virus, and thus inhibits hepatic carcinoma (McPartland 1996). These flavonoids may synergize with CBN, which also down-regulates NF-κB (Herring and Kaminski 1999), thereby counteracting the effects of THC, which may increase NF-κB activity (Daaka et al. 1997).

Cannflavin A is one of a pair of prenylated flavones apparently unique to cannabis (Barrett et al. 1986). The yield of cannflavin A is 0.02 percent of dry herb. This compound is a potent inhibitor of prostaglandin E$_2$ in human rheumatoid synovial cells, with an IC_{50} of 31 ng/mL, about 30 times more potent than aspirin in that system (Barrett et al. 1986). Cannflavin A inhibits cyclooxygenase (COX) enzymes and lipoxygenase (LO) enzymes more potently than THC (Evans et al. 1987). However, these assays were done with alcohol-extracted cannflavin; we question whether cannflavin is sufficiently volatile. Other phenols related to flavonoids are volatile and apparently retain pharmacological activity in cannabis smoke, such as eugenol and *p*-vinylphenol (Burstein et al. 1976).

β-Sitosterol was demonstrated in significant concentrations in the red oil extract of cannabis (Fenselau and Hermann 1972). In animal assays, this phytosterol reduced acute inflammation 65 percent and chronic edema 40.6 percent (Gomez et al. 1999). This agent has been the subject of most interest as the active ingredient of *Serenoa repens,* the saw palmetto, and *Urtica dioica,* the nettle, wherein β-sitosterol acts as a 5-α-reductase inhibitor. In numerous trials (Wilt et al. 1998; McPartland and Pruitt 2000), standardized extracts of saw palmetto have proven equivalent or superior to finasteride in treatment of benign prostatic hyperplasia.

CONCLUSIONS

Does the body absorb noncannabinoids in physiologically relevant concentrations? In the absence of experimental data, we can estimate, using limonene as an example of AChE inhibition. According to Ross and ElSohly (1996), fresh female flowering tops consist of 0.29 percent essential oil. Air drying of female flowering tops decreases their moisture content (MC) from approximately 85 to 15 percent, with a concomitant loss in water weight (McPartland and Pruitt 1997). Although some essential oil is volatilized and lost in the drying process, the remaining terpenoids become concentrated. The concentration of essential oil in air-dried cannabis is 0.8 percent, and limonene consists of 17.2 percent of the essential oil (Ross and ElSohly 1996). Thus, air-dried cannabis consists of 0.14 percent limonene; therefore a 500 mg cannabis cigarette (which is half the size of a standard tobacco cigarette) would contain 0.7 mg limonene. If we assume the systemic bioavailability of limonene from smoking cannabis is 18 percent, the same as THC (Ohlsson et al. 1980), then 0.13 mg would be absorbed. Distributing this dose evenly in the total body water of a 70 kg man, without metabolism or sequestration, would produce a maximum tissue concentration of 1.3 μM. This concentration is an order of magnitude below the IC_{50} concentration of limonene's inhibition of AChE (Miyazawa et al. 1997). Hence, limonene *must* synergize with other AChE inhibitors in order to be effective.

Vaporizer technology may improve the bioavailability of limonene and other compounds, which volatilize around the same temperature as THC (see Tables 9.1 to 9.3). Vaporizers are smoking apparati that heat cannabis to 185°C (365°F), which vaporizes THC but is below the ignition point of combustible plant material. Vaporized cannabis emits a thin gray vapor, whereas combusted cannabis produces a thick smoke. Thus, vaporizers deliver a better cannabinoid-to-tar ratio than cigarettes or water pipes (Gieringer 1996). In a recent study, traces of THC were vaporized at temperatures as low as 140°C (284°F) and the majority of THC vaporized by 185°C (365°F); benzene and other carcinogenic vapors did not appear until 200°C (392°F), and cannabis combustion occurred around 230°C (446°F) (Gieringer 2001).

Concerning bioavailability, it should be mentioned that cannabis compounds need not be absorbed systemically through the lungs to produce CNS activity. Inhaled compounds may reach receptors in the olfactory bulb, sending mood-altering messages via olfactory nerves directly to the limbic region and hippocampus. This route may be responsible for some sedative effects of terpenoids upon inhalation (Buchbauer et al. 1993).

The paucity of research concerning non-THC synergists in cannabis is periodically criticized (Mechoulam et al. 1972; McPartland and Pruitt 1999; Russo 2000). We have highlighted several cannabinoids, terpenoids, and flavonoids that deserve further attention regarding their contributions to the effects of clinical cannabis. Most of the data we present here are based on in vitro experiments or animal studies. Clearly the next step should involve human clinical trials of each constituent, alone or in combination with THC, or combined with a cocktail of cannabis compounds.

REFERENCES

Abrahamov, A., and R. Mechoulam. 1995. An efficient new cannabinoid antiemetic in pediatric oncology. *Life Sci* 56(23-24):2097-2102.

Achiron, A., S. Miron, V. Lavie, R. Margalit, and A. Biegon. 2000. Dexanabinol (HU-211) effect on experimental autoimmune encephalomyelitis: Implications for the treatment of acute relapses of multiple sclerosis. *J Neuroimmunol* 102(1): 26-31.

Agrawal, A.K., P. Kumar, A. Gulati, and P.K. Seth. 1989. Cannabis-induced neuro-toxicity in mice: Effects on cholinergic (muscarinic) receptors and blood brain barrier permeability. *Res Commun Subst Abuse* 10:155-168.

Anderson, P.F., D.M. Jackson, and G.B. Chesher. 1974. Interaction of delta-9-tetrahydrocannabinol and cannabidiol on intestinal motility in mice. *J Pharm Pharmacol* 26(2):136-137.

Aydin, S., T. Demir, Y. Ozturk, and K.H. Baser. 1999. Analgesic activity of *Nepeta italica* L. *Phytother Res* 13(1):20-23.

Baek, S.H., Y.O. Kim, J.S. Kwag, K.E. Choi, W.Y. Jung, and D.S. Han. 1998. Boron trifluoride etherate on silica-A modified Lewis acid reagent (VII). Antitumor activity of cannabigerol against human oral epitheloid carcinoma cells. *Arch Pharmacol Res* 21:353-356.

Banerjee, S.P., S.H. Snyder, and R. Mechoulam. 1975. Cannabinoids: Influence on neurotransmitter uptake in rat brain synaptosomes. *J Pharmacol Exper Therap* 194:74-81.

Barrett, M.L., A.M. Scutt, and F.J. Evans. 1986. Cannflavin A and B, prenylated flavones from *Cannabis sativa* L. *Experientia* 42:452-453.

Basile, A.C., J.A. Sertie, P.C. Freitas, and A.C. Zanini. 1988. Anti-inflammatory activity of oleoresin from Brazilian *Copaifera*. *J Ethnopharmacol* 22(1):101-109.

Biegon, A., and A.B. Joseph. 1995. Development of HU-211 as a neuroprotectant for ischemic brain damage. *Neurol Res* 17(4):275-280.

Bisset, N.G. and M. Wichtl. 1994. *Herbal drugs and phytopharmaceuticals: A handbook for practice on a scientific basis.* Stuttgart, Boca Raton: Medpharm Scientific Publishers, CRC Press.

Bornheim, L.M., K.Y. Kim, J. Li, B.Y. Perotti, and L.Z. Benet. 1995. Effect of cannabidiol pretreatment on the kinetics of tetrahydrocannabinol metabolites in mouse brain. *Drug Metab Dispos* 23:825-831.

Boucher, F., M. Paris, and L. Cosson. 1977. Mise en évidence de deux type chimques chez le *Cannabis sativa* originaire d'Afrique du Sud. *Phytochem* 16:1445-1448.

British Medical Association. 1997. *Therapeutic uses of cannabis.* Amsterdam: Harwood Academic Publishers.

Brodkin, J., and J.M. Moerschbaecher. 1997. SR141716A antagonizes the disruptive effects of cannabinoid ligaands on learning in rats. *J Pharmacol Exper Therap* 282:1526-1532.

Browne, R.G., and A. Weissman. 1981. Discriminative stimulus properties of delta 9-tetrahydrocannabinol: Mechanistic studies. *J Clin Pharmacol* 21(8-9 Suppl): 227S-234S.

Buchbauer, G., L. Jirovetz, W. Jager, C. Plank, and H. Dietrich. 1993. Fragrance compounds and essential oils with sedative effects upon inhalation. *J Pharm Sci* 82(6):660-664.

Buckingham, J. (ed.) 1992. *Dictionary of natural products.* London: Chapman & Hall.

Burits, M., and F. Bucar. 2000. Antioxidant activity of *Nigella sativa* essential oil. *Phytoth Res* 14(5):323-328.

Burnette-Curley, D., and G.A. Cabral. 1995. Differential inhibition of RAW264.7 macrophage tumoricidal activity by Δ^9-tetrahydrocannabinol. *Proc Soc Exp Biol Med* 210:64-76.

Burstein, S., E. Levin, and C. Varanelli. 1973. Prostaglandins and *Cannabis*—II. Inhibition of biosynthesis by the naturally occurring cannabinoids. *Biochem Pharmacol* 22:2905-2910.

Burstein, S., P. Taylor, F.S. El-Feraly, C. Turner. 1976. Prostaglandins and *Cannabis*—V. Identification of p-vinylphenol as a potent inhibitor of prostaglandin synthesis. *Biochem Pharmacol* 25:2003-2004.

Burstein, S., C. Varanelli, and L.T. Slade. 1975. Prostaglandins and *Cannabis*—III. Inhibition of biosynthesis by essential oil components of marihuana. *Biochemical Pharmacology* 24:1053-1054.

Campbell, W.E., D.W. Gammon, P. Smith, M. Abrahams, and T.D. Purves. 1997. Composition and antimalarial activity in vitro of the essential oil of *Tetradenia riparia*. *Planta Med* 63(3):270-272.

Carlini, E.A., and J.M. Cunha. 1981. Hypnotic and antiepileptic effects of cannabidiol. *J Clin Pharmacol* 21:417S-427S.

Carlini, E.A., I.G. Karniol, P.F. Renault, and C.R. Schuster. 1974. Effects of marihuana in laboratory animals and man. *Brit J Pharmacol* 50:299-309.

Carson, C.F., and T.V. Riley. 1995. Antimicrobial activity of the major components of the essential oil of *Melaleuca alternifolia*. *J Appl Bacter* 78(3):264-269.

Carta, G., F. Nava, and G.L. Gessa. 1998. Inhibition of hippocampal acetylcholine release after acute and repeated Δ^9-tetrahydrocannabinol in rats. *Brain Res* 809:1-4.

Cheney, D.L., A.V. Revuelta, and E. Costa. 1981. Marijuana and cholinergic dynamics. In G. Pepeu and H. Ladinsky (eds.), *Cholinergic mechanisms: Phylogenetic aspects, central and peripheral synapses, and clinical significance* (pp. 825-832). New York: Plenum Press.

Clarke, R.C. 1998. *Hashish!* Los Angeles, CA: Red Eye Press.

Compton, D.R., K.C. Rice, B.R. DeCosta, R.K. Razdan, L.S. Melvin, M.R. Johnson, and B.R. Martin. 1993. Cannabinoid structure-activity relationships: Correlation of receptor binding and in vivo activities. *J Pharmacol Exp Therap* 265:218-226.

Consroe, P. 1998. Brain cannabinoid systems as targets for the therapy of neurological disorders. *Neurobiol Dis* 5:534-551.

Costa, T.R., O.F. Fernandes, S.C. Santos, C.M. Oliveira, L.M. Liao, P.H. Ferri, J.R. Paula, H.D. Ferreira, B.H. Sales, and M.R. Silva. 2000. Antifungal activity of volatile constituents of *Eugenia dysenterica* leaf oil. *J Ethnopharmacol* 72(1-2):111-117.

Crowell, P.L. 1999. Prevention and therapy of cancer by dietary monoterpenes. *J Nutr* 129:775S-778S.

Daaka, Y., W. Zhu, H. Friedman, and T.W. Klein. 1997. Induction of interleukin-2 receptor α gene by Δ^9-tetrahydrocannabinol is mediated by nuclear factor κB and CB1 cannabinoid receptor. *DNA Cell Biol* 16:301-309.

Dalterio, S., D. Mayfield, A. Bartke, W. Morgan. 1985. Effects of psychoactive and non-psychoactive cannabinoids on neuroendocrine and testicular responsiveness in mice. *Life Sci* 36:1299-1306.

Davis, W.M., and N.S. Hatoum. 1983. Neurobehavioral actions of cannabichromene and interactions with Δ^9-tetrahydrocannabinol. *Gen Pharmacol* 14(2):247-252.

De Oliveira, A.C., L.F. Ribeiro-Pinto, J.R. Paumgartten. 1997. In vitro inhibition of CYP2B1 monooxygenase by beta-myrcene and other monoterpenoid compounds. *Toxicol Lett* 92:39-46.

Devane, W.A., F.A. Dysarz, M.R. Johnson, L.S. Melvin, A.C. Howlett. 1988. Determination and characterization of a cannabinoid receptor in rat brain. *Molecular Pharmacol* 34:605-613.

Di Marzo, V. and A. Fontana. 1995. Anandamide, an endogenous cannabinomimetic eicosanoid: "Killing two birds with one stone." *Prostagland Leukotr Essent Fatty Acids* 53:1-11.

Domino, E.F. 1976. Effect of Δ^9-terahydrocannabinol and cannabinol on rat brain acetylcholine. In Nahas G.G., Panton W.D.M., Idanpaan-Heikkila J.E. (eds.), *Marijuana: chemistry, biochemistry, and cellular effects* (pp. 407-413). New York: Springer-Verlag.

ElSohly, M.A., S. Feng, T.P. Murphy, S.A. Ross, A. Nimrod, Z. Mehmedic, and N. Fortner. 1999. Delta-9-tetrahydrocannabivarin (delta-9-THCV) as a marker for the ingestion of cannabis versus Marinol. *J Analyt Toxicol* 23(3):222-224.

ElSohly, H.N., C.E. Turner, A.M. Clark, and M.A. ElSohly. 1982. Synthesis and antimicrobial activities of certain cannabichromene and cannabigerol related compounds. *J Pharmaceut Sci* 71:1319-1323.

Evans, A.T., E.A. Formukong, and F.J. Evans. 1987. Actions of cannabis constituents on enzymes of arachidonate metabolism: Anti-inflammatory potential. *Bioch Pharmacol* 36:2035-2037.

Evans, F.J. 1991. Cannabinoids: the separation of central from peripheral effects on a structural basis. *Planta Med* 57(Suppl 1):S60-S67.

Fairbairn, J.W., and J.T. Pickens. 1981. Activity of cannabis in relation to its delta[1]-trans-tetrahydro-cannabinol content. *British J Pharmacol* 72:401-409.

Falk, A.A., M.T. Hagberg, A.E. Lof, E.M. Wigaeus-Hjelm, and Z.P. Wang. 1990. Uptake, distribution and elimination of alpha-pinene in man after exposure by inhalation. *Scand J Work Envir Health* 16(5):372-378.

Falk-Filipsson, A., A. Löf, M. Hagberg, E.W. Hjelm, and Z. Wang. 1993. *d*-Limonene exposure to humans by inhalation: Uptake, distribution, elimination, and effects on the pulmonary function. *J Toxicol Envir Health* 38:77-88.

Faubert, B.L., and N.E. Kaminski. 2000. AP-1 activity is negatively regulated by cannabinol through inhibition of its protein components, c-fos and c-jun. *J Leukocyte Biol* 67:259-266.

Fenselau, C., and G. Hermann. 1972. Identification of phytosterols in red oil extract of cannabis. *J Forens Sci* 17(2):309-312.

Foletta, V.C., D.H. Segal, and D.R. Cohen. 1998. Transcriptional regulation in the immune system: all roads lead to AP-1. *J Leukocyte Biol* 63:139-152.

Formukong, E.A., A.T. Evans, and F.J. Evans. 1988. Inhibition of the cataleptic effect of tetrahydrocannabinol by other constituents of *Cannabis sativa* L. *J Pharm Pharmacol* 40:132-134.

Fournier, G., C. Richez-Dumanois, J. Duvezin, J.P. Mathieu, and M. Paris. 1987. Identification of a new chemotype in *Cannabis sativa*: Cannabigerol-dominant plants, biogenetic and agronomic prospects. *Planta Med* 53:277-280.

Franchomme, P., and Pénoël. 1990. *L'aromathérapie exactement*. Limoges, France: Roger Jallois.

Fuhr, U. 1998. Drug interactions with grapefruit juice. Extent, probable mechanism and clinical relevance. *Drug Safety* 18:251-272.

Gadow, A von, E. Joubert, and C.G. Hansmann. 1997. Comparison of the antioxidant activity of aspalathin with that of other plant phenols of rooibos tea (*Aspalathus linearis*), α-tocopherol, BHT, and BHA. *J Agricult Food Chem* 45: 632-638.

Gallily, R., A. Yamin, Y. Waksmann, H. Ovadia, J. Weidenfeld, A. Bar-Joseph, A. Biegon, R. Mechoulam, and E. Shohami. 1997. Protection against septic shock and suppression of tumor necrosis factor alpha and nitric oxide production by dexanabinol (HU-211), a nonpsychotropic cannabinoid. *J Pharm Exper Therap* 283(2):918-924.

Gerritsen, M.E., W.W. Carley, G.E. Ranges, C.-P. Shen, S.A. Phan, G.F. Ligon, and C.A. Perry. 1995. Flavonoids inhibit cytokine-induced endothelial cell adhesion protein gene expression. *Am J Path* 147:278-292.

Gieringer, D. 1996. Marijuana research: Waterpipe study. *MAPS [Multidisciplinary Association for Psychedelic Studies] Bull* 6(3):59-66.

Gieringer, D. 2001. NORML study shows vaporizers reduce marijuana smoke toxins. *California NORML Reports* 25(1):2.

Gil, M.L., J. Jimenez, M.A. Ocete, A. Zarzuelo, and M.M. Cabo. 1989. Comparative study of different essential oils of Bupleurum gibraltaricum Lamarck. *Pharmazie* 44(4):284-287.

Gill, E.W., W.D.M. Paton, and R.G. Pertwee. 1970. Preliminary experiments on the chemistry and pharmacology of *Cannabis*. *Nature* 228:134-136.

Gomez, M.A., M.T. Saenz, M.D. Garcia, and M.A. Fernandez. 1999. Study of the topical anti-inflammatory activity of *Achillea ageratum* on chronic and acute inflammation models. *Zeitscrift fur Naturforsch [C]* 54 (11):937-941.

Greene-McDowelle, D.M., B. Ingber, M.S. Wright, H.J. Zeringue, D. Bhatnagar, and T.E. Cleveland. 1999. The effects of selected cotton-leaf volatiles on growth, development and aflatoxin production of *Aspergillus parasiticus*. *Toxicon* 37:883-893.

Greenspan, H.C. 1993. The role of reactive oxygen species, antioxidants and phytopharmaceuticals in human immunodeficiency virus activity. *Med Hypoth* 40:85-92.

Grinspoon, L., J.B. Bakalar. 1997. *Marihuana, the forbidden medicine,* Revised edition. New Haven, CT: Yale University Press.

Guenther, E. 1948. *The essential oils: Individual essential oils of the plant families*. New York: D. Van Nostrand.

Gwanzura, L., W. McFarland, D. Alexander, R. L. Burke, and D. Katzenstein. 1998. Association between human immunodeficiency virus and herpes simplex virus type 2 seropositivity among male factory workers in Zimbabwe. *J Infect Dis* 177(2):481-484.

Hammerschmidt, F.J., A.M. Clark, F.M. Soliman, E.S. el-Kashoury, M.M. Abd el-Kawy, and A.M. el-Fishawy. 1993. Chemical composition and antimicrobial activity of essential oils of *Jasonia candicans* and *J. montana. Planta Med* 59(1):68-70.

Hampson, A.J., M. Grimaldi, J. Axelrod, and D. Wink. 1998. Cannabidiol and (−) Δ^9-tetrahydrocannabinol are neuroprotective antioxidants. *Proc Natl Acad Sci* 95:8268-8273.

Hardcastle, I.R., M.G. Rowlands, A.M. Barber, R.M. Grimshaw, M.K. Mohan, B.P. Nutley, and M. Jarman. 1999. Inhibition of protein prenylation by metabolites of limonene. *Biochem Pharmacol* 57:801-809.

Hatoum, N.S., W.M. Davis, M.A. ElSohly, and C.E. Turner. 1981. Cannabichromene and of Δ^9-tetrahydrocannabinol: Interactions relative to lethality, hypothermia, and hexobarbital hypnosis. *Gen Pharmacol* 12:357-362.

Herring, A.C., N.E. Kaminski. 1999. Cannabinol-mediated inhibition of nuclear factor-κB, cAMP response element-binding protein, and interleukin-2 secretion by activated thymocytes. *J Pharmacol Exp Therap* 291:1156-1163.

Heyser, C.J., R.E. Hampson, and S.A. Deadwyler. 1993. Effects of Δ^9-tetrahydrocannabinol on delayed match to sample performance in rats: Alterations in short-term memory associated with changes in task specific firing of hippocampal cells. *J Pharmacol Exp Therap* 264:294-307.

Hollister, L.E. 1974. Structure-activity relationships in man of cannabis constituents, and homologs and metabolites of delta-9-tetrahydrocannabinol. *Pharmacol* 11(1):3-11.

Hudson, B.J.F., and S.E.O. Mahgoub. 1981. Synergism between phospholipids and naturally-occurring antioxidants in leaf lipids. *J Sci Food Agricult* 32:208-210.

Iversen, L.L. 2000. *The science of marijuana.* Oxford, UK: Oxford University Press.

Jones, C.L.A. 1999. Monoterpenes: Essence of a cancer cure. *Nutr Sci News* 4 (4):190.

Kapeghian, J.C., A.B. Jones, J.C. Murphy, M.A. Elsohly, and C.E. Turner. 1983. Effect of cannabichromene on hepatic microsomal enzyme activity in the mouse. *Gen Pharmacol* 14:361-363.

Klein, T.W., H. Friedman, and S. Specter. 1998. Marijuana, immunity and infection. *J Neuroimmunol* 83:102-105.

Klein, T.W., C. Newton, and H. Friedman. 1987. Inhibition of natural killer cell function by marijuana components. *J Toxicol Envir Health* 20:321-332.

Klingeren, B.V., and M.T. Ham. 1976. Antibacterial activity of Δ^9-tetrahydrocannabinol and cannabidiol. *Antonie van Leeuwenhoek* 42:9-12.

Komori, T., R. Fujiwara, M. Tanida, J. Nomura, and M.M. Yokoyama. 1995. Effects of citrus fragrance on immune function and depressive states. *Neuroimmunomod* 2:174-180.

Kovar, K.A., B. Gropper, D. Friess, and H.P. Ammon. 1987. Blood levels of 1,8-cineole and locomotor activity of mice after inhalation and oral administration of rosemary oil. *Planta Med* 53(4):315-318.

Kubena, R.K., and H. Barry. 1972. Stimulus characteristics of marihuana components. *Nature* 235:397-398.

Lawless, J. 1995. *The illustrated encyclopedia of essential oils: The complete guide to the use of oils in aromatherapy and herbalism.* Shaftesbury, Dorset, UK: Element.

Liu, S.L. 1990. [Therapeutic effects of borneol-walnut oil in the treatment of purulent otitis media]. *Chung Hsi I Chieh Ho Tsa Chih* 10(2):93-95, 69.

Lorenzetti, B.B., G.E.P. Souza, S.J. Sarti, D. Santos Filho, and S.H. Ferreira. 1991. Myrcene mimics the peripheral analgesic activity of lemongrass tea. *J Ethnopharmacol* 34:43-48.

Malfait, A.M., R. Gallily, P.F. Sumariwalla, A.S. Malik, E. Andreakos, R. Mechoulam, and M. Feldman. 2000. The nonpsychoactive cannabis constituent cannabidiol is an oral anti-arthritic therapeutic in murine collagen-induced arthritis. *Proc Natl Acad Sci* 97:9561-9566.

Malingré, T., H. Hendriks, S. Batterman, R. Bos, and J. Visser. 1973. The essential oil of *Cannabis sativa*. *Planta Med* 28:56-61.

Marcihac, A., N. Dakine, N. Bourhim, V. Guillaume, M. Grino, K. Drieu, and C. Oliver. 1998. Effect of chronic administration of *Ginkgo biloba* extract or kinkgolide on the hypothalamic-pituitary-adrenal axis in the rat. *Life Sci* 62:2329-2340.

Martin, L., D.M. Smith, and C.G. Farmilo. 1961. Essential oil from fresh *Cannabis sativa* and its use in identification. *Nature* 191:774-776.

Mathew, R.J., and W.H. Wilson. 1993. Acute changes in cerebral blood flow after smoking marijuana. *Life Sci* 52:757-767.

McPartland, J.M. 1984. Pathogenicity of *Phomopsis ganjae* on *Cannabis sativa* and the fungistatic effect of cannabinoids produced by the host. *Mycopathologia* 87: 149-153.

McPartland, J.M. 1996. Viral hepatitis treated with *Phyllanthus amarus* and milk thistle (*Silybum marianum*): A case report. *Complement Med Internat* 3(2):40-42.

McPartland, J.M. 1997. *Cannabis* as a repellent crop and botanical pesticide. *J Internat Hemp Assoc* 4(2):89-94.

McPartland, J.M., R.C. Clarke, and D.P. Watson. 2000. *Hemp diseases and pests: Management and biological control.* Wallingford: UK. CABI.

McPartland, J.M., and P.P. Pruitt. 1997. Medical marijuana and its use by the immunocompromised. *Altern Therap* 3(3):39-45.

McPartland, J.M., and P.P. Pruitt. 1999. Side effects of pharmaceuticals not elicited by comparable herbal medicines: The case of tetrahydrocannabinol and marijuana. *Altern Therap* 5(4):57-62.

McPartland, J.M., and P.L. Pruitt. 2000. Benign prostatic hyperplasia treated with saw palmetto: A literature search and an experimental case study. *J Amer Osteopath Assoc* 100(2):89-96.

Mechoulam, R., and S. Ben-Shabat. 1999. From gan-zi-gun-nu to anandamide and 2-arachidonoylglycerol: The ongoing story of cannabis. *Nat Prod Rep* 16(2):131-143.

Mechoulam, R., Z. Ben-Zvi, A. Shani, H. Zemler, and S. Levy. 1972. Cannabinoids and Cannabis activity. In W.D.M Paton and J. Crown (eds.), *Cannabis and its derivatives* (pp. 1-13). London: Oxford University Press.

Mechoulam, R., and Y. Gaoni. 1965. Hashish–IV. The isolation and structure of cannabinolic, cannabidiolic, and cannabigerolic acids. *Tetrahedr* 21:1223-1229.

Mechoulam, R., and Y. Gaoni. 1967. Recent advances in the chemistry of hashish. *Fortschritte der Chemie Organischer Naturstoffe* 25:175-213.

Mediavilla, V., and S. Steinemann. 1997. Essential oil of *Cannabis sativa* L. strains. *J Internat Hemp Assoc* 4(2):82-84.

Meier, C., Mediavilla, V. 1998. Factors influencing the yield and the quality of hemp (*Cannabis sativa* L.) essential oil. *J Internat Hemp Assoc* 5(1):16-20.

Merkus, F.W.H.M. 1971. Cannabivarin and tetrahydrocannabivarin, two new constituents of hashish. *Nature* 232:580-581.

Meschler, J.P., and A.C. Howlett. 1999. Thujone exhibits low affinity for cannabinoid receptors but fails to evoke cannabimimetic responses. *Pharmacol Biochem Behav* 62:473-480.

Misner, D.L., and J.M. Sullivan. 1999. Mechanism of cannabinoid effects on long-term potentiation and depression in hippocampal CA1 neurons. *J Neurosci* 19(16): 6795-6805.

Miyazawa, M., H. Watanabe, and H. Kameoka. 1997. Inhibition of acetylcholinesterase activity by monoterpenoids with a *p*-methane skeleton. *J Agricult Food Chem* 45:677-679.

Musonda, C.A., and J.K. Chipman. 1998. Quercetin inhibits hydrogen peroxide-induced NF-κB DNA binding activity and DNA damage in HepG2 cells. *Carcinogen* 19:1583-1589.

Musty, R.E., I.G. Karniol, I. Shirakawa, N. Takahshi, and E. Knobel. Interactions of Δ^9-THC and cannabinol in man. In: *Pharmacology of marihuana*, MC Braude and S. Szara, eds. Raven Press, NY. Vol. 2:559-563.

Nasel, C., B. Nasel, P. Samec, E. Schindler, and G. Buchbauer. 1994. Functional imaging of effects of fragrances on the human brain after prolonged inhalation. *Chem Senses* 19:359-364.

Nigam, M.C., K.L. Handa, I.C. Nigam, and L. Levi. 1965. Essential oils and their constituents. XXIX. The essential oil of marihuana: composition of the genuine Indian *Cannabis sativa* L. *Canad J Chem* 43:3372-3376.

Offord, E.A., K. Macé, O. Avanti, and A.M.A. Pfeifer. 1997. Mechanisms involved in the chemoprotective effects of rosemary extract studied in human liver and bronchial cells. *Cancer Lett* 114:275-281.

Ohlsson, A., J.E. Lindgren, A. Wahlen, S. Agurell, L.E. Hollister, and H.K. Gillespie. 1980. Plasma Δ9-tetrahydrocannabinol concentrations and clinical effects after oral and intravenous administration and smoking. *Clin Pharmacol Therap* 28:409-416.

Onawunmi, G.O., W.A. Yisak, and E.O. Ogunlana. 1984. Antibacterial constituents in the essential oil of *Cymbopogon citratus* (DC.) Stapf. *J Ethnopharmacol* 12(3): 279-286.

O'Neil, J.D., W.S. Dalton, and R.B. Forney. 1979. The effect of cannabichromene on mean blood pressure, heart rate, and respiration rate responses to tetrahydrocannabinol in the anesthetized rat. *Toxicol Appl Pharmacol* 49:265-270.

Ortiz de Urbina, A.V., M.L. Martin, M.J. Montero, A. Moran, and L. San Roman. 1989. Sedating and antipyretic activity of the essential oil of *Calamintha sylvatica* subsp. *ascendens*. *J Ethnopharmacol* 25(2):165-171.

Paris, R.R., E. Henri, and M. Paris. 1976. Sur les c-flavonoïdes du *Cannabis sativa* L. *Plantes Médicinales et Phytothérapie* 10:144-154.

Parry, E.J. 1918. *The chemistry of essential oils and artificial perfumes.* 2 vols. London: Scott, Greenwood and Son.

Pate, D. 1994. Chemical ecology of cannabis. *J Internat Hemp Assoc* 2:32-37.

Pate, D. 1999. Anandamide structure-activity relationships and mechanisms of action on intraocular pressure in the normotensive rabbit model. Doctoral thesis, University of Kuopio, Finland, 99 pp.

Perry, N., G. Court, N. Bidet, J. Court, and E. Perry. 1996. European herbs with cholinergic activity: Potential in dementia therapy. *Internat J Geriatr Psych* 11: 1063-1069.

Perry, N.S., P.J. Houghton, A. Theobald, P. Jenner, and E.K. Perry. 2000. In-vitro inhibition of human erythrocyte acetylcholinesterase by salvia lavandulaefolia essential oil and constituent terpenes. *J Pharm Pharmacol* 52(7):895-902.

Petitet, F., B. Jeantaud, A. Imperato, and M.C. Dubroeucq. 1998. Complex pharmacology of natural cannabinoids: Evidence for partial agonist activity of Δ^9-tetrahydrocannabinol and antagonist activity of cannabidiol on rat brain cannabinoid receptors. *Life Sci* 63:PL1-PL6.

Pitts, J.E., J.D. Neal, and T.A. Gough. 1992. Some features of Cannabis plants grown in the United Kingdom from seeds of known origin. *J Pharm Pharmacol* 44(12): 947-951.

Poddar, M.K., and W.L. Dewey. 1980. Effects of cannabinoids on catecholamine uptake and release in hypothalamic and striatal synaptosomes. *J Pharmacol Exper Therap* 214:63-67.

Poirier, J., M.C. Delisle, R. Quirion, I. Aubert, M. Farlow, D. Lahiri, S. Hui, P. Bertrand, J. Nalbantoglu, B.M. Gilfix, and S. Gauthier. 1995. Apolipoprotein E4 allele as a predictor of cholinergic deficits and treatment outcome in Alzheimer's disease. *Proc Natl Acad Sci* 92:12260-12264.

Raman, A., U. Weir, and S.F. Bloomfield. 1995. Antimicrobial effects of tea-tree oil and its major components on *Staphylococcus aureus, Staph. epidermidis* and *Propionibacterium acnes. Lett Appl Microbiol* 21(4):242-245.

Rao, V.S.N., A.M.S. Menezes, and G.S.B. Viana. 1990. Effect of myrcene on nociception in mice. *J Pharm Pharmacol* 42:877-878.

Rodríguez de Fonseca, F., P. Rubio, F. Menzaghi, E. Merlo-Pich, J. Rivier, G.F. Koob, and M. Navarro. 1996. Corticotropin-releasing factor (CRF) antagonist (D-Phe[12], Nle[21], CαMeLeu[37]) CRF attenuates the acute actions of the highly potent cannabinoid receptor agonist HU-210 on defensive-withdrawal behavior in rats. *J Pharm Exp Therap* 276:56-64.

Rose, J.E., and F.M. Behm. 1994. Inhalation of vapor from black pepper extract reduces smoking withdrawal symptoms. *Drug Alcohol Dep* 34(3):225-229.

Ross, S.A., and M.A. ElSohly. 1996. The volatile oil composition of fresh and air-dried buds of *Cannabis sativa. J Natl Prod* 59:49-51.

Russo, E.B. 2000. *Handbook of psychotropic herbs: A scientific analysis of herbal remedies for psychiatric conditions.* Binghamton, NY: The Haworth Press, Inc.

Russo, E.B. 2001. Hemp for headache: an in-depth historical and scientific review of cannabis in migraine treatment. *J Cann Therap* 1(2):21-92.

Russo, E., C.M. Macarah, C.L. Todd, R.S. Medora, and K.K. Parker. 2000. Pharmacology of the essential oil of hemp at 5-HT$_{1A}$ and 5-HT$_{2a}$ receptors. Poster at 41st Annual Meeting of the American Society of Pharmacognosy, July 22-26, Seattle, WA.

Salgueiro, J.B., P. Ardenghi, M. Dias, M.B.C. Ferreira, I. Izquierdo, and J.H. Medina. 1997. Anxiolytic natural and synthetic flavonoid ligands of the central benzodiazepine receptor have no effect on memory tasks in rats. *Pharmacol Biochem Behav* 58:887-891.

Santos, F.A., and V.S. Rao. 2000. Antiinflammatory and antinociceptive effects of 1,8-cineole a terpenoid oxide present in many plant essential oils. *Phytother Res* 14(4):240-244.

Sauer, M.A., S.M. Rifka, R.L. Hawks, G.B. Cutler, and D.L. Loriaux. 1983. Marijuana: Interaction with the estrogen receptor. *J Pharm Exper Therap* 224:404-407.

Setzer, W.N., M.C. Setzer, D.M. Moriarity, R.B. Bates, and W.A. Haber. 1999. Biological activity of the essential oil of *Myrcianthes* sp. *nov.* "black fruit" from Monteverde, Costa Rica. *Planta Med* 65(5):468-469.

Shen, M., and S.A. Thayer. 1999. Δ^9-tetrahydrocannabinol acts as a partial agonist to modulate glutamatergic synaptic transmission between rat hippocampal neurons in culture. *Molec Pharmacol* 55:8-13.

Shimizu, E., Y.P. Tang, C. Rampon, and J.Z. Tsien. 2000. NMDA receptor-dependent synaptic reinforcement as a crucial process for memory consolidation. *Science* 290:1170-1173.

Shivers, S.C., C. Newton, H. Friedman, and T.W. Klein. 1994. Δ^9-Tetrahydrocannabinol (THC) modulates IL-1 bioactivity in human monocyte/macrophage cell lines. *Life Sci* 54:1281-1289.

Showalter, V.M., D.R. Compton, B.R. Martin, and M.E. Abood. 1996. Evaluation of binding in a transfected cell line expressing a peripheral cannabinoid receptor (CB2): Identification of cannabinoid receptor subtype selective ligands. *J Pharm Exper Therap* 278:989-999.

Small, E. 1979. *The species problem in cannabis.* Volume 1: *Science.* Ottawa: Corpus Information Services Limited.

Sparacino, C.M., P.A. Hyldburg, and T.J. Hughes. 1990. Chemical and biological analysis of marijuana smoke condensate. *NIDA Res Monogr* 99:121-140.

Tambe, Y., H. Tsujiuchi, G. Honda, Y. Ikeshiro, and S. Tanaka. 1996. Gastric cytoprotection of the nonsteroidal anti-inflammatory sesquiterpene, beta-caryophyllene. *Planta Med* 62(5):469-470.

Tashkin, D.P., S. Reiss, B.J. Shapiro, B. Calvarese, J.L. Olsen, and W. Lodge. 1977. Bronchial effects of aerosolized Δ^9-tetrahydrocannabinol in healthy and asthmatic subjects. *Am Rev Resp Dis* 115:57-65.

Thompson, G.R., H. Rosenkrantz, U.H. Schaeppi, and M.C. Braude. 1973. Comparison of acute oral toxicity of cannabinoids in rats, dogs and monkeys. *Toxicol Appl Pharmacol* 25:363-373.

Tisserand, R., and T. Balacs. 1995. *Essential oil safety: A guide for health care professionals.* Edinburgh: Churchill Livingstone.

Turner, C.E., M.A. Elsohly, and E.G., Boeren. 1980. Constituents of *Cannabis sativa* L. XVII. A review of the natural constituents. *J Nat Prod* 43:169-304.

Veszki, P., G. Verzár-Petri, and S. Mészáros. 1980. Comparative phytochemical study on the cannabinoid composition of the geographical varieties of *Cannabis sativa* L. under the same condition. *Herba Hungarica* 19:95-102.

Vigushin, D.M., G.K. Poon, A. Boddy, J. English, G.W. Halbert, C. Pagonis, M. Jarman, and R.C. Coombes. 1998. Phase I and pharmacokinetic study of D-limonene in patients with advanced cancer. Cancer Research Campaign Phase I/II Clinical Trials Committee. *Cancer Chemother Pharmacol* 42(2):111-117.

Walton, R.P. 1938. *Marihuana, America's new drug problem.* J.B. Lippincott Co., Philadelphia.

Wang, C., and M.S. Kurzer. 1998. Effects of phytoestrogens on DNA synthesis in MCF-7 cells in the presence of estradiol or growth factors. *Nutr Cancer* 31: 90-100.

Wilt, T.J., A. Ishani, G. Stark, R. MacDonald, J. Lau, and C. Mulrow. 1998. Saw palmetto extracts for treatment of benign prostatic hyperplasia: a systematic review. *J Amer Med Assoc* 280(18):1604-1609.

Wirth, P.W., E.S. Watson, M. ElSohly, C.E. Turner, and J.C. Murphy. 1980. Anti-inflammatory properties of cannabichromene. *Life Sci* 26:1991-1995.

Zuardi, A.W., S.L. Morais, F.S. Guimarães, and R. Mechoulam. 1995. Antipsychotic effect of cannabidiol. *J Clin Psychiatr* 56:485-486.

Zuardi, A.W., I. Shirakawa, E. Finkelfarb, and I.G. Karniol. 1982. Action of cannabidiol on the anxiety and other effects produced by Δ^9-THC in normal subjects. *Psychopharmacol* 76:245-250.

UPDATE

Ethan B. Russo

The key contribution of "minor components" to the activity of cannabis has become a topic of more widespread interest over time, while some (Wachtel et al. 2002; Varvel et al. 2005) continue to maintain or imply that THC is "the only game in town."

Recent reviews certainly highlight the medicinal value of cannabidiol (Mechoulam et al. 2002; Parker et al. 2002; Pertwee 2004; Russo 2006). Clinical studies utilizing cannabis extracts including CBD content are accruing rapidly to the body of literature (Carroll et al. 2004; Fox et al. 2004; Teare et al. 2005; Zajicek et al. 2003, 2004; Berman et al. 2004; Brady et al. 2004; Notcutt et al. 2004; Nicholson et al. 2004; Wade et al. 2004, 2005, 2003).

The genetics work of Etienne de Meijer (de Meijer 2004; de Meijer et al. 2003), and Karl Hillig (Hillig 2004a,b; Hillig and Mahlberg 2004) have done a great deal to illuminate the biochemical mysteries of this plant but also highlight how many remain, and how much yet requires elucidation through additional research.

Another exciting discovery surrounds the propyl cannabinoids and the recent finding that tetrahydrocannabivarin (THCV) is a powerful antagonist at CB_1 (Pertwee et al. 2004), making it possible that cannabis extracts of THCV-rich strains may be harnessed to treat obesity, substance dependency, and other ills.

The authors hope to publish additional information on the medicinal effects of phytocannabinoids, cannabis terpenoids, flavonoids, and sterols in due course.

REFERENCES

Berman, J.S., C. Symonds, and R. Birch. 2004. Efficacy of two cannabis based medicinal extracts for relief of central neuropathic pain from brachial plexus avulsion: results of a randomised controlled trial. *Pain* 112 (3):299-306.

Brady, C.M., R. DasGupta, C. Dalton, O.J. Wiseman, K.J. Berkley, and C.J. Fowler. 2004. An open-label pilot study of cannabis based extracts for bladder dysfunction in advanced multiple sclerosis. *Multiple Sclerosis* 10:425-433.

Carroll, C.B., P.G. Bain, L. Teare, X. Liu, C. Joint, C. Wroath, S.G. Parkin, P. Fox, D. Wright, J. Hobart, and J. P. Zajicek. 2004. Cannabis for dyskinesia in Parkinson disease: A randomized double-blind crossover study. *Neurology* 63 (7): 1245-1250.

de Meijer, E. 2004. The breeding of cannabis cultivars for pharmaceutical end uses. In G.W. Guy, B.A. Whittle and P. Robson (eds.), *Medicinal uses of cannabis and cannabinoids* (pp. 55-70). London: Pharmaceutical Press.

de Meijer, E.P., M. Bagatta, A. Carboni, P. Crucitti, V.M. Moliterni, P. Ranalli, and G. Mandolino. 2003. The inheritance of chemical phenotype in *Cannabis sativa* L. *Genetics* 163(1):335-346.

Fox, P., P. G. Bain, S. Glickman, C. Carroll, and J. Zajicek. 2004. The effect of cannabis on tremor in patients with multiple sclerosis. *Neurology* 62 (7):1105-1109.

Hillig, K.W. 2004. A chemotaxonomic analysis of terpenoid variation in *Cannabis. Biochemical Systematics and Ecology* 32:875-891.

Hillig, K.W. 2005. Genetic evidence for speciation in *Cannabis* (Cannabaceae). *Genetic Resources and Crop Evolution* 53:161-180.

Hillig, K.W., and P.G. Mahlberg. 2004. A chemotaxonomic analysis of cannabinoid variation in *Cannabis* (Cannabaceae). *American Journal of Botany* 91(6):966-975.

Mechoulam, R., L.A. Parker, and R. Gallily. 2002. Cannabidiol: An overview of some pharmacological aspects. *J Clin Pharmacol* 42(11 Suppl):11S-19S.

Nicholson, A.N., C. Turner, B.M. Stone, and P.J. Robson. 2004. Effect of delta-9-tetrahydrocannabinol and cannabidiol on nocturnal sleep and early-morning behavior in young adults. *J Clin Psychopharmacol* 24(3):305-313.

Notcutt, W., M. Price, R. Miller, S. Newport, C. Phillips, S. Simmonds, and C. Sansom. 2004. Initial experiences with medicinal extracts of cannabis for chronic pain: Results from 34 "N of 1" studies. *Anaesthesia* 59:440-452.

Parker, L.A., R. Mechoulam, and C. Schlievert. 2002. Cannabidiol, a non-psychoactive component of cannabis and its synthetic dimethylheptyl homolog suppress nausea in an experimental model with rats. *Neuroreport* 13 (5):567-570.

Pertwee, R.G. 2004. The pharmacology and therapeutic potential of cannabidiol. In V. DiMarzo (ed.), *Cannabinoids* (pp. 32-83). Dordrecht, Netherlands: Kluwer Academic Publishers.

Pertwee, R.G., L.A. Stevenson, R.A. Ross, M.R. Price, K.N. Wease, and A. Thomas. 2004. The phytocannabinoid, THCV, potently antagonizes WIN55212-2 and anandamide in the mouse isolated vas deferens. In *Proceedings of the British Pharmacology Society* 21(4): Abstract 1P. British Pharmacology Society.

Russo, E.B., and G.W. Guy. 2006. A tale of two cannabinoids: The therapeutic rationale for combining tetrahydrocannabinol and cannabidiol. *Medical Hypotheses* 60(2):234-246.

Teare, L.J., J.P. Zajicek, D. Wright, and L.J. Priston. 2005. What is the relationship between serum levels of cannabinoids and clinical effects in patients with multiple sclerosis and does it explain the differences between Δ9-tetrahydrocannabinol and whole extract of cannabis? Paper read at Conference on the cannabinoids, June 26, Clearwater, FL.

Varvel, S.A., D.T. Bridgen, Q. Tao, B. Thomas, B. Martin, and A. Lichtman. 2005. {Delta}9-Tetrahydrocannabinol accounts for the antinociceptive, hypothermic, and cataleptic effects of marijuana in mice. *J Pharmacol Exp Ther* 314(1):329-337.

Wachtel, S.R., M.A. ElSohly, R.A. Ross, J. Ambre, and H. de Wit. 2002. Comparison of the subjective effects of delta9-tetrahydrocannabinol and marijuana in humans. *Psychopharmacology* 161:331-339.

Wade, D.T., P. Makela, H. House, C. Bateman, and P.J. Robson. 2006. Long-term use of a cannabis-based medicine in the treatment of spasticity and other symptoms in multiple sclerosis. *Multiple Sclerosis* (in press).

Wade, D.T., P. Makela, P. Robson, H. House, and C. Bateman. 2004. Do cannabis-based medicinal extracts have general or specific effects on symptoms in multiple sclerosis? A double-blind, randomized, placebo-controlled study on 160 patients. *Mult Scler* 10 (4):434-441.

Wade, D.T., P. Robson, H. House, P. Makela, and J. Aram. 2003. A preliminary controlled study to determine whether whole-plant cannabis extracts can improve intractable neurogenic symptoms. *Clinical Rehabilitation* 17:18-26.

Zajicek, J., P. Fox, H. Sanders, D. Wright, J. Vickery, A. Nunn, and A. Thompson. 2003. Cannabinoids for treatment of spasticity and other symptoms related to multiple sclerosis (CAMS study): Multicentre randomised placebo-controlled trial. *Lancet* 362(9395):1517-1526.

Zajicek, J., P. Fox, H. Sanders, D. Wright, J. Vickery, A. Nunn, and A. Thompson. 2004. The cannabinoids in MS study—Final results from 12 months follow-up. *Mult Scler* 10(suppl.):S115.

PART III:
ENDOCANNABINOIDS
AND CANNABINOID RECEPTORS

Chapter 10

The Endocannabinoid System: Can It Contribute to Cannabis Therapeutics?

Vincenzo Di Marzo

THE ENDOCANNABINOID SYSTEM

Research on the mechanism of action of the psychoactive components of *Cannabis sativa,* the cannabinoids, culminated in the early 1990s with the finding of cannabinoid receptors and of their possible endogenous agonists (see Matsuda 1997 and Di Marzo 1998 for reviews) (Figure 10.1). These molecules, together with the proteins that regulate their activity and/or levels, constitute the "endocannabinoid system." The first subtype of cannabinoid receptors, named CB_1, is widely distributed in both nervous and nonnervous tissues, and is responsible for most of the central actions, and also for some of the peripheral ones, of plant and synthetic cannabinoids. The second subtype of cannabinoid receptors, named CB_2, has been found to date in high levels only in immune tissues and cells and may mediate some of the immune-modulatory effects of the cannabinoids, although little direct evidence for this possibility has been found so far. Evidence for CB_2-like receptors in peripheral nerves has been also described (Griffin et al. 1997). The finding of selective CB_1 and, more recently, CB_2 receptor antagonists (Rinaldi-Carmona et al. 1994, 1998; Felder et al. 1998), and the development of cannabinoid receptor knockout mice (Ledent et al. 1999; Zimmer et al. 1999; Buckley et al., 1999) will soon provide a definitive answer as to which of the typical pharmacological actions of cannabinoids are mediated

The work of the author was funded by the Human Frontier Science Program Organization, the INTAS, the MURST and the CNR, and could not have been carried out without the valuable help of Drs. T. Bisogno, L. De Petrocellis and D. Melck.

Handbook of Cannabis Therapeutics

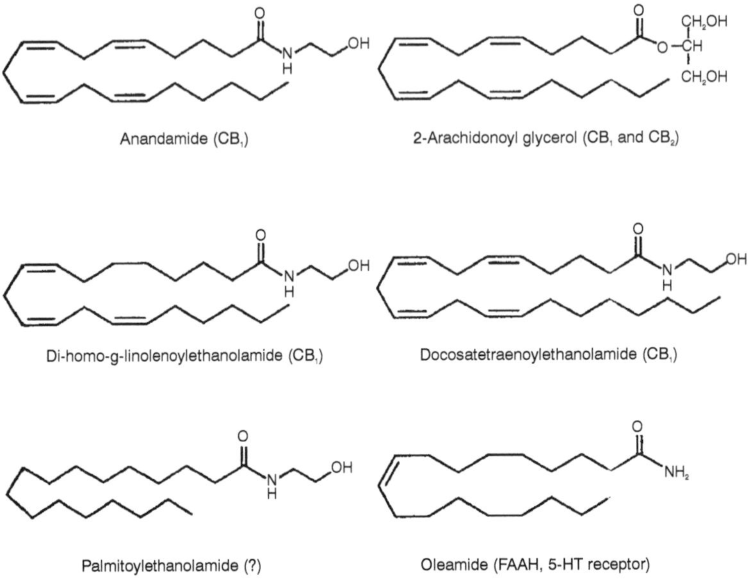

Anandamide (CB₁)

2-Arachidonoyl glycerol (CB₁ and CB₂)

Di-homo-g-linolenoylethanolamide (CB₁)

Docosatetraenoylethanolamide (CB₁)

Palmitoylethanolamide (?)

Oleamide (FAAH, 5-HT receptor)

FIGURE 10.1. Chemical structures and likely molecular targets of the endocannabinoids and other cannabimimetic fatty acid derivatives.

by either receptor subtype, and may even support the hypothetical presence of further molecular targets for these compounds. As to the possible endogenous counterparts of the cannabinoids, over the last seven years several fatty acid derivatives have been found to mimic the properties of Δ^9-tetrahydrocannabinol (THC), cannabis's major psychoactive principle. Not all of these substances, however, have the capability to displace high affinity cannabinoid ligands from selective binding sites in membrane preparations containing the CB_1 or the CB_2 receptor. Anandamide (Devane et al. 1992), the amide of arachidonic acid with ethanolamine, was the first of such compounds to be isolated and received its name from the Sanskrit word for "internal bliss," *ananda*. Next came two polyunsaturated congeners of anandamide (Hanus et al. 1993), and a glycerol ester, 2-arachidonoyl glycerol (2-AG) (Mechoulam et al. 1995; Sugiura et al. 1995). These compounds share the ability to bind to and activate CB_1 and (particularly in the case of 2-AG) CB_2 receptors. Therefore, they induce a series of pharmacological effects in vitro and in vivo that are, to some extent, similar to those exerted by THC (Hillard and Campbell 1997; Di Marzo 1998; Mechoulam et al. 1998). Hence the name "endocannabinoids" was proposed for anandamide and 2-AG. Other fatty acid derivatives (Figure 10.1), such as palmitoylethanolamide and *cis*-9-octadecenoamide (oleamide), do not have high affinity for either of the two cannabinoid receptor subtypes discovered so far, and yet they exhibit pharmacological actions that in some cases are cannabis-like (see Lambert and Di Marzo 1999 for review). The molecular mode of action of these latter compounds that cannot be referred to as endocannabinoids, is currently being debated and is possibly due in part to the modulation of either the action or the metabolism of anandamide and 2-AG (Mechoulam et al. 1997; Lambert and Di Marzo 1999).

The study of the pharmacological properties of the endocannabinoids was not limited to confirm for these compounds the same spectrum of activities previously described for THC. Indeed, qualitative and quantitative differences between the action of classical and endogenous cannabinoids became evident since the first studies on these new metabolites (Hillard and Campbell 1997; Di Marzo 1998; Mechoulam et al. 1998). The chemical structure of anandamide and 2-AG (Figure 10.1), with the presence of hydrolysable amide or ester bonds and of an arachidonate moiety, raises the possibility that these substances may be metabolized to other bioactive compounds through the several oxidizing enzymes of the arachidonate cascade (Burstein et al. 2000). Moreover, the lack of chiral centers contributes to making these molecules capable, in principle, of interaction with many molecular targets. The endocannabinoids, therefore, are ideal templates for the development of new drugs. Three different pieces of information are necessary in order to understand whether an endogenous substance can represent the starting point for the design of therapeutic agents. First, its pharmacological activity in vitro and in vivo needs to be thoroughly assessed. Next, the biochemical bases for the biosynthesis, action and degradation of the substance need to be fully understood. Finally, a correlation between the occurrence of particular physiological and pathological conditions and the levels of this metabolite in tissues must be investigated. In this chapter, I briefly describe the landmarks in these three aspects of the research on endocannabinoids. I also provide a few examples of how endocannabinoid-derived molecules might turn out to be useful in the alleviation and cure not only of those illnesses traditionally treated with cannabis preparations, such as inflammation, nausea, diarrhea, and chronic pain, but also for cancer, mental disorders and immune diseases.

ENDOCANNABINOID PHARMACOLOGY: MORE THAN MEETS THE EYE

As mentioned, anandamide, in some cases, exhibits effects qualitatively and quantitatively different from those of the classical cannabinoids. This may be partly due to the rapid metabolism of this compound both in vitro and in vivo (Deutsch and Chin 1993; Willoughby et al. 1997) but also to the fact that anandamide is a partial agonist in some functional assays of CB_1 and CB_2 activity (Mackie et al. 1993; Breivogel et al. 1998). Moreover, recent studies seem to suggest that this compound is able to adapt to binding sites within other receptors (Hampson et al. 1998; Kimura et al. 1998; Zygmunt et al. 1999). The selective antagonists developed so far for cannabinoid receptors (Rinaldi-Carmona et al. 1994, 1998) have been and still are useful tools to understand when and where anandamide effects are mediated by these proteins. It is still difficult at this stage to distinguish, among these effects, those with a physiological or therapeutic relevance. However, it is possible to speculate based on the range of concentrations necessary to observe a certain effect as compared to the usually low tissue concentrations of anandamide. Thus, in the brain, this metabolite was shown to exert inhibitory actions on learning and memory (Mallet and Beninger 1996; Castellano et al. 1997), to modulate the extra-pyramidal control of motor behavior (Romero et al. 1995) and to protect astrocytes against inflammatory stress (Molina-Holgado et al. 1997). These effects are probably due to the capability of anandamide to induce, via activation of CB_1 receptors, a series of intracellular events resulting in the modulation of neurotransmitter release, action and reuptake (see Di Marzo, Meleck, et al. 1998 for review). This neuromodulatory action may also underlie anandamide regulation of hormone release at the level of the hypothalamus-pituitary-adrenal axis (Fernandez-Ruiz et al. 1997), as well as the antinociceptive effects of the compound through both spinal and supraspinal mechanisms (reviewed by Martin and Lichtman 1998). In peripheral tissues, anandamide regulates the heartbeat and vascular blood pressure and produces vasodilator effects through several possible mechanisms (recently reviewed by Kunos et al. 2000). The endocannabinoid also relaxes smooth muscle in the gastrointestinal system and reproductive/urinary tract (Pertwee and Fernando 1996; Izzo et al. 1999). Regulation of reproduction also occurs at the level of the sperm acrosome reaction (Schuel et al. 1994) and embryo development and implantation (Paria et al. 1995, 1998). As most of these findings were obtained after the development of the CB_1 receptor antagonist SR141716A (Rinaldi-Carmona et al. 1994), it was possible to demonstrate the intermediacy of this receptor in most of the above effects. Conversely, the involvement of CB_2 receptors in the immune-regulatory effects of anandamide is yet to be fully established (for a recent review see Parolaro 1999), probably due to the only very recent availability of a selective antagonist for these receptors, SR144528 (Rinaldi-Carmona et al. 1998). Finally, anandamide was also found to regulate some key cell functions such as cell proliferation and energy metabolism (De Petrocellis et al. 1998; Guzman and Sanchez 1999), but only in the first case by activating CB_1 receptors. As to 2-AG, only a few pharmacological studies have been performed to date on this compound, possibly because of its limited commercial availability until recently. Apart from its activity in the mouse "tetrad" of tests for cannabimimetic compounds (i.e., analgesia in the "hot-plate" or "tail-flick" test, immobility on a ring, hypothermia and inhibition of spontaneous activity in an open field [Mechoulam et al. 1995]), this compound shares with THC an immune-modulatory action (Ouyang et al. 1998) and an inhibitory effect on embryo development (Paria et al. 1998) and breast and prostate cancer cell proliferation (De Petrocellis et al. 1998; Melck et al. 2000). 2-AG also induces calcium transients in neuroblastoma × glioma cells and HL-60 cells (via CB_1 and CB_2 receptors, respectively), an effect that is not efficaciously exerted by anandamide (Sugiura et al. 1999, 2000). Therefore, different pharmacological actions can be observed not only for *endo*cannabinoids and *exo*cannabinoids but also for anandamide and 2-AG.

LEVELS OF ENDOCANNABINOIDS IN TISSUES: PHYSIOLOGY AND PATHOLOGY

Biochemical pathways for anandamide and 2-AG biosynthesis and inactivation by intact cells have been identified (see Hillard and Campbell 1997; Di Marzo 1998; Di Marzo, Melck, et al. 1998 for reviews) (Figure 10.2). Mechanisms for the regulation by both physiological and pathological stimuli of the enzymes involved in these pathways have also been found. On stimulation with calcium ionophores, or other calcium-mobilizing stimuli, anandamide is produced by neurons and leukocytes from the hydrolysis of a membrane phospholipid precursor, *N*-arachidonoyl phosphatidyl ethanolamine (NArPE). The reaction is catalyzed by a phospholipase D specific for NArPE and other homologous phospholipids. Notably, phospholipase D enzymes are known to be subject to regulation by intracellular mediators (e.g., the diacylglycerols). NArPE, in turn, is produced by the transfer of arachidonic acid from the *sn*-1 position of phospholipids onto phosphatidylethanolamine. The enzyme involved in this case is a *trans*-acylase regulated by calcium and cAMP-induced protein phosphorylation. 2-AG is produced in intact neurons from the hydrolysis of diacylglycerols catalyzed by the *sn*-1 selective diacylglycerol lipase. Diacylglycerols serving as 2-AG precursors are in turn formed from the hydrolysis of either phosphatidylinositol or phosphatidic acid. The enzymes catalyzing these two reactions are a phospholipase C and a phosphatidic acid hydrolase, respectively. There is no evidence that these two enzymes are different from enzymes of the same type responsible for the formation of intracellular

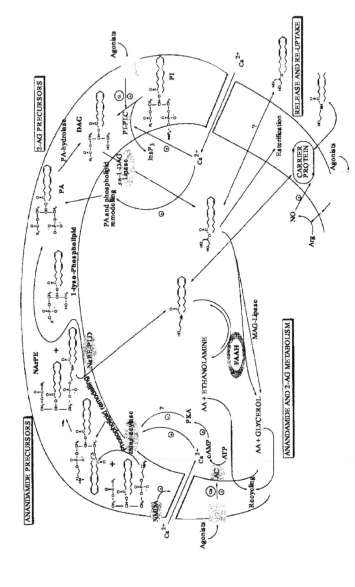

FIGURE 10.2. Schematic representation of endocannabinoid biosynthetic and metabolic pathways described so far in intact cells. (*Source*: Adapted from Di Marzo, Melck, et al., 1998). Abbreviations: NMDA, *N*-Methyl-*D*-Aspartate; NaPE-PLD, *N*-acylphosphatidylethanolamine-selective phospholipase D; PI-PLC, phosphatidylinositol-selective phospholipase C; PA, phospatidic acid; DAG, diacylglycerol; AC, adenylyl cyclase; PKA, protein kinase A; MAG, mono-acylglycerol; NO, nitric oxide; AA, arachidonic acid; FAAH, fatty acid amide hydrolase.

mediators, and therefore it is likely that they are subject to several regulative mechanisms.

Also the routes leading to endocannabinoid degradation are likely to be tightly regulated (Hillard and Campbell 1997; Di Marzo 1998; Di Marzo, Melck, et al. 1998). The major enzyme responsible for anandamide hydrolysis, fatty acid amide hydrolase (FAAH), has been cloned from four species (Cravatt et al. 1996; Giang and Cravatt 1997; Goparaju et al. 1999) and found to contain a proline-rich domain necessary for enzymatic activity (Arreaza and Deutsch, 1999). This domain contains a consensus sequence for recognition by regulatory proteins that may target FAAH to its subcellular location, thereby regulating its activity. FAAH also recognizes as a substrate 2-AG (Goparaju et al. 1998), for which, however, other hydrolytic enzymes have been described. One of these hydrolases, present in rat platelets and macrophages, is down-regulated by lipopolysaccharides (LPS) exposed by bacterial walls (Di Marzo et al. 1999).

As the hydrolytic enzymes responsible for the degradation of endocannabinoids seem to be located in intracellular sites (Giang and Cravatt 1997), the internalization of these compounds is necessary for their degradation to occur. A mechanism for the facilitated diffusion of anandamide across the cell membrane has been identified in several cell types. This "carrier" is temperature-dependent, saturable, quite selective for anandamide and some of its analogues, and sensitive to specific inhibitors (Beltramo et al. 1997; Hillard et al. 1997; Di Marzo, Bi Sogno, et al. 1998a; Melck et al. 1999). More important, the anandamide carrier is activated by nitric oxide (Maccarrone et al. 1998, 2000), a finding that creates the possibility of regulatory loops between the action of some mediators or pathological stimuli and anandamide inactivation.

The observations described above suggest that the levels of pharmacologically active endocannabinoids in tissues may change during a certain physiological or pathological response and, therefore, that substances interfering with anandamide or 2-AG biosynthesis, action and metabolism may be used as therapeutic agents. However, over the last six years, only a few studies have attempted to correlate endocannabinoid levels with particular physiopathological conditions. Pioneering studies have been carried out in peripheral tissues. Anandamide was produced in the highest levels in the mouse uterus when this tissue is least receptive to the embryo (Schmid et al. 1997). This finding and the observation that anandamide inhibits embryo implantation (Paria et al. 1995, 1998) suggest that a defective regulation of endocannabinoid levels in the uterus may underlie early pregnancy failures. If this is proven to be the case, inhibitors of anandamide synthesis, or CB_1 receptor antagonists, could be used to prevent this clinical problem. Formation of 2-AG in platelets and of both 2-AG and anandamide in macrophages was correlated with septic shock-induced hypotension in rats (Varga et al. 1998). In fact, macrophages and platelets from rats treated with LPS were shown to induce CB_1-mediated hypotension in untreated rats. Likewise, macrophages from rats undergoing hemorrhagic shock produce anandamide and induce hypotension in untreated rats in a fashion sensitive to the CB_1 antagonist SR141716A (Wagner et al. 1997). In this case, THC treatment was found to improve the chances of survival of rats after hemorrhagic shock, whereas SR141716A appeared to rescue the animals from septic shock. These data underlie the importance of studies on the endogenous cannabinoid system for the development of alternative therapeutic approaches.

In the brain, anandamide but not 2-AG was found to be released from the dorsal striatum of freely moving rats and shown to counteract the motor-inducing action of the dopamine D2 receptor agonist quinpirole (Giuffrida et al. 1999). This finding is in agreement with data suggesting for anandamide a role in the extrapyramidal control of locomotion, possibly at the level of dopamine action (Romero et al. 1995). A more recent study showed that endocannabinoid levels in the external layer of the globus pallidus are inversely correlated with spontaneous motor activity in the reserpine-treated rat, an animal model of Parkinson's disease (Di Marzo, Hill, et al. 2000). Out of the six brain regions analyzed, only the globus pallidus-an area which receives CB_1-containing GABAergic terminals from the striatum, and where both classical and endogenous cannabinoids potentiate GABA inhibitory action on movement (Wickens and Pertwee 1993)—was found to contain *increased* amounts of 2-AG concomitantly to the akinesia induced by reserpine-mediated catecholamine depletion in the striatum. Both anandamide and 2-AG levels in the globus pallidus were *reduced* concomitantly to the administration to reserpine-treated rats of dopamine receptor agonists and the subsequent partial recovery of motor behavior. Finally, coadministration to rats of quinpirole and the CB_1-antagonist SR141716A almost totally restored normal locomotion. On the other hand, it was also found that the dyskinesia induced in MTPT-treated monkeys after prolonged treatment with L-dopa, a typical consequence of curing Parkinson's disease in humans with this drug, was alleviated by SR141716A (Fox et al. 1999). These studies suggest that agonists and antagonists of CB_1 receptors may be used advantageously in the future for the treatment of parkinsonian patients. Furthermore, these data reveal the existence of a complex regulatory interplay between the dopaminergic and endocannabinoid systems, according to which activation of dopamine receptors may either activate or inhibit endocannabinoid signaling, and endocannabinoids would either counteract or reinforce dopamine action, depending on the brain region and the pathophysiological situation. Indeed, this interplay may occur also at the level of the limbic system and underlie a role of endocannabinoids in the reinforcement of, or the recovery from, the effects of prolonged drug abuse. In fact, a recent study showed that chronic treatment of rats with THC results in the down-regulation of cannabinoid receptor binding and signaling in all brain regions analyzed except for the limbic forebrain, where these two parameters were not altered (Di Marzo, Berrendero, et al. 2000). This region was also the only one exhibiting higher amounts of anandamide with respect to vehicle-treated rats. It is possible that dopamine released in the nucleus accumbens following chronic administration with THC (or more potent drugs of abuse, such as morphine and alcohol) (Tanda et al. 1997) stimulates the formation of anandamide in this region, by analogy to what was previously found for the dorsal striatum (Giuffrida et al. 1999). In any event, this finding may suggest the involvement of the endocannabinoid system in motivation and reward, thus opening the way also to the possibility that drugs derived from anandamide and 2-AG be used in the treatment of depression, and related nervous disturbances.

The finding of anandamide and 2-AG in the hypothalamus of rats (Gonzales et al. 1999) and of CB_1 receptors in some nuclei such as the arcuate nucleus and the medial preoptic area (Fernandez-Ruiz et al. 1997) supports the notion, based on the well-known appetite-stimulating, antiemetic and hypothermic properties of THC, that the endocannabinoid system may be involved in the control of hypothalamic functions. Further studies are now required to understand whether endocannabinoid levels can be associated with hyperphagia or anorexia, and be tuned by the several transmitter systems that intervene in the regulation of food intake.

Finally, a possible correlation between anandamide release from neurons of the periaqueductal grey (PAG), a region of the brainstem, and antinociception was recently described (Walker et al. 1999). Electrical stimulation of the PAG results in CB_1-mediated analgesia and the release of anandamide in microdialysates from this region. Small amounts of the endocannabinoid were released from the PAG also following a nociceptive stimulus such as the injection of formalin into the hindpaw (Walker et al. 1999). The same stimulus does not lead to the local formation of anandamide, 2-AG or palmitoylethanolamide in the hindpaw (Beaulieu et al. 2000). Therefore, it is possible that anti-nociceptive endocannabinoids are formed at a supraspinal level following noxious stimuli. However, it is not clear how the low concentration of anandamide found in PAG microdialysates (~180 pM) can be consistent with the weak analgesic effect observed with this compound following intrathecal, systemic and, particularly, intracerebroventricular administration (Calignano et al., 1998; Martin and Lichtman 1998), or with the high nM concentrations required for this compound to activate CB_1 receptors (Hillard and Campbell 1997).

NEW DRUGS FROM THE ENDOCANNABINOID SYSTEM: CURATIVE OR PALLIATIVE?

From the findings described in the previous sections, it is clear that the discovery of endocannabinoids opens several unprecedented possibilities for the development of new drugs. First, the finding that a novel class of compounds derived from fatty acids and different from classical canna-binoids and aminoalkyl-indoles could activate the cannabinoid receptors stimulated the synthesis of several new endocannabinoid-based com-pounds (see Martin et al. 1999 for a comprehensive review). Some of these compounds (Figure 10.3) are several-fold more potent than anandamide and 2-AG at CB_1 receptors, while others are more resistant to enzymatic hydrolysis and can exert longer-lasting pharmacological actions. Second, when a cause and effect relationship is established between certain patho-logical conditions and the levels of endocannabinoids (measured by sensi-tive analytical techniques as in some of the studies described in the previous section), the application of endocannabinoid-based drugs for the cure of these disorders will be possible. In fact, these studies should provide indis-pensable hints as to what pathological state can be treated with CB_1 and

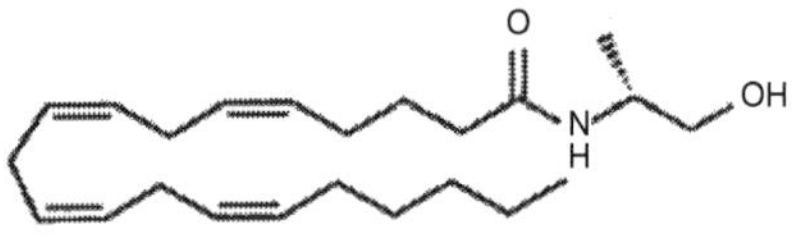

(R)-methanandamide

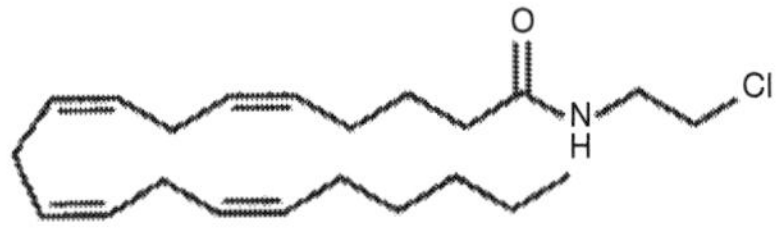

chloro-anandamide

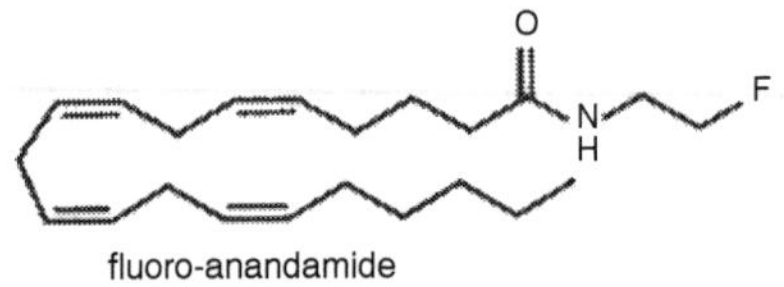

fluoro-anandamide

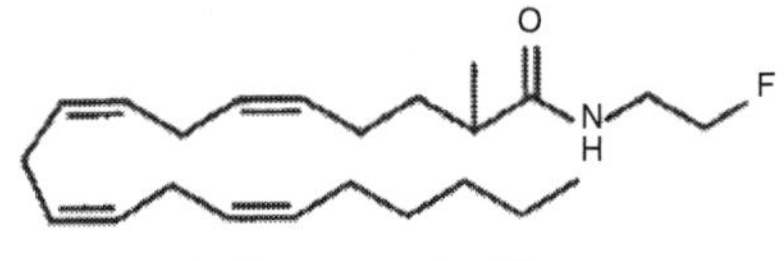

a-methyl-fluoro-anandamide

FIGURE 10.3. Chemical structures of potent synthetic anandamine analogues with high affinity for CB_1 receptors and/or enhanced metabolic stability.

CB_2 agonists or antagonists. Third, our knowledge of the enzymes regulating endocannabinoid levels will allow us to develop selective inhibitors to be used for those disorders for which a correlation with defective endocannabinoid synthesis or inactivation is clearly demonstrated. Indeed, a few such substances are already available, as in the case of the rather selective inhibitors of FAAH and the anandamide carrier shown in Figure 10.4. Some of these compounds, such as AM404 and linvanil (two carrier inhibitors) and AM374 (a FAAH inhibitor), have been shown to lower the concentration threshold for anandamide activity both in vivo and in vitro (Beltramo et al. 1997; Gifford et al. 1999; Maccarrone et al. 2000). These compounds may be useful for those yet-to-be discovered pathological states arising from excessive degradation of endogenous anandamide. Moreover, if ways to target them selectively to peripheral tissues are devised, these compounds may render locally active doses of exogenous anandamide analogues that are devoid of undesired psychotropic activity.

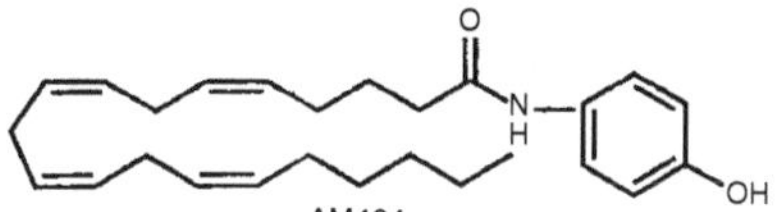

AM404
(Anandamide carrier)

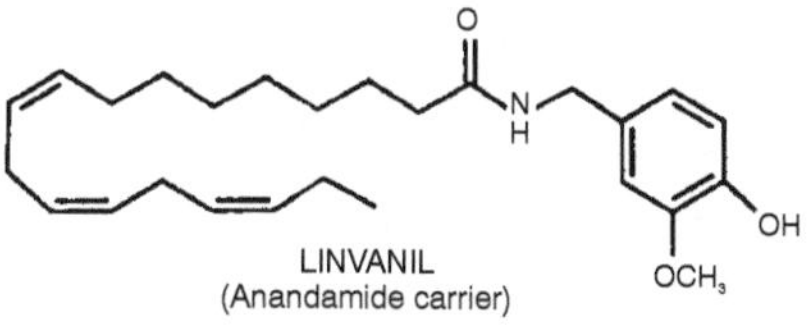

LINVANIL
(Anandamide carrier)

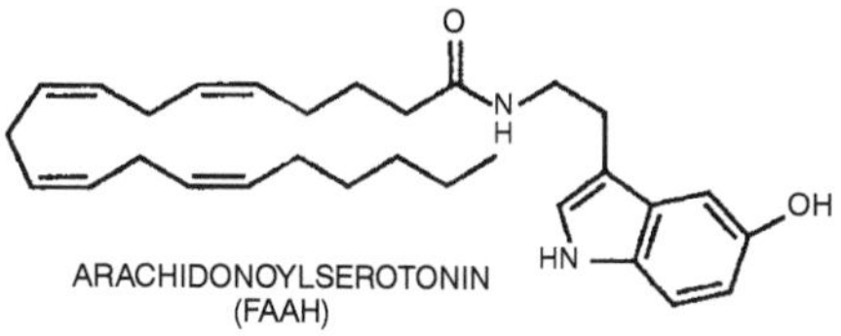

ARACHIDONOYLSEROTONIN
(FAAH)

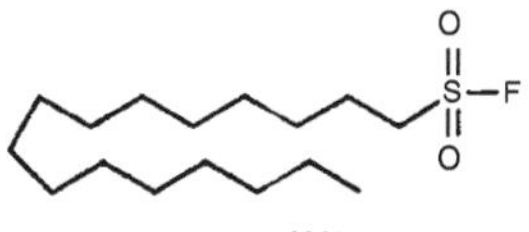

AM374
(FAAH)

FIGURE 10.4. Chemical structures of synthetic inhibitors of anandamide inactivation (i.e., facilitated transport into cells or fatty acid amide hydrolase-catalyzed hydrolysis).

Indeed, the development of new therapeutic agents from the endo-cannabinoids may provide a way out of the social and legal implications arising from the prescription of medical cannabis, at the center of heated de-bates in the United Kingdom and the United States. In fact, given the nu-merous differences found so far between the pharmacological effects of the endogenous compounds and THC, it is likely that endocannabinoid-like drugs may have beneficial effects by simply compensating for possible malfunctions in the endogenous system, without causing the "high" typical of marijuana intoxication. Indeed, a recent study showed that both ananda-mide and its metabolically stable analogue (*R*)-methanandamide (Figure 10.3) do not cause dependence in rats (Aceto et al. 1998).

Finally, one last issue that should be addressed in the future is whether these putative therapeutic agents will be used simply as palliatives, as the history of medicinal cannabis would suggest, or instead as curative drugs. The answer to this question may come from studies attempting to establish a causative role of a defective endocannabinoid system in some disorders such as, for example, those arising from exaggerated or disrupted immune responses (inflammation, allergy, autoimmune diseases), or from the hyper- or hypoactivity of the dopaminergic or other neurotransmitter systems (schizo-phrenia, Tourette's syndrome, anorexia, depression) (Consroe 1998). Were such a causative role to be found, metabolically stable endocannabinoids analogues and/or inhibitors of endocannabinoid degradation may contrib-ute to the cure of these diseases. On the other hand, there may be a case for the use of exogenous endocannabinoids also in the treatment of those pathological states that are not necessarily related to altered endocan-nabinoid levels and action. One example may be the recent finding of anandamide derivatives with potent antiproliferative activity against growth factor-dependent breast and prostate cancer cell proliferation (De Petro-cellis et al. 1998; Melck et al. 2000; Di Marzo, Melck, et al. 2000). One of these compounds, arvanil (Figure 10.5 and [Melck et al. 1999]) is a struc-tural "hybrid" between anandamide and the widely used pharmacological tool capsaicin (the active principle of hot chiles), and exerts also very potent analgesic actions. Last but not least, the capability of endocannabinoids to synergize with opioids and opiates in the treatment of hyperalgesia and chronic pain is being debated (Manzanares et al. 1999).

In conclusion, the road to novel drugs from the endocannabinoid system is still long and unpaved. Although much progress has been done toward the understanding of the chemical bases underlying anandamide molecular rec-ognition by cannabinoid receptors and inactivating proteins, thus leading to new pharmacologically active substances (Figures 10.3 to 10.5), a multi-

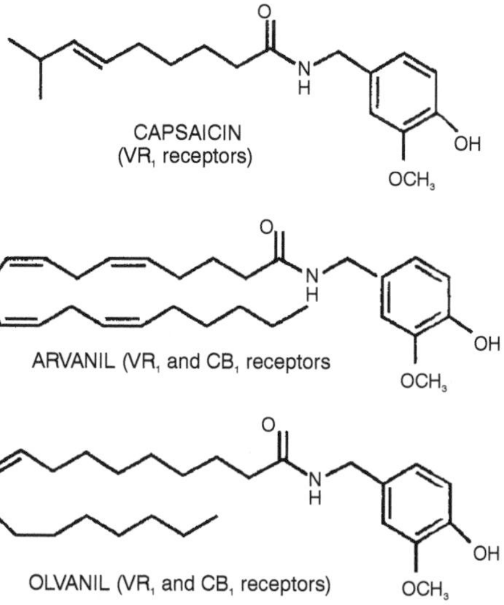

FIGURE 10.5. Chemical structures and properties of cannabinoid-vanilloid "hybrids."

disciplinary effort will be now required from biochemists, physiologists, pharmacologists and clinicians in order to understand whether and for what disorders these new chemicals can be used as therapeutic agents.

REFERENCES

Aceto, M.D., S.M. Scates, R.K. Razdan, and B.R. Martin. 1998. Anandamide, an endogenous cannabinoid, has very low physical dependence potential. *J Pharmacol. Exp Ther* 287:598-605.

Arreaza, G. and D.G. Deutsch. 1999. Deletion of a proline-rich region and a transmembrane domain in fatty acid amide hydrolase. *FEBS Lett* 454:57-60.

Beaulieu, P., T. Bisogno, S. Punwar, W.P. Farquhar-Smith, G. Ambrosino, V. Di Marzo et al. 2000. Role of the endogenous cannabinoid system in the formalin test of persistent pain in the rat, *Eur J Pharmacol,* 396:85-92.

Beltramo, M., N. Stella, A. Calignano, S.Y. Lin, A. Makriyannis, and D. Piomelli. 1997. Functional role of high-affinity anandamide transport, as revealed by selective inhibition. *Science* 277:1094-1097.

Breivogel, C.S., D.E. Selley, and S.R. Childers. 1998. Cannabinoid receptor agonist efficacy for stimulating [35S]GTP-Δ-S binding to rat cerebellar membranes correlates with agonist-induced decreases in GDP affinity. *J Biol Chem* 273:16865-16873.

Buckley, N.E., K.L. McCoy, E. Mezey, T. Bonner, A. Zimmer, C.C. Felder, M. Glass. 2000. Immunomodulation by cannabinoids is absent in mice deficient for the cannabinoid CB (2) receptor. *Eur J Pharmacol* 396:141-149.

Burstein, S.H., R.G. Rossetti, B. Yagen, and R.B. Zurier. 2000. Oxidative metabolism of anandamide. *Prostagl Other Lipid Med* 61(1-2):29-41.

Calignano, A., G. La Rana, A. Giuffrida, and D. Piomelli. 1998. Control of pain initiation by endogenous cannabinoids. *Nature* 394:277-281.

Castellano, C., S. Cabib, A. Palmisano, V. Di Marzo, and S. Puglisi-Allegra. 1997. The effects of anandamide on memory consolidation in mice involve both D1 and D2 dopamine receptors. *Behav Pharmacol* 8:707-712.

Consroe, P. 1998. Brain cannabinoid systems as targets for the therapy of neurological disorders, *Neurobiol Dis* 5:534-551.

Cravatt, B.F., D.K. Giang, S.P. Mayfield, D.L. Boger, R.A. Lerner, and N.B. Gilula. 1996. Molecular characterization of an enzyme that degrades neuromodulatory fatty-acid amides. *Nature* 384:83-87.

De Petrocellis, L., D. Melck, A. Palmisano, T. Bisogno, C. Laezza, M. Bifulco, and V. Di Marzo. 1998. The endogenous cannabinoid anandamide inhibits human breast cancer cell proliferation. *Proc Natl Acad Sci USA* 95:8375-8380.

Deutsch, D.G. and S.A. Chin. 1993. Enzymatic synthesis and degradation of anandamide, a cannabinoid receptor agonist. *Biochem Pharmacol* 46:791-796.

Devane, W.A., L. Hanus, A. Breuer, R.G. Pertwee, L.A. Stevenson, G. Griffin, D. Gibson, A. Mandelbaum, A. Etinger, and R. Mechoulam 1992. Isolation and structure of a brain constituent that binds to the cannabinoid receptor. *Science* 258:1946-1949.

Di Marzo, V. 1998. "Endocannabinoids" and other fatty acid derivatives with cannabimimetic properties: biochemistry and possible physiopathological relevance. *Biochim Biophys Acta* 1392:153-175.

Di Marzo, V., F. Berrendero, T. Bisogno, S. Gonzalez, P. Cavaliere, J. Romero, M. Cebeira, J.M. Ramos, and J.J. Fernandez-Ruiz 2000. Enhancement of anandamide formation in the limbic forebrain and reduction of endocannabinoid contents in the striatum of Δ^9-tetrahydrocannabinol-tolerant rats. *J Neurochem* 74:1627-1635.

Di Marzo, V., T. Bisogno, L. De Petrocellis, D. Melck, P. Orlando, J.A. Wagner et al. 1999. Biosynthesis and inactivation of the endocannabinoid 2-arachidonoyl glycerol in circulating and tumoral macrophages. *Eur J Biochem* 264:258-267.

Di Marzo, V., T. Bisogno, D. Melck, R. Ross, H. Brockie, L. Stevenson et al. 1998. Interactions between synthetic vanilloids and the endogenous cannabinoid system. *FEBS Lett* 436:449-454.

Di Marzo, V., M.P. Hill, T. Bisogno, A.R. Crossman, and M. Brotchie. 2000. Enhanced levels of endogenous cannabinoids in the globus pallidus are associated with a reduction in movement in an animal model of Parkinson's disease. *FASEB J* 14:1432-1438.

Di Marzo, V., D. Melck, T. Bisogno, and L. De Petrocellis. 1998. Endocanna-binoids: Endogenous cannabinoid receptor ligands with neuromodulatory action. *Trends Neurosci* 21:521-528.

Di Marzo, V., D. Melck, L. De Petrocellis, and T. Bisogno. 2000. Cannabimimetic fatty acid derivatives in cancer and inflammation. *Prostaglandins Other Lipid Mediat* 61:43-61.

Felder, C.C., K.E. Joyce, E.M. Briley, M. Glass, K.P. Mackie, K.J. Fahey et al. 1998. LY320135, a novel cannabinoid CB1 receptor antagonist, unmasks coupling of the CB1 receptor to stimulation of cAMP accumulation. *J Pharmacol Exp Ther* 284:291-297.

Fernandez-Ruiz, J.J., R.M. Munoz, J. Romero, M.A. Villanua, A. Makriyannis, and J.A. Ramos. 1997. Time course of the effects of different cannabimimetics on prolactin and gonadotrophin secretion: evidence for the presence of CB1 receptors in hypothalamic structures and their involvement in the effects of canna-bimimetics, *Biochem Pharmacol* 53:1919-1927.

Fox, S.H., M.P. Hill, A.R. Crossman, and J.M. Brotchie. 1999. On the role of endocannabinoids in L-dopa-induced dyskinesia. *Soc Neurosci Abstr* 25:585.17.

Giang, D.K. and B.F. Cravatt. 1997. Molecular characterization of human and mouse fatty acid amide hydrolases. *Proc Natl Acad Sci U S A* 94:2238-2242.

Gifford, A.N., M. Bruneus, S. Lin, A. Goutopoulos, A. Makriyannis, N.D. Volkow et al. 1999. Potentiation of the action of anandamide on hippocampal slices by the fatty acid amide hydrolase inhibitor, palmitylsulphonyl fluoride. *Eur J Pharmacol* 383:9-14.

Giuffrida, A., L.H. Parsons, T.M. Kerr, F. Rodriguez de Fonseca, M. Navarro, and D. Piomelli. 1999. Dopamine activation of endogenous cannabinoid signaling in dorsal striatum. *Nat Neurosci* 2:358-363.

Gonzalez, S., J. Manzanares, F. Berrendero, T. Wenger, J. Corchero, T. Bisogno et al. 1999. Identification of endocannabinoids and cannabinoid CB_1 receptor mRNA in the pituitary gland. *Neuroendocrinology* 70:137-145.

Goparaju, S.K., Y. Kurahashi, H. Suzuki, N. Ueda, and S. Yamamoto. 1999. Anandamide amidohydrolase of porcine brain: cDNA cloning, functional expression and site-directed mutagenesis(1). *Biochim Biophys Acta* 1441:77-84.

Goparaju, S.K., N. Ueda, H. Yamaguchi, and S. Yamamoto. 1998. Anandamide amidohydrolase reacting with 2-arachidonoyl glycerol, another cannabinoid receptor ligand. *FEBS Lett* 422:69-73.

Griffin, G., S.R. Fernando, R.A. Ross, N.G. McKay, M.L. Ashford, D. Shire, J.W. Huffman, S. Yu, J.A. Lainton, and R.G. Pertwee. 1997. Evidence for the presence of CB2-like cannabinoid receptors on peripheral nerve terminals. *Eur J Pharmacol* 339:53-61

Guzman, M. and C. Sanchez. 1999. Effects of cannabinoids on energy metabolism. *Life Sci* 65:657-664.

Hampson, A.J., L.M. Bornheim, M. Scanziani, C.S. Yost, A. T. Gray, B.M. Hansen, D.J. Leonoudakis, and P.E. Bickler 1998. Dual effects of anandamide on NMDA receptor-mediated responses and neurotransmission. *J Neurochem* 70:671-676.

Hanus, L., A. Gopher, S. Almog, and R. Mechoulam. 1993. Two new unsaturated fatty acid ethanolamides in brain that bind to the cannabinoid receptor. *J Med Chem* 36:3032-3034.

Hillard, C.J. and W. B. Campbell. 1997. Biochemistry and pharmacology of arachidonyl ethanolamide, a putative endogenous cannabinoid. *J Lipid Res* 38:2383-2398.

Hillard, C.J., W. S. Edgemond, A. Jarrahian, and W.B. Campbell. 1997. Accumulation of N-arachidonoyl ethanolamine (anandamide) into cerebellar granule cells occurs via facilitated diffusion. *J Neurochem* 69:631-638.

Izzo, A.A., N. Mascolo, R. Capasso, M.P. Germano, R. De Pasquale, and F. Capasso. 1999. Inhibitory effect of cannabinoid agonists on gastric emptying in the rat. *Naunyn Schmiedebergs Arch Pharmacol* 360:221-223.

Kimura, T., T. Ohta, K. Watanabe, H. Yoshimura, and I. Yamamoto. 1998. Anandamide, an endogenous cannabinoid receptor ligand, also interacts with 5-hydroxytryptamine (5-HT) receptor. *Biol Pharm Bull* 21:224-226.

Kunos, G., Z. Járai, K. Varga, J. Liu, L. Wang, and J. Wagner. 2000. Cardiovascular effects of endocannabinoids-The plot thickens. *Prostagl Other Lipid Med* 61(1-2):71-84.

Lambert, D.M. and V. Di Marzo. 1999. The palmitoylethanolamide and oleamide enigmas: are these two fatty acid amides cannabimimetic? *Curr Med Chem* 6:757-773.

Ledent, C., O. Valverde, G. Cossu, F. Petitet, J.F. Aubert, F. Beslot, G.A. Bohme, A. Imperato, T. Pedrazzini, B.P. Roques, G. Vassart, W. Fratta, and M. Parmentier. 1999. Unresponsiveness to cannabinoids and reduced additive effects of opiates in CB1 receptor knockout mice. *Science* 283:401-404.

Maccarrone, M., M. Bari, T. Lorenzon, T. Bisogno, V. Di Marzo, and A. Finazzi-Agrò. 2000. Anandamide uptake by human endothelial cells and its regulation by nitric oxide. *J. Biol. Chem.* 275:13484-13492.

Maccarrone, M., M. van der Stelt, A. Rossi, G.A. Veldink, J.F. Vliegenthart, and A. Finazzi-Agrò. 1998. Anandamide hydrolysis by human cells in culture and brain. *J Biol Chem* 273:32332-32339.

Mackie, K., W.A. Devane, and B. Hille. 1993. Anandamide, an endogenous cannabinoid, inhibits calcium currents as a partial agonist in N18 neuroblastoma cells. *Mol Pharmacol* 44:498-503.

Mallet, P.E. and R.J. Beninger. 1996. The endogenous cannabinoid receptor agonist anandamide impairs memory in rats. *Behav Pharmacol* 7:276-284.

Manzanares, J., J. Corchero, J. Romero, J.J. Fernandez-Ruiz, J.A. Ramos, and J.A. Fuentes. 1999. Pharmacological and biochemical interactions between opioids and cannabinoids. *Trends Pharmacol Sci* 20:287-294.

Martin, B.R. and A.H. Lichtman. 1998. Cannabinoid transmission and pain perception. *Neurobiol Dis* 5:447-461.

Martin, B.R., R. Mechoulam, and R.K. Razdan. 1999. Discovery and characterization of endocannabinoids. *Life Sci* 65:573-595.

Matsuda, L.A. 1997. Molecular aspects of cannabinoid receptors. *Crit Rev Neurobiol* 11:143-166.

Mechoulam, R., S. Ben-Shabat, L. Hanus, M. Ligumsky, N.E. Kaminski, A.R. Schatz et al. 1995. Identification of an endogenous 2-monoglyceride, present in canine gut, that binds to cannabinoid receptors. *Biochem Pharmacol* 50:83-90.

Mechoulam, R., E. Fride, and V. Di Marzo. 1998. Endocannabinoids. *Eur J Pharmacol* 359:1-18.

Mechoulam, R., E. Fride, L. Hanus, T. Sheskin, T. Bisogno, V. Di Marzo et al. 1997. Anandamide may mediate sleep induction. *Nature* 389:25-26.

Melck, D., T. Bisogno, L. De Petrocellis, H.H. Chuang, D. Julius, M. Bifulco et al. 1999. Unsaturated long-chain N-acyl-vanillyl-amides (N-AVAMs): vanilloid receptor ligands that inhibit anandamide-facilitated transport and bind to CB1 cannabinoid receptors. *Biochem Biophys Res Commun* 262:275-284.

Melck, D., L. De Petrocellis, P. Orlando, T. Bisogno, C. Laezza, M. Bifulco, and V. Di Marzo. 2000. Suppression of *trk* and prolactin receptor levels by endocannabinoids leads to inhibition of human breast and prostate cancer cell proliferation. *Endocrinology* 141:118-126.

Molina-Holgado, F., A. Lledo, and C. Guaza, C. 1997. Anandamide suppresses nitric oxide and TNF-alpha responses to Theiler's virus or endotoxin in astrocytes, *Neuroreport* 8:1929-1933.

Ouyang, Y., S.G. Hwang, S.H. Han, and N.E. Kaminski. 1998. Suppression of interleukin-2 by the putative endogenous cannabinoid 2-arachidonyl-glycerol is mediated through down-regulation of the nuclear factor of activated T cells. *Mol Pharmacol* 53:676-683.

Paria, B.C., S.K. Das, and S.K. Dey. 1995. The preimplantation mouse embryo is a target for cannabinoid ligand-receptor signaling. *Proc Natl Acad Sci USA* 92: 9460-9464.

Paria, B.C., W. Ma., D.M. Andrenyak, P.C. Schmid, H.H. Schmid, D.E. Moody, H. Deng, A. Makriyannis, and S.K. Dey. 1998. Effects of cannabinoids on preimplantation mouse embryo development and implantation are mediated by brain-type cannabinoid receptors. *Biol Reprod* 58:1490-1495.

Parolaro, D. 1999. Presence and functional regulation of cannabinoid receptors in immune cells. *Life Sci* 65:637-644.

Pertwee, R.G. and S.R. Fernando. 1996. Evidence for the presence of cannabinoid CB1 receptors in mouse urinary bladder. *Br J Pharmacol* 118:2053-2058.

Rinaldi-Carmona, M., F. Barth, M. Héaulme, D. Shire, B. Calandra, C. Congy, S. Martinez, J. Marvani, G. Neliat, D. Caput et al. 1994. SR 141716A, a potent and selective antagonist of the brain cannabinoid receptor. *FEBS Lett* 350:240-244.

Rinaldi-Carmona, M., F. Barth, J. Millan, J.M. Derocq, P. Casellas, C. Congy, D. Oustrio, M. Sarran, M. Bouaboula, B. Calendra, M. Portier, D. Shire, J.C. Brelier, and G.L. LeFur. 1998. SR 144528, the first potent and selective antagonist of the CB2 cannabinoid receptor. *J Pharmacol Exp Ther* 284:644-650.

Romero, J., R. de Miguel, E. Garcia-Palomero, J.J. Fernandez-Ruiz, and J.A. Ramos. 1995. Time-course of the effects of anandamide, the putative endogenous cannabinoid receptor ligand, on extrapyramidal function. *Brain Res* 694: 223-232.

Schmid, P.C., B.C. Paria, R.J. Krebsbachm, H.H. Schmid, and S.K. Dey. 1997. Changes in anandamide levels in mouse uterus are associated with uterine receptivity for embryo implantation, *Proc Natl Acad Sci USA* 94:4188-4192.

Schuel, H., E. Goldstein, R. Mechoulam, A.M. Zimmerman, and S. Zimmerman. 1994. Anandamide (arachidonylethanolamide), a brain cannabinoid receptor agonist, reduces sperm fertilizing capacity in sea urchins by inhibiting the acrosome reaction. *Proc Natl Acad Sci USA* 91:7678-7682.

Sugiura, T., T. Kodaka, S. Nakane, T. Miyashita, S. Kondo, Y. Suhara, H. Takayama, K. Waku, C. Seki, N. Baba, and Y. Isima. 1999. Evidence that the cannabinoid CB1 receptor is a 2-arachidonoylglycerol receptor. Structure-activity relationship of 2-arachidonoylglycerol, ether-linked analogues, and related compounds. *J Biol Chem* 274:2794-2801.

Sugiura, T., S. Kondo, S. Kishimoto, T. Miyashita, S. Nakane, T. Kodaka, Y. Suhara, H. Takayama, and K. Waku. 2000. Evidence that 2-arachidonoylglycerol but not *N*-palmitoylethanolamine or anandamide is the physiological ligand for the cannabinoid CB2 receptor. *J Biol Chem* 275:605-612.

Sugiura, T., S. Kondo, A. Sukagawa, S. Nakane, A. Shinoda, K. Itoh, A. Yamashita, and K. Waku. 1995. 2-Arachidonoylglycerol: A possible endogenous cannabinoid receptor ligand in brain, *Biochem Biophys Res Commun* 215:89-97.

Tanda, G., F.E. Pontieri, and G. Di Chiara. 1997. Cannabinoid and heroin activation of mesolimbic dopamine transmission by a common mu 1 opioid receptor mechanism, *Science* 276:2048-2050.

Varga, K., J.A. Wagner, D.T. Bridgen, and G. Kunos. 1998. Platelet- and macrophage-derived endogenous cannabinoids are involved in endotoxin-induced hypotension, *FASEB J* 12:1035-1044.

Wagner, J.A., K. Varga, E.F. Ellis, B.A. Rzigalinski, B.R. Martin, and G. Kunos. 1997. Activation of peripheral CB1 cannabinoid receptors in haemorrhagic shock. *Nature* 390:518-521.

Walker, J.M., S.M. Huang, N.M. Strangman, K., Tsou, and M.C. Sanudo-Pena. 1999. Pain modulation by release of the endogenous cannabinoid anandamide. *Proc Natl Acad Sci USA* 96:12198-12203.

Wickens, A.P. and R.G. Pertwee. 1993. Δ^9-tetrahydrocannabinol and anandamide enhance the ability of muscimol to induce catalepsy in the globus pallidus of rats. *Eur J Pharmacol* 250:205-208.

Willoughby, K.A., S.F. Moore, B.R. Martin, and E.F. Ellis. 1997. The biodisposition and metabolism of anandamide in mice. *J Pharmacol Exp Ther* 282:243-247.

Zimmer, A., A.M. Zimmer, A. Hohmann, M. Herkenham, and T. Bonner. 1999. Increased mortality, hypoactivity and hypoalgesia in cannabinoid CB1 receptor knockout mice. *Proc Natl Acad Sci USA* 96:5780-5785.

Zygmunt, P.M., J. Petersson, D.A. Andersson, H. Chuang, M. Sørgard, V. Di Marzo et al. 1999. Vanilloid receptors on sensory nerves mediate the vasodilator action of anandamide. *Nature* 400:452-457.

UPDATE

Ethan B. Russo

The past and present contributions of Vincenzo Di Marzo and his research team are incomparable. Interested readers are requested to search with his name at the PubMed/National Library of Medicine Web site: http://www.ncbi.nlm.nih.gov/entrez/query.fcgi. His recent article (Di Marzo et al. 2004) and book (Di Marzo 2004) are highly recommended supplements to this landmark chapter.

REFERENCES

Di Marzo, V. 2004. *Cannabinoids*. New York: Springer.
Di Marzo, V.D., M. Bifulco, and L.D. Petrocellis. 2004. The endocannabinoid system and its therapeutic exploitation. *Nat Rev Drug Discov* 3 (9):771-784.

Chapter 11

Cannabinoids and Feeding:
The Role of the Endogenous
Cannabinoid System As a Trigger
for Newborn Suckling

Ester Fride

Cannabis is well-known appetite stimulant (Abel 1971; Mattes et al. 1994; Fride 2002b). It is possible that the enhancement of appetite is selective for snack foods (Foltin et al. 1986; Mattes, Shaw, and Engelman 1994). A role of the endocannabinoid system in the primitive invertebrate *Hydra vulgaris* has been demonstrated (De Petrocellis et al. 1999), thus pointing at a very widespread stimulatory role for cannabinoids in feeding. This, for most cannabis users, undesirable "side effect" has been clinically utilized for a number of years to combat a reduction in appetite and consequent weight reduction and wasting, as seen in conditions including AIDS and cancer (Mechoulam et al. 1998). However, few controlled clinical studies have been performed (Bennett and Bennett 1999). In open pilot studies, dronabinol (Δ^9-THC) caused weight gain in the majority of subjects (Plasse et al. 1991). A relatively low dose of dronabinol, 2.5 mg twice daily, enhanced appetite and stabilized body weight in AIDS patients suffering from anorexia (Beal et al. 1997) for at least seven months. In another study on AIDS patients, no weight gain was reported over the course of 12 weeks of dronabinol administration (2.5 mg twice a day), whereas a dose of 750 mg/day of megestrol acetate (a synthetic progestational drug), effected significant weight gain (Timpone et al. 1999). In that study, a high dose of megestrol (with potential adverse effects including dyspnea and hypertension) and a low dose of dronabinol were used. Higher doses of dronabinol

This work was supported in part by a grant from the Danone Research Institute in Israel.

Handbook of Cannabis Therapeutics
doi:10.1300/5741_12

may be more effective, although side effects such as weakness, confusion, memory impairment and anxiety are a concern.

When dronabinol was administered to healthy volunteers, an increase in caloric intake was recorded after twice-daily administrations for three days, when rectal suppositories were used, rather than the oral route (Mattes, Engleman, et al. 1994). When the effects of cannabis smoking by healthy volunteers on the intake of various types of food were compared, a selective increase in snack foods was observed (Foltin et al. 1986). Thus the use of higher doses of cannabinoids as well as different routes of administration, including the rectal (Bennett and Bennett 1999) or the sublingual (Whittle et al. 2001) route, should be further investigated.

Studies in laboratory animals have confirmed the human data and unequivocally shown that cannabinoid 1 (CB_1) receptors mediate cannabinoid-induced increase in food ingestion (Williams and Kirkham 2002), especially of palatable foods (Koch and Matthews 2001). Thus both exogenous cannabinoids (Δ^9-THC) and the endocannabinoid anandamide-induced enhancement of appetite were reversed by the specific CB_1 antagonist SR141716A (Williams et al. 1998; Williams and Kirkham 2002). SR141716A injected by itself reduced appetite and body weight. Whether palatability is required for the antagonist's anorectic effect is controversial (Colombo et al. 1998; Freedland et al. 2000; Arnone et al. 1997). In a chronic study in mice, very low doses of anandamide (0.001 mg/kg) were effective in enhancing food intake (Hao et al. 2000), in according with a stimulatory effect of very low doses of anandamide in a series of cannabimimetic assays (Sulcova et al. 1998).

INTERACTIONS OF THE ENDOCANNABINOID SYSTEM WITH HORMONES REGULATING FOOD INTAKE

CB_1 receptors have been located in the hypothalamus (Herkenham et al. 1991; Mailleux and Vanderhaeghen 1992), a brain structure which is important in weight regulation. Although the precise mechanism by which cannabinoid receptors enhance appetite and food intake is not known, progress has been made in recent years to uncover such mechanisms (Mechoulam and Fride 2001). Thus Arnone et al. (1997) showed that the neuropeptide Y (NPY)-induced increase in sucrose drinking was inhibited by SR141716A, possibly linking this hormone, which is known to enhance food intake (Mechoulam and Fride 2001), to cannabinoid-stimulated appetite.

The hormone leptin is produced by fat tissue and is considered to be a key signal through which the hypothalamus senses the nutritional state of the body and helps maintain weight within a narrow range (Friedman 2000; Schwartz et al. 2000).

Within the hypothalamus, the arcuate nucleus contains neurons with receptors for two appetite-stimulating peptides (neuropeptide Y and agouti-related protein), as well as receptors for two peptides that reduce appetite (α-melanocyte-stimulating hormone and cocaine-and-amphetamine-regulated transcript). Leptin directly suppresses the activity of the two appetite-stimulating peptides, and stimulates the activity of the appetite-reducing ones, thereby decreasing appetite. Other molecules indirectly affected by leptin include melanin-concentrating hormone and a family of neuropeptides called orexins, which enhance appetite, as well as corticotropin- releasing hormone and oxytocin, which cause mice to eat less and to lose weight.

Di Marzo et al. (2001) have demonstrated that the endocannabinoid receptor system is an additional factor in this already complex weight-regulating system. Thus, when they administered leptin, the levels of the endocannabinoids anandamide and 2-arachidonylglycerol in the hypothalamus of normal rats were reduced. Further evidence strengthens the idea that leptin down-regulates endocannabinoids. In a strain of obese rats in which leptin activity is impaired, the levels of endocannabinoids are higher than normal (Di Marzo et al. 2001). The same is true of obese *ob/ob* mice, which have an inherited lack of leptin, and of obese *db/db* mice, which have defective leptin receptors. Endocannabinoid levels are not affected in the cerebellum (which is commonly associated with motor coordination, but not with feeding) in these mice.

Taking the human and animal studies together, the effects of the cannabinoid system on food intake and appetite are significant, representing one of a multitude of players involved in this vital function.

ENDOCANNABINOIDS IN FOOD SUBSTANCES

The discovery of anandamide in chocolate (di Tomaso et al. 1996) raised the possibility that endocannabinoids contribute to the attractiveness of, and perhaps the intense craving for, this desirable food. Indeed, orally administered endocannabinoids (anandamide and 2-AG), albeit in very high doses, induced cannabimimetic effects in mice (Di Marzo et al. 1998). The very low amounts of anandamide found in cocoa powder and even lower concentrations in unfermented cocoa beans would suggest the possibility that the anandamide in chocolate may be an artifact of processing (Di Marzo et al. 1998). Anandamide congeners that do not bind CB_1 receptors, including linoleoyl ethanolamide, oleoyl ethanolamide and oleamide ("sleep factor," Cravatt et al. 1995), all display cannabiminetic effects when applied in vivo, probably by inhibiting the fatty acid amide hydrolase (FAAH) enzyme which breaks down anandamide (see Fride 2002b). Oleamide, when given orally, displayed cannabimimetic effects in mice at doses several magnitudes higher than those present in chocolate, similar to orally administered anandamide (Di Marzo et al. 1998). Taken together, these results suggest that anandamide in chocolate, whether present in cocoa beans or as an artifact of processing, could be responsible for any cannabinoid contribution to "chocolate craving." Future studies, testing anandamide and its congeners in more subtle behavioral assays such as "drug discrimination" or "place preference" designs may shed further light on the putative role for endocannabinoids in the rewarding effects of chocolate.

Interestingly, in the same study, and in a more recent one, relatively high concentrations of the endocannabinoid 2-AG but very low quantities of anandamide were detected in various types of milk (for instance, $8.7 \pm 2.8\,\mu g$ 2-AG/g extracted lipids from "mature" human milk). These concentrations of 2-AG were much higher than those found in other foods such as soybeans, hazelnuts and oatmeal (Di Marzo et al. 1998; Fride, Ginzburg, et al. 2001).

DEVELOPMENTAL ASPECTS
OF THE ENDOCANNABINOID-CB_1 RECEPTOR SYSTEM

Based on the findings described, it is suggested that as 2-AG is found in milk in significant amounts, this endocannabinoid must be of importance for the development of the newborn mammal. Several observations on developmental aspects of the endocannabinoid system in the central nervous system support such a hypothesis.

First, "atypical distribution patterns" of CB_1 receptors (i.e., a transient presence during development in regions where none are found at adulthood) were detected in white matter regions including the corpus callosum and anterior commissure (connecting neuronal pathways between the left and right hemispheres) between gestational day 21 and postnatal day 5, suggesting a role for endocannabinoids in brain development (Romero et al. 1997).

Further, although initial reports studying the development of the cannabinoid receptor system during the first weeks of postnatal life in the rat described a gradual increase in brain CB_1 receptor mRNA (McLaughlin and Abood 1993) and in the density of CB_1 receptors (Belue et al. 1995; Rodriguez de Fonseca et al. 1993), in later studies CB_1 receptor mRNA was also detected from gestational day 11 in the rat (Buckley et al. 1998). Additional studies have uncovered more complex developmental patterns. Thus, whereas the highest levels of mRNA expression of the CB_1 receptor are seen at adulthood in regions such as the caudate-putamen and the cerebellum, other areas such as the cerebral cortex, the hippocampus and the ventromedial hypothalamus display the highest mRNA CB_1 receptor levels on the first postnatal day (Berrendero et al. 1999; Fernandez-Ruiz et al. 2000). Finally, endocannabinoids were also detected from the gestational period in rodents, 2-AG at 1000 fold higher concentrations than anandamide. Interestingly, while anandamide displayed a gradual increase, constant levels of 2-AG were measured throughout development except for a single a peak on the first postnatal day (Berrendero et al. 1999).

Is it therefore possible that the high levels of CB_1 receptor mRNA and 2-AG which have been observed on the first day of life in structures including the hypothalamic ventromedial nucleus (which is associated with feeding behavior) comprise a major stimulus for the first episode of milk suckling in the newborn?

BLOCKADE OF CB_1 RECEPTORS IN NEWBORN MICE

Over the last few years, our group has investigated a role for the endocannabinoid system immediately after birth in mice. Administration of the specific CB_1 receptor antagonist SR141716A to the nursing mother had no effect on maternal weight, pup growth and development, or on maternal behavior (Fride, Ginzburg and Mechoulam, unpublished observations). However, when CB_1 receptors were blocked by SR141716A in one-day-old pups by a single subcutaneous injection of SR141716A, a complete growth arrest and death within the first week of life was observed in virtually all SR141716A-treated pups (Fride, Ginzburg, et al. 2001; Figure 11.1).

This devastating effect of SR141716A on the pups was dose-dependent (between 5-20 mg/kg). Furthermore, for the complete (almost 100 percent mortality) effect to take place, the antagonist had to be injected within the first 24 hours of life. Coadministration of Δ^9-THC almost completely reversed the effect, thus strongly suggesting that the SR141716A-induced effects were CB_1 receptor mediated. Co-administration of the endocannabinoid 2-AG did not reverse the SR141716A-induced mortality, presumably due to its rapid breakdown. However, 2-AG injected together with its "entourage" (fatty acid esters which are always coreleased with 2-AG, but which do not bind CB_1 receptors, and which counteract the breakdown and reuptake of 2-AG; see Ben-Shabat et al. 1998) significantly antagonized the growth-arresting effects of SR141716A on the pups (Figure 11.2). Subsequent experiments designed to further support the specificity of the CB_1 receptor in the mediation of the antagonist-induced pup mortality indicated

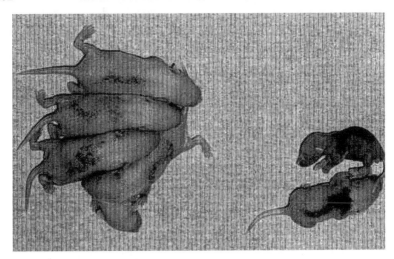

FIGURE 11.1. Five-day-old vehicle-injected (left) and SR141716A-injected (right) mouse pups. Pups, from the same litter, were injected subcutaneous (10 μL/g) within 24 hours after birth with vehicle (ethanol:emulphor:saline = 1:1:18), or SR141716A (20 mg/kg).

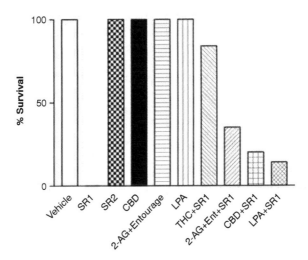

FIGURE 11.2. Summary of survival rates in pups one week after birth after various treatments on day 1 of life. SR1 = SR141716A (20 mg/kg), SR2 = SR144528 (20 mg/kg), CBD = cannabidiol (20 mg/kg), Entourage = palmityl glycerol (5 mg/kg) and lineoyl glycerol (10 mg/kg); these were added to the injection of 2-AG (1 mg/kg). LPA = lysophosphatidic acid (18:1, n-9, 20 mg/kg). All compounds were injected subcutaneously in the neck or flank in volumes of 10 μL/g.

that cannabidiol (CBD), the nonpsychoactive, non-CB_1 receptor-binding cannabinoid, did not reverse the effects of SR141716A (Fride, Ginzburg, et al. 2001; Figure 11.2), while the CB_2 receptor antagonist, SR144528, did not affect pup growth (unpublished observations).

MECHANISMS OF THE CB_1 RECEPTOR BLOCKADE-INDUCED GROWTH-STUNTING EFFECTS

An initial investigation of possible mechanisms involved in sequelae of CB_1 receptor blockade in pups suggested that maternal behavior toward SR141716A-injected pups was not adversely affected. On the contrary, the dams spent significantly more time "licking" and nursing the antagonist-treated pups (Fride, Ginzburg, et al. 2001). Rather, the CB_1 receptor blockade on day 1 of life disables the ability of the newborns to initiate milk suckling, as their stomachs were empty of milk (Fride, Ginzburg, et al. 2001).

More recent evidence for the role of CB_1 receptors in milk suckling is derived from CB_1 receptor-deficient ($CB_1^{-/-}$ knockout) mice, where it was observed that the CB_1 receptor antagonist had significantly less severe effects on the $CB_1^{-/-}$ pups, as compared to the effects on wild type mice (Fride et al., in preparation).

Lysophosphatidic acid (LPA) is a multifunctional lipid mediator with growth factor-like properties. LPA occurs in brain in considerable concentrations and is structurally similar to the endocannabinoid 2-AG. The LPA and CB_1 receptors display substantial (30 percent) homology. LPA, with 2-arachidonic acid as the acyl moiety, differs only by the absence of a phosphate group from 2-AG while a related lysophosphatidic acid (with 1-arachidonic acid as the acyl moiety) has been detected in rat brain (Sugiura et al. 1999). A defective suckling response was reported in neonatal mice that have a targeted deletion of the gene for the LPA receptor (lp_{A1}) (Contos et al. 2000). Our group therefore investigated the possibility that LPA and 2-AG may interact at their receptors. If the inhibition of milk ingestion in our experiments were due to an interaction of the CB_1 antagonist at the LPA receptor, or alternatively, if LPA interacts with the CB_1 receptor, then co-application of LPA with SR141716A on newborn pups should reverse the antagonist inhibition of pup development. This was not the case in our experiments. Thus, when LPA was coinjected with SR141716A, only a temporary delay in mortality, with borderline significance ($p = 0.09$), was observed (Fride, Rosenberg, and Mechoulam 2001). Moreover, LPA did not bind to CB_1 receptors (Hanus and Fride, unpublished observations). Since the LPA employed contained oleic acid as the acyl moiety and not arachidonic acid (which cannot be obtained commercially), further investigation of the interaction between the LPA and CB_1 receptor systems is warranted.

Several neuroactive substances have been implicated in milk suckling. For example, Smotherman and colleagues (Petrov, Varlinskaya, and Smotherman 1998) have demonstrated an inhibition of several components of the suckling response after injection of naloxone into the cerebral ventricles of rat pups. When effects of intracisternal injections of a specific μ opiate receptor antagonist on weight gain were recorded, only a slight, transient reduction was seen; similar injections into the cerebral ventricles did not have any effect on body weight (Petrov, Varlinskaya, Becker, and Smotherman 1998).

Taken together, our studies argue for a critical role for CB_1 receptor activation in milk suckling in the newborn, presumably by 2-AG produced by the neonatal brain. As far as is known, the endocannabinoid-CB_1 receptor system is the first neural system discovered thus far that seems to display complete control over milk ingestion and neonatal survival.

CONCLUSIONS

Our data have indicated that the CB_1 receptor antagonist had to be injected within 24 hours after birth of mouse pups in order to produce a virtual 100 percent mortality effect (injection on day 2 resulted in less than 50 percent mortality). It is proposed that without CB_1 receptor activation by 2-AG (or another as yet undefined endocannabinoid) within the first 24 hours of life, the first suckling episode is not initiated. As the pups have not suckled yet, the source of this 2-AG must be the pup's brain, and not maternal milk. This is compatible with the surge of 2-AG and CB_1 receptor mRNA in the one-day old rat brain (Berrendero et al. 1999; Fernandez-Ruiz et al. 2000). The lower levels of 2-AG and CB_1 receptors present from day 2 onward are apparently too low, or too late, to allow the suckling response to be initiated on subsequent days.

These observations further suggest that the enhancement in appetite and food intake induced by cannabinoids in the adult organism may only be the tip of the iceberg of the vital role for the cannabinoid system in milk suckling immediately after birth (Fride, Ginzburg, et al. 2001). The comparatively more partial control of the endocannabinoid system of appetite and food intake by the mature organism should not diminish our efforts to develop cannabis-based medicines for appetite stimulation in conditions involving cachexia. Rather, it does suggest that treatment of children suffering such conditions may benefit at least as much as adults from cannabinoids to combat anorexia (Fride 2002a). Further, treating infants suffering from a failure to thrive with cannabinoid-derived medicines deserves future research.

REFERENCES

Abel, E.L. 1971. Effects of marihuana on the solution of anagrams, memory and appetite. *Nature* 231(5300):260-261.

Arnone, M., J. Maruani, F. Chaperon, M.H. Thiebot, M. Poncelet, P. Soubrie, and G. Le Fur. 1997. Selective inhibition of sucrose and ethanol intake by SR 141716, an antagonist of central cannabinoid (CB_1) receptors. *Psychopharmacology (Berl)* 132(1):104-106.

Beal, J.E., R. Olson, L. Lefkowitz, L. Laubenstein, P. Bellman, B. Yangco, J.O. Morales, R. Murphy, W. Powderly, T.F. Plasse, et al. 1997. Long-term efficacy and safety of dronabinol for acquired immunodeficiency syndrome-associated anorexia. *J Pain Symptom Manage* 14(1):7-14.

Belue, R.C., A.C. Howlett, T.M. Westlake, and D.E. Hutchings. 1995. The ontogeny of cannabinoid receptors in the brain of postnatal and aging rats. *Neurotoxicol Teratol* 17(1):25-30.

Bennett, W.A., and S.S. Bennett. 1999. Marihuana for AIDS wasting. In G.G. Nahas, K.M. Sutin, D. Harvey, and S. Agurell (eds.), *Marihuana and Medicine* (pp. 717-721).Totowa, NJ: Humana Press.

Ben-Shabat, S., E. Fride, T. Sheskin, T. Tamiri, M.H. Rhee, Z. Vogel, T. Bisogno, L. De Petrocellis, V. Di Marzo, and R. Mechoulam. 1998. An entourage effect: Inactive endogenous fatty acid glycerol esters enhance 2-arachidonoyl-glycerol cannabinoid activity. *Eur J Pharmacol* 353(1):23-31.

Berrendero, F., N. Sepe, J.A. Ramos, V. Di Marzo, and J.J. Fernandez-Ruiz. 1999. Analysis of cannabinoid receptor binding and mRNA expression and endogenous cannabinoid contents in the developing rat brain during late gestation and early postnatal period. *Synapse* 33(3):181-191.

Buckley, N.E., S. Hansson, G. Harta, and E. Mezey. 1998. Expression of the CB_1 and CB_2 receptor messenger RNAs during embryonic development in the rat. *Neuroscience* 82(4):1131-1149.

Colombo, G., R. Agabio, G. Diaz, C. Lobina, R. Reali, and G. L. Gessa. 1998. Appetite suppression and weight loss after the cannabinoid antagonist SR 141716. *Life Sci* 63(8):L113-117.

Contos, J.J., N. Fukushima, J.A. Weiner, D. Kaushal, and J. Chun. 2000. Requirement for the lpA1 lysophosphatidic acid receptor gene in normal suckling behavior. *Proc Natl Acad Sci USA* 97(24):13384-13389.

Cravatt, B.F., O. Prospero-Garcia, G. Siuzdak, N.B. Gilula, S.J. Henriksen, D.L. Boger, and R.A. Lerner. 1995. Chemical characterization of a family of brain lipids that induce sleep. *Science* 268(5216): 1506-1509.

De Petrocellis, L., D. Melck, T. Bisogno, A. Milone, and V. Di Marzo. 1999. Finding of the endocannabinoid signalling system in Hydra, a very primitive organism: Possible role in the feeding response. *Neuroscience* 92(1):377-387.

Di Marzo, V., S.K. Goparaju, L. Wang, J. Liu, S. Batkai, Z. Jarai, F. Fezza, G.I. Miura, R.D. Palmiter, T. Sugiura, and G. Kunos. 2001. Leptin-regulated endocannabinoids are involved in maintaining food intake. *Nature* 410(6830):822-825.

Di Marzo, V., N. Sepe, L. De Petrocellis, A. Berger, G. Crozier, E. Fride, and R. Mechoulam. 1998. Trick or treat from food endocannabinoids? *Nature* 396 (6712):636-637.

di Tomaso, E., M. Beltramo, and D. Piomelli. 1996. Brain cannabinoids in chocolate. *Nature* 382(6593):677-678.

Fernandez-Ruiz, J., F. Berrendero, M.L. Hernandez, and J.A. Ramos. 2000. The endogenous cannabinoid system and brain development. *Trends Neurosci* 23(1): 14-20.

Foltin, R.W., J.V. Brady, and M.W. Fischman. 1986. Behavioral analysis of marijuana effects on food intake in humans. *Pharmacol Biochem Behav* 25(3):577-582.

Freedland, C.S., J.S. Poston, and L.J. Porrino. 2000. Effects of SR141716A, a central cannabinoid receptor antagonist, on food-maintained responding. *Pharmacol Biochem Behav* 67(2):265-270.

Fride, E. 2002a. Cannabinoids and cystic fibrosis: A novel approach to etiology and therapy. *J Cannabis Therapeutics* 2(1):59-71.

Fride, E. 2002b. Endocannabinoids in the central nervous system—An overview. *Prostaglandins, Leukotrienes and Essential Fatty Acids* 66(2-3):221-233.

Fride, E., Y. Ginzburg, A. Breuer, T. Bisogno, V. Di Marzo, and R. Mechoulam. 2001. Critical role of the endogenous cannabinoid system in mouse pup suckling and growth. *Eur J Pharmacol* 419(2-3):207-214.

Fride, E., E. Rosenberg, and R. Mechoulam. 2001. Role of endocannabinoids in newborn food intake and development: Interaction with lysophopspatidic acid? 2001 Symposium on the Cannabinoids, Burlington, Vermont, International Cannabinoid Research Society.

Friedman, J.M. 2000. Obesity in the new millennium. *Nature* 404(6778):632-634.

Hao, S., Y. Avraham, R. Mechoulam, and E.M. Berry. 2000. Low dose anandamide affects food intake, cognitive function, neurotransmitter and corticosterone levels in diet-restricted mice. *Eur J Pharmacol* 392(3):147-156.

Herkenham, M., A.B. Lynn, M.R. Johnson, L.S. Melvin, B.R. de Costa, and K.C. Rice. 1991. Characterization and localization of cannabinoid receptors in rat brain: A quantitative in vitro autoradiographic study. *J Neurosci* 11(2):563-583.

Koch, J.E., and S.M. Matthews. 2001. Delta9-tetrahydrocannabinol stimulates palatable food intake in Lewis rats: Effects of peripheral and central administration. *Nutr Neurosci* 4(3):179-187.

Mailleux, P., and J.J. Vanderhaeghen. 1992. Distribution of neuronal cannabinoid receptor in the adult rat brain: A comparative receptor binding radioautography and in situ hybridization histochemistry. *Neuroscience* 48(3):655-668.

Mattes, R.D., K. Engelman, L.M. Shaw, and M.A. Elsohly. 1994. Cannabinoids and appetite stimulation. *Pharmacol Biochem Behav* 49(1):187-195.

Mattes, R.D., L.M. Shaw, and K. Engelman. 1994. Effects of cannabinoids (marijuana) on taste intensity and hedonic ratings and salivary flow of adults. *Chem Senses* 19(2):125-140.

McLaughlin, C.R., and M.E. Abood. 1993. Developmental expression of cannabinoid receptor mRNA. *Brain Res Dev Brain Res* 76(1):75-78.

Mechoulam, R., and E. Fride. 2001. Physiology. A hunger for cannabinoids. *Nature* 410(6830):763, 765.

Mechoulam, R., L. Hanus, and E. Fride. 1998. Toward cannabinoid drugs—Revisited. *Prog Med Chem* 35:199-243.

Petrov, E.S., E.I. Varlinskaya, L.A. Becker, and W.P. Smotherman. 1998. Endogenous mu opioid systems and suckling in the neonatal rat. *Physiol Behav* 65(3): 591-599.

Petrov, E.S., E.I. Varlinskaya, and W.P. Smotherman. 1998. Endogenous opioids and the first suckling episode in the rat. *Dev Psychobiol* 33(2):175-183.

Plasse, T.F., R.W. Gorter, S.H. Krasnow, M. Lane, K.V. Shepard, and R.G. Wadleigh. 1991. Recent clinical experience with dronabinol. *Pharmacol Biochem Behav* 40(3):695-700.

Rodriguez de Fonseca, F., J.A. Ramos, A. Bonnin, and J.J. Fernandez-Ruiz. 1993. Presence of cannabinoid binding sites in the brain from early postnatal ages. *Neuroreport* 4(2):135-138.

Romero, J., E. Garcia-Palomero, F. Berrendero, L. Garcia-Gil, M.L. Hernandez, J.A. Ramos, and J.J. Fernandez-Ruiz. 1997. Atypical location of cannabinoid receptors in white matter areas during rat brain development. *Synapse* 26(3):317-323.

Schwartz, M.W., S.C. Woods, D. Porte, Jr., R.J. Seeley, and D.G. Baskin. 2000. Central nervous system control of food intake. *Nature* 404(6778):661-671.

Sugiura, T., S. Nakane, S. Kishimoto, K. Waku, Y. Yoshioka, A. Tokumura, and D.J. Hanahan. 1999. Occurrence of lysophosphatidic acid and its alkyl ether-linked analog in rat brain and comparison of their biological activities toward cultured neural cells. *Biochim Biophys Acta* 1440(2-3):194-204.

Sulcova, E., R. Mechoulam, and E. Fride. 1998. Biphasic effects of anandamide. *Pharmacol Biochem Behav* 59(2):347-352.

Timpone, J.G., D.J. Wright, N. Li, M.J. Egorin, M.E. Enama, J. Mayers, and G. Galetto. 1999. The safety and pharmacokinetics of single-agent and combination therapy with megestrol acetate and dronabinol for the treatment of HIV wasting syndrome. In G.G. Nahas, K.M. Sutin, D. Harvey, and S. Agurell (eds.), *Marihuana and Medicine* (pp. 701-710). Totowa, NJ: Humana Press.

Whittle, B.A., G.W. Guy, and P. Robson. 2001. Prospects for new cannabis-based prescription medicines. *J Cannabis Therapeutics* 1(3-4):183-205.

Williams, C.M., and T.C. Kirkham. 2002. Reversal of delta 9-THC hyperphagia by SR141716 and naloxone but not dexfenfluramine. *Pharmacol Biochem Behav* 71(1-2):333-340.

Williams, C.M., P.J. Rogers, and T.C. Kirkham. 1998. Hyperphagia in pre-fed rats following oral delta9-THC. *Physiol Behav* 65(2):343-346.

UPDATE

Ethan B. Russo

This therapeutic area is one of extreme interest at the current time, as it has become increasingly apparent that the endocannabinoid system is one of many regulators/modulators of appetite and feeding behavior throughout the life span.

Dr. Fride has updated her own work (Fride et al. 2005), and an additional current review (Di Marzo and Matias 2005) that advocates the concept of an overactive endocannabinoid system in obesity is most helpful. The drug SR141716A (Rimonabant/Acomplia) is in advanced Phase III clinical trials for the indication of weight loss (Le Fur 2004), but phytocannabinoids such as cannabidiol (CBD)(Pertwee 2004) and tetrahydrocannabivarin (THCV) (Pertwee et al. 2004) may also be clinically applicable.

Further investigation reveals that serum anandamide levels are elevated in anorexia nervosa patients and binge eaters, but not those with bulima-rexia (Monteleone et al. 2005). It is apparent that a great deal of practically useful information of clinical value will result from this research in the near future.

REFERENCES

Di Marzo, V., and I. Matias. 2005. Endocannabinoid control of food intake and energy balance. *Nat Neurosci* 8 (5):585-589.

Fride, E., T. Bregman, and T.C. Kirkham. 2005. Endocannabinoids and food intake: Newborn suckling and appetite regulation in adulthood. *Exp Biol Med (Maywood)* 230 (4):225-234.

Le Fur, G. 2004. Clinical results with Rimonabant in obesity. Paper read at Conference on the Cannabinoids, June 25, Paestum, Italy.

Monteleone, P., I. Matias, V. Martiadis, L. De Petrocellis, M. Maj, and V. Di Marzo. 2005. Blood levels of the endocannabinoid anandamide are increased in anorexia nervosa and in binge-eating disorder, but not in bulimia nervosa. *Neuropsychopharmacology* 30(6):1216-1221.

Pertwee, R.G. 2004. The pharmacology and therapeutic potential of cannabidiol. In V. Di Marzo (ed.), *Cannabinoids* (pp. 32-83). Dordrecht, Netherlands: Kluwer Academic Publishers.

Pertwee, R.G., L.A. Stevenson, R.A. Ross, M.R. Price, K.N. Wease, and A. Thomas. 2004. The phytocannabinoid, THCV, potently antagonizes WIN55212-2 and anandamide in the mouse isolated vas deferens. In *Proceedings of the British Pharmacology Society:* Abstract P1. British Pharmacology Society.

PART IV:
MEDICINAL USES

Chapter 12

Marijuana (Cannabis) As Medicine

Leo E. Hollister

INTRODUCTION

Marijuana has been used medically for millennia and in the United States for over 150 years. It was in the U.S. Pharmacopoeia until 1942 when it was removed because of federal legislation making the drug illegal. The number of potential indications ranged so widely as to rival those of patent medicines of the time (Exhibit 12.1). Like the latter, all the proposed indications were based on anecdote and folklore. A few studies of the medical utility of a material thought to be similar to the active component of marijuana, synhexyl (parahexyl), were made during the 1940s and 1950s (Himmelsbach et al. 1944; Loewe 1946; Stockings 1947; Pond 1948; Parker 1950; Thompson and Proctor 1953). However, it was not until the isolation and synthesis of delta-9-tetrahydrocannabinol (THC) as the active component during the mid 1960s that more formal pharmacologically based studies became possible (Gaoni and Mechoulam 1964; Isbell et al. 1967). Nonetheless, a comparison of synhexl and THC revealed them virtually identical in clinical effects, except that synhexyl was less potent and slower in onset of action (Hollister et al. 1968). Curiously, almost all studies of medical marijuana have employed THC or its homologs rather than smoked marijuana. This oversight has created the current climate of controversy about the medical uses of marijuana.

During the past 25 years, a number of reviews have appeared touching upon the therapeutic aspects of marijuana (Nahas 1973; Bhargava 1978; Zinberg 1979; AMA Council 1980; AMA Council 1981; Ungerleider and Andrysiak 1985; Hollister 1986; Hall et al. 1994; Grinspoon and Bakalar

The author acknowledges Steven C. Markoff who provided valuable assistance in searching the literature.

Handbook of Cannabis Therapeutics
doi:10.1300/5741_13

EXHIBIT 12.1.
Proposed Therapeutic Indications of Marijuana

Antiemetic*	Melancholia
Appetite stimulation*	Neuralgia
Antispasmodic, muscle relaxant*	Antitussive
Analgesic*	Antineoplastic
Bronchodilator*	Antipyretic
Anticonvulsant*	Topical antibiotic
Sedative-hypnotic	Anti-inflammatory
Opiate, alcohol withdrawal	Obsessive-compulsive
Antihypertensive	Dysmenorrhea

*Some suggestive evidence for efficacy.

1995; Voth and Schwartz 1997). As with most issues surrounding use of marijuana, interpretation of the medical literature has been filled with controversy, ranging from those who believed it to be a panacea provided by nature to alleviate the ills of humankind to those who believe that any acceptance of medical use will send the wrong message to young people, for whom marijuana is considered to be a menace and a stepping-stone to the use of more dangerous drugs. This reviewer will try assiduously to avoid bias as well as to place the possible medical uses of marijuana in the context of currently available alternative treatments for the same indication.

The present chapter will focus primarily on clinical studies evaluating proposed medical uses of marijuana published in refereed medical journals. The various indications will be discussed in the order of the amount of evidence currently available to support each. Readers may then form their own opinion regarding the overall quality of the evidence. Medical indications are divided into two categories, those with enough available evidence to merit further study and those for which evidence is so lacking or so poor as to merit little serious further consideration. Most studies will involve THC rather than smoked marijuana. The argument has been made that smoked marijuana, which contains almost 300 chemicals, few of which have been studied, might therefore have superior utility over the pure material. Although a number of cannabinoids have been found in marijuana, most with similar effects to those of THC itself, they are uniformly weaker and far less abundant than THC. Thus, customarily doses of raw marijuana have been calibrated to their THC content (Hollister 1974).

INDICATIONS WITH EVIDENCE
FOR MEDICAL EFFICACY

Antiemetic Action

The antiemetic action of marijuana was not anticipated despite anecdotal reports over the years. The story is that a young patient being treated with chemotherapy for leukemia reported to his oncologists that smoking a marijuana cigarette before and during the chemotherapy ameliorated the nausea and vomiting which is routinely produced. These side effects of cancer chemotherapy are so noxious that patients may refuse life-saving treatment rather than endure them. Over time, repeated experiences of nausea and vomiting may be conditioned so that this adverse effect is evoked by the mere anticipation of a round of chemotherapy.

Although an antiemetic effect of THC had been suggested as early as 1972, the first report of a placebo-controlled trial came in 1975 from one of the top oncology centers in the USA. THC in the form of gelatin capsules, in which the drug was dissolved in sesame seed oil, was given in doses of 15 to 20 mg to 20 patients undergoing cancer chemotherapy. Three doses were given, 2 h before and 2 and 4 h after chemotherapy. Fourteen of the 20 patients in whom an evaluation could be made reported a definite antiemetic effect from the THC, while none was observed from placebo during 22 courses (Sallan et al. 1975).

Another comparison of THC with placebo was made in 15 patients with 11 acting as their own control. Fourteen of the 15 patients given THC obtained more relief of nausea and vomiting than from placebo during a course of high-dose methotrexate chemotherapy (Chang et al. 1979). Best results were obtained when plasma concentrations of THC were more than 12 mg/mL. Such concentrations would ordinarily be expected to produce rather definite mental effects (Hollister et al. 1981).

A larger uncontrolled study was done several years later confirming these results. Fifty-three patients refractory to other treatments were studied in an uncontrolled fashion. Ten had complete control of vomiting when THC was administered before chemotherapy and for 24 h thereafter. Twenty-eight had 50 percent or more reduction in vomiting, and only 15 patients showed no therapeutic effect whatsoever. However, four patients were dropped from the study because of adverse effects (Lucas and Laszlow 1980).

In yet another comparison of THC and placebo, the former treatment was superior, but the side effects were so profound that the patients preferred avoiding treatment. However, doses were far in excess of what might be needed for efficacy, obtaining plasma concentration of 300 ng/mL of THC, several times those required (Kluin-Neleman et al. 1979).

Several studies followed with the next logical step, a comparison of THC with prochlorperazine, which was then the favored antiemetic. One of the first was by the group making the original controlled trial. Doses of 15 mg of THC were compared with 10 mg doses of prochlorperazine in a controlled crossover trial in 84 patients. THC produced complete response in 36 of 79 courses, while prochlorperazine was effective in only 16 of 78 courses. Twenty-five patients received both drugs, of whom 20 preferred THC. Of the 36 courses of THC that resulted in complete antiemetic response, 32 were associated with mental effects characterized as a "high" (Sallan et al. 1978).

Another comparison between THC in 15 mg doses and prochlorperazine in 10 mg doses versus a placebo control was made in 116 patients who received oral doses 3 times a day. The THC regimen was equal to prochlorperazine, and both were superior to placebo. However, many patients who received THC found it unpleasant (Frytak et al. 1979). When THC was compared with prochlorperazine and placebo, the latter two treatments were found to differ, but THC was superior to either one (Orr et al. 1980). A controlled crossover design compared oral doses of THC 7.5 to 12 mg with oral doses of prochlorperazine in 214 patients and concluded that the two treatments were equal (Ungerleider et al. 1982).

Comparisons with other antiemetics have also been made. THC was found to be superior to either prochloperazine or metoclopramide in pediatric cancer patients. An increase in drowsiness, appetite and "high" were reported in patients treated with THC (Ekert et al. 1979). A crossover comparison of THC and haloperidol for treatment of 52 patients with nausea and vomiting from cancer chemotherapy compared oral doses of 10 mg/day of THC with 2 mg/day of haloperidol given alternately in two-week courses. Both drugs were equally effective. Some patients who did not respond to one drug responded to the other. Although no serious side effects were reported, THC toxicity was less well tolerated than that of haloperidol (Neidhart et al. 1981).

An uncontrolled study used 56 patients undergoing cancer chemotherapy that had not responded to standard treatment for prevention of nausea and vomiting. After being allowed four marijuana cigarettes daily during the course of chemotherapy, 78 percent benefited. Young age and previous experience with cannabis were predictors of good response. Sedation and dry mouth were the only side effects (Vinciguerra et al. 1988).

A review of dronabinol (oral THC) cancer chemotherapy patients treated for nausea and vomiting indicated that combination with prochloperazine was more effective than either drug alone. Among 750 courses of therapy with THC, about one-third each of patients had considerable response, partial response or no response. In open studies of appetite stimulation among patients with either cancer or symptomatic HIV infections, doses of 2.5 mg twice daily were effective in stabilizing weight and improving appetite (Plasse et al. 1991).

Although smoked marijuana is often preferred, whether it is superior to orally administered THC has not been tested in controlled comparisons. It may very well be those pharmacokinetic differences between orally administered THC and smoked marijuana might explain the preference for the latter route. Orally administered THC is slow in onset of action though longer in duration. Smoked marijuana produces a THC concentration that mimics the pattern of intravenously administered THC (Agurell et al. 1986). This immediate effect might be perceived by patients as more desirable. For those patients who have this perception, smoked marijuana may be the drug of choice. Smoking marijuana cigarettes, even at street prices, would certainly be less expensive than using conventional antiemetic drugs.

An oral preparation of THC (Marinol, dronabinol) has attained approval for two indications. Nausea and vomiting associated with cancer chemotherapy are still something of a problem with usual anti-nauseants and THC has been shown to be an effective treatment compared with prochlorperazine (Lane et al. 1991). Severe weight loss associated with the wasting syndrome experienced by patients with AIDS is another indication less well established. No comparisons have been made with other possible treatments, either 5-HT_3 receptor antagonists or anabolic steroids, such as testosterone.

A survey that questioned members of the American Society of Clinical Oncology obtained responses from 1,035 members. About 44 percent of the responders told of using illegal marijuana for the treatment of at least one patient and almost one-half would prescribe marijuana were it to be made legal. Respondents also were of the opinion that marijuana itself was more effective than THC or semisynthetic cannabinoids (Doblin and Kleiman 1991).

A later survey of oncologists in 1993 by means of questionnaire obtained replies from 141 physicians. The major question was how they would rank available antiemetics for such use (Schwartz 1994). The four favored drugs were metoclopramide, lorazepam, dexamethasone or other corticosteroids, and prochlorperazine or promethazine. Marijuana or oral THC (dronabinol) was rated sixth in preference. Of those oncologists who had prescribed marijuana or THC for their patients, the drug was considered efficacious in about 50 percent of patients. However, one in four patients complained of bothersome side effects. By the time of the survey, prescriptions for marijuana had declined. Few oncologists reckoned that they would prescribe the drug more frequently were it made legal and freely available. This survey was completed before the availability of 5-HT$_3$ antagonists, such as ondansetron, which would currently be the first choice in treatment. Neither did it consider the efficacy of combinations of antiemetics, which have often surpassed the efficacy of single drugs.

In summary, one can conclude that marijuana, both taken orally as THC or smoked, is effective in controlling nausea and vomiting associated with cancer chemotherapy being comparable in efficacy to some currently used antiemetics. As this indication is already approved for the oral form, and as no evidence indicates that the effects from smoking are qualitatively different, one might accept the use of smoked marijuana for the same indication. The choice of dosage form could then be made based on whether a rapid-acting short-lived effect was preferable to a slow-onset, longer duration of action. One might even imagine scenarios in which both dosage forms might be used together. Although evidence for efficacy of the smoked form is less than optimal, in part due to less opportunity for such studies, it is now at least as convincing as was the evidence for orally administered THC. The admission of smoked marijuana as an acceptable treatment for this specific indication would be justified on the basis of present knowledge and would save both much effort and expense by avoiding the need for their elegant proof of efficacy demanded for drugs with the less well-known efficacy and safety.

Very likely, the major drawback would be the psychoactive effects, which, while sought out by those who use marijuana socially, are unwanted effects when the drug is used therapeutically. This difficulty might be met if one could find a cannabinoid that retained the antiemetic action without causing any mental changes. As isomer of the synthetic cannabinoid, 7-hydroxy-delta-6-tetrahydrocannabinol, is devoid of psychoactivity. Yet, in pigeons treated with the anticancer drug cisplatin, a drug most likely to cause vomiting, it showed antiemetic effects (Feigenbaum et al. 1989). Thus, the goal of separating these effects may be within reach. However, the number of drugs now shown useful for control of vomiting has increased greatly since cannabinoids were first considered as useful. The issue may have become moot, unless such cost considerations prevail more in the future than they have in the past.

Appetite Stimulation

Frequent anecdotal reports by users of cannabis testify to the development of a ravenous appetite with a craving for sweets, especially chocolate. An experimental study, using a standardized chocolate milkshake, tested this idea. Subjects were treated with oral doses of THC 0.5 mk/kg, as well as placebo, alcohol and dextroamphetamine as a negative control. Of 12 fasted subjects, 7 who received THC increased their intake, 2 showed no change and 3 consumed less as compared with placebo. As expected, dextroamphetamine decreased intake. Alcohol, despite the calories provided, produced little change. When 12 subjects were fed before the test, 7 increased food intake, and 5 showed no change. Results were inconstant, both within and between subjects (Hollister 1971).

After 21 days of inpatient marijuana smoking, both body weight gain and caloric consumption were higher in casual and heavy users than in the control subjects (Greenberg et al. 1994). The psychological toxicological effects of chronic administration (0.1-0.34 mg/kg po qid) of THC were studied in cancer patients on in-and-out patient bases. The clinical observations demonstrated that THC slows or reverses weight loss and possesses some antiemetic and analgesic properties (Regelson et al. 1976).

The wasting syndrome associated with AIDS has made the search for drugs that might stimulate appetite more meaningful. THC in the form of dronabinol has been most often studied. An open pilot study of dronabinol in patients with AIDS-associated cachexia showed it effective in increasing weight as well as being well tolerated. Ten men received doses of 2.5 mg three times daily for periods of 4 to 20 weeks. Eight patients gained weight an average of 0.6 kg/month while 2 showed no gain. Initially, patients had been losing weight at the rate of 0.93 kg/month. Increasing the dose to 5 mg three times daily did not enhance weight gain (Plasse et al. 1991).

A randomized double-blind comparison of dronabinol 2.5 mg twice daily with placebo over a 6-week period was completed in 88 patients. Before the study, patients were at least 2.3 kg below their ideal weight. Among the dronobinol-treated patients, the mean weight gain was 0.1 kg from baseline compared with a loss of 0.4 kg among the placebo group. Side effects were not severe enough to merit discontinuation of treatment (Beal et al. 1995). Following the controlled study, patients entered an open study of one year's duration. Doses could vary between 2.5 and 20 mg/day according to response. A weight gain of 2 kg was found in those patients who completed three months of treatment. No evidence of the development of tolerance was noted. Side effects were not a major problem.

A phase 2 study of dronabinol in patients with cancer-associated anorexia and weight loss, revealed that low doses (2.5 mg twice daily after meals) improved appetite. Despite the low dose, 22 percent of patients withdrew from therapy because of side effects (Nelson et al. 1994). In a letter concerning this subject, the authors responded that dronabinol was safe and effective for appetite stimulation during chemotherapy, but that they considered metoclopramide, megestrol and dexamethasone better (Nelson and

Walsh 1995). As the latter drugs are mainly used as antiemetics, one wonders whether whatever weight gain they might have provided was due to that action.

Four studies explored the role of age, gender, satiety state, and route of drug administration and dose on appetite stimulation in normal men. Increased food intake was found only after chronic dosing with rectally administered THC 2.5 mg three times daily for 3 days. Orally administered THC in the same dose did not increase appetite. Nor did inhalation of marijuana smoke. The conclusion was that appetite stimulation from cannabinoids was highly variable (Mattes et al. 1994).

An experimental approach to determine the effect of marijuana smoking on appetite used seven men who were sequestered during observation. A single marijuana cigarette smoked during a period of isolation and work had no effect. However, two to three cigarettes smoked during a period of socialization increased caloric intake. The intake was largely in the form of snacks rather than increased consumption at mealtime (Foltin et al. 1986).

Testosterone enanthate, a long-acting injectable form, given in doses of 200 mg IM every 3 weeks, increased weight gain in AIDS patients, most particularly in the form of increased lean body mass. It should be noted that all these patients showed a low serum testosterone level at baseline, which may limit this beneficial effect to such patients (Grinspoon et al. 1998). Nonetheless, testosterone, other anabolic steroids, and human growth hormone might be reasonable competitors of THC for this indication.

Spasticity

It is said around our hospital if you want to know what marijuana smoke smells like, you should drop by the spinal cord injury ward. Such patients think that marijuana is helpful for relieving the pain and muscle spasm secondary to spinal cord injuries.

Ten patients who admitted using marijuana after spinal cord injury perceived a decrease in pain and spasticity as reported on a questionnaire (Dunn and Davis 1974). Another questionnaire given to 43 patients also with spinal cord injury reported decreased spasticity following marijuana use. Current use was related to past use and to use by peers, suggesting some possible bias in reporting (Hanigan et al. 1986).

The effects of oral THC 35 mg/day on muscle resistance, deep tendon reflexes and spasticity was evaluated in 5 patients with traumatic paraplegia. Two patients showed beneficial effects of THC, two had no real benefit and the fifth withdrew from the study because of the mental side effects (Malec et al. 1982).

A double-blind study was performed comparing 5 mg of THC orally, 50 mg codeine orally, and placebo in a patient with spasticity and pain due to spinal cord injury. The three conditions were applied 18 times each in a randomized and balanced order. THC and codeine both had an analgesic effect in comparison with placebo. Only THC showed a significant beneficial effect on spasticity. In the dosage used, no altered consciousness occurred (Maurer et al. 1990).

An antispastic action of THC was confirmed by the first clinical study. Oral doses of 5 and 10 mg of THC were compared with placebo in patients multiple sclerosis. The 10 mg dose reduced spasticity by clinical measurement (Petro and Ellenberger 1989).

A short-term trial of oral THC in 13 patients with multiple sclerosis and spasticity refractory to standard drugs revealed that a dose of 7.5 mg/day was the minimally effective dose. At this dose, subjective spasticity scores were less for THC than placebo. However, on objective measurements, there were no differences. A dose of 7.5 g/day was also highest tolerated; none of the patients in the trial requested continuation after the blind condition was abandoned (Meinck et al. 1989). A study of one patient with multiple sclerosis and another with spinal cord injury showed that doses of 5 mg/day of THC produced some relief of symptoms. Improvement in a 30-year-old man with multiple sclerosis after smoking a marijuana cigarette was confirmed by electromyography of the flexor muscles of the leg and measurement of hand action tremor (Ungerleider et al. 1987). Administration of oral THC 5 to 10 mg to eight severely disabled multiple sclerosis patients yielded mild subjective improvement in tremor and sense of well being among two patients (Clifford 1983). The overall impression is that THC has some beneficial effect on spasticity, but tolerance to the side effects of the drug may be idiosyncratic.

On the other hand, a group that started with the premise that marijuana would reduce the spasticity of patients with multiple sclerosis and permit better postural control found the opposite. Ten adult patients with that disease were compared with 10 normal volunteers after smoking a marijuana cigarette. Both groups suffered a decrease in posture and balance as measured by a computer-controlled dynamic posturographic platform. No differences were observed between them (Greenberg et al. 1994). The medical treatment of spasticity with drugs such as diazepam, cyclobenzaprine, baclofen and dantrolene leaves much to be desired. In this case, smoking marijuana, which produces a sudden rise of THC levels, might not be the best route of administration. Further studies with oral dosing are required before this indication is written off.

A questionnaire concerning the effects of marijuana in 122 patients with multiple sclerosis revealed a generally beneficial profile of perceived effects. In descending order, the following symptoms were reported as being relieved: spasticity (97 percent), chronic pain in extremities, acute paroxysmal phenomenon, tremor, emotional dysfunction, anorexia/weight loss, fatigue, double vision, sexual, bowel and bladder dysfunction, and visual dimness (30 percent). Thus, we are faced with a substantial conflict between patients' perceptions and objective studies (Consroe et al. 1997).

Cannabidiol, another naturally occurring cannabinoid, was given in doses increasing from 100 to 600 mg/day to five patients with idiopathic dystonias, along with previously administered treatments. Dose-related improvement ranging from 20 percent to 50 percent was noted in all patients. However, in two patients with coexisting Parkinson syndromes, doses of over 300 mg/day exacerbated the hypokinesia and resting tremor, indicating an aggravating action in such patients (Consroe et al. 1986).

Analgesic Effects

Preclinical evidence of an analgesic effect of cannabinoids is strong. THC and the synthetic homologues, nantradol, and nabilone, shared some properties with morphine in the chronic spinal dog model. Latency of the skin twitch reflex was increased, and withdrawal abstinence was suppressed. Naltrexone did not antagonize these actions, suggesting that they are not mediated through opiate receptors which might suggest the eventual combination of opiate and cannabinoids (Gilbert 1981).

Both THC and a synthetic cannabinoid induced an antinociceptive effect in spinally transected rats, indicating a supraspinal mechanism of analgesia. Previously the same investigators had found evidence of a spinal site mediated through spinal alpha-adrenergic receptors (Lichtman and Martin 1991).

There is clinical support for an analgesic action as well. Single oral doses of 10 mg and 20 mg of THC compared with codeine (60 mg and 120 mg) in patients with cancer pain. A 20 mg dose of THC was comparable to both doses of codeine. The 10 mg dose, which was better tolerated, was less effective than either dose of codeine (Noyes et al. 1975). THC given IV in doses of 44 ng/kg to patients undergoing dental extraction produced an analgesic effect, which was less than that achieved from intravenous doses of 157 µg of diazepam. Several of these patients actually preferred placebo to the dose of 22 mg of THC per kg because of anxiety and dysphoria from the latter drug (Raft et al. 1977). Intramuscular levonantradol was compared with placebo in postoperative pain, and a significant analgesic action was confirmed. No dose-response relationship was observed, and the number of side effects from levonantradol was rather high (Jain et al. 1981).

Paradoxically, smoking of material estimated to deliver 12 mg of THC increased sensitivity to an electric shock applied to the skin of normal volunteers (Hill et al. 1974). The apparent paradox is that the biphasic action of THC (initial stimulation followed by sedation) both increases and decreases pain. Traditionally, aspirin-like drugs, which work peripherally by inhibiting the synthesis of prostaglandins, are used to treat pain derived from the integument. The initial mental stimulation from THC might increase sensitivity to this kind of pain. Visceral pain, such as that of cancer patients, is usually treated by opiates having both peripheral and central sites of action. Recent evidence suggests that opiates may act directly on pain pathways in the spinal cord as well as reducing the affective response that accompanies pain. Thus, when the two types of pain are distinguished from each other and viewed in the context of the sequential biphasic action the apparent paradox is solved.

Because THC and other cannabinoids seem to be relatively safe (no deaths from overdose) and produce at best only a mild form of dependence, the notion of producing a synthetic cannabinoid with few other actions than analgesia has stimulated a great deal of interest on the part of various pharmaceutical companies. While it seems unlikely that THC itself will ever be used as an analgesic, synthetics may ultimately fulfill this role. Such drugs might be expected to act primarily on peripheral cannabinoid receptors rather than on those abundant in the CNS.

INDICATIONS WITH SPARSE EVIDENCE OF EFFICACY

Glaucoma

Discovery of the ability of cannabis to lower intraocular pressure (IOP) was more or less fortuitous. Intraocular pressure was measured as part of a multifaceted study of the effects of chronic smoking of large amounts of cannabis. IOP was found to decrease as much as 45 percent in 9 of 11 subjects, 30 min after smoking (Hepler and Frank 1971). Lowered intraocular pressure lasted 4 to 5 h after smoking a single cigarette. Its magnitude was unrelated to the total number of cigarettes smoked. The maximal effect on IOP was produced by the amount of THC absorbed in a single cigarette containing 19 mg of THC. When patients with ocular hypertension or glaucoma were tested, 7 of 11 showed a fall of intraocular pressure of 30 percent. Confirmatory evidence was obtained from a trial in which intravenous injection of THC in doses of 22 µg/kg and 44 µg/kg produced an average fall in IOP of 37 percent, with some decreases as much as 51 percent (Cooler and Gregg 1977).

The effects of intravenously administered cannabinoids on IOP were measured in 12 normal volunteers. Half received intravenous doses of THC, cannabidiol and cannabinol, the other half received doses of delta-8-THC, 11-hydroxy-THC, and 8-beta-hydroxy-delta-9-THC. Total dose of THC and its 11-hydroxy metabolite was 3 mg; delta-8-THC was given in total dose of 6 mg, 8-beta-hydroxy-THC to a total of 9 mg, cannabinol and cannabidiol to total of 20 mg. Significant reductions in IOP were produced by the THC, delta-8-THC, and 11-hydroxy-THC, all of which are psychoactive compounds while the other cannabinoids had little or no such activity. Thus, it seemed impossible to separate mental effects, which were considerable for the effective drugs, from lowering of IOP (Perez-Reyes et al. 1976).

Orally administered THC (20 or 25 mg) lowered IOP about 8 mm Hg among 17 patients with heterologous glaucomas. No such lowering was found in patients who received only 5 or 10 mg doses. All patients who received the higher doses experienced severe mental effects. One patient, who received only a 5 mg dose, experienced severe tachycardia and orthostatic hypotension (Merritt, Crawford, et al. 1980).

Similar findings were reported from the same group after having 16 patients smoke marijuana cigarettes weighing 900 mg (amount of THC unspecified). Compared with placebo, IOP was lowered for 3-4 hours following the smoke. However, rapid heart rate and lowering of blood pressure which preceded this action were quite large and would not be tolerated by many patients among the age group who suffer glaucoma (Merritt, McKinnon, et al. 1980).

As treatment for glaucoma is a lifetime proposition, systemic therapy has never been seriously considered. Topical therapy, properly used, has been generally satisfactory. Unfortunately, attempts to make a tolerable topical preparation of THC or other cannabinoids have been impossible to date. One hears tales of patients with glaucoma whose vision is spared only by smoking marijuana cigarettes; remarkably, no case reports, along with objective measurements, even of a few such patients, have appeared. As glaucoma occurs most often in older patients, one has difficulty imagining such patients embracing a lifetime of possible marijuana intoxication. This possible indication has elicited no literature during the past 12 years.

Anticonvulsant

One of the therapeutic uses suggested for cannabis was as an anticonvulsant. Such an effect was documented experimentally many years ago (Loewe and Goodman 1947). Studies in various animal species have shown cannabidiol effective in many animal-screening tests for anticonvulsants (Wada et al. 1973; Turkanis et al. 1974).

Clinical testing has been rare, despite all these various lines of evidence supporting an anticonvulsant effect of cannabinoids. Better control of seizures following regular marijuana smoking was reported in a not very convincing single case (Consroe et al. 1975).

Cannabidiol (CBD), a non-psychoactive cannabinoid, was tested in 15 epileptic patients poorly controlled by usual drugs. Patients were randomly assigned to a dose of 300 mg of CBD or placebo and treated for as long as 4½ months, while continuing their past anticonvulsant drugs. Of eight CBD-treated patients, four remained free of seizures, three showed partial improvements and one showed no response. Of seven placebo-treated patients, only one showed improvement. The drug was well tolerated (Cunha et al. 1980). As cannabidiol has little if any psychoactivity, it is a good candidate for this use.

The number of effective anticonvulsants has increased since the original interest in cannabidiol. Consequently, no further clinical studies have been reported.

Bronchial Asthma

A general study of the effects of marijuana on respiration revealed a bronchodilating action in normal volunteer subjects. Marijuana smoke delivered by smoking cigarettes containing 2.6 percent THC caused fall of 38 percent in airway resistance and an increase of 44 percent in airway conductance, with less change when a 1 percent THC cigarette was smoked. The low-dose group showed lesser changes, but they were still significant as compared with baseline (Vachon et al. 1973).

Asthma was deliberately induced by either inhalation or methacholine or exercise in asthmatic patients. They were then treated with inhalation of placebo marijuana, of saline, of isoproterenol, or of smoke derived from 500 mg of marijuana containing 2 percent THC. Both marijuana smoke and isoproterenol aerosol effectively reversed both methacholine- and exercise-induced asthma while saline and placebo marijuana had no effect (Tashkin et al. 1975).

Aerosols of placebo-ethanol, THC (200 µg) in ethanol, or of salbutamol (100 µg) were tested in another study of 10 stable asthmatic patients. Forced expiratory volume in 1 s, forced vital capacity, and peak flow rates were measured on each occasion. Both salbutamol and THC significantly improved ventilatory function. Improvement was more rapid with salbutamol, but two treatments were equally effective at the end of 1 h (Williams et al. 1972).

While it is conceivable that an aerosol preparation could be made, those currently used (corticosteroids and beta-adrenergic agonists) are well established. Although treatment of asthma in the past has employed smoked drugs (stramonium [*Datura* spp.] cigarettes known as cubebs were used until 60 to 70 years ago), it seems intuitively wrong to treat a pulmonary condition with a method of drug administration that increases inflammation. As treatment of bronchial asthma has shifted toward emphasis on alleviating the inflammatory aspects, there is little support for using smoked marijuana. Consequently, interest in the indication is currently nonexistent.

Insomnia

THC does not differ from conventional hypnotics in reducing rapid eye movement (REM) sleep (Pivik et al. 1972). THC in doses ranging from 61 to 258 µg/kg produces in normal subjects increments in stage four sleep and decrements in REM sleep, but without the characteristic REM rebound which follows chronic treatment with an hypnotic. When THC was administered orally as a hydroalcoholic solution in doses of 10, 20 and 30 mg, subjects fell asleep faster after having mood alterations consistent with a "high." Some degree of "hangover" the day following was noted from larger doses (Cousens and Dimascio 1973). Another sleep laboratory study showed that a dose of 2 mg of THC given orally decreased REM sleep. After four to six nights of use, abrupt discontinuation of THC produced a mild insomnia but not marked REM rebound (Freemon 1974). REM rebound may not be apparent after low doses of THC; however, very high doses (70 to 210 mg) reduced REM sleep during treatment and were followed by marked REM rebound after withdrawal (Feinberg et al. 1976). The sleep produced by THC does not seem to differ much from that of most currently used hypnotics. Side effects before sleep induction as well as hangover effects make the drug less acceptable than currently popular benzodiazepines. No further studies have been reported.

Early on, synthetic cannabinoids were tried as antianxiety and antidepressant drugs. Diazepam 5 mg was superior to the synthetic cannabinoid nabilone 2 mg for treating experimentally induced anxiety in highly anxious people. Thus, even aside from the marijuana-like effects of nabilone, it was not acceptable (Nakano et al. 1978). Following a favorable report from use of synexyl for treatment of depression, a further study found it to be of no benefit (Parker 1950). Again, cannabinoid-like drugs were of little use in these psychiatric conditions. Nor has there been any attempt to exploit them in this fashion over the succeeding decades.

DISCUSSION

Among the many possible therapeutic uses of marijuana, a few have enough supporting evidence to justify further studies. Greatest support has been elicited for using the drug, mainly in the form of orally administered THC, for the control of nausea and vomiting. This use has been further legalized by the switch of synthetic oral THC to Schedule III of the Controlled Substances Act. Capsules (Marinol or dronabinol) containing THC dissolved in oil have been marketed for this purpose. Demand for such preparations has not been great, however, probably because of the reluctance of physicians to prescribe a drug that so recently was considered illegal and possibly also to the fact that many other antiemetics have been developed during the past decade which obviate the mental side effects of THC. The remaining issue is whether smoked marijuana might be superior, as such administration permits rapid and close titration of dose. This issue has not been resolved and would take a large, expensive clinical trial to settle. Thus far, no support has been offered for such a trial.

As appetite stimulants are not very effective, this possible action of marijuana is certainly worth consideration. Data suggest that stimulation is inconstant and mild. All of the studies have involved oral THC, which would seem to be the most appropriate route for this purpose, its slower but more prolonged duration of action being consonant with the aims of treatment. Anabolic steroids offer another approach to this indication. Comparisons between these and THC would be required.

Available medications to relieve muscle spasticity are generally somewhat disappointing. Whether the few reports of benefit from marijuana improve the situation is questionable. The incoordinating effects of this drug might aggravate the underlying neurological condition.

Development of cannabinoids as analgesics is attractive, but it seems obvious that neither oral THC nor smoked marijuana is the best approach. If synthetic cannabinoids could be developed which retain the analgesic action but minimize the mental effects, this indication would be more promising.

Other potential medical uses, such as treatment for glaucoma, asthma, seizures and insomnia or anxiety, not only have very little experimental support but also would seem adequately treated with existing drugs. During the past dozen years, little interest in exploring these is apparent in the medical literature.

A major unresolved issue is the comparison between orally administered THC and smoked marijuana. Many users aver that smoke marijuana may have active ingredients other than THC, as perhaps 300 or so chemicals are present in the plant or in the smoke. As few of these have ever been studied alone (nor will they be), the argument cannot be settled directly. On the other hand, except for some THC-like structures, which are present in marijuana in much smaller amounts, and with far less potency than that of THC, no other active material has been found. Thus, it appears unlikely that some panacea is being missed. As for the kinetic advantages of smoking, immediate effects might be desirable for situations in which immediate action is preferable; most drugs are used for longer-lived conditions in which sustained effects are more essential.

CONCLUSION

It is surprising that more than 35 years after the synthesis of THC, and the resulting capability of clinical pharmacological studies, little published literature has tested various potential therapeutic uses of the drug. Earliest studies were more concerned with the actions of the drug on various organ systems and were not concerned with therapeutic actions. For part of the past 15 years, an increasing literature explored this aspect but has recently dropped off. Therapeutic use has become entwined with the political and legal moves that have polarized investigators. The consequence is that legal steps have been taken which are poorly supported by medical evidence.

For those of us who like to have new treatments accepted on the basis of evidence rather than plebiscite, it has been a discouraging period. The solutions proposed by the recent Institute of Medicine report would seem to be even more discouraging than those which were obtained before. In view of the fact that marijuana and its constituents may be among the safest materials one can be exposed to, it would seem reasonable to make its testing less, rather than more difficult.

Meanwhile, we must ponder the question, "Are we missing a therapeutic advance or is the lore of the past only folklore that has no place in modern science?" Innovation is desperately needed if we are to settle the question before all chances for proper appraisals are lost.

REFERENCES

Agurell S., H. Halldin, JE. Lindgren, A. Ohlsson, M. Widman, H. Gillespie and LE. Hollister. 1986. Pharmacokinetics and metabolism of delta-1-tetrahydrocannabinol and other cannabinoids with emphasis on man. *Pharmacological Rev* 38:21-43.

AMA Council on Scientific Affairs. 1980. Marihuana reconsidered: Pulmonary risks and therapeutic potentials. *Conn Med* 44:521-523.

AMA Council on Scientific Affairs. 1981. Marijuana. Its health hazards and therapeutic potentials. *J Amer Med Assoc* 248:1823-1827.

Beal J.E., R. Olson, L. Laubenstein, J.O. Morales, P. Bellamen, B. Yangco. 1995. Dronabinol as a treatment for anorexia associated with weight loss in patients with AIDS. *J Pain Symptom Manage* 10:89-97.

Bhargava H.N. 1978. Potential therapeutic application of naturally occurring and synthetic cannabinoids. *General Pharmacol* 9:195-213.

Chang, A.E., D.J. Shiling, R.C. Stillman, N. Goldberg, C. Seipp, Z. Barofsky, P. Simon, and S. Rosenberg. 1979. Delta-9-tetrahydrocannabinol as antiemetic in cancer patients receiving high-dose methotrexate: A prospective, randomized evaluation. *Ann Int Med* 91:819-824.

Clifford, D.B. 1983. Tetrahydrocannabinol for tremor in multiple sclerosis. *Annals Neurol* 13(6), 669-671.

Consroe, P., R. Musty, J. Rein, W. Tillery and R. Pertwee. 1997. The perceived effects of smoked cannabis on patients with multiple sclerosis. *European Neurology* 38(1):44-48.

Consroe, P., R. Sandyk and S.R. Snider. 1986. Open label evaluation of cannabidiol in dystonic movement disorder. *Intern J Neuroscience* 30:277-282.

Consroe, P., G.C. Wood and H. Buchsbaum. 1975. Anticonvulsant effect of marihuana smoking. *J Amer Med Assoc* 234:306-307.

Cooler, P. and J.M. Gregg. 1977. Effect of delta-9-tetrahydrocannabinol on intraocular pressure in humans. *South Med J* 70:951-954.

Cousens, K. and A. Dimascio. 1973. Delta-9-THC as an hypnotic. An experimental study of 3 dose levels. *Psychopharmacologia* 33:355-364.

Cunha, J.M., E.A. Carlini, A.E. Periera, O.L. Ramos, C. Pimental, R. Gagliardi, W.L. Snavito, N. Lander and R. Mechoulam. 1980. Chronic administration of cannabidiol to healthy volunteers and epileptic patients. *Pharmacology* 21: 175-185.

Doblin, R.E. and M.A.R. Kleiman. 1991. Marijuana as antiemetic medicine: A survey of oncologist's experiences and attitudes. *J Clin Oncol* 313-319.

Dunn, M. and R. Davis. 1974. The perceived effects of marijuana on spinal cord injured males. *Paraplegia* 12(3):175-178.

Ekert, H., K.D. Waters, I.A. Julik, J. Mobina and P. Lougnnan. 1979. Amelioration of cancer chemotherapy-induced nausea and vomiting by delta-9-tetrahydrocannabinol. *Med J Aust* 2:657-659.

Feigenbaum, J.J., S.A. Richmond, Y. Wiessman and R. Mechoulam. 1989. Inhibition of cisplatin-induced emesis in the pigeon by a non-psychotropic synthetic cannabinoid. *European J Pharmacol* 169:159-165.

Feinberg, I., R. Jones, J. Walker, C. Caveness and E. Floyd. 1976. Effects of marijuana extract and tetrahydrocannabinol on electroencephalographic sleep patterns. *Clin Pharmacol Ther* 19:782-794.

Foltin, R.W., J.V. Brady and M. Fischman. 1986. Behavioral analysis of marijuana effect on food intake in normals. *Pharmacology Biochemistry Behavior* 25:573-582.

Freemon, F.R. 1974. The effect of delta-9-tetrahydrocannabinol on sleep. *Psychopharmacology* 35:39-44.

Frytak, S., C. Moertel, J. O'Fallon, J. Rubin, E. Creagan, M. O'Nell, A. Schutt and N. Schwarau. 1979. Delta-9-tetrahydrocannabinol as an antiemetic for patients receiving cancer chemotherapy. *Ann Int Med* 91:825-830.

Gaoni, Y. and R. Mechoulam. 1964. Isolation, structure and partial synthesis of an active constituent of hashish. *J Am Chem Soc* 86: 646-648.

Gilbert, P.E. 1981. A comparison of THC, nantradol, nabilone and morphine on chronic spinal dog. *J Clin Pharmacol* 21:311S-319S.

Greenberg, H.S., S.A. Werness, J.E. Pugh, R.O. Andrus, D.J. Anderson and E.F. Domino. 1994. Short-term effects of smoking marihuana on balance in patients with multiple sclerosis and normal volunteers. *Clin Pharm Ther* 55: 324-328.

Grinspoon, S., C. Corcoran, H. Askari, D. Schoenfeld, L. Wolf, B. Burrows, M. Walsh, D. Hayden, K. Parlman, E. Anderson, N. Basgoz, and A. Klibanski. 1998. Effects of androgen administration in men with the AIDS wasting syndrome. A randomized, double-blind, placebo-controlled trial. *Ann Intern Med* 129(1):18-26.

Hanigan, W.C., R. Destree, and X.T. Truong. 1986. The effect of delta-9-THC on human spasticity. *J Amer Soc Clin Pharmacol Therap* 39(Feb.):198.

Hepler, R.S., and I.R. Frank. 1971. Marihuana smoking and intraocular presssure. *J Amer Med Assoc* 217(10):1392.

Hill, S.Y., R. Schwin, D.W. Goodwin, and B.J. Powell. 1974. Marihuana and pain. *J Pharmacol Exp Ther* 188(2):415-418.

Himmelsbach, C.K. 1944. Treatment of the morphine-abstinence syndrome with a synthetic cannabis-like compound. Southern M J 37:26-29.

Hollister, L.E. 1971. Hunger and appetite after single doses of marihuana, alcohol and dextroamphetamine. *Clin Pharmacol Ther* 12:44-49.

Hollister, L.E. 1974. Structure activity relationship in man of cannabis constituents and homologues of delta-9-tetrahydrocannabinol. *Pharmacology* 11:3-11.

Hollister, L.E. 1986. Health aspects of cannabis. *Pharmacol Rev* 6:38:2-20.

Hollister, L.E., H.K. Gillespie, A. Ohlsson, J.E. Lindgren, A. Whalen and S. Agurell. 1981. Do plasma concentrations of delta-9-hydrocannabinol reflect the degree of intoxication? *J Clin Pharmacol* 21: 171S-177S.

Hollister, L.E., R.K. Richards and H.K. Gillespie. 1968. Comparison of tetrahydrocannabinol and synhexl in man. *Clin Pharmacol Ther* 9:783-791.

Isbell, H., G.W. Gorodetzy, D. Jasinski, V. Claussen, F.V. Spulak and F. Korte. 1967. Effects of (*) delta-trans-tetrahydrocannabinol in man. *Psychopharmacologia* 11:184-188.

Jain, A.K., J.R. Ryan, F.G. McMahon and G. Smith. 1981. Evaluation of intramuscular levonantradol and placebo in acute postoperative pain. *J Clin Pharmacol* 21:320S-326S.

Kluin-Neleman, J.C., F.A. Neleman, O.J. Meuwissen and R.A. Maes. 1979. Delta-9-tetrahydrocannabinol (THC) as an antiemetic in patients treated with cancer chemotherapy: a double-blind cross-over trial against placebo. *Vet Hum Toxicol* 21:338-340.

Lane, M., C.L. Vogal, J, Ferguson, S. Dransow, J.L. Saiers, J. Hamm, K. Slava, P.H. Wiernik, C.P. Holroyde, S. Hammil, K. Sheppard and T. Plasse. 1991. Dronabinol and prochlorperazine in combination for treatment of cancer. *J Pain Symptom Manage* 16:352-359.

Lichtman, A.H. and B.R. Martin. 1991. Spinal and supraspinal components of cannabinoid-induced antinociception. *J Pharmacol Exp Ther* 258:517-523.

Loewe, S. 1946. Studies on the pharmacology and acute toxicity of compounds with marijuana activity. *J Pharmacol Exper Therap* 88:154-161.

Loewe, S. and L.S. Goodman. 1947. Anticonvulsant action of marijuana-active substances. *Fed Proc* 6:352.

Lucas, V.S., Jr. and J. Laszlo. 1980. Delta-9-tetrahydrocannabinol for refractory vomiting induced by cancer chemotherapy. *J Amer Med Assoc* 243:1241-1243.

Malec, J., R.F. Harve and J.J. Cayner. 1982. Cannabis effect on spasticity in spinal cord injury. *Arch Phys Med Rehabil* 63(3):116-118.

Mattes, R.D., K. Engelman, L.M. Shaw and M.A. Elsohly. 1994. Cannabinoids and appetite stimulation. *Pharmacol Biochem Behav* 49:187-195.

Maurer, M., V. Henn, A. Dittrich and A. Hofmann. 1990. Delta-9-Tetrahydrocannabinol shows antispastic and analgesic effects in a single case double-blind trial. *Eur Arch Psychiatry Clin Neurosci* 240 (1): 1-4.

Meinck, H.M., P.W. Schonie and B. Conrad. 1989. Effect of cannabinoids on spasticity and ataxia in multiple sclerosis. *J Neurol* 236:120-2.

Merritt, J.C., W. Crawford, P. Alexander, A. Anduze and S. Gelbart. 1980. Effect of marijuana on intraocular and blood pressure in glaucoma. *Ophthalmol* 87:222-228.

Merritt, J.C., S. McKinnon, J.R. Armstrong, G. Hatem and L.A. Reid. 1980. Oral delta-9-tetrahydrocannabinol in heterogeneous glaucomas. *Ann Ophthamol* 12: 947-950.

Nahas, G.G. 1973. The medical use of cannabis. In G.G. Nahas (ed.), *Marijuana in Science and in Medicine* (pp. 247-261). New York: Raven Press.

Nakano, S., H.K. Gillespie and L.E. Hollister. 1978. A model for evaluation of antianxiety drugs with the use of experimentally-induced stress: Comparison of nabilone and diazepam. *Clin Pharmacol Ther* 23:54-62.

Neidhart, J., M.M. Gagen, H.E. Wilson and D.C. Young. 1981. Comparative trial of the antiemetic effects of THC and haloperidol. *J Clin Pharmacol* 21:385S-342S.

Nelson, K. and D. Walsh. 1995. Appetite effect of dronabinol. *J Clin Oncol* 12: 1524-1525.

Nelson K., D. Walsh, P. Deeter and F. Sheehan. 1994. A phase II study of delta-9-tetrahydrocannabinol for appetite stimulation in cancer-associated anorexia. *J Palliat Care* 10:14-18.

Noyes, R., S.T. Brunk, D.H. Avery and A. Canter. 1975. The analgesic properties of delta-9-tetrahydrocannabinol and codeine. *Clin Pharmacol Ther* 18:84-89.

Orr, L.E., J.F. McKerran and B. Bloome. 1980. Antiemetic effect of tetrahydrocannabinol compared with placebo and prochlorperazine in chemotherapy-associated nausea and emesis. Arch Int Med 140:1411-1433.

Parker, C.S. 1950. Synthetic cannabis preparations in psychiatry. Synhexyl. *J Ment Sc* 96:276-279.

Perez-Reyes M, Wagner D, Wall ME, Davis KH. 1976. Intravenous administration of cannabinoids and intraocular pressure. In *Pharmacology of marihuana*, edited by M. Braude and S. Szara. New York: Raven Press. Pg. 829-832.

Petro, D.J. and C.E. Ellenberger. 1989. Treatment of human spasticity with delta-9-tetrahydrocannabinol. *J Neurol* 236:120-122.

Pivik, R.T., V. Zarcone, W.C. Dement and L.E. Hollister. 1972. Delta-9-tetrahydrocannabinol and synhexyl; effects on human sleep patterns. *Clin Pharmacol Ther* 13:426-435.

Plasse, T.F., R.W. Gorter, S.H. Krasnow, M. Lane, K.V. Shepard and R.G. Wadleigh. 1991. Recent clinical experiences with dronabinol. *Pharmacol Biochemistry Behavior* 40:695-700.

Pond, D.A. 1948. Psychological effects in depressive patients of the marijuana homologue, synhexyl. *Neurol Neurosurg Psychiatr* 11:271-279.

Raft, D., J. Gregg, J. Ghia and L. Harris. 1977. Effect of intravenous tetrahydrocannabinoids on experimental and surgical pain. *Clin Pharmacol Ther* 21:26-33.

Regelson, W., J.R. Butler, J. Schulz, T. Kirk, L. Peek, M.L. Green and M.O. Zalis. 1976. Delta-9-tetrahydrocannabinol as an effective antidepressant and appetite stimulating agent in advanced cancer patients. In M.C. Braude, S. Szara (eds.), *Pharmacology of marijuana,* vol. 2 (pp. 763-776). New York: Raven Press.

Sallan, S.E., C. Cronin, M. Zelen and N.E. Ainberg. 1980. Antiemetics in patients receiving chemotherapy for cancer: A randomized comparison of delta-9-tetrahydrocannabinol and prochlorperazine. *N Engl J Med* 302:135-138.

Sallan, S.E., N.E. Zinberg and E. Frei. 1975. Antiemetic effect of delta-9-tetrahydrocannabinol in patients receiving cancer chemotherapy. *N Engl J Med* 293:795-797.

Schwartz, R.H. 1994. Marijuana as an antiemetic drug: How useful is it? Opinions from clinical oncologists. *J Addictive Dis* 13(1):53-65.

Stockings, G.T. 1947. New euphoriant for depressive mental states. *Brit M J* 1:918-922.

Tashkin, D.P., B.J. Shapiro and V.E. Lee. 1975. Effects of a smoked marihuana in experimentally induced asthma. *Am Rev Respir Dis* 112:377-385.

Thompson, L.J. and R.C. Proctor. 1953. Continued use of pyrahexyl in treatment of alcoholic and drug withdrawal conditions. *North Carolina M J* 14:520-523.

Turkanis, S.A., W. Cely, D.M. Olson and R. Karler. 1974. Anticonvulsant properties of cannabidiol. *Res Commun Chem Pathol Pharm* 8:231-246.

Ungerleider, J.T. and T. Andrysiak. 1985. Therapeutic issues of marijuana and THC (tetrahydrocannabinol). *Int J Addictions* 5:20:691-699.

Ungerleider, J.T., T. Andrysiak, L. Fairbanks, G.W. Ellison and L.W. Myers. 1987. Delta-9-THC in the treatment of spasticity associated with multiple sclerosis. *Advances in Alcohol & Substance Abuse* 7(1):39-50.

Ungerleider, J.T., T. Andrysiak, L. Fairbanks, O. Goodnight, G. Sarna and K. Jamison. 1982. Cannabis and cancer chemotherapy: A condition of oral delta-9-tetrahydrocannabinol and prochlorperazine. *Cancer* 50:636-645.

Vachon, L., N.X. Fitzgerald, N.H. Solliday, L.A. Gould and E.A. Gaensler. 1973. Bronchial dynamics and respiratory-center sensitivity in normal subjects. *N Eng J Med* 288:985-989.

Vinciguerra, V., T. Moore and E. Brennan. 1988. Inhalation marijuana as an antiemetic for cancer chemotherapy. *New York State J Med* 88:525-528.

Voth, E.A. and R.H. Schwartz. 1997. Medicinal Applications of delta-9-tetrahydro-cannabinol and marijuana. *Ann Int Med* 126:791-798.

Wada, J.A., M. Sato and M.E. Corcoran. 1973. Antiepileptic properties of delta-9-tetrahydrocannabinol. *Exp Neurol* 39:157-165.

Williams, S.J., J.P.R. Hartley and J.D.P. Graham. 1972. Bronchodilator effect of delta-9-tetrahydrocannabinol administered by aerosol to asthmatic patients. *Thorax* 331:720-723.

Zinberg, N.E. 1979. On cannabis and health. *J Psychedel Drugs* 11:135-144.

UPDATE

Ethan B. Russo

Unbeknownst to us at the time, Dr. Leo Hollister died in December 2000, just a few weeks before the official publication of the prior entry. It was the last article he ever wrote, in a career output of several hundred. He admitted to me in a letter that it was the most difficult of his career (perhaps beset by a demanding editor, and the challenges of a malignant computer virus on his diskette, *inter alia*). His death was unheralded in the media, and perhaps that is the manner in which he preferred it to be, but no one involved in clinical cannabis research will fail to recognize his name and contributions. Though a conservative gentleman of the old school, he had a very open mind, and also contributed to investigation of LSD, being the researcher who introduced the popular cult icon and author Ken Kesey to the drug during clinical trials in the early 1960s.

We are truly proud to have had Dr. Hollister's input on the topic of the potential for cannabis therapeutics at the end of his career and at a critical juncture, just on the cusp of a renaissance of applied research. We would love to know his thoughts now on the spectacular advances of the intervening six years.

Chapter 13

Effects of Smoked Cannabis and Oral Δ⁹-Tetrahydrocannabinol on Nausea and Emesis After Cancer Chemotherapy: A Review of State Clinical Trials

Richard E. Musty
Rita Rossi

The first study comparing oral Δ^9-tetrahydrocannabinol (THC) to placebo capsules and marijuana to marijuana placebo cigarettes was published by Chang et al. (1979). In this study 15 patients were given oral doses of THC over several courses of chemotherapy. Each subject received a 10 mg THC capsule beginning two hours prior to chemotherapy and every three hours subsequently. In the event of a breakthrough vomiting episode, those patients were given marijuana cigarettes to smoke for the remaining administrations rather than oral THC. When measured THC blood levels were < 5 ng/mL, 44 percent of subjects vomited, between 5 ng/mL and 10 ng/mL, 21 percent vomited, and > 10 ng/mL, 6 percent vomited. After smoking marijuana, the incidence of vomiting for the same blood levels ranges were 83 percent, 38 percent and 0 percent. Vomiting rates after placebo capsules or smoked placebo marijuana were 72 percent and 96 percent, respectively.

In a marijuana-only trial, Vinciguerra et al. (1988) tested 56 patients, nonrandomized, who acted as their own controls. Patients rated themselves via subjective assessment of nausea and vomiting. Thirty-four percent of the patients rated smoked marijuana as being very effective, 44 percent moderately effective, and 22 percent ineffective. The authors did not report the frequency of nausea and vomiting when marijuana was not smoked.

Richard E. Musty was supported by an individual project fellowship from the Open Society Institute.

Technical reports were obtained from six states, in which inhaled marijuana was used in patients undergoing cancer chemotherapy. The states had passed legislation to make these studies legal. Usually, studies were designed by researchers in collaboration with State Departments of Health. Each state was required to write a protocol for the research (which was submitted to the Food and Drug Administration [FDA] for approval). Subsequently, a Schedule I license was obtained from the Drug Enforcement Administration (DEA). Finally, rolled marijuana cigarettes and capsules of THC (in sesame oil) were obtained from the National Institute on Drug Abuse (NIDA). These studies will be reviewed individually in this article.

In 1999, the Institute of Medicine (IOM) recommended that marijuana be made available for patients refractory to other medications (Joy et al. 1999). This review provides further support to the Chang and Vinciguerra studies.

TENNESSEE

Background

The State of Tennessee conducted this trial after legislative action in April 1981 (Board of Pharmacy, 1983).

Treatment Method

Patients (all of whom were refractory to other antiemetics) were referred for treatment by the patient's personal physician. Patient records were reviewed by a Patient Qualification Review Board of the State of Tennessee. Those approved were randomized to 3 age groups: less than 20 years old, 20 to 40 years old, and over 40 years old. Those not having conditions precluding oral administration were administered the THC capsule and those unable to ingest capsules were treated with smoked marijuana cigarettes. Most of the patients had previously been treated with the THC capsule. Thus the report focused on the effects of use of marijuana cigarettes.

Measures

A patient treatment evaluation form was completed for each day of treatment. Recording forms included a record of dose and notes, the patient's assessment of nausea and vomiting, appetite and food intake, physical state, and (marijuana) "high." Forty-three patients were enrolled in the study. Sixteen patients were excluded for various reasons: missing data, abusive drug use, premature death, those who could not tolerate smoking, or patients who declined treatment.

Results

The results of the study are shown in Table 13.1. Treatment success by method was also discussed. Success was defined as partially, moderately, or very effective. For those under age 40 years of age, 100 percent success was achieved with marijuana cigarettes. For those over 40, 83.3 percent success was achieved. Only 6 patients used the THC capsule alone, and 100 percent success occurred in those under 40 years of age, and in 33 percent for those over 40. Side effects were predominantly mild, and appetite improved in about one out of five patients.

MICHIGAN

Background

Michigan conducted a study under the direction of the Michigan Department of Public Health after legislative action in 1979. John R. Ingall of the Detroit Metropolitan Comprehensive Cancer Center was the study coordinator, and the report was complied by the Michigan Cancer Foundation (Department of Social Oncology, Evaluation Unit 1982).

Treatment Method

In order to be eligible for the trial, patients had to meet these criteria: be under active cancer chemotherapy treatment, have a satisfactory medical status such that potential side effects of marijuana or a phenothiazine deriv-

TABLE 13.1. Tennessee trial: Patient assessment of the effects of smoked marijuana on nausea and vomiting, side effects and appetite.

	Marijuana effect			Side effects			Appetite	
	n	%		n	%		n	%
Very effective	11	40.1	Mild	23	85	Above average	5	18.5
Moderately effective	11	40.1	Moderate	3	11.1	Normal	16	59.3
Partially effective	1	0.04	Severe	1	0.04	Below normal	5	18.5
Slightly effective	4	15						
Poor	1	0.04						

ative, thiethylperazine (Torecan), were not life-threatening or likely to evoke serious mental/behavioral effects, and be free of serious mental or organic disease. Patients were randomly assigned to a marijuana cigarette or thiethylperazine therapy group. If the treatment failed in a 24-hour trial, patients were then crossed over to the other treatment group. For the marijuana group, patients took one puff per minute until they felt "high" 30 minutes prior to chemotherapy. The smoking procedure continued until sometime after chemotherapy was completed. One hundred sixty-five patients completed this trial (78 male and 86 female).

Measures

Measures were recorded by patient self-report as well as physician/nurse observations.

Results

The results for this study are shown in Table 13.2. Marijuana was marginally more effective as compared to thiethylperazine in controlling nausea and vomiting/retching. As in the previous study, reported side effects were mild.

GEORGIA

Background

The State of Georgia and Emory University collaborated to conduct this trial after legislative action in 1980 (Kutner 1983).

Treatment Method

Cancer patients who were unresponsive to usual anti-emetics, but who were able to employ the oral route of administration were eligible for this trial. Patients were randomly assigned to one of three treatment groups by age: less than 20 years old, 20 to 40 years old, and over 40. The treatment groups were oral THC capsules, standardized cannabis smoking, or patient-controlled smoking.

Measures

At each treatment a form was completed containing information on effectiveness of treatment, side effects and the patient's assessment of nausea,

TABLE 13.2. Michigan trial: Frequency of nausea, vomiting/retching and side effects.

Nausea

Frequency	Marijuana		Torecan[a]	
	No.	%	No.	%
None	14	15.0	8	15.7
Mild	31	33.3	16	31.4
Moderate	22	23.7	14	27.5
Severe	19	20.0	12	23.5
Unknown	7	7.5	1	0.02

Vomiting/retching after chemotherapy

Frequency	Marijuana		Torecan[a]	
	No.	%	No.	%
None	19	18.1	10	14.9
Less than 4 h	25	23.8	19	28.4
Between 4-12 h	25	23.8	19	28.4
Between 12-24 h	14	13.3	10	14.9
Over 24 h	9	8.6	4	6.0
Unknown	13	12.4	5	7.5

Side effects of marijuana smoking (n = 113)

Side effect	No.	%
Sleepiness	21	18.5
Sore throat	13	11.5
Headache	7	6.2

[a]Thiethylperazine (Torecan).

vomiting, appetite, physical status, mood and "high." One hundred nineteen patients completed the study.

Observations included patient self-reports and physician summaries. Patient satisfaction was assessed for each treatment. Success was judged by the patient reporting as to whether he or she was satisfied or very satisfied with the treatment. If the patient was not sure of effectiveness on the first cycle of treatment but was satisfied or very satisfied on subsequent cycles, this was also considered to be a success. Failure was defined when the patient was dissatisfied on the initial cycle, the patient dropped out of the study, or changed treatment method.

Results

The overall results are shown in Table 13.3 and by age group in Table 13.4. Examining the data (in percentages) by age groups reveals success rates were very similar across age groups. These data show success rates were about the same for oral THC and patient-controlled smoking, but standardized smoking yielded somewhat inferior outcomes.

Reasons for failure in patients who failed treatment with oral THC were as follows: eight patients experienced severe nausea and vomiting, six had adverse reactions, two were dissatisfied, one had breakthrough vomiting, and one had no effect. For those who smoked marijuana, six patients experienced smoking intolerance, one had an adverse reaction, one had severe nausea and vomiting, two had breakthrough vomiting, and four had other side effects.

NEW MEXICO (1983)

Background

This program of research was conducted by the Lynn Pierson Therapeutic Research Program for the New Mexico Health and Environment Department after authorization by the legislature in 1978 (Behavioral Science Division, 1983).

TABLE 13.3. Georgia trial: Overall success with all treatments by age.

	Age			
	< 20	**20-40**	**> 40**	**Total**
Success	10 (71.4%)	30 (75%)	47 (72.3%)	87 (73.1%)
Failure	4 (28.6%)	10 (25%)	18 (27.7%)	32 (26.9%)
Total	14	40	65	119

TABLE 13.4. Georgia trial: Success by treatment with oral THC (PO), standardized smoking (SS) and patient-controlled smoking (PCS) of marijuana.

	PO	**SS**	**PCS**	**Total**
Success	57 (76%)	17 (65.4%)	13 (72.2%)	87 (73.1%)
Failure	18 (24%)	9 (34.6%)	5 (27.8%)	32 (26.9%)
Total	75	26	18	119

Treatment Method

Patients were enrolled in the program, randomly assigned to treatment groups (n=180), but complete data were available for 140 patients. They were assigned to one of two treatment groups: THC capsule or marijuana cigarettes. Doses were matched so that each patient received approximately 15 mg of THC. Patients were administered the treatment before a cycle of chemotherapy. After this they were allowed to continue treatment for 5 days.

Measures

Observations were made by patients with a self-report scale called the Target Problem Rating Scale. For nausea and vomiting, improvement was defined when patients reported less nausea or vomiting compared with previous antiemetics. No improvement was defined as no change compared with previous antiemetics.

Results

The data are shown in Table 13.5. Patients who smoked marijuana achieved improvement overprevious antiemetic drugs, with those smoking the drug with a 90 percent success, while about 60 percent achieved improvement with oral administration.

NEW MEXICO (1984)

Background

The Lynn Pierson Therapeutic Research Program continued in 1984 (Behavioral Science Division 1984).

TABLE 13.5. New Mexico trial (1983).

Group	Oral THC	Inhaled marijuana
Improvement	46 (>60%)	58 (>90%)
No improvement	30 (<40%)	6 (<10%)

Note: Percentages are stated as approximate due to rounding issues.

Treatment Method

The program was similar to that in 1983, with the exception that some patients received only one treatment and others received an average of six treatments after chemotherapy. Patients were randomly assigned to the same treatment groups as in the 1983 protocol. The protocol also allowed patients options to begin in one treatment group and switch to another, to refuse to be in the smoking group, or to try both routes of administration sequentially. Success was defined as a reduction in nausea and vomiting, and failure was defined as no reduction. Table 13.6 shows the results. It is important to note that few patients continued with the oral THC treatment, while those who smoked marijuana achieved over 90 percent success. Summarizing side effects of both THC and marijuana reported over the two years, treated patients often fell asleep. Of those who did not (approximately 90 patients), 50 percent reported sleepiness and 45 percent felt "high." No other side effects were noted in the report.

CALIFORNIA

Background

After legislation passed by the State of California Legislature in 1979, a cannabis therapeutic program was carried out between 1983 and 1989 under the supervision of the California Research Advisory Panel (1989).

Treatment Method

Over the years, several protocols were used. Essentially, the early protocols were conservative, e.g., patients were required to have failed treatment with conventional antiemetic drugs. Later, a more relaxed protocol was used in which the patient and the physician decided whether to try the THC capsule or smoke marijuana.

TABLE 13.6. New Mexico trial (1984): Treatment success after the first treatment with inhaled marijuana or oral THC.

Group	Oral THC	Inhaled marijuana	Combined
Success	6 (54.5%)	79 (95.2%)	79 (98.8%)
Failure	5 (45.5%)	4 (4.8%)	1 (1.2%)

Measures

Physicians used 5-point rating scales to record nausea and vomiting.

Results

Table 13.7 shows the combined results of the various protocols combined. In this study, smoked marijuana was consistently more effective than oral THC in blocking vomiting except in the most severe cases (greater than six times). Control of nausea was about the same for both groups. The pattern of side effects did not differ, to any extent, between smoked marijuana and oral THC.

NEW YORK

Background

The New York Department of Health study conducted a large scale (Phase III type) cooperative clinical trial (Randall, 1990).

Treatment Method

The central question addressed was how effective inhaled marijuana was in preventing nausea and vomiting due to chemotherapy in patients who failed to respond to previous anti-emetic therapy. Patients undergoing chemotherapy were allowed to use marijuana distributed through three centers: North Shore Hospital (NSH), Columbia Memorial Hospital (CMH), and a triad of the Upstate Medical Center, St. Joseph's Hospital and Jamestown

TABLE 13.7. California trials: Ratings of nausea and vomiting for smoked marijuana or the THC capsule.

Nausea	Smoked marijuana	THC capsule	Vomiting	Smoked marijuana	THC capsule
None	9 (9.2%)	38 (14.8%)	None	19 (19.4%)	89 (34.6%)
Mild	34 (34.7%)	85 (33.1%)	1-3 times	36 (36.7%)	69 (26.9%)
Moderate	36 (36.7%)	73 (28.4%)	4-6 times	18 (18.4%)	35 (13.6%)
Severe	17 (17.3%)	55 (21.4%)	> 6 times	24 (24.5%)	59 (23.0%)
Missing	2 (2%)	6 (2.3%)	Missing	1 (1%)	5 (1.9%)

Note: Side effects (combined ratings from mild to severe) are shown in Table 13.8.

TABLE 13.8. California trials: Side effects reported by patients.

	Smoked marijuana		THC alone	
	n = 98	%	*n* = 257	%
Dry mouth	53	54.1	112	43.6
Tachycardia	6	6.1	25	9.7
Ataxia	16	16.3	31	12.1
Dizziness	31	31.6	67	26.1
Orthostatic	7	7.1	32	12.5
Anxiety	19	19.4	47	18.3
Sedation	49	50.0	160	62.3
Elated mood	25	25.5	61	23.7
Confusion	23	23.4	79	30.7
Perceptual	15	15.3	57	22.2
Fantasizing	10	10.2	29	11.3
Depressed	17	17.3	33	12.8
Panic/fear	7	7.1	9	3.5

General Hospital (JGH). By 1985, the New York program provided marijuana therapy to 208 patients through 55 practitioners. Of those, data on 199 patients were evaluated. These patients had received a total of 6,044 NIDA-supplied marijuana cigarettes provided to patients during 514 treatment episodes.

Measures

Observations were made by patient self-report.

Results

North Shore Hospital reported marijuana was effective at reducing emesis 92.9 percent of the time; Columbia Memorial Hospital reported efficacy of 89.7 percent; the triad of Upstate Medical Center, St. Joseph's Hospital and Jamestown General Hospital reported 100 percent of the patients smoking marijuana gained significant benefit.

Analyzing patient evaluations, the report concluded that approximately 93 percent of marijuana inhalation treatment episodes were effective or highly effective when compared with other antiemetics. The New York study reported no serious adverse side effects. No patient receiving marijuana required hospitalization or any other form of medical intervention.

DISCUSSION

Even though slightly different methods and different research designs were used in these studies, it is clear that inhaled marijuana was effective in reducing or eliminating nausea and vomiting following cancer chemotherapy. In those studies which compared the inhalation route to oral THC, inhalation was equal to or better than oral administration. In almost all of these studies, patients were admitted only after they failed treatment with standard antiemetics, suggesting the patients may have been under fairly aggressive treatment for their cancers.

With regard to side effects, short-term use of marijuana leads to sedation, a high, and smoke intolerance in some patients. At this point in time there is no conclusive evidence that marijuana smoke seriously affects the immune system or is associated with cancer (Joy et al. 1999).

In a 1991 survey, Doblin and Kleiman reported that more than 70 percent of responding oncologists ($n = 1,035$) reported at least one of their patients had used marijuana as an antiemetic, and that they had also either observed or discussed the patients' use. In addition, 44 percent of the respondents reported recommending marijuana to at least one patient. Two hundred seventy-seven respondents felt they had clinical experience with both marijuana and Marinol (oral THC): (44 percent thought marijuana was more effective, 43 percent thought they were about equally effective, and 13 percent thought Marinol was more effective). These data suggest that physicians at that time continued to discuss or recommend marijuana use to some patients. In this sample of oncologists, it seems they understood the potential efficacy of marijuana use. Whether this situation has changed since 1991 is unknown, but one might argue that the introduction of the antiemetics of the selective serotonin-3 antagonist class may have changed this practice.

While there have been no studies which have compared smoked marijuana or Marinol with the serotonin receptor type-3 antagonists (granisetron or ondansetron), it is instructive to review published clinical trials with these compounds for the sake of comparison. In 9 clinical trials with ondansetron, antiemesis was obtained in 40 to 81 percent (mean 63.5 percent) of patients (Beck et al. 1993; Buser et al. 1993; Crucitt et al. 1996; Hainsworth et al. 1991; Herrstedt et al. 1993; Kaasa et al. 1990; Marty et al. 1990; Olver et al. 1996; Roila et al. 1991). In 5 clinical trials with granisetron, 37.7 to 93 percent (mean 56.6 percent) antiemesis was reported (Italian Group for Antiemetic Research 1995; Markman et al. 1996; Perez et al. 1997; Ritter et al. 1998; Sekine et al. 1996). It is generally known that combining antiemetic drugs with different mechanisms of action often improves efficacy (Jones et al. 1991). This suggests that future research should consider combining cannabinoids with other antiemetics.

The data reviewed here suggest that the inhalation of THC appears to be more effective than the oral route. In order to achieve the IOM recommendation to allow patients access to marijuana, both state and federal governments would need to reschedule marijuana from Schedule I to Schedule II, or reinstate the Compassionate Use Program. The development of smokeless inhalation devices would certainly be an advance in the use of THC as an anti-emetic medication. Finally, a large number of synthetic cannabinoid and endocannabinoid agonist analogs have been developed. It would seem that testing of these compounds as potential anti-emetics would also be worthwhile.

REFERENCES

Beck TH, AA Ciociola, SE Jones, WH Harvey, NS Tehekmedian, A Chang, D Galvin, and NE Hart and the Ondansetron Study Group. 1993. Efficacy of oral ondansetron in the prevention of emesis in outpatients receiving cyclophosphamide-based chemotherapy. *Ann Intern Med* 118:407-413.

Behavioral Health Sciences Division. 1983. *The Lynn Pierson Therapeutic Research Program.* Santa Fe, NM: Health and Environment Department.

Behavioral Health Sciences Division. 1984. *The Lynn Pierson Therapeutic Research Program.* Santa Fe, NM: Health and Environment Department.

Board of Pharmacy, State of Tennessee. 1983. *Annual Report: Evaluation of marijuana and tetrahydrocannabinol in the treatment of nausea and/or vomiting associated with cancer therapy unresponsive to conventional anti-emetic therapy: Efficacy and toxicity.* Nashville, TN: Author.

Buser KS, RA Joss, D Piquet, MS Aapro, F Cavalli, JM Haefliger, WF Jungi, J Bauer, R Obnst, and KW Brunner. 1993. Oral ondansetron in the prophylaxis of nausea and vomiting induced by cyclophosphamide, methotrexate and 5-fluorouracil (CMF) in women with breast cancer. Results of a prospective, randomized, double-blind, placebo-controlled study. *Ann Oncol* 4:475-479.

Chang AE, DJ Shiling, RC Stillman, et al. 1979. Delta-9-tetrahydrocannabinol as an antiemetic in cancer patients receiving high-dose methotrexate. A prospective, randomized evaluation. *Ann Intern Med* 91:819-824.

Crucitt MA, W Hyman, T Grote, W Tester, S Madajewicz, S Yee, A Wentz, D Griffin, TV Parasuraman, and J Brysor. 1996. Efficacy and tolerability of oral ondansetron versus prochlorperazine in the prevention of emesis associated with cyclophosphamide-based chemotherapy and maintenance of health-related quality of life. *Clin Ther* 18(4):778-788.

Department of Social Oncology, Evaluation Unit. 1982. State of Michigan, *Marihuana Therapeutic Research Project.*

Doblin, R and M Kleiman. 1991. Marijuana as antiemetic medicine: A survey of oncologists' experiences and attitudes *J Clin Oncol* 9(5):1314-1319.

Hainsworth, J, W Harvey, K Pendergrass, B Kasimis, D Oblon, G Monaghan, D Gandara, P Hesketh, A Khojasteh, G Harker, et al. 1991. A single-blind comparison of intravenous ondansetron, a selective serotonin antagonist, with intravenous metoclopramide in the prevention of nausea and vomiting associated with high-dose cisplatin chemotherapy. *J Clin Oncol* 9 (5):721-728.

Herrstedt J, T Sigsgaard, M Boesgaard, T Jensen, and P Dombernowski. 1993. Ondansetron plus metopimazine compared with ondansetron in patients receiving moderately emetogenic chemotherapy. *N Engl J Med* 328(15):1076-1080.

Italian Group for Antiemetic Research. 1995. Dexamethasone, granisetron, or both for the prevention of nausea and vomiting during chemotherapy for cancer. *New Engl J Med* 332(1):1-5.

Jones AL, AS Hill, M Soukop, AW Hutcheon, J. Cassidy, SB Kaye, K Sikora, DN Carney, and D Cunningham. 1991. Comparison of dexamethasone and ondansetron in the prophylaxis of emesis induced by moderately emetogenic chemotherapy. *Lancet* 338:483-487.

Joy J, SJ Watson, and JA Benson. 1999. *Marijuana as medicine: Assessing the science base.* Washington DC: National Academy Press.

Kaasa S, S Kvaløy, MA Dicato et al., and the International Emesis Study Group. 1990. A comparison of ondansetron with metoclopramide in the prophylaxis of chemotherapy-induced nausea and vomiting: A randomized, double-blind study. *Eur J Cancer* 26(3):311-314.

Kutner, MH. 1983. *Evaluation of the use of both marijuana and THC in cancer patients for the relief of nausea and vomiting associated with cancer chemotherapy after failure of conventional anti-emetic therapy: Efficacy and toxicity, as prepared for the Composite State Board of Medical Examiners, Georgia Department of Health, by physicians and researchers at Emory University, Atlanta.*

Markman M, A Kennedy, K Webster et al. 1996. Control of carbonplatin-induced emesis with a fixed low dose of granisetron (0.5 mg) plus dexamethasone. *Gynecol Onco* 60:435-437.

Marty M, P Pouillart, S Scholl, JP Droz, M Azab, N Brion, E. Pujade-Lauraine, B Paule, D Paes, and J Bons. 1990. Comparison of the 5-hydroxytryptamine$_3$ (serotonin) antagonist ondansetron (GR 38032F) with high-dose metoclopramide in the control of cisplatin-induced emesis. *N Engl J Med* 322(12):816-821.

Michigan Cancer Foundation, Department of Social Oncology, Evaluation Unit. 1992. *Michigan Department of Public Health Marijuana Therapeutic Research Project, Trial A 1980-81.*

Olver I, W Paska, A Depierre, JF Seitz, DJ Stewart, L. Goedhals, B McQuade, J McRae, and JR Wilkinson. 1996. A multicentre, double-blind study comparing placebo, ondansetron and ondansetron plus dexamethasone for the control of cisplatin-induced delayed emesis. *Ann Oncol* 7:945-952.

Perez EA, RM Navari, HG Kaplan, RJ Gralla, SM Grunberg, RH Palmer, and D Fitts. 1997. Efficacy and safety of different doses of granisetron for the prophylaxis of cisplatin-induced emesis. *Support Care Cancer* 5:31-37.

Randall RC. 1990. *Cancer Treatment & Marijuana Therapy.* Washington DC: Galen Press, 1990.

Research Advisory Panel. 1989. *Cannabis Therapeutic Research Program. Report to the California Legislature.*

Ritter HL, Jr., RJ Gralla, SW Hall, JK Wada, C Friedman, L Hand and D Fitts. 1998. Efficacy of intravenous granisetron to control nausea and vomiting during multiple cycles of cisplatin-based chemotherapy. *Cancer Invest* 16(2):87-93.

Roila F, M Tonato, F Cognettti, E Cortesi, G Faralli, M Marangolo, D Amadori, MA Bella, V Gramazio, et al. 1991. Prevention of cisplatin-induced emesis: A double-blind multicenter randomized crossover study comparing ondansetron and ondansetron plus dexamethasone. *J Clin Oncol* 9(4):675-678.

Sekine I, Y Nishiwaki, R Kakinuma, K Kubota, F Hojo, T Matsumoto, H. Omatsu, M Yokozaki, and T Kodama. 1996. A randomized cross-over trial of granisetron and dexamethasone versus granisetron alone: The role of dexamethasone on day 1 in the control of cisplatin-induced delayed emesis. *Jp J Clin Oncol* 26(3):164-168.

Vinciguerra V, T Moore, E Brennan. 1988. Inhalation marijuana as an antiemetic for cancer chemotherapy. *NY State J Med* 88:525-527.

UPDATE

Ethan B. Russo

Surprisingly little clinical work has been done of late in the area of cannabinoid treatments for nausea and vomiting associated with cancer chemotherapy. However, this portends to be an important indication for such drugs in the future. This prospect has been bolstered by a great deal of corroboratory basic science experimentation. Both THC and CBD have proven efficacious in animal models of nausea (Parker et al. 2002) and vomiting (Parker and Mechoulam 2003). Cannabidiol is virtually absent, however, from drugs strains of cannabis in North America (ElSohly et al. 2000). Marinol (synthetic THC) has been approved for this indication in the United States since 1985 but remains little utilized due to difficulties with adverse event profiles (Calhoun et al. 1998), and the questionable ability to employ an oral agent in the context of this clinical challenge. The hypothetical logic in employing alternative delivery systems of cannabis-based medicines for such situations is compelling. Sativex, an oromucosal cannabis-based medicine with a prominent CBD complement now approved for treatment of central neuropathic pain in multiple sclerosis, has yet to receive formal investigation for this problem.

REFERENCES

Calhoun, S.R., G.P. Galloway, and D.E. Smith. 1998. Abuse potential of dronabinol (Marinol). *J Psychoactive Drugs* 30(2):187-196.

ElSohly, M. A., S. A. Ross, Z. Mehmedic, R. Arafat, B. Yi, and B. F. Banahan, III. 2000. Potency trends of delta9-THC and other cannabinoids in confiscated marijuana from 1980-1997. *J Forensic Sci* 45(1):24-30.

Parker, L. A., and R. Mechoulam. 2003. Cannabinoid agonists and antagonists modulate lithium-induced conditioned gaping in rats. *Integr Physiol Behav Sci* 38(2): 133-145.

Parker, L. A., R. Mechoulam, and C. Schlievert. 2002. Cannabidiol, a non-psychoactive component of cannabis and its synthetic dimethylheptyl homolog suppress nausea in an experimental model with rats. *Neuroreport* 13(5):567-570.

Chapter 14

Hyperemesis Gravidarum
and Clinical Cannabis:
To Eat or Not to Eat?

Wei-Ni Lin Curry

The ideal pregnant woman radiates the image of a full-fleshed, well-nourished femininity whose presence glows of maternal well-being and ripeness. She is commonly encouraged by her family and friends to eat in increased proportions because the accepted consensus is that she is "eating for two." Her circle of loved ones will often assist her in fulfilling her food cravings. It matters not that she fancies strange foods, demands unappealing concoctions, or eats during the most unpredictable and indiscriminate times of the day (Murcott 1988). What matters is that she eats well. However, what happens when she is *unable* to eat for two? What happens when she *cannot eat for even one?*

While such a debilitating illness does not often occur, it happens to pregnant women who suffer from a disease known as hyperemesis gravidarum (HG) (Erick 1997; Van de Ven 1997). HG to a pregnant woman is similar to the wasting syndrome of an AIDS sufferer or a cancer chemotherapy patient whose body becomes severely emaciated, dehydrated, and malnourished due to persistent, uncontrollable vomiting and the inability to eat and drink (Grinspoon and Bakalar 1997). A striking difference, however, is that the survivor of HG carries the added responsibility of sustaining another life within her womb. While she perishes from hunger, her baby in utero continues to absorb any remains of stored fat, muscle tissue, and nutrients from her body in order to survive. Compared to the weight loss endured by those undergoing AIDS or cancer chemotherapy, the HG woman's shedding of pounds is deceptively unsparing, as her baby's continual growth and weight gain disguises the actual body mass she is really losing. In essence, a pregnant woman with hyperemesis does not come anywhere near eating for two; she is more accurately *starving* for two.

Handbook of Cannabis Therapeutics
© 2006 by The Haworth Press, Inc. All rights reserved.
doi:10.1300/5741_15

HG, ITS MEDICALIZATION, AND THE SURVIVORS

Hyperemesis gravidarum is conservatively defined in *The Harvard Guide to Women's Health* (Carlson 1996) as a debilitating condition of severe nausea and vomiting during pregnancy, resulting in malnutrition, dehydration, and weight loss. While women experience various degrees of HG, the prolonged retching and starvation often trigger the onset of other physically disabling ailments such as, but not limited to, partial paralysis, failed muscle coordination, ruptured esophagus, bloody emesis and/or stool, hemorrhage of the retina, inflamed pancreas, and/or wasting of muscle tissue. In rare cases, HG has also been associated with coma, temporary blindness, and even death (Hillborn et al. 1999; Tesfaye et al. 1998).

The following personal anecdotes of real women bring into perspective the devastation and symptoms of starvation caused by HG: "Sarah" stated, "I lost a total of thirty pounds and I was skinny to begin with. I was a walking skeleton with a belly. I looked like death and smelled like poison." "Sofia" said, "With my son [first pregnancy], I just got very ill from the point the sperm met the egg. I lost thirty pounds within the first two months, and I stayed in bed the whole nine months, only getting up to use the restroom." She also observed, "During my [second pregnancy] I was throwing up first the acid in my stomach, which is yellow, then it's orange because it's the outer layer, and then you get to the green bile which is [from] your intestines. Then once you're past that, you go straight blood."

With her first pregnancy, Sofia was at least able to swallow and digest one burrito as her entire weekly sustenance. By her second pregnancy, however, food was definitely not an option. Sofia explains:

> I knew within one week of the conception that I was pregnant. Immediately vomiting and loss of appetite. *I couldn't swallow my own spit* for the first five months of my pregnancy . . . Within the first two weeks of my pregnancy, [I was hospitalized] twice. I would have five days that I could survive at home, then I would get so dehydrated that I'd have to go to the hospital to the ER so that I could get hydrated. I'd stay in the hospital one to two days. They'd get me fully hydrated, and then they'd send me home.

Also, Sofia's attempt at the traditional folk remedy of soda and crackers resulted in vomiting: "The doctors thought that it was all in my head—thought that I was *bulimic*." The doctors intravenously injected units of fluid into her body in an attempt to increase her caloric intake. She grimaces: "They were feeding me lard. It *smelled* like lard. It *smelled* like grease."

One who physically experiences the starvation and nausea of hyper-emesis gravidarum will often encounter psychological and emotional distress. The hormonal changes and mood fluctuations that are often associated with a normal pregnancy inevitably become more severe with the onset of HG (Simpson et al. 2001). In struggling to bear her child, the HG mother must also brace herself through such symptoms as depression, unnatural fatigue, amnesia, apathy, distorted body image, fear, and/or guilt (Erick 1997; Hillborn et al. 1999; Tesfaye et al. 1998). Some even contemplate suicide, as each living moment is excruciatingly taxing and painful:

> *I wanted to die every waking hour.* I thought I was in hell. Doctors told me that I was trying to orally vomit my baby out, that the pregnancy was not wanted. They sent me to psychiatrists claiming that all this was "in my head." Nobody understood me. My husband even left me. I was all alone with my tortured body, praying to God to give me strength to go on. (Sarah)

> *I . . . just wanted to die every minute that I was awake.* I still consider it a miracle that I and (more importantly) my two healthy children survived. I was *depressed* throughout the pregnancies as well as from not being able to take care of my two-and-a-half-year-old when I was pregnant with the second. I shudder when I think about it. . . . (Julia)

> *I'd cry every night.* . . . I feel that I'm a very strong individual, but this was no time to be strong. I'd cry every night, telling my husband how it hurt so bad. (Sofia)

A substantial number of HG survivors are also left with no choice but to cease employment and, if needed, temporarily relinquish the custody of their children to a more capable caregiver, such as a relative or a friend. Sofia solemnly recalls that when she was pregnant with her second child, she had to drop out of college where she was a student; she also had to give her mother legal guardianship of her seven-year-old son for the entire pregnancy, "because I couldn't even cook or clean my own body, I couldn't do it to my own child. *And I wouldn't want him to be subjected to see me the way that I was.*"

Sadly enough, physical disability and the continual and frequent visits to the hospital for vital replenishment often isolate the HG woman from the warmth and comfort of her family and home during a time when she needs support the most.

While general nausea and vomiting, better known as morning sickness, is experienced by 70 to 80 percent of all pregnancies, only 1 to 2 percent are affected by the pernicious emesis and distress associated with hyperemesis gravidarum. Of this HG populace, 5 percent endure the debilitating symptoms for the entire nine-month period of their infant's gestation (Van de Ven 1997). Statistics taken in 1993 reveal that within one year, 42,000 women in the United States sought the help of a health care professional in an effort to counteract their symptoms of HG. In Britain, a study also shows that 2 of every 100 HG mothers will opt for abortion, most likely as a last resort to terminate their unbearable suffering and not the lives of their often much-wanted unborn babies (Erick 1997). Sarah, who aborted against her will, grieves:

> Two weeks ago, I terminated my very much wanted pregnancy because of hyperemesis gravidarum. This disease is so disgusting and nightmarish, I don't know how I was able to do it the first time around. *I regret the abortion,* but I just have to think about HG and remember the ordeal I went through and don't want to go through again. . . . Before my abortion, I was prescribed Diclectin [a Canadian combination of vitamin B$_6$ and the antihistamine doxylamine], four doses a day. It didn't help. I just wish there was a cure for this disease because *I want my baby back!*

Sofia chose not to abort, even at the strong recommendation of medical professionals and loved ones:

> [When] I was five months, three weeks pregnant sitting in the medical center for the umpteenth time, I had the chief of staff, my personal ob/gyn was a chief resident, and three other specialists—whether they be the gastrointestinal specialist and a couple of other ones—there'd be around six or seven other specialists standing around my bed. They all came to the conclusion that I needed to abort. . . . I just told them I've survived five months and three weeks, why couldn't I survive two more months?

Other women adamantly refuse to consider abortion on grounds of their moral paradigm.

While many women and infants throughout history have died due to HG, prenatal mothers in industrialized, metropolitan areas are usually spared such a fatal outcome with the assistance of approved medical modalities. Western physicians prescribe antiemetic pharmaceutical drugs, such as metaclopramide (Reglan), prochlorperazine (Compazine), promethazine (Phenergan), and ondansetron (Zofran), to help mothers keep their nausea at bay and nourish themselves and their fetuses. The drugs, which are also commonly given to AIDS and cancer chemotherapy patients, are taken orally, intravenously, or as rectal suppositories. While the long-term risks to the human child in utero remains unknown, the general consensus from the medical establishment is that the risks to the mother and fetus of severe morning sickness warrant possible risks of using these drugs during pregnancy (Carlson et al. 1996). At the very least, the babies who have ingested these medications via the placenta have been born comparatively healthy; none have emerged from the womb with birth defects, as did the infant casualties of thalidomide, the pharmaceutical drug given to mothers in the 1950s to alleviate indications of morning sickness and HG.

Nevertheless, the drugs are not fail proof. According to the Summary of Data on Hyperemesis Gravidarum (Schoenberg 2000), some of the most common antiemetic medications and the safety ratings that were assigned to them by the Food and Drug Administration (FDA) are listed as follows: ten drugs (scopolamine, promethazine, prochlorperazine, chlorpromazine, trimethobenzamide, cisapride, droperidol, coricosteroids, ondansetron, and hydoxyzine) received the rating of C, six drugs (doxylamine, diphenhydramine, cyclizine, meclizine, dimenhydrinate, and metaclopramide) received the rating of B, and one drug (pyridoxine, vitamin B6) received the rating of A. A C rating means "animal studies show risk but human studies are lacking, or there are no studies in humans or animals." A B rating means "animal studies show no risk but human studies are inadequate, or animal studies show some risk but the risk is not supported by human studies." An A rating signifies "no fetal risk" (Schoenberg 2000). Apparently, all the drugs listed, with the exception of one, a vitamin, are questionable in their safety, posing a potential threat to the fetus. Unsurprisingly, these pharmaceutical drugs threaten the mother, if not the baby, with many side effects and harmful allergic reactions. Sofia recounts her experience with the antiemetic drugs—prochloperazine, metaclopramide, and promethazine, before she had to suspend her student status at her university due to HG:

> Well, the second week [of pregnancy] I was taking all three [medications]. I was sitting in lecture hall, and my body began to convulse. And literally, like an *epileptic seizure,* my tongue was upside down, my back was out of whack, [and I] couldn't control my legs or my arms. My husband conveniently was visiting me that day, and was in lecture hall with me. He had to pick me up and take me to the ER.

From that point onward, Sofia was unable to take any medications for her nausea and vomiting. It was not until she was in her sixth month of pregnancy that she was given another, ondansetron. She was discouraged from taking the drug any earlier because the doctors were uncertain of the possible side effects. Another fellow student and HG survivor, Nora, has also professed to me that if she ever became pregnant again, she would not want to take any medications because they made her feel "drugged out" and "like a zombie" all day.

Because the modern antiemetic medications have not succeeded in eliminating all symptoms of vomiting and nausea, and fail to stimulate the woman's appetite, mothers with hyperemesis continue to struggle with eating and maintaining (if not gaining) weight. Hence, within the framework of modern medicine, a crucial part of the women's survival relies on intake of liquid nutrition through tubes: intravenously, nasogastrically, or enterally, and often without the use of anesthesia. In certain situations, a gastrostomy tube is required for the purpose of drainage and decompression. Some may suffer from what Sofia calls a "collapsed digestive system." She noted, "[The doctors] were worried that all my organs were going to shut down, because I wasn't using them. I . . . [was having] bowel movements maybe once every two months. . . . I had no food. I had no intake. I just didn't need to go."

To this day, six years after the birth of her daughter, Sofia is unable to digest a regular meal; unless she divides a single portion into two or three smaller servings, and unless she avoids anything too meaty, greasy, or rich, she will vomit shortly after consuming the food.

Sofia also braved the tortures of having intravenous tubes continually inserted and reinserted into her body due to life-threatening blood clots that periodically developed as a result of being fed liquid nutrition. Sofia said that even though the nurses were administering heparin through her IV to achieve anticoagulation, the blood clots continued to recur. She recounts:

> I was around seven months pregnant when that one [about the eighth tube inserted] went bad with a blood clot close to my neck. [The doctors] immediately said, "We need to take it out." But they didn't know what they had done inside. There were roots growing all along, all around the tubes inside of my chest because all the scar tissue that had formed. And the doctor, when he was taking it out, was literally pulling it—mind you, I had *no anesthesia,* and I was in *pain!*

At this point, I could not resist interrupting her to make sure I was hearing correctly, asking: "So he basically *tore your flesh?*"

> *Yes.* And when it didn't come out, he had to stick scalpels in through these bottom holes, and try to tear away the scar tissue underneath. Yeah. And my husband had to sit there and tell me everything is "okay—don't worry, it doesn't look that bad." But after the fact, he was like, "I was just trying to give you moral support. That *asshole* was tearing you apart and I was watching every minute of it."

Sofia emphasizes that throughout her pregnancy she had "really bad scabs everywhere." She said she looked like a "druggy." Just the one surgical procedure left an open, gaping wound "about the size of a quarter" above her chest for nearly a month. Unfortunately, these scars will remain with her for the rest of her life, physically and emotionally.

Sofia is one of many women whose flesh and blood are sacrificed at the price of HG medical treatments. Another hyperemesis sufferer ("Mary") is highlighted in a dietician's case study that explains the woman's struggles with receiving liquid nutrition throughout her pregnancy (Erick 1997). I have paraphrased the case.

When Mary was first admitted to the hospital, she was severely malnourished and dehydrated due to HG. The hospital began medical treatments by administering an IV feeding tube for her, but it was unsuccessful due to continued malnutrition. A nasogastric tube followed. Mary vomited three of the tubes in a two-day period, so she refused further replacements. The doctors then tried a different route via a jejunostomy and gastrostomy tube, one for feeding and the other for drainage. This method remained until the time of her delivery. However, for the entire pregnancy, Mary continued to vomit in spite of antiemesis medications. The smell of the liquid formula used for her enteral feedings also increased her nausea. Mary also continued suffering from insomnia, pancreatitis, increased bloating, abdominal pain, chest pain, thick phlegm, depression, and a distorted body image. Her partner was said to have shown disgust with the presence of the tubes sticking out of her body. Finally, she threatened suicide if she was not delivered immediately. A cesarean operation was performed before the expected date of delivery, as well as a permanent sterilization, done at her request. The baby was born relatively healthy at 6.45 pounds.

The story of Mary's struggles to feed herself and her baby through the devastating symptoms of HG cries for empathy and compassion. Though her doctors were most likely sincere in their intentions to keep her sickness under control, and though they succeeded in saving the life of the infant, I wonder if they realize how truly horrific their treatments really were. To what extent did they help Mary and to what extent did they hurt her, physically and psychologically? How much did they contribute to her experience of a healthy and dignified pregnancy, one that every woman deserves? Alternatives are in dire need.

Because many HG patients have shown that their nausea and vomiting are "linked to the consumption of food," the administration of liquid nutrition via feeding tubes is justified by doctors; it is argued that in sparing HG women from the physical act of smelling, masticating, and swallowing their meals, their nausea and vomiting will decrease (Van de Ven

1997). Unfortunately, in the case of both Sofia and Mary, their vomiting was triggered by the smell of the liquid formula.

The causes of hyperemesis have provoked heated speculation, but no substantial evidence has been discovered or acknowledged within the Western medical hegemony. Some scientists hypothesize the following as factors that often lead to and/or are connected to HG: hormones, increased estrogen level, nutrition, thiamine deficiency, psychological factors (Simpson et al. 2001), and the sex of the child, higher concentration of human chorionic gonadotropin level associated with a female fetus (Askling et al. 1999; Panesar et al. 2001). As none of the factors offer a satisfactory answer, HG remains a perplexing female mystery for the present-day medical establishment. The frustration is mostly felt by women who are survivors of HG, desperately searching for a cure and increased understanding of this harrowing disease:

> I have suffered through two pregnancies with this debilitating condition. . . . In both pregnancies, it started at six weeks and continued until the baby was born. I was induced early both times because I was so sick. I tried everything: hypnosis, homeopathic treatment, acupuncture, sea sick bands, IVs, smelling ginger and lemons, Compazine, Reglan, Phenergan, Atavan, Unisom, Zofran (to name a few). Nothing worked. I threw up constantly, including a lot of bile and dry heaving, could barely walk and just wanted to die every minute. . . . It is extremely frustrating how little research and ideas exist on the topic, and I feel quite confident that if men could experience the condition, there would be a remedy for it. (Julia)

The medical establishment must begin to realize that even though the HG woman is unable to eat, the only thing she really wants *is* to eat.

The HG sufferer is not simply a lifeless, unfeeling, docile body (Foucault 1995) that robotically pumps vitamins and minerals into her growing child. She is a human being who needs to eat to live. Her ability to savor her meal, to salivate, to masticate, to swallow, to digest, is a primal and essential part of her existence. The woman with hyperemesis needs more than feeding tubes and synthetic liquid nutrition. She craves and requires real food, just like her baby needs a mother, and not a machine.

CANNABIS, PREGNANCY, AND HG

I, too, am a survivor of hyperemesis gravidarum. While I suffered through severe morning sickness my first pregnancy, it was not until my second pregnancy that I experienced the merciless symptoms of life-threatening HG.

Within two weeks of my daughter's conception, I became desperately nause-ated and vomited throughout the day and night. Every time I attempted to eat or drink *anything,* even water, I would immediately throw it up. Because nothing would stay in my stomach, I lost 21 pounds within the first two weeks of hyperemesis, which was over 20 percent of my normal body weight at the time (105 pounds). I vomited bile of every shade, and soon began retching blood. I was also bleeding out of my vagina due to the pressures from vomit-ing and owing to the fact that my vulva was still weak from two surgeries to remove cervical cancer after my first pregnancy.

I felt so helpless and distraught that I went to the abortion clinic twice, but both times I left without going through with the procedure. My partner and my three-year-old son feared for my life. My son would often ask me, with tears streaming down his face, "Mommy, are you going to die?" Each time, I reassured him that Mommy would be okay soon, but he was not con-vinced. Could I blame him? I felt as if my whole world was falling apart, and that the ones I loved most were being dragged down with me. I tried desperately to function as usual—to work, cook, clean, care for my son—but all of my usual duties had to be sacrificed as I spent my entire day retch-ing into the toilet, where I would often pass out because I had no energy to walk to and from the bathroom.

When I went to an obstetrician in search of help, the options he gave me were the usual: hospitalization, intravenous feedings, and antiemesis phar-maceutical drugs that had unknown long-term side effects with the potential of affecting my child negatively. Instead, I tried ginger, raspberry tea, soda and crackers, acupressure, meditation—all the recommended home reme-dies—but nothing worked. Finally, I decided to try medical cannabis. The medical cannabis initiative, the Compassionate Use Act of 1996, which had been passed by the voters of California, permits the legal use of cannabis for the severely ill. If cannabis had been so effective in alleviating the nausea and vomiting for AIDS and cancer chemotherapy patients, then why would it not work for pregnant HG patients? I asked a Harvard physician, Lester Grinspoon, who had been studying the therapeutic properties of cannabis for the past thirty-some years. He said that other women throughout history and in modern times have used cannabis for HG and experienced positive results. With his reassurance, I felt more confident in attempting to remedy my sickness with the herb.

Because I had never smoked before, I first had to learn to take the medi-cine, but that was a welcome task, seeing that the herb worked wonders. Just one to two little puffs at night, and if needed in the morning, resulted in an entire day of wellness. I went from not eating, not drinking, not functioning, and continually vomiting and bleeding from two orifices to being com-pletely cured. The only HG symptom that persisted was my acute sense of smell which, in the absence of nausea and vomiting, was tolerable. Not only did I eat and drink, I consumed food with a hearty and open appetite.

The cannabis worked so miraculously that at first I thought my mind was playing tricks on me, as if I was being deceived by some placebo effect. In order to test, I stopped taking the cannabis three times, and each time the uncontrollable and violent retching returned. Finally, my son, who was three years old at the time, begged me, "Mommy, *please* go take your medicine!" That was when I knew that cannabis is truly an efficacious medicine, and that, yes, I could look forward to enjoying a well-nourished and dignified pregnancy.

Not only did the cannabis save my son from not having a mother during the duration of my hyperemesis, it saved the life of my child within my womb. Every day, I am grateful for her bright and vivacious existence. Developmentally, she has proven to be very advanced for her age. She began walking at eight and a half months (norm eleven to thirteen months), and she began expressing herself quite articulately at a year and a half. Her teachers at her children's center frequently comment on her maturity and the advancement of her motor, social, and cognitive abilities. I was told by one of her teachers that the university pediatricians who frequent the school to conduct research in child development were also highly impressed by her accelerated abilities. So for my situation, it is safe for me to conclude that my choice to use cannabis as a therapeutic "folk" remedy for my HG symptoms was a positive and beneficial decision with healthful and quite amazing results for my daughter.

And no, I am *not* a "drug addict," as the stigma dictates. As soon as my symptoms of HG passed, I no longer needed to use the cannabis. My Taiwanese medical obstetrician who helped deliver my daughter informed me that since ancient times the Chinese have used cannabis to treat HG, and the smoke that is inhaled does not go to the fetus, but rather directly to the brain of the mother to help counteract her nausea and stimulate her appetite. Studies also confirm that "only relatively small amounts" of the psychoactive cannabinoid ingredient-delta-9-THC "actually cross the placenta barrier to the fetus" (Dreher 1997, p. 160). While medication in the form of pills is easily vomited by one who is susceptible to nausea, smoking/inhaling in this situation is actually a preferred route of administration. The HG mom more accurately and readily gauges the dosage of each treatment according to how she feels each time, unlike pills and suppositories that often leave one feeling "knocked out" all day. As a result, I am in disbelief at how our government has kept such a valuable medicine from so many ailing women. If I had not experienced the cannabis myself, I would not have believed its truly effective and gentle therapeutic powers.

While I am not one to condone the use of illicit drugs during pregnancy, I strongly believe that in the case of women suffering from HG, an exception must be made in regards to the use of cannabis. In *Mothers and Illicit Drug Use: Transcending the Myths,* Susan Boyd (1999, p. 4) states:

> Critical researchers acknowledge that "crime" is a political construct . . . where selective criminalization takes place. In North America the most dangerous drugs are legal. Tobacco and alcohol are more lethal than the more benign drugs, such as marijuana, and both heroin and cocaine. The so-called dangers of illicit drugs are widely depicted by both government and the media. But the real dangers of legal drugs, including alcohol, tobacco, and pharmaceutical, are viewed differently.

She also emphasizes that of all the illicit drugs, cannabis is the most benign (Boyd 1999).

Personally, I did not appreciate my ability to use this herb until I learned of the extreme suffering experienced by other women with HG while at the hands of the well-intentioned medical community. How can one justify the extreme methods discussed previously as being less criminal than condoning women to use an herb that does not harm the fetus but simply offers the HG mother the chance to eat, drink, function normally, and experience the positive pregnancy she deserves?

Do I dare suggest that the medical hegemony and the pharmaceutical companies are suspect for not prioritizing the best interest of the mothers but rather their immense profit margins? For instance, while the cost for cannabis treatment, even at expensive street prices, might not exceed $400 for the entire duration of one's HG pregnancy, the medical cost of ondansetron, the antiemetic pharmaceutical drug commonly used by HG women, is sometimes charged at $600 for each intravenous dose. Hypothetically, even if an HG sufferer took only three doses a day for sixteen weeks (the usual duration of HG, though some experience HG their entire pregnancy), the cost would be more than $200,000 (Grinspoon and Bakalar 1997, p. 42).

When I share my story with others, the reaction is either one of sincere enthusiasm and curiosity or apprehensive disapproval and skepticism. One HG woman, upon hearing of my self-remedy, instantly said, "No, no, no . . . I wouldn't trust it. What about the side effects? And besides, maybe your symptoms of HG were not as severe, and that's why you were okay without getting hospital treatment."

It is not surprising that my suffering was belittled and my cure denounced. Most view the use of illicit drugs, especially during pregnancy, to be deviant, threatening, and something to avoid at all costs (Boyd 1999). Murphy and Rosenbaum (1999, p. 1) state, "In modern society the use of illegal drugs during pregnancy is commonly defined as the antithesis of responsible behavior and good health. The two statuses, pregnant woman and drug user, simply do not go together."

This stigma, while serving its purposes to discourage careless behavior during pregnancy, is counterproductive in isolated situations that permit the medical use of cannabis by HG sufferers. In the United States and Canada, medical research on cannabis in relation to mothers and their offspring has produced reports that are fear-inducing and negative, often because the pregnant subjects involved use multiple drugs, come from low-income and disadvantaged situations, endure domestic violence, suffer from poor nutrition, and/or have preexisting psychological disorders (Dreher 1997). However, propaganda and the media often conveniently exclude the latter details, misinforming the public into believing inaccurate and sensationalized perinatal risk factors caused by the side effects of the stigmatized "killer weed." These studies more accurately reveal the results of a dysfunctional lifestyle, and not the actual side effects of cannabis use. They marginalize the herb as a psychoactive, recreational drug rather than a therapeutic agent.

In the book chapter "Cannabis and Pregnancy," Melanie Dreher (1997) writes that much historical and cross-cultural evidence has been uncovered on the therapeutic uses of cannabis during pregnancy, labor, delivery, and nursing. In fact, archaeological and written records substantiate that the plant was often used to treat female ailments, such as to treat dysmenorrhea, ease labor, alleviate morning sickness/hyperemesis gravidarum, and/or facilitate childbirth in places such as Ancient Egypt, Judea, and Assyria (Mathre 1997), ancient China (Grinspoon and Bakalar 1997; Mathre 1997, p. 36), historical Europe (Benet 1975), rural Southeast Asia, specifically Cambodia, Thailand, Laos, and Vietnam (Martin 1975), Jamaica (Dreher 1975), Africa (Du Toit 1980), and colonial and contemporary America (Grinspoon and Bakalar 1997; Mathre 1997; Wright 1862; www.folkmed.ucla.edu). Dreher's anthropological study reconfirms many of the historical and contemporary findings. Conducted in Jamaica amongst Rastafarians who highly esteem cannabis as a sacred herb and therapeutic agent for a wide spectrum of ailments, the researchers in the study were stunned to discover that babies whose mothers used cannabis throughout their pregnancy (whether or not they had the symptoms of nausea and vomiting) were healthier, more advanced, more alert, and less irritable than infants whose mothers did not use cannabis. What the team revealed through time-consuming, labor-intensive research and observation, Jamaican women knew all along, claiming that

> smoking and drinking *ganja* [cannabis] was good for the mother and the baby because it relieved the nausea of pregnancy, increased appetite, gave them strength to work, helped them relax and sleep at night, and in general, relieved the "bad feeling" associated with pregnancy. (Dreher 1997, p. 164)

From personal experience with my own "cannabis baby," I can attest to the validity of these conclusions. Similar to the results of the study, my daughter is "healthier, more advanced, more alert, and less irritable" than other infants her age.

TWO WOMEN'S STORIES
OF USING FOLK, ALTERNATIVE MEDICINE

In winter 2000, when I discovered through various parenting and childbirth Web sites the pervasiveness of HG, I decided to post a short message in a midwifery Internet site, sharing with others that I had discovered a nonpharmaceutical, natural cure and that anyone interested could contact me at my e-mail address. I felt that unless I shared my experiential knowledge, I would be withholding valuable information from women who could otherwise benefit from this rediscovered ancient folk remedy. Due to its controversial and illicit nature, I purposely posted a message that was vague, suppressing the fact that I was referring to cannabis. Only when I received an electronic-mail query did I reveal to the person the actual name of the herb, along with an option to request more detailed information if they were still interested. Of over 50 people who wrote to me in the following months to learn more about the herbal medicine, 2 women followed through, deciding to use cannabis medicinally for their hyperemesis. They both had negative experiences with mainstream medical procedures and pharmaceutical drugs during their previous pregnancies and were determined to find alternatives. When they first corresponded with me they were not pregnant, but after months of researching further into the prospect of using cannabis they eventually felt secure enough to conceive, hoping that the herb would work as efficaciously for them as it did for me. Although I did not interview them in the traditional sense, insights into their personal lives and profiles slowly emerged through correspondence.

The first woman, "Gina," is an elementary school teacher living in Southern California. When Gina first e-mailed me, she wrote:

> I had HG with my sons, now aged 19 and 17, and I had my most severe HG with my last pregnancy, which ended in a fetal demise at 14 weeks. I want to try again very much for another child (this is my second marriage, and my husband has no children). But I am deathly afraid of the HG. . . . I am so glad you are researching this disease. It is a crime that so many women have to suffer.

The second woman, "Didi," shared similar feelings. In her first correspondence, she wrote:

> I would love to hear about a natural cure [other] than [pharmaceutical] medicine. I just lost a baby at 5 months [when] I was on Reglan pump and IV Picc line. I started to feel better, then the baby just died with no reason. I lost another baby two years ago at 13 weeks. Any advice is welcomed. . . . My husband does not want to try again because of my condition. I should tell you I do have a 7-year-old son. I was sick with him but not as sick as I get now. I think it is because I am older now too (32 years old).

The challenges that Gina and Didi faced in considering cannabis as a therapeutic option were similar. The first obstacle was the lack of social and medical support that they felt in considering the use of a stigmatized therapy. Although open-minded, they still experienced feelings of fear and guilt, especially while using cannabis. For instance, although Gina repeatedly stated in many of her correspondences to me that she felt "very comfortable" with the thought of treating her HG with cannabis, her confidence level was soon undermined by others: women on the Internet chastised her, her husband discouraged her from relying upon it as the sole medicine, and her obstetrician was "very curt and uninterested" even before she could share with him her newly discovered medical choice. Although Gina lives in California and could logistically use medical cannabis under the protection of the Compassionate Use Act of 1996, she decided that it was best that she kept her "secret remedy" to herself, stating that she was "afraid to say anything," but was "not afraid to do it" in the privacy of her own home.

Didi also had fears in contemplating the use of the herb. When she asked her obstetrician if he could help her research the medicinal benefits of cannabis for pregnant women, he told his nurse to tell Didi that he was "too busy" and that she should do the research on her own. She followed his instruction, investigated the topic, and sent him her findings on the use of cannabis as a viable treatment for HG; in response, he refused further discussion, and sent her "pamphlets on the dangers of drugs" without additional comment. The doctor's callousness and lack of understanding and support deeply angered Didi. She later confided her feelings: "You would think that after everything I went through [losing two children due to HG], he would look into it harder with an open mind. This leads me to question . . . When I do find my next doctor [whether] to say nothing at all." Didi became more discouraged when she heard through her "sister's friend's aunt who is a nurse" that "doctors still check for drugs without your consent." In one of her e-mails, she asked me, "This is Michigan—is that possible? Will they send the social workers after me? Or is this a scare tactic?" Although I replied to her that by law, a woman has the right to not sign the consent form, she replied through e-mail with the proof of her findings:

> There was this one [woman's story posted on cannabisculture.com] that scared the SHIT out of me—by a woman named Aislinn who used cannabis throughout her pregnancy (recreationally) and they tested her baby for drugs [cannabis only]. Now they are taking her newborn away. What they said was she signed a consent form for treatment. They can test her for whatever they want. But who would think drugs? I am really scared now. I don't want to take any chances of losing my son and my new baby (whenever that happens).

A few weeks after this correspondence, Didi ceased relying on the Internet as a source of communicating, opting to use the telephone for the purpose of privacy and legal safety. She reasoned that the few sites that discussed cannabis usage during pregnancy were "shut down" simultaneously and all too "coincidentally," as if the government was censoring data being exchanged over the Internet and "making it harder for women" to openly exchange information. Whether this was a valid conclusion or an unfounded hypothesis I am not sure, but of certainty is the element of fear that continued to linger in Didi's consciousness.

According to researchers who have studied the properties of cannabinoids, two factors that are crucial to consider when a person uses a "psychoactive drug" such as cannabis are the "set and setting." Mathre explains in *Cannabis in Medical Practice* that "*set* refers to the mood and expectations of the user and *setting* refers to the environment in which the drug is used" (Mathre 1997, p. 175). Hence, if a person is already sensing "fear, guilt, and paranoia," these same feelings will become more exaggerated after the intake of cannabis, which can prevent the therapeutic properties from taking effect. Possibly, Gina and Didi's fear-laden set and setting took away from the women's abilities to allow the medicine to completely alleviate their symptoms. Gina stated in one of her correspondences:

> I started using [the herb] between weeks 5 and 6, when the symptoms started. It helps enormously! I still don't feel wonderful—I still don't have an appetite for food, I have to make myself eat, but at least it stays down, and I can keep my liquids up. . . . I know the nutrition part is really gonna bring this thing together.

Although the cannabis actually helped her achieve the relief that no other pharmaceutical drug had offered, she confessed that she continued to feel "nervous" and "guilty." In order to hide the fact that she was using cannabis for her nausea, she also took Diclectin to explain her relief without exposing her "secret remedy" to her obstetrician. She explained: "Still taking the Diclectin. Doctor said he'll order as much as I need. But it is really the cannabis that is saving me, because some days I am too sick to swallow the pills, so I smoke about two hits, wait a while, then I am able to eat and drink a little." Therefore, even though cannabis provided the true relief, she took the Diclectin to prevent suspicion from her obstetrician. The cannabis she obtained simply did not do much for her. It made her sleep a lot, counteracted her nausea and vomiting only slightly, and made her feel "paranoid and afraid." Its unsatisfactory effects could be traced to a number of possibilities: (1) the particular strain of the cannabis, (2) her psychological and physiological state, the "set," and (3) her environmental situation, the "setting." For the first point, both Gina and I have concluded through sharing our experiences that strains of *Cannabis indica,* while more potent, were less effective for us than *Cannabis sativa* strains in counteracting the nausea and vomiting of HG. *Indica* seemed to render the patient more vulnerable to paranoia, while *sativa* alleviated nausea/vomiting without the residual feelings of "getting high." In response to the second and third points: the controversial and illicit nature of the drug, along with the government's unwillingness to conduct further research, make situations even more difficult for women who could truly benefit from comprehensive guidelines and medical endorsement.

Procuring the illicit herb proved to be a challenge for both women. Gina had an easier time in Southern California. Didi had more difficulty acquiring good product in Michigan. It was no surprise to me when she later told me that she was not getting much, if any, relief from her cannabis. By the time I committed the risky and illicit act of sending some higher quality *sativa* via the mail, it was already too late and she had turned to the hospitalized treatment of HG, where her doctor started her on an intravenous line to receive liquid nutrition and ondansetron to curb her nausea and vomiting.

For Gina, cannabis was effective enough to keep her out of the hospital. Through experimentation, she found she was able to "autotitrate" (Mathre 1997, p. 146) according to what her body demanded:

> I haven't been getting sick in the middle of the night, which is great, because I can get some sleep. The times I have felt sick, I just get up and take a hit, then I'm fine. Sometimes I have to take up to 6 hits a day, 2 in the early morning, 2 in the afternoon, and 2 at night. But usually, it is about 4 hits, 2 in am, 2 in pm. I am no longer worried about it—because the alternatives are to be in the hospital again, or not go through with the pregnancy. The cannabis is really what is saving me—because I am able to eat and drink some, I can still work, although it is far from pleasant.

Unfortunately, in December 2000, I received the sad news that Gina miscarried as in her previous pregnancy. She stated: "The doctor said the fetus appeared to be about 13-14 weeks old, so I do not believe for a second that the cannabis or the Diclectin caused the fetal demise. There's something else going on." She said that her obstetrician was going to follow up with different chromosome and blood tests so that she could see why her body was "rejecting the fetuses." In spite of the tragic ending, Gina wrote to me: "I want to thank you for your support. I still believe in the medicinal value of cannabis for hyperemesis." I mourned Gina's miscarriage not because I had lost a potential candidate to study the use of cannabis for HG, but because she had lost a much-wanted child, a heartbreaking process that many, many mothers with HG too often endure. Fortunately, Didi's baby was birthed in health and wellness.

CONCLUSION

In retrospect, I wonder if my home-based, underground, pilot study on HG and cannabis was more depressing than it was encouraging. While my findings revealed some promise, I am left feeling deeply frustrated by the social and legal impossibilities of engaging in a formal clinical study in present-day America. What grieves me most is the knowledge that women with HG continue to suffer with no medically (and legally) efficacious treatment when I am convinced that we already have the cure. The stories I have been privileged to know have left me with images that continue to haunt me: of Sofia with her thighs dwindled to the width of my thin arms, interchangeably crying and vomiting as she watches the food channel on television because she wants so much to be able to eat, but cannot in the devastation of hyperemesis; of Maria threatening suicide because she is given no choice but to be bound to endless machinery with tubes surgically inserted into her abdomen for feeding and drainage for the sake of keeping her baby alive; of Sarah, whose husband deserted her because she appeared "skeletal with a belly," looking like "death," smelling like "poison," and wanting to die every waking hour; of Gina, devastated with the discovery that she had lost a much-wanted baby for the second time. These real-life tragedies bombard me with a dispirited, *"Why?"* Why do HG women continue to suffer, even amidst pharmaceutical and hospitalized treatments that can cost over hundreds of thousand of dollars of insurance money per pregnancy?

Why was I so blessed to have found a cure, one that cost no more than $90 for the entire duration of my HG? If it were not for the study of Jamaican pregnant women who used cannabis safely with positive effects on their babies, and if it were not for my Taiwanese obstetrician who reassured me that birthing women in China have commonly used cannabis to alleviate their nausea and vomiting, and if it were not for Dr. Grinspoon at Harvard Medical School, with his extensive research on the medicinal properties of cannabis, who found credibility and value in my anecdote, I would definitely be filled with self-doubt in the face of surrounding fear, persecution, and paranoia. While I should simply let the issue pass, a part of me is unwilling to give up so easily, partially because cannabis is an important, but lost, part of my cultural heritage. Having experienced severe hyperemesis, I can empathize with all the women who also endure its debilitating effects. If one could imagine surviving the nausea and retching of food poisoning combined with vertigo and motion sickness nonstop for four to nine months straight, night and day, then one could possibly begin fathoming the physical and psychological trauma of living with HG.

In summary, it is relevant to ask: What are the rites and rights of birth offered to a woman with hyperemesis within the realm of modern medicine? The rites are obvious: *the ritual of isolation,* when the woman is attached to tubes and machines in the hospital, sometimes for the entire nine month duration, torn from her community of family and friends; *the ritual of sacrifice,* when the woman's body, viewed as an "object" rather than a "subject," is poked and prodded, severed and bloodied as she is merely treated as the container who must somehow "produce" the baby, the "product" (Davis-Floyd 1992, pp. 160-161); *the ritual of denial,* when the woman's incessant and tenacious nausea and vomiting is downplayed as being "all in the head," or accused as a way for her to "vomit out her baby" or disguise her "bulimia" disorder; *the ritual of suffering,* when the woman is expected to withstand the tortures of highly gruesome medical procedures that involve the surgical cutting and ripping of flesh without anesthesia, bear the pangs of long-term starvation, and endure the end result of a "chronically collapsed digestive system"; *the ritual of silence,* when the woman's voice is not heard, in spite of her cries for help, and her body is not acknowledged, in spite of its emaciation. And finally, within these rites is simply her right to give birth with much medical intervention but no real cure.

BIBLIOGRAPHY

Abel, E.L. 1980. *Marihuana: The first 12,000 years.* New York: Plenum Press.

Abel, E.L. 1982. *A marihuana dictionary: Words, terms, events, and persons relating to cannabis.* Westport, CT: Greenwood Press.

Arms, S. 1975. *Immaculate deception: A new look at women and childbirth in America.* New York: Bantam Books.

Arms, S. 1994. *Immaculate deception II: Myth, magic, and birth.* Berkeley, CA: Celestial Arts.

Askling, J., G. Erlandsson, M. Kaijser, O. Akre, and B. Anders. 1999. Sickness in pregnancy and sex of child. *Lancet* 354(9195):2053-2055.

Benet, S. 1975. Early diffusion and folk uses of hemp. In V. Rubin (ed.), *Cannabis and culture* (pp. 39-49). Chicago: Mouton Publishers.

Boyd, S.C. 1999. *Mothers and illicit drug use: Transcending the myths.* Toronto: University of Toronto Press.

Brady, E. (Ed.). 2001. *Healing logics: Culture and medicine in modern health belief systems.* Logan, UT: Utah State University Press.

Browner, C.H. and N. Press. 1997. The production of authoritative knowledge in American prenatal care. In R.E. Davis-Floyd and C. Sargent (eds.), *Childbirth and authoritative knowledge: Cross-cultural perspectives* (pp. 113-131). Berkeley: University of California Press.

Carlson, K.J., S.A. Eisenstat, and T. Ziporyn. 1996. *The Harvard guide to women's health.* Cambridge: Harvard University Press.

Chêng, T.-K.. 1959. *Archaeology in China,* Volume 1: *Prehistoric China.* Cambridge, UK: W. Heffer and Sons.

Christ, C.P. 1997. *Rebirth of the goddess: Finding meaning in feminist spirituality.* New York: Routledge Press.

Christy, C.P. 1978. Why women need the goddess: Phenomenological, psychological, and political reflections. *Heresies* (spring):273-287.

Davis-Floyd, R.E. 1992. *Birth as an American rite of passage.* Berkeley: University of California Press.

Davis-Floyd, R.E. and C.F. Sargent (eds.). 1997. *Childbirth and authoritative knowledge: Cross-cultural perspectives.* Berkeley: University of California Press.

Dick-Read, G. 1959. *Childbirth without fear: The principals and practice of natural childbirth.* New York: Harper and Brothers.

Dreher, M.C. 1997. Cannabis and pregnancy. In M.L. Mathre (ed.), *Cannabis in medical practice: A legal, historical and pharmacological overview of the therapeutic use of marijuana* (pp. 159-170). Jefferson, NC: McFarland.

Du Toit, B.M. 1980. *Cannabis in Africa: A survey of its distribution in Africa, and a study of cannabis use and users in multi-etnic [sic] South Africa.* Rotterdam, Netherlands: A.A. Balkema.

England, P. and R. Horowitz. 1998. *Birthing from within: An extra-ordinary guide to childbirth preparation.* Albuquerque, NM: Partera Press.

Erick, M. 1997. Nutrition via jejunostomy in refractory hyperemesis gravidarum: A case report. *J Amer Dietetic Assoc* 97(10):1154-1156.

Fleming, M.P. and R.C. Clarke. 1998. Physical evidence for the antiquity of *Cannabis sativa* L. (Cannabaceae). *J Internat Hemp Assoc* 5(2):80-92.

Foucault, M. 1973. *The birth of the clinic: An archeology of medical perception.* New York: Vintage Books.

Foucault, M. 1980. *Power/knowledge: Selected interviews and other writings 1972-1977.* Edited/translated by C.G.L. Marshall, J. Mepham, K. Soper. New York: Pantheon Books.

Foucault, M. 1995. *Discipline and punishment: The birth of the prison.* New York: Vintage Books.

Gaskin, I.M. 1990. *Spiritual midwifery,* Third edition. Summertown, TN: The Book Publishing Company.

Ginsburg, F.D. and R. Rapp. 1991. The politics of reproduction. *Annual Review Anthropol* 20:311-343.

Ginsburg, F.D. and R. Rapp (eds.). 1995. *Conceiving the new world order: The global politics of reproduction.* Berkeley: University of California Press.

Glenn, E.N., G. Chang, and L.R. Forcey (eds.). 1994. *Mothering: Ideology, experience, and agency.* New York: Routledge.

Grinspoon, L., and J.B. Bakalar. 1997. *Marihuana: The forbidden medicine.* New Haven: Yale University Press.

Hillborn, M.J., V. Pylvenen, and K. Sotaniemi. 1999. Pregnant, vomiting, and coma (Wernicke's encephalopathy): Case report. *Lancet* 353(9164):1584.

Hufford, D.J. 1994. Folklore and medicine. In M.O. Jones (ed.), *Putting folklore to use* (pp. 117-135). Lexington: University Press of Kentucky.

Jordan, B. 1993. *Birth in four cultures: A cross-cultural investigation of childbirth in Yucatan, Holland, Sweden, and the United States,* Fourth edition. Prospect Heights, IL: Waveland Press.

Jordan, B. 1997. Authoritative knowledge and its construction. In R. Davis-Floyd and C.F. Sargent (eds.), *Childbirth and authoritative knowledge: Cross-cultural perspectives* (pp. 55-79). Berkeley: University of California Press.

Lamaze, F. 1956. *Painless childbirth.* Translated by L.R. Celestin. Chicago: H. Regnery Company.

Leavitt, J.W. 1986. *Brought to bed: Childbearing in America 1750-1950.* New York: Oxford University Press.

Leboyer, F. 1975. *Birth without violence.* New York: Alfred A Knopf.

Li, H.-L. 1975. The origin and use of cannabis in Eastern Asia: Their linguistic-cultural implications. In V. Rubin (ed.), *Cannabis and culture* (pp. 51-62). Chicago: Mouton Publishers.

Jones, M.O. (Ed.). 1994. *Putting folklore to use.* Lexington: University Press of Kentucky.

Mallon, C.L. 1997. Unnatural childbirth: A feminist sociology of birth in America. PhD dissertation in comparative culture, University of California, Irvine.

Mathre, M.L. 1997. *Cannabis and medical practice: A legal, historical, and pharmaceutical overview of the therapeutic use of marijuana.* Jefferson, NC: McFarland & Co., Inc.

Meltzer, D.I. 2000. Complementary therapies for nausea and vomiting in early pregnancy. *Fam Pract* 17(6):570-573.

Murcott, A. 1988. On the altered appetites of pregnancy: Conceptions of food, body and person. *Sociological Rev* 36(4):733-764.

Murphy, S., and M. Rosenbaum. 1999. *Pregnant women on drugs: Combating stereotypes and stigma.* New Brunswick, NJ: Rutgers University Press.

Panesar, N.S., C.-Y. Li, and M.S. Rogers. 2001. Are thyroid hormones or hCG responsible for hyperemesis gravidarum? A matched paired study in pregnant Chinese women. *Acta Obstetricia et Gynecologica Scandinavica* 80:519-524.

Peterson, A. and R. Bunton (Eds.). 1997. *Foucault, health, and medicine.* New York: Routledge.

Rubin, V. (ed.). 1975. *Cannabis and culture.* The Hague, Netherlands: Mouton Publishers.

Schoenberg, F.P. 2000. Summary of data on hyperemesis gravidarum. *The Birthkit* (spring):4-8.

Schultes, R.E., and A. Hofmann. 1979. *Plants of the gods: Origins of hallucinogenic use.* New York: McGraw-Hill Book Company.

Simpson, S.W., T. M. Goodwin, S.B. Robins, A.A. Rizzo, R.A. Howes, D.K. Buckwalter, and J.G. Buckwalter. 2001. Psychological factors and hyperemesis gravidarum. *J Women's Health and Gender-Based Med* 10(5):471-477.

Tesfaye, S., V. Achari, Y.C. Yang, S. Harding, A. Bowden, and J.P. Vora. 1998. Pregnant, vomiting, and going blind. *Lancet* 352(9140):1594.

Thompson, L. 1999. *The wandering womb: A cultural history of outrageous beliefs about women.* Amherst, NY: Prometheus Books.

University of California, Los Angeles. 2001. Folk Medicine Archive. Web site: http:// www.folkmed.ucla.edu.

Van de Ven, C.J.M. 1997. Nasogastric enteral feeding in hyperemesis gravidarum. *Lancet* 349(9050):445-446.

W.B. Saunders Dictionary Staff. 1994. *Dorland's illustrated medical dictionary,* Twenty-eighth edition. Philadelphia: W.B. Saunders Company.

Wright, T.L. 1862. Correspondence. *Cincinatti Lancet and Observer* 5(4):246-247.

UPDATE

Ethan B. Russo

Although cannabis usage in pregnancy remains one of the great "forbidden areas" (Russo 2003), morning sickness and hyperemesis gravidarum remain important clinical imperatives accounting for a great deal of morbidity, and even maternal and fetal mortality. A recent publication has provided very strong anecdotal corroboratory evidence of benefit of cannabis in context (Westphal et al. 2005), with the vast majority of women who had utilized cannabis to treat nausea of pregnancy obtaining good to excellent relief of symptoms. At some point, utilization of a standardized, nonsmoked cannabis-based medicine in a controlled clinical trial seems warranted.

REFERENCES

Russo, E.B. 2003. Future of cannabis and cannabinoids in therapeutics. *Journal of Cannabis Therapeutics* 3 (4):163-174.

Westphal, R., P. Janssen, P. Lucas, and R. Capler. 2006. Survey of medicinal cannabis use among childbearing women: Patterns of its use in pregnancy and retroactive self-assessment of tis efficacy against "morning sickness." *Complementary Therapies in Clinical Practice* 12:27-33.

Chapter 15

Therapeutic Cannabis (Marijuana) As an Antiemetic and Appetite Stimulant in Persons with Acquired Immunodeficiency Syndrome

Richard E. Bayer

AIDS IN THE UNITED STATES

The history of acquired immunodeficiency syndrome (AIDS) began in 1981 when the first five cases of AIDS were reported in the United States. Shortly thereafter, the disease was categorized as an epidemic. In 1984, the etiology of AIDS was found to be an RNA virus dubbed human immunodeficiency virus (HIV). In 1985, a sensitive enzyme-linked immunosorbent assay (ELISA) was developed, and clinical testing for antibodies to HIV became possible.

By 1993, the United States Department of Health and Human Services (DHHS) listed AIDS as the most common cause of death among men aged 25 to 44 years (US DHHS 1995). By the end of 1998, the United States Centers for Disease Control and Prevention (CDC) estimated that nearly one million Americans had contracted HIV infection, one-third of whom were unaware of their affliction (CDC 1999).

By the end of 1999, a total of 733,374 cases of affected persons with AIDS (PWAs) had been reported to the CDC. Demographics revealed that 82 percent were men, and 18 percent were women. Only 1 percent were children less than 13 years of age. Forty-three percent of persons with AIDS were white, 37 percent black, 18 percent Hispanic, < 1 percent Asians and Pacific Islanders, and < 1 percent American Indians and Alaska Natives. Forty-seven percent of persons with AIDS were men who have sex with men, 25 percent were injection drug users, 10 percent were persons infected

Handbook of Cannabis Therapeutics
© 2006 by The Haworth Press, Inc. All rights reserved.
doi:10.1300/5741_16

heterosexually, and 2 percent were persons infected through blood or blood products (CDC 1999).

HIV destroys CD4+ T lymphocytes, and laboratory measurements of T cells indicate immune system damage. More recently, the technology of polymerase chain reaction has allowed the actual measurement of HIV RNA blood levels or viral load, and this parameter is increasingly utilized clinically to help determine when to initiate and modify antiretroviral therapies (Saag et al. 1996).

The surveillance conditions for diagnosis of severe HIV disease or AIDS were originally defined by the CDC prior to the identification of HIV as the etiologic agent. Although surveillance criteria have changed over the years, the clinician should view HIV disease as a spectrum of illness that ranges from a primary infection to the asymptomatic infected to advanced disease or AIDS, which causes marked morbidity and mortality (Fauci and Lane 2000).

For surveillance purposes, AIDS is defined by indicator diseases such as the AIDS wasting syndrome, *Pneumocystis carinii* pneumonia, or Kaposi's sarcoma in young adults. AIDS is identified in asymptomatic persons by laboratory tests such as CD4+ T lymphocyte counts of less than 200/mcL or a CD4+ T lymphocyte percent of total lymphocytes less than 14 (CDC 1992). Since 1992, scientists have estimated that about half the people with HIV develop AIDS within ten years after infection, but this time varies greatly from person to person (CDC 2000).

AIDS wasting syndrome is an AIDS-defining condition, identified when a patient manifests involuntary weight loss of more than 10 percent associated with intermittent or constant fever and diarrhea or fatigue for more than 30 days in the absence of a non-HIV explanation. It is the initial AIDS-defining illness in 9 percent of patients with AIDS in the United States and thus is currently the leading initial clinical indication of AIDS (Fauci and Lane 2000).

Standard antiretroviral treatments for HIV infection, such as zidovudine (AZT or ZVD) or lamivudine (3TC) can cause significant nausea. Treated patients often have difficulty maintaining baseline weight. In 1996, the United States Food and Drug Administration (FDA) approved the use of protease inhibitors, which when taken in combination with standard antiretroviral drugs can reduce viral load and markedly slow the progression of HIV/AIDS disease (CDC 1998).

A concern for many who take protease inhibitors is that the side effects can be more severe than those associated with standard antiretroviral drugs. As occurs with some persons receiving chemotherapy for cancer, patients with AIDS often find that the medicines they need to sustain their lives can produce side effects so intolerable that they become reluctant to maintain their treatments, or fail to take treatment regularly. This can be dangerous, for failure to maintain a regular medication schedule can lead to the development of treatment-resistant strains of HIV (CDC 2000).

CANNABINOIDS AS ANTIEMETIC
AND APPETITE STIMULANT IN AIDS WASTING SYNDROME

Ethnobotany documents important medical uses of herbs, including cannabis (Russo 2000), but the first modern placebo-controlled trial that demonstrated efficacy of THC as an antiemetic in cancer chemotherapy was published in 1975 (Sallan et al. 1975). In the 1970s and 1980s, six American states engaged in clinical trials of smoked cannabis and oral THC to control nausea and emesis from cancer chemotherapy. These trials involved 748 persons who smoked cannabis and 345 patients who used oral THC capsules, and demonstrated that smoked marijuana can be a very successful treatment for nausea and vomiting following cancer chemotherapy (Musty and Rossi 2001). A synergistic relationship of the combination of THC and the antiemetic prochloperazine was more effective than either drug alone, as suggested by past studies (Hollister 2001). These are important findings, because our most efficacious modern antiemetics, including well-tolerated serotonin antagonists such as ondansetron (Zofran), promise only about 80 percent efficacy (Zofran 2000). In other words, in one out of every five treatment episodes, our best antiemetics demonstrate no efficacy. Although no studies have been done comparing ondansetron to cannabis, patients would be well served by studying efficacy of cannabinoids alone, or in combination with other antiemetics in persons who currently cannot control nausea and emesis with modern serotonin antagonists like ondansetron.

In 1992, the FDA approved the use of Marinol (dronabinol or synthetic THC) for the treatment of AIDS wasting syndrome. Dronabinol has been shown to stimulate appetite, promote weight gain and improve mood in persons with AIDS in short-term studies (Beal et al. 1995), while maintaining effectiveness and safety over during a longer (12-month) study (Beal et al. 1997). Marinol is usually prescribed at a dose of 2.5 mg by mouth 2 to 3 times daily before meals to improve appetite (Roxane Labs 1999). Although the Drug Enforcement Administration (DEA) originally listed dronabinol as a Schedule II drug, it was recently moved to Schedule III, which may increase the likelihood of American physicians prescribing it.

While dronabinol is the only cannabinoid that physicians can legally prescribe in the United States, it remains extremely expensive (often US$600 to $1200 each month), has a slow onset of action because it can only be taken orally and has a relatively high incidence of side effects (particularly dysphoria), so that many patients prefer herbal cannabis. As is the case in many cancer patients, people with AIDS frequently expressed a preference for smoked cannabis over dronabinol because it provides results with smaller doses and fewer undesirable side effects. In addition, some persons report better symptom control consuming cannabis rather than dronabinol, which may be related to the additional cannabinoids, such as cannabidiol, that are found in cannabis but not in dronabinol (Grinspoon and Bakalar 1997).

Other agents used to treat AIDS wasting include anabolic steroid hormones such as the progesterone megestrol acetate (Megace), tested alone and in combination with dronabinol (Timpone et al. 1997), and androgenic steroids such as oral oxandrolone (Berger et al. 1996), or intramuscular testosterone enanthate (Grinspoon et al. 1998). More extreme options include human growth hormone, which can cost more than $150 daily, and total parenteral nutrition, which is expensive, invasive, and medically risky (Krampf 1997). These treatments have shown some successes, but all have drawbacks, and thus treatment must be individualized to meet each patient's needs.

For a more comprehensive discussion of cannabis as antiemetic and appetite stimulant, readers are referred to Leo Hollister's review, "Marijuana (Cannabis) as Medicine" in the charter issue of *Journal of Cannabis Therapeutics* (Hollister 2001). For a comprehensive clinical discussion of HIV disease, readers are referred to an internal medicine textbook such as *Harrison's Principles of Internal Medicine* (Fauci and Lane 2000).

CASE REPORTS (THE PATIENTS' PERSPECTIVE)

There are many case reports from persons with AIDS who benefit from adjunctive use of cannabis to stimulate appetite, control pain, and improve quality of life (Zimmerman et al. 1998; Grinspoon and Bakalar 1997; Krampf 1997).

Patient S.C. describes:

> Within eight months, beginning in 1995, I was hospitalized three times for pneumonia and sinus infection. I'd been feeling pain and congestion in my chest, and then I began having trouble breathing. I was still taking AZT and they put me on antibiotics and prednisone for the pneumonia. It was so difficult for me to swallow the pills. Almost immediately after taking them, a violent nausea would set in. I couldn't eat or hold down any food. After a few weeks of this, my weight dropped down from 150 to 115 pounds.

I did what I could during that time to get relief. That's when I realized, almost coincidentally, that marijuana alleviated my nausea. When I took a few hits of marijuana, I felt better within five to fifteen minutes. It also gave me back my appetite. In a short time, I gained back almost all my weight, and I began feeling much healthier.

Just as importantly, my marijuana use would help me deal with the new drugs I'd soon be taking. They began combining AZT and another antiviral drug, called 3TC, with a protease inhibitor called Crixivan. I did notice a gradual improvement in my health, and my T-cell count started coming up. But the nausea I experienced was worse than anything I had felt with AZT alone. It was indescribable. It didn't seem like I had many choices though. I knew I needed these medicines to stay alive, even though the nausea they caused me was unbearable. So, I kept taking them, along with marijuana to control the nausea.

I have to tell you that I sincerely doubt I could have continued the treatment without marijuana. This is very important because, while there is no cure for AIDS, I believe these medications have actually reversed my disease and saved my life. What marijuana did, aside from making me feel better, was make these drugs tolerable for me.

Right now, my weight is up to 148 pounds. I take 16 pills a day, and I smoke marijuana before each meal to quell the nausea and stimulate my appetite. About one-half hour before I want to eat, I take three or four puffs. Usually, in about 20 minutes, I get the munchies and then I want to eat. It's still a struggle sometimes, but I'm healthier, stronger, and I enjoy living. (Zimmerman et al. 1998, pp. 48-49)

Patient G.S. summarizes his experience:

Even if I was not recovering [from AIDS], the relief would have been worth any bad effect the marijuana might have had. I could keep down food, and I could stop the aching. Also, I'm convinced that one of the worst things for my immune system was the stress my sickness caused me. Marijuana reduced my stress and it calmed my soul. It made me not worry so much about the difficult regimen of pills I had to take, or how I was going to get to the grocery store because I didn't think I'd be able to walk. Marijuana allowed me to accept the possibility that I might die, and yet, I believe, because I smoked marijuana, I lived. (Zimmerman et al. 1998, p. 53)

In the United States, many persons with AIDS use cannabis daily to control nausea, increase appetite, decrease pain, and improve mood. Although case reports like those above are frequent, the federal drug bureaucracy has kept a virtual stranglehold on all clinical research into the safety and effectiveness of cannabis (Doblin 2000).

RECENT CLINICAL RESEARCH ON CANNABINOIDS, IMMUNITY, AND WEIGHT GAIN

After a Byzantine ordeal that lasted the better part of a decade (Doblin 2000), University of California—San Francisco (UCSF) researcher Donald Abrams was finally able to do a study to compare the effectiveness of dronabinol (Marinol) versus smoked cannabis versus placebo in persons with AIDS.

The results of Dr. Abrams's study, "Marijuana Does Not Appear to Alter Viral Loads of HIV Patients Taking Protease Inhibitors," were released July 13, 2000, by UCSF (Abrams 2000). The study found that patients with HIV infection taking protease inhibitors do not experience short-term (three-week) adverse virologic effects from using cannabinoids.

Of the 62 subjects who completed the inpatient study, values for 36 with undetectable HIV RNA levels remained unchanged through the trial. All 26 subjects with detectable HIV RNA levels experienced declines in those levels. Of those, the subjects who smoked cannabis or took oral dronabinol experienced slightly greater decreases in HIV RNA levels than did subjects who took the placebo, but there was no statistical difference between the three groups.

All three groups gained weight, thanks to regularly scheduled meals and available snacks. However, the subjects in the placebo arm gained an average of 1.30 kg, while those who took oral dronabinol gained an average of 3.18 kg, and those who smoked cannabis gained an average of 3.51 kg. These results should alleviate some concerns about the effects of THC as dronabinol and smoked herbal cannabis on immunity,

CANNABIS AND HARM REDUCTION STRATEGIES FOR PERSONS WITH AIDS

There is concern about risk of potential respiratory and lung infection in immunocompromised persons from smoking cannabis because underground market sources may be contaminated with bacteria or fungal spores. Some patients minimize this risk by cultivating their own cannabis, while others are careful to obtain cannabis only from trusted sources. Some persons heat the cannabis in a toaster oven for several minutes to reach the temperature used to pasteurize milk, 71°C (160°F), but keep the heat much lower than the 140°C to 190°C (284°F to 374°F), at which temperature the cannabinoids "vaporize" or "volatize" causing significant degradation of source material (Rosenthal et al. 1997; Gieringer 2001).

These are descriptions of some patients' strategies, but there are no controlled trials demonstrating increased risk for infection in cannabis-only smokers versus nonsmokers among persons with AIDS or any documented clinical benefit from attempting to sterilize the cannabis as described above.

Some patients try to reduce the risk of using contaminated cannabis by alternately smoking cannabis and cooking it in food. Some books on medical use of cannabis contain recipes (Rosenthal et al. 1997), or alternatively, patients may use a standard search engine on the Internet. Patients sometimes rely on smoked cannabis when the symptoms of nausea are so severe they are incapable of oral intake, but at other times they bake it into brownies or put in other food. In this way, the patient may get the immediate and effective relief that smoking provides, but when the need is less pressing, minimize the risk of smoking potentially contaminated cannabis through oral intake.

Oral ingestion of cannabis resolves the issues of smoking toxicity, but the harm-reduction issue is complicated by the United States' War on Drugs, which causes a "prohibition tariff" and increases cost by a factor of about ten. Estimates are that without cannabis prohibition, production costs would be $30 to $40 per ounce (Grinspoon 1997), but current street prices are about $300 to $400 per dry ounce for high-quality female flowers ("bud"). Eating cannabis or making tea is expensive, and as for dronabinol, it has a slower onset of action. Oral THC also produces lower blood levels and is less effective in controlling nausea when compared to smoked THC cigarettes (Chang 1979).

Inhalation of therapeutic drugs, such as treatment of asthma using metered dose inhalers, provides rapid onset of action and dose titration using the minimum effective dose (which minimizes drug side effects). Medical inhalation of cannabis provides similar advantages, but without vaporization, carries the risk of inhaling smoke. Therefore, one method to reduce harm from smoking is for patients to use only high quality medical cannabis, so there is a greater concentration of therapeutic cannabinoids per mass ingested.

Promising initial results from a study by California NORML (National Organization to Reform Marijuana Laws) and the Multidisciplinary Association for Psychedelic Studies (MAPS) demonstrate that patients may be able to protect themselves from harmful toxins in cannabis smoke by inhaling their medicine using an electric vaporizer (Gieringer 2001). Vaporization involves releasing cannabinoids by heating cannabis to temperature short of combustion, thereby eliminating or substantially reducing harmful toxics that are present in cannabis smoke. Gieringer reports traces of THC appearing at temperatures as low as 140°C (284°F) while significant amounts of benzene did not appear until 200°C (392°F) and combustion did not appear until around 230°C (446°F) or above. An aromatherapy device called the Volatizer (www.volatizer.com) consisting of an electric heating element similar to an automobile cigarette lighter on a metal wand produces a temperature of 185°C (385°F) and is placed over the bowl of cannabis that sits inside the top of a 0.5 liter side-arm Erlenmeyer flask. Vapors are inhaled through a rubber tube connected to the side-arm of the flask. The Volatizer reduced measured toxins (benzene, a known carcinogen, plus toluene and naphthalene), carbon monoxide, and tars when compared to combusting the cannabis by flame. More research is indicated, but vaporizers appear to substantially reduce what is widely perceived as the leading health hazard of cannabis, namely respiratory damage from smoking. Drawbacks to vaporization include cost (a complete Volatizer unit costs US$250), and portability. Competing aromatherapy devices include using a thermocouple heat gun blown across the cannabis and collecting vapors in a chamber or bag (www.mystifier.com) or placing cannabis in one end of a small (pencil size) glass tube with the other end of the glass tube connected to a plastic tube for inhalation. The glass end with cannabis is then inserted in an "oven" that looks like an automobile oil filter and vapors are inhaled through the plastic tube (www.vaportechco.com). These two units are less expensive (about US$150) than the Volatizer but have not yet been laboratory tested. Other units are available, but until paraphernalia laws are relaxed and mass production of vaporizers is possible (e.g., using small batteries), vaporization remains an attractive but expensive harm reduction tool.

Simpler devices such as water pipes or "bongs" that combust the cannabis and draw the smoke through water before inhalation serve to cool the inhaled smoke, but there is no evidence that they reduce the ratio of tar and particulate matter to therapeutic cannabinoids (Gieringer 1994). There may be undiscovered health advantages from cooling the inhaled smoke or filtering out certain gases, but any advantage of a water pipe or bong over a joint to deliver smoked cannabis remains undocumented.

A medical records review of 452 daily cannabis smokers who never smoked tobacco showed a slight increase in clinic visits for colds, flu, and bronchitis over a two-year period when compared to demographically similar group of nonsmokers of either substance (Polen 1993). Although heavy cannabis smokers report "smokers' cough" (chronic bronchitis), there is no evidence that cannabis smokers who do not smoke tobacco will develop small airways disease, such as emphysema (Tashkin et al. 1997).

Patients should be advised to stop holding their breath after inhaling smoke, for this technique does not increase benefits from cannabis, but rather appears to increase risks of potentially dangerous deposits in the airways. Probably because the lifetime quantity of smoke consumed by cannabis smokers is typically far less than for tobacco smokers, there exists no clinical evidence that typical cannabis smokers have higher rates of respiratory cancer (Zimmer and Morgan 1997). However, recent reports from the United States (Zhang et al. 1999) and Europe (Carriot and Sasco 2000) suggest heavy cannabis smokers may increase risk of head and neck cancer with a strong dose-response pattern.

CONCLUSION

Many patients report that cannabis helped prolong their lives by enabling them to cope with some of the difficult symptoms and treatments associated with AIDS. In spite of a need for more rigorous scientifically controlled research, an increasing number of persons with AIDS are using cannabis because they find it controls nausea, increases appetite, promotes weight gain, decreases pain, and improves mood.

REFERENCES

Abrams, D. 2000. Marijuana does not appear to alter viral loads of HIV patients taking protease inhibitors. University of California at San Francisco press release. ©1999 Regents of the University of California. Alice Trinkl, News Director. Source: Jeff Sheehy (415) 597-8165. http://www.ucsf.edu/pressrel/2000/07/071302.html.

Beal, J. R., L. Olson, J. Laubenstein, J. Morales, P. Bellman, B. Yangco, L. Lefkowitz, T. Plasse, and K. Shepard. 1995. Dronabinol as a treatment for anorexia associated with weight loss in patients with AIDS. *J Pain Sympt Manag* 10(2):89-97.

Beal, J.R., L. Olson, L. Lefkowitz, L. Laubenstein, P. Bellman, B. Yangco, J. Morales, R. Murphy, W. Powderly, T. Plasse, K. Mosdell, and K. Shepard. 1997. Long-term efficacy and safety of dronabinol for acquired immunodeficiency syndrome-associated anorexia. *J Pain Sympt Manag* 14(1):7-14.

Berger J., L. Pall, C. Hall, D. Simpson, P. Berry, and R. Dudley. 1996. Oxandrolone in AIDS-wasting myopathy. *AIDS* 10(14):1657-1662.

Carriot, F. and Sasco, A. 2000. Cannabis and cancer. *Revue d'Épidémiologie et de Santé Publique* 48(5):473-483.

Centers for Disease Control and Prevention. 1992. 1993 revised classification system for HIV infection and expanded surveillance case definition for AIDS among adolescents and adults. *MMWR Morb Mortal Wkly Rep* 41(51):961-962. http://www. cdc.gov/mmwr/preview/mmwrhtml/00018179.htm.

Centers for Disease Control and Prevention. 1999. CDC guidelines for national human immunodeficiency virus case surveillance, including monitoring for human immunodeficiency virus infection and acquired immunodeficiency syndrome.

MMWR Morb Mortal Wkly Rep 48(RR-13). http://www.cdc.gov/mmwr/PDF/ RR/RR4813.pdf.

Centers for Disease Control and Prevention. National Center for HIV, STD, and TB Prevention, Divisions of HIV/AIDS Prevention. 1998. *Trends in the HIV and AIDS Epidemic, 1998.* http://www. cdc.gov/hiv/stats/trends98.pdf.

Centers for Disease Control and Prevention. National Center for HIV, STD, and TB Prevention, Divisions of HIV/AIDS Prevention. 1999. *HIV/AIDS Surveillance Report* 11(2):5. http://www.cdc.gov/hiv/stats/hasr1102.htm or www.cdc.gov/ hiv/stats/hasr1102.pdf.

Centers for Disease Control and Prevention. National Center for HIV, STD, and TB Prevention, Divisions of HIV/AIDS Prevention. 2000. *Guidelines for the use of antiretroviral agents in HIV-infected adults and adolescents.* http://www.cdc. gov/ hiv/treatment.htm.

Chang, A. 1979. Delta-9-tetrahydrocannabinol as an antiemetic in cancer patients receiving high-dose methotrexate. *Ann Intern Med* 91(6):819-824. http://www. teleport.com/~omr/omr chang.html.

Doblin, R. 2000. Multidisciplinary Association for Psychedelic Studies (MAPS) website with additional references: http://www.maps.org/mmj/mjabrams.html.

Fauci, A.S. and H.C. Lane. 2000. *Harrison's Principles of Internal Medicine. Harrison's Online Edition.* New York: McGraw Hill, Inc.

Gieringer, D. 1994. The MAPS/California NORML marijuana waterpipe/vaporizer study. *MAPS Bull* 5(1):19-22. http://www.maps.org/news-letters/v06n3/06359 mj1.html.

Gieringer, D. 2001. *NORML-MAPS study shows vaporizers reduce toxins in marijuana smoke.* California NORML press release. ©2001 California NORML. (415) 563-5858. http://www.canorml.org/research/vaporizerstudy1.html.

Grinspoon, L. 1997. Testimony of Lester Grinspoon, M.D. before the Crime Subcommittee of the Judiciary Committee, U.S. House of Representatives on October 1, 1997. http://www.rxmarihuana.com/testimony.htm.

Grinspoon, L. and J. Bakalar. 1997. *Marihuana: The forbidden medicine.* New Haven, CT: Yale University Press.

Grinspoon S., C. Corcoran, H. Askari, D. Schoenfeld, L. Wolf, B. Burrows, M. Walsh, D. Hayden, K. Parlman, E. Anderson et al. 1998. Effects of androgen administration in men with the AIDS wasting syndrome. A randomized, double-blind, placebo-controlled trial. *Ann Intern Med* 129(1):18-26.

Hollister, L.E. 2001. Marijuana (cannabis) as medicine. *Journal of Cannabis Therapeutics* 1(1):5-27.

Krampf, W. 1997. AIDS and the wasting syndrome. In M.L. Mathre (ed.), *Cannabis in medical practice: A legal, historical, and pharmacological overview of the therapeutic use of cannabis* (pp. 84-93). Jefferson, N.C: McFarland & Co.

Musty, R.E., and R. Rossi. 2001. Effects of smoked cannabis and oral delta-9-tetrahydrocannabinol on nausea and emesis after cancer chemotherapy: A review of state clinical trials. *Journal of Cannabis Therapeutics* 1(1):29-42.

Polen, M.R., S. Sidney, I. Tekawa, M. Sadler, and G. Friedman. 1993. Health care use by frequent marijuana smokers who do not smoke tobacco. *West J Med* 158(6):596-601.

Rosenthal, E., D. Gieringer, and T. Mikuriya. 1997. *Marijuana medical use handbook: A guide to therapeutic use.* Oakland, CA: Quick American Archives.

Roxane Laboratories package insert with full prescribing information for Marinol brand of dronabinol. Revised 1999. http://hiv.roxane.com/prodinfo/marinol.html.

Russo, E. 2000. *Handbook of psychotropic herbs: A scientific analysis of herbal remedies for psychiatric conditions.* Binghamton, NY: The Haworth Press, Inc.

Saag M.S., M. Holodniy, D. Kuritzkes, et al. 1996. HIV viral load markers in clinical practice: recommendations of an International AIDS Society-USA Expert Panel. *Nature Med* 2:625-629.

Sallan, S.E., N.E. Zinberg and E. Frei. 1975. Antiemetic effect of delta-9-tetrahydrocannabinol in patients receiving cancer chemotherapy. *New Eng J Med* 293:795-797.

Tashkin, D., M. Simmons, D. Sherrill, and A. Coulson. 1997. Heavy habitual marijuana smoking does not cause an accelerated decline in FEV1 with age. *Am J Respir Crit Care Med* 155:141-148.

Timpone, J., D. Wright, N. Li, M. Egorin, M. Enama, J. Mayers, and G. Galetto. 1997. The safety and pharmacokinetics of single-agent and combination therapy with megestrol acetate and dronabinol for the treatment of HIV wasting syndrome. *AIDS Res Hum Retroviruses.* 13(4):305-315.

United States Department of Health and Human Services. 1995. National Center for Health Statistics. *Health United States 1995.* http://www.cdc.gov/nchs/data/hus_95.pdf.

Zhang Z.F., H. Morgenstern, M. Spitz, D. Tashkin, G. Yu, J. Marshall, T. Hsu, and S. Schantz. 1999. Marijuana use and increased risk of squamous cell carcinoma of the head and neck. *Cancer Epidemiol Biomarkers Prevent* 8(12):1071-1078.

Zimmer, L. and J.P. Morgan. 1997. *Marijuana myths: Marijuana facts. A review of the scientific evidence.* New York and San Francisco: The Lindesmith Center.

Zimmerman B., R. Bayer, and N. Crumpacker. 1998. *Is marijuana the right medicine for you? A factual guide to medical uses of marijuana.* New Canaan, CT: Keats Publishing, Inc.

Zofran, brand of ondansetron, package insert. 2000. Glaxo-Welcome Inc. http: //www.glaxowellcome.com/pi/zofran.pdf.

UPDATE

Ethan B. Russo

Since this article was first published, a couple of key studies from San Francisco have appeared, noting a lack of obvious immunological sequelae to cannabis use in HIV/AIDS (Bredt et al. 2002), and significant weight gain with cannabis or THC compared to placebo (Abrams et al. 2003). In addition, cannabis may enhance HIV/AIDS patients' ability to adhere to antiretroviral drug regimens (de Jong et al. 2005). Alternative delivery techniques with standardized cannabis-based medicines should serve to mitigate associated pulmonary risks.

REFERENCES

Abrams, D. I., J.F. Hilton, R.J. Leiser, S.B. Shade, T.A Elbeik, F.T. Aweeka, N.L. Benewitz, B.M. Bredt, B. Kosel, J.A. Aberg, et al. 2003. Short-term effects of cannabinoids in patients with HIV-1 infection. A randomized, placcbo-controlled clinical trial. *Ann Intern Med* 139:258-266.

Bredt, B. M., D. Higuera-Alhino, S. B. Shade, S. J. Hebert, J. M. McCune, and D. I. Abrams. 2002. Short-term effects of cannabinoids on immune phenotype and function in HIV-1-infected patients. *J Clin Pharmacol* 42 (11 Suppl):82S-89S.

de Jong, B. C., D. Prentiss, W. McFarland, R. Machekano, and D. M. Israelski. 2005. Marijuana use and its association with adherence to antiretroviral therapy among HIV-infected persons with moderate to severe nausea. *J Acquir Immune Defic Syndr* 38 (1):43-46.

Chapter 16

Cannabis Treatments
in Obstetrics and Gynecology:
A Historical Review

Ethan B. Russo

INTRODUCTION

For much of history the herbal lore of women has been secret. As pointed out in John Riddle's book, *Eve's Herbs* (Riddle 1997), botanical agents for control of reproduction have been known for millennia, but have often been forgotten over time or lost utterly, as in the case of the Greek contraceptive, *sylphion*. The same is true for other agents instrumental in women's health, frequently due to religious constraints. One botanical agent that exemplifies this lost knowledge is cannabis. As will be discussed, its role as an herbal remedy in obstetric and gynecological conditions is ancient, but will surprise most by its breadth and prevalence. Cannabis appears in this role across many cultures, Old World and New, classical and modern, among young and old, in a sort of herbal vanishing act. This study will attempt to bring some of that history to light, and place it in a modern scientific context.

THE ANCIENT WORLD
AND MEDIEVAL MIDDLE AND FAR EAST

The earliest references to cannabis in female medical conditions probably originate in Ancient Mesopotamia. In the seventh century BCE, Assyrian

The author would like to thank the dedicated women of the Interlibrary Loan office at the Mansfield Library of the University of Montana, whose continued assistance has helped to revitalize lost medical knowledge. Dr. John Riddle provided valuable guidance, while Drs. Indalecio Lozano, David Deakle, and Daniel Westberg translated key passages.

King Ashurbanipal assembled a library of manuscripts of vast scale, including Sumerian and Akkadian medical stone tablets dating to 2000 BCE. Specifically according to Thompson, *azallû,* as hemp seeds were mixed with other agents in beer for an unspecified female ailment (Thompson 1924). *Azallû* was also employed for difficult childbirth, and staying the menses when mixed with saffron and mint in beer (Thompson 1949). Usage of cannabis rectally and by fumigation was described for other indications.

Cannabis has remained in the Egyptian pharmacopoeia since pharaonic times (Mannische 1989), administered orally, rectally, vaginally, on the skin, in the eyes, and by fumigation. The Ebers Papyrus has been dated to the reign of Amenhotep I, circa 1534 BCE, while some hints suggest an origin closer to the first Dynasty in 3000 BCE (Ghalioungui 1987). One passage (Ebers Papyrus 821) describes use of cannabis as an aid to childbirth (p. 209): "Another: *smsm-t* [shemshemet]; ground in honey; introduced into her vagina *(iwf).* This is a contraction."

The *Zend-Avesta,* the holy book of Zoroastrianism, survives only in fragments dating from around 600 BCE in Persia. Some passages clearly point to psychoactive effects of *Banga,* which is identified as hempseed by the translator (Darmesteter 1895). Its possible role as an abortifacient is noted as follows (Fargard XV, IIb., 14 [43], p. 179):

> And the damsel goes to the old woman and applies to her for one of her drugs, that she may procure her miscarriage; and the old woman brings her some Banga, or Shaêta ["another sort of narcotic"], a drug that kills in womb or one that expels out of the womb, or some other of the drugs that produce miscarriage.

Physical evidence to support the presence of medicinal cannabis use in Israel/Palestine was found by Zias et al. (1993) in a burial tomb, where the skeleton of a 14-year-old girl was found along with fourth-century bronze coins. She apparently had failed to deliver a term fetus due to cephalopelvic disproportion. Gray carbonized material was noted in the abdominal area (Figure 16.1). Analysis revealed phytocannabinoid metabolites. The authors stated (p. 363), "We assume that the ashes found in the tomb were cannabis, burned in a vessel and administered to the young girl as an inhalant to facilitate the birth process."

Budge (1913) noted Syriac use of cannabis to treat anal fissures, as might occur postpartum.

Dwarakanath (1965) described a series of Ayurvedic and Arabic tradition preparations containing cannabis indicated as aphrodisiacs and treatments for pain. It was noted that cannabis was employed in Indian folk medicine onwards from the fourth to third centuries BCE.

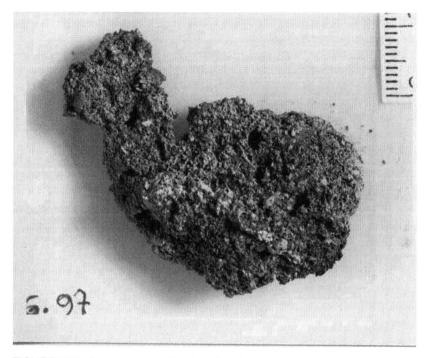

FIGURE 16.1. Carbonized residue from fourth-century Judea, containing phyto-cannabinoid elements, as a presumed obstetrical aid. (*Source:* Permission Courtesy of the Israel Antiquities Authority.)

In the ninth century, Sabur ibn Sahl in Persia cited use of cannabis in the *Al-Aqrabadhin Al-Saghir,* the first *materia medica* in Arabic (Kahl 1994). According to the translation of Indalecio Lozano of the Universidad de Granada, Spain (personal communication, February 4, 2002), an intranasal base preparation of juice from cannabis seeds was mixed with a variety of other herbs to treat migraine, calm uterine pains, prevent miscarriage, and preserve fetuses in their mothers' abdomens.

In the eleventh century, Andalusian physician Ibn Wafid al-Lajmi indicated that drying qualities of hemp seeds would inhibit maternal milk production. Tabit ibn Qurra claimed that they would reduce female genital lubrication when mixed in a potion with lentils and vinegar (Lozano 1993).

In the thirteenth century, famous Persian physician Avicenna (ibn Sina 1294) recommended seeds and leaves of cannabis to resolve and expel uterine gases (Lozano 1998).

According to Lozano (2001), Ibn al-Baytar prescribed hemp seed oil for treatment of hardening and contraction of the uterus (al-Baytar 1291).

In the *Makhzan-ul-Adwiya,* a seventeenth-century Persian medical text, it was claimed that cannabis leaf juice (Dymock 1884, p. 606) "checks the discharge in diarrhoea and gonorrhoea, and is diuretic."

Farid Alakbarov has recently brought to light the amazing richness of cannabis therapeutics of medieval Azerbaijan (Alakbarov 2001). Four citations are pertinent. Muhammad Riza Shirwani employed hemp seed oil in the seventeenth century to treat uterine tumors. Contemporaneously, another author advised likewise (Mu'min 1669). Tibbnama recommended a poultice of cannabis stems and leaves to treat hemorrhoids, and the leaves mixed with asafetida for "hysteria" (*Tibbnama* 1712).

In China, the *Pen T'sao Kang Mu*, or *Bencao Gang Mu* was compiled by Li Shih-Chen in 1596 based on ancient traditions. This was later translated as Chinese *Materia Medica* (Stuart 1928). In it, cannabis flowers were recommended for menstrual disorders. Seed kernels were employed for postpartum difficulties. It was also observed (p. 91), "The juice of the root is . . . thought to have a beneficial action in retained placenta and post-partum hemorrhage."

EUROPEAN AND WESTERN MEDICINE

The earliest European references to the use of cannabis in women's medicine may derive from Anglo-Saxon sources. In the eleventh century *Old English Herbarium* (Vriend 1984, CXVI, p.148), *haenep,* or hemp is recommended for sore breasts. This was translated as follows (Crawford 2002, p. 74): "Rub [the herb] with fat, lay it to the breast, it will disperse the swelling; if there is a gathering of diseased matter it will purge it."

The Österreichische Nationalbibliothek in Vienna, Austria displays a manuscript of the *Codex Vindobonensis 93,* said to be a thirteenth-century southern Italian copy of a work produced in previous centuries, or even earlier Roman sources (Zotter 1996). Plate 108 depicts a clearly recognizable cannabis plant above the figure of a bare-breasted woman (Figure 16.2). According to a translation of Drs. David Deakle and Daniel Westberg (personal communication 2002), the Latin inscription describes the use of cannabis mixed into an ointment and rubbed on the breasts to reduce swelling and pain.

A translation in Old Catalan of Ibn Wafid's work above, interpreted it differently, indicating that hemp seeds, when eaten in great quantity, liberate maternal milk and treat the pain of amenorrhea (Lozano 1993; personal communication 2002).

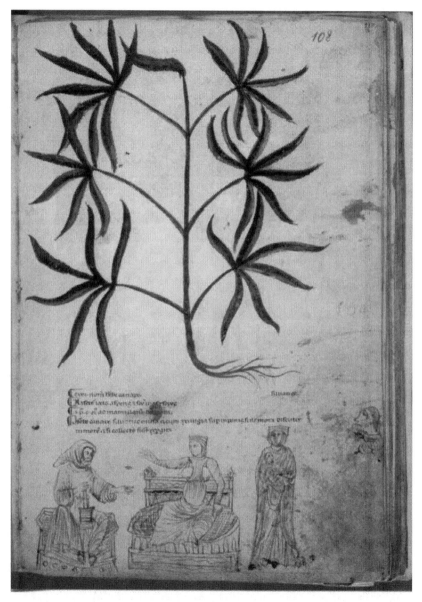

FIGURE 16.2. Plate from the *Codex Vindobonensis 93* from the thirteenth century or earlier, depicting use of cannabis to allay breast swelling and pain. (*Source:* From Bildarchiv d., with permission of the Österreichishe National-bibliothek, Vienna, Austria.)

Citing the *Kräuterbuch* of Tabernaemontanus in 1564, it was noted (Kabelik et al. 1960, p. 7), "Women stooping due to a disease of the uterus were said to stand up straight again after having inhaled the smoke of burning cannabis."

In England, in the *Theatrum Botanicum* (Parkinson et al. 1640), John Parkinson noted (p. 598) "Hempe is cold and dry . . . the Emulsion or decoction of the seede, stayeth laskes and fluxes that are continuall."

In 1696, Georg Eberhard Rumpf (Rumphius), a German physician in the service of the Dutch crown, reported on the use of cannabis root in Indonesia to treat gonorrhea (Rumpf and Beekman 1981, p. 197): "the green leaves of the female plant, cooked in water with Nutmeg, to drink to folks who felt a great oppression in their breasts, along with stabs, as if they had Pleuritis too."

According to Hamilton (1852), Valentini recommended hemp seed emulsion in the previous century to treat *furor uterinus,* a loosely defined malady of the era frequently associated with nymphomania, melancholia or other ills, more fully discussed by Dixon (1994).

In his book, *Medicina Britannica,* Short (1751) employed cannabis for treatment of obstruction of the menses, even of chronic duration. In one case, he stated (pp. 137-138), "I once ordered only the Hemp alone, where they [menses] had been obstructed not only Months, but some Years, with Success; and, when it could not break the Uterine or Vaginal Vessels, the Woman threw up Blood from the Lungs, but had them naturally the next Time."

Short (1751) also described a combination of hemp in "New-wort" (steeped crushed grain used in brewing beer) with feverfew *(Tanacetum parthenium)* and pennyroyal *(Mentha pulegium)* employed on three successive nights to (p. 137) "bring down the *Menses minime fallax*." Feverfew has anti-inflammatory effects, while pennyroyal is a known abortifacient (Riddle 1997). Thus, this treatment may well have induced miscarriage.

Finally, Short (1751, p. 138) noted this of a complex herbal mixture with hemp: "Some pretend the following a great Secret against Pissing the Bed."

In 1794, the *Edinburgh New Dispensatory* noted use of a hemp seed oil emulsion in milk, useful for "heat of urine," "incontinence of urine," and "restraining venereal appetites" (Lewis 1794, p. 126).

After the reintroduction of cannabis to Western medicine in the form of solid oral extracts and tinctures by O'Shaughnessy (1842), its spectrum of activity quickly extended to many conditions. The first citation of its use for uterine hemorrhage in modern medicine is probably from Churchill (1849), and its discovery for this indication was apparently serendipitous (p. 512):

> We possess two remedies for these excessive discharges, at the time of the menses going off, which were not in use in Dr. Fothergill's time [eighteenth century]. I mean *ergot of rye,* and *tincture of Indian hemp* . . .

The property of Indian hemp, of restraining uterine hemorrhage, has only been known to the profession a year or two. It was accidentally discovered by my friend, Dr Maguire of Castleknock, and since then it has been extensively tried by different medical men in Dublin, and by myself, with considerable success. The tincture of the resin is the most efficacious preparation, and it may be given in doses of from five to fifteen or twenty drops three times a day, in water. Its effects, in many cases, are very marked, often instantaneous, but generally complete after three or four doses. In some few cases of ulceration in which I have tried it on account of the hemorrhage, it seemed to be equally beneficial.

Alexander Christison extended the work of Churchill and applied Indian hemp to the problem of childbirth (Christison 1851), offering the following (pp. 117-118):

Indian hemp appears to possess a remarkable power of increasing the force of uterine contraction during labour. . . .

One woman, in her first confinement, had forty minims of the tincture of cannabis one hour before the birth of the child. The os uteri was then of the size of a shilling, the parts very tender, with induration around the os uteri. The pains quickly became very strong, so much so as to burst the membranes, and project the liquor amnii to some distance, and soon the head was born. The uterus subsequently contracted well.

Another, in her first confinement, had one drachm of the tincture, when the os uteri was rigid, and the size of a half-crown; from this the labour became very rapid.

Another, in her first confinement, had also one drachm of the tincture, when the os uteri was the size of a half-crown. Labour advanced very rapidly, and the child was born in an hour and a-half. There were severe after-pains.

Subsequently, Christison (1851) studied the oxytocic effects of cannabis tincture systematically in seven cases. He made several conclusions:

Shortening of the [pain] interval was in general a more conspicuous phenomenon than prolongation of the pain. . . .

It is worthy of remark, that in none of these cases were the ordinary physiological effects produced; there was no excitement or intoxicating action, and there did not seem to be the least tendency to sleep in any of them. . . .

While the effect of ergot does not come on for some considerable time, that of hemp, if it is to appear, is observed within two or three minutes. Secondly, the action of ergot is of a lasting character, that of hemp is confined to a few pains shortly after its administration. Thirdly, the action of hemp is more energetic, and perhaps more certainly induced, than that of ergot.

There appears little doubt, then, that the Indian hemp may often prove of essential service in promoting uterine contraction in tedious labours. (pp. 120-121)

Grigor (1852) also examined the role of tincture of *Cannabis indica* in facilitation of childbirth. In nine cases, little was noticeable, but in seven, including five primiparous women (p. 125),

> I have noticed the contractions acquire great increase of strength and frequency immediately on swallowing the drug, and have seen four or five minutes ere the effect ensued; . . . when effectual it is capable of bringing the labour to a happy conclusion considerably within a half of the time that would other have been required. . . .
>
> I have not observed it to possess any anaesthetic effects. . . .
>
> I consider the expulsive action of the cannabis to be stronger than that of ergot, but less certain in its effect. . . .
>
> Nor have unpleasant consequences, so far as I have seen, appeared afterwards.

By 1854, the first uses of therapeutic cannabis were acknowledged in the *Dispensatory of the United States* (Wood and Bache 1854), and these effects of cannabis to hasten childbirth without anesthesia were noted (p. 339).

Willis (1859) reviewed past literature on therapeutic cannabis and then described his own experience, which was frequently cited subsequently (p. 176):

> I have used the Indian hemp for some time and in many diseases, especially in those connected with the womb, in neuralgic dysmenorrhoea, in menorrhagia, in cessation of menstruation where the red discharge alternates with uterine leucorrhoea of long continuance, in repeated attacks of uterine hemorrhage, in all cases of nervous excitability, and in tedious labor, where there is restlessness of the patient, with ineffectual propulsive action of the uterus. . . .
>
> I was led to the use of hemp in puerperal convulsions, having also seen its beneficial effects in convulsions in general, after all the common remedies had been tried without relief.

Willis opined, based on literature and experience (p. 178), "It is a safe conclusion, from the many facts which have been published, that Indian hemp deserves further trial; in all cases making sure that the preparation used is good."

McMeens (1860) headed an Ohio State Commission that examined medical effects of cannabis. In addition to many references cited above, he reported on a Dr. M.D. Mooney of Georgia, who noted that a mixture of milk sugar and *Cannabis indica* extract (20 mg) taken every 3 to 4 h to treat gonorrhea was (p. 90) "successful in every case in from five to seven days."

That same year, a popular text (Stillé 1860) cited many contemporary authorities, noted irregular effects, and opined (Volume 2, p. 88), "From some experiments, cannabis would appear to excite contractions of the uterus."

Wright (1862) specifically noted the benefit of cannabis in relieving vomiting of pregnancy. In an initial letter, he discussed the case of a woman where all other available remedies had failed (pp. 246-247): "In a patient of mine, who was suffering to an extent that threatened death, with vomiting, I found the vomiting completely arrested by cannabis indica, given in repeated doses of three grains every four hours, until several doses were taken." He later revisited the issue in a subsequent article (Wright 1863), and explained (p. 75), "*Cannabis indica* does not paralyze the nerves, but strengthens them directly. It does not *constipate* by paralysis—it *cures* by beneficent virtues."

Silver (1870) devoted an entire article to the use of cannabis to treat menorrhagia and dysmenorrhea, reporting five cases in detail, all relieved nicely with cannabis within a few doses. He also referred to a colleague who had never failed in over a hundred cases to control pain and discomfort in these disorders within three doses. When flow was not checked after early treatment, Silver felt this diagnostic of "organic mischief" (p. 60) due to uterine fibroids, cervical carcinoma or other cause.

Grailey Hewitt authored a comprehensive textbook of obstetrics and gynecology. Cannabis was endorsed as a hemostatic treatment for menorrhagia, analgesic in dysmenorrhea and uterine cancer (Hewitt 1872). He compared it to other available remedies for the latter, including belladonna, hyoscyamus, opium and chloroform, remarking (p. 416), "The Indian hemp is, however, better entitled to consideration, and in many cases undoubtedly exercises a marked influence in allaying or preventing pain."

In another contemporary text (Scudder 1875), the author observed (p. 100), "I have employed the Cannabis specially to relieve irritation of the kidneys, bladder and urethra. It will be found especially beneficial in vesical and urethral irritation, and is an excellent remedy in the treatment of gonorrhoea."

Cannabis was also popular in France for such indications. Racime (1876) described medical usage of hashish and Indian hemp (p. 443 [translation EBR]): "In women, hemp has a most manifest action on the uterus; this action translates itself into a contraction of the uterine muscular fibers."

A selection from a broad French review follows (Michel 1880, pp. 111-112 [translation EBR]):

> Illnesses of the genito-urinary organs.-Indian hemp has been employed in a large number of uterine affections, but principally in the diverse disturbances of menstruation. The tendency of authors is to administer it while the pain element predominates. . . .
>
> We have ourselves administered it often and in diverse cases of uterine hemorrhage: we have always seen success as well in post-partum hemorrhages, cases in which we employ it today in preference to the ergot of rye. . . .
>
> The reader would well permit us to affirm that but one first spoonful of the potion against menorrhagia (see the formula) has almost always succeeded in sufficiently diminishing the flow of blood. Rarely, the patient has had to take 4 spoonfuls. What has certainly struck us in its proper action is that its influence seems to have an effect on the following cycles; the Indian hemp acts, according to our observation and the remarks of Churchill himself, like a regulator of the catamenial function. Administered, in effect, during one sole period, sometimes two, rarely three, the menses return henceforth to just proportions and all medication becomes unnecessary. I know not of a similar effect that has been reported with ergotine or ergot of rye.

Michel also endorsed cannabis treatment for blennorrhagia, or bloody uterine mucous discharge.

In 1883, two consecutive letters to the *British Medical Journal* attested to the benefits of extract of *Cannabis indica* in menorrhagia, treating both pain and bleeding successfully with a few doses. In the first, cannabis was termed "a valuable remedy" (Brown 1883, p. 1002):

> Indian hemp has such specific use in menorrhagia—there is no medicine which has given such good results. . . . A few doses—commencing with 5 minims of tincture—are sufficient. . . . The failures are so few, that I venture to call it a specific in menorrhagia. The drug deserves a trial.

The second letter also extolled the benefits of cannabis (Batho 1883, p. 1002):

> Considerable experience of its employment in menorrhagia, more especially in India, has convinced me that it is, in that country at all events, one of the most reliable means at our disposal. I feel inclined to go further, and state that it is par excellence the remedy for that condition, which, unfortunately, is very frequent in India.
> I have ordered it, not once, but repeatedly, in such cases and always with satisfactory results. The form used has been the tincture, and the dose ten to twenty minims, repeated once or twice in the twenty-four hours. It is so certain in its power of controlling menorrhagia, that it is a valuable aid to diagnosis in cases where it is uncertain whether an early abortion may or may not have occurred. Over the hemorrhage attending the latter condition, it appears to exercise but little force. I can recall one case in my practice in India, where my patient had lost profusely at each period for years, until the tincture was ordered; subsequently, by commencing its use, as a matter of routine, at the commencement of each flow, the amount was reduced to the ordinary limits, with corresponding benefit to the general health. Neither in this, nor in any other instance in which I prescribed the drug, were any disagreeable physiological effects observed.

One dissenting voice of the era was that of Oliver (1883) who felt that cannabis was not useful in dysmenorrhea since (p. 905) "its action seems so variable and the preparation itself so unreliable, as to be hardly worthy of a place on our list of remedial agents at all." Quality control problems with cannabis were a frequent concern throughout its reign in Western medicine.

Sydney Ringer, the British pioneer of intravenous fluid therapy, observed the following of *Cannabis indica* extract (Ringer 1886, p. 563):

> It is said to relieve dysuria, and strangury, and to be useful in retention of urine, dependent on paralysis from spinal disease. It is used occasionally in gonorrhoea. It is very useful in menorrhagia, or dysmenorrhoea. Half a grain to a grain thrice daily, though a grain every two hours, or hourly, is sometime required in those who can tolerate so large a dose, often relieve the pain of dysmenorrhoea. It is said to increase the energy of the internal contractions.

In India, it was reported of *Cannabis indica* (McConnell 1888, p. 95), "its powerful effect in controlling uterine hemorrhage (menorrhagia, &c.) has been repeatedly recorded by competent observers, and its employment for the relief of such affections is well understood and more or less extensively resorted to."

Farlow (1889) penned a treatise on the use of rectal preparations of cannabis describing its use in young women before marriage to alleviate premenstrual symptoms and subsequent dysmenorrhea (p. 508):

> If the excitement can be moderated, if the pelvic organs can be made less irritable, there will be less pain, less hemorrhage, less weakness, and consequently a much longer period of health between the catamenia. This, I feel sure, can often be very successfully done by the rectal use of belladonna and cannabis indica, beginning a few days before the menstrual symptoms or prodromes appear.

Farlow continued by describing another setting in sexually active but nulliparous women (p. 508):

> After marriage and before childbirth, the uterus and pelvis, especially the left ovary, are very liable to be tender and irritable, even when there is no evident organic disease. The backache, bearing down, pain in the side, groin and legs, the frequent micturition, painful coitus, constipation and headache are often much relieved by the suppositories.

Finally, Farlow mentioned another cannabis indication (p. 580): "At the menopause the well-known symptoms, the various reflexes, the excitement, the irritability, and pain in the neck of the bladder, flashes of heat, and cold, according to my experience, can frequently be much mitigated, by the suppositories."

Farlow employed low doses of these agents, 1/4 grain each (15 mg) or extracts of belladonna and *Cannabis indica,* administered by rectal suppository at night, or bid. Apparently no intoxication was necessary for therapeutic benefit (p. 509): "I do not think there is anything to be gained by pushing the drugs to their physiological action."

Aulde (1890) recommended cannabis extract for dysmenorrhea, sometimes combined with gelsemium (pp. 525-526):

> The majority of these cases uncomplicated by displacements, such as seen in young girls and married women, will be promptly benefited, and the menstrual flow appears, when there is no further trouble until the next period. . . .
>
> Cannabis has been highly recommended for the relief of *menorrhagia,* but is not curative in the true sense of the term.

Sir John Russell Reynolds was personal physician to Queen Victoria, and it has been widely acknowledged that she received monthly doses of *Cannabis indica* for menstrual discomfort throughout her adult life. In 1890, after more than thirty years' experience with the agent, Reynolds reported (Reynolds 1890, p. 38), "Indian hemp . . . is of great service in cases of simple spasmodic dysmenorrhoea."

Another textbook of the era noted the following therapeutic indications for *Cannabis indica* (Cowperthwaite 1891, p. 188): "Said to be especially useful in gonorrhoea when the chordee is well marked. Uterine colic."

J.B. Mattison wrote extensively on therapeutic cannabis. He noted the following among several gynecological conditions reviewed (Mattison 1891, p. 268): "In genito-urinary disorders it often acts kindly—the renal pain of Bright's disease; and it calms the pain of clap equal to sandal or copaiva, and is less unpleasant."

The Indian Hemp Drugs Commission of 1893-1894 exhaustively examined the uses and abuses of cannabis, noting its indication for prolonged labor and dysmenorrhea (Kaplan 1969; Commission 1894).

In this era, patent medicines containing cannabis were very common. One preparation, named "Dysmenine," contained cannabis with a variety of other herbal tinctures, "Indicated for Dysmenorrhea, Menstrual Colic, and Cramps" (Figure 16.3). Interestingly, one component was capsicum, raising the possibility of synergistic action on cannabinoid and vanilloid receptors.

An 1898 text opined of the fluidextract of cannabis (Lilly 1898, p. 32), "Its anodyne power is marked in chronic metritis and dysmenorrhea."

Shoemaker (1899) reported a case of endometritis with metrorrhagia, that required surgery, but in which (p. 481) "Marked relief of symptom was afforded, however, by the administration of Indian hemp. It relieved pain and diminished hemorrhage, and was highly valued by the patient."

Lewis (1900) observed the following (p. 251):

> Dysmenorrhea, not due to anatomical or inflammatory causes, is, in my opinion, one of the principal indications for indian hemp. No other drug acts so promptly and with fewer after effects.
>
> From my own personal observation, I am convinced that cannabis indica does exert a powerful influence on muscular contraction, particularly of the uterus. It may not, as Bartholow says, have the power of initiating uterine contraction, but I have demonstrated time and time again to my own satisfaction that the presence of the merest contractile effort is enough to permit its fullest effects. It is therefore of some service in uterine hemorrhage, but since its action is much slower than that of ergot, it is not as useful in those sudden hemorrhages great enough to require immediate check. I have noticed,

however, that ergot is considerably quicker and more prolonged in its action when combined with cannabis indica.

The drug is very useful in profuse menstruation, decreasing the flow nicely without completely arresting it, as ergot very frequently and improperly does.

Felter and Lloyd (1900) described numerous ob-gyn indications for cannabis (pp. 426-427):

> The pains of *chronic rheumatism, sciatica, spinal meningitis, dysmenorrhea, endometritis, subinvolution,* and the vague pains of *amenorrhoea,* with depression, call for cannabis. Owing to a special action upon the reproductive apparatus, it is accredited with averting *threatened abortion.* . . .
>
> Cannabis is said in many cases to increase the strength of the uterine contractions during parturition, in atonic conditions, without the unpleasant consequences of ergot, and for which purpose it should be used in the form of tincture (see below), 30 drops, or specific cannabis, 10 drops, in sweetened water or mucilage, as often as required. In *menorrhagia,* the tincture in doses of 5 or 10 drops, 3 or 4 times a day, has checked the discharge in 24 or 48 hours.
>
> The greatest reputation of cannabis has been acquired from its prompt results in certain disorders of the genito-urinary tract. In fact, its second great keynote or indication is irritation of the genito-urinary tract, and the indication is even of more value when associated with general nervous depression.
>
> It is therefore useful in *gonorrhoeas, chronic irritation of the bladder, in chronic cystitis,* with painful micturition, and in *painful urinary affections generally.* It makes no difference whether a urethritis be specific or not, or whether it is acute or chronic, the irritation is a sufficient guide to the selection of cannabis. Use it in *gonorrhoea* to relieve the *ardor urinae,* and to prevent urethral spasm and avert chordee, and in *gleet,* to relive the irritation and discharge; employ it also in *spasm of the vesical sphincter,* in *dysuria* and in *strangury,* when spasmodic. Burning and scalding in passing urine, with frequent desire to micturate, are always relieved by cannabis.

The authors clearly understood that the potency of the preparation directly affected clinical results. While both Indian hemp and American hemp were said to be effective, much higher doses of the latter were said to be required.

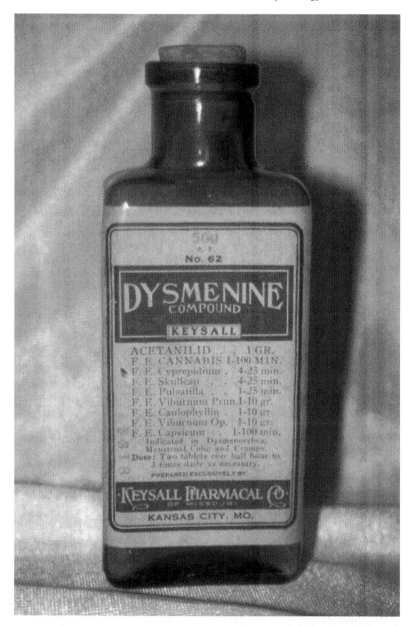

FIGURE 16.3. Photo of Dysmenine, a late-nineteenth-century patent medicine for menstrual cramps, containing cannabis. (*Source:* Photo by Ethan Russo, with permission of Michael Krawitz, the Cannabis Museum.)

In a popular American text of the era, Bartholow (1903) noted :

> It is well established that hemp has the power to promote uterine contractions. It can not initiate them, but increased their energy when action has begun. It may be given with ergot. In consequence of this power which it possesses to affect the muscular tissue of organic life, hemp is used successfully in the treatment of *menorrhagia*. It is said to be especially useful in that form of *menorrhagia* which occurs in the climacteric period (Churchill). It has, more recently, been shown to possess the power to arrest *hemorrhage* from any point, but it is chiefly in menorrhagia that much good is accomplished. . . .
>
> This agent has also been used with success in the treatment of *gonorrhoea*. It diminishes the local inflammation, allays chordee, and lessens the pain and irritation, with accompanying restlessness. (p. 557)

In Ceylon, Ratnam (1916, p. 37) defended use of therapeutic cannabis against legislative challenges: "I and other medical practitioners have used it extensively in the treatment of tetanus, asthma and uterine disorders, especially dysmenorrhea and menorrhagia."

In a text of the era, cannabis was deemed useful in menopausal headaches (Hare 1922), as well as the following (p. 182):

> In cases of *uterine subinvolution, chronic inflammation,* and *irritation* cannabis is of great value, and it has been found of service in *metrorrhagia* and *nervous and spasmodic dysmenorrhea*. Not only does it relieve pain, but it also seems to act favorably upon the muscular fibers of the uterus.

Another popular text (Sajous and Sajous 1924) cited cannabis as an analgesic for menopause, uterine disturbances, dysmenorrhea, menorrhagia and impending abortion, and postpartum hemorrhage.

In 1928, in *Pharmacotherapeutics, Materia Medica and Drug Action,* the authors remarked on the ability of cannabis to counteract "painful cramps" and its "particular influence over visceral pain" (Solis-Cohen and Githens 1928, p. 1702). More specifically, they noted (p. 1705):

> Cannabis acts favorably upon the uterine musculature and may be used as a synergist to ergot in sluggish labor. It is useful also in relieving the pain of chronic *metritis* and *dysmenorrhea* and reduces the flow in *menorrhagia*. It is employed as a symptomatic remedy in *gonorrhea* in doses of 1/4 grain (0.015 Gm.) of the extract four times a day, relieving the pain, dysuria, and chordee.

An anonymous editor (probably Morris Fishbein) noted the ability of cannabis to achieve a labor with pain burden substantially reduced or eliminated, followed by a tranquil sleep (Anonymous 1930, p. 1165):

> Hence a woman in labor may have a more or less painless labor. If a sufficient amount of the drug is taken, the patient may fall into a tranquil sleep from which she will awaken refreshed. . . . As far as is known, a baby born of a mother intoxicated with cannabis will not be abnormal in any way.

The *British Pharmaceutical Codex* retained an indication for cannabis in treatment of dysmenorrhea in 1934 (Pharmaceutical Society of Great Britain 1934).

Despite the fact that cannabis had been dropped from the *National Formulary* the previous year, Morris Fishbein, the editor of the *Journal of the American Medical Association,* continued to recommend cannabis in migraine associated with menstruation (Fishbein 1942, p. 326):

> In this instance the patient may be given either sodium bromide or fluidextract of cannabis three days before the onset of the menstrual period, continued daily until three days after the menstrual period. . . . The dose of fluidextract of cannabis is five drops three times daily, increased daily by one drop until eleven drops, three times daily, are taken. Then the dosage is reduced by one drop daily until 5 drops are taken three times daily and so on.

Medical investigation of cannabis persisted in Czechoslovakia. One group noted success in use of a cannabis extract in alcohol and glycerine to treat rhagades, or fissures, on the nipples of nursing women to prevent staphylococcal mastitis (Kabelik et al. 1960).

MODERN ETHNOBOTANY OF CANNABIS IN OBSTETRICS AND GYNECOLOGY

In the folk medicine of Germany, in the late nineteenth century (Rätsch 1998, p. 122), a cannabis preparation was "laid on the painful breasts of women who have given birth; hemp oil is also rubbed onto these areas; hempseed milk is used to treat bladder pains and dropsy."

Although the carminative properties of cannabis seeds had been noted since the time of Galen, Lozano (2001) notes that al-Mayusi (1877) claimed similar properties for the leaves, and to treat uterine gases.

In nineteenth-century Persia, Schlimmer (1874) reported his observations on usage of *Cannabis indica* leaves as a treatment for urethritis associated with the practice of prostitution. In modern Iran, Zargari (1990) notes continued use of *Cannabis sativa* seed oil rubbed on the breasts to diminish or even completely prevent lactation.

Cannabis or *nasha* was employed medicinally despite Soviet prohibition in Tashkent in the 1930s (Benet 1975, pp. 46-47): "A mixture of lamb's fat with *nasha* is recommended for brides to use on their wedding night to reduce the pain of defloration." In the same culture (p. 47), "An ointment made by mixing hashish with tobacco is used by some women to shrink the vagina and prevent fluor alvus [leukorrhea]." More fancifully, Benet noted that in German folk medicine (p. 46), "sprigs of hemp were placed over the stomach and ankles to prevent convulsions and difficult childbirth."

Nadkarni (1976) reported the use in India of a poultice of cannabis for hemorrhoids and "The concentrated resin exudate (resinous matters) extracted from the leaves and flowering tops or agglutinated spikes of C. sativa, and known as *nasha* or *charas* . . . is valuable in preventing and curing . . . dysuria and in relieving pain in dysmenorrhea and menorrhagia. . ." (p. 263).

In a book about medicinal plants of India (Dastur 1962), we see the following: "Charas [hashish] . . . is of great value in-dysuria . . . it is also used as an anaesthetic in dysmenorrhea . . . . Charas is usually given in one-sixth to one-fourth grain doses" (p. 67). A seed infusion was also employed to treat gonorrhea.

Aldrich (1977) has extensively documented the Tantric use of cannabis in India from the seventh century onward as an aid to sexual pleasure and enlightenment:

> The Kama Sutra and Ananga Ranga eloquently detail Hindu sexual techniques, and the Tantras transform such sexual practices into a means of meditational yoga. . . . In Hindu Tantrism, the female energy (shakti) is dynamic and paramount: the male is passive and takes all his vitality from the shakti. . . . In Buddhist Tantra it is just the opposite: the male is active and assumes the dynamic role of compassion, while the female is the passive embodiment of wisdom. (p. 229)

We have little modern research to document a biochemical basis to these claims, which persist, nonetheless. In his inimitable prose, Ott (2002, p. 29) has stated of cannabis, "many women I have known are effusively enthusiastic about its aphrodisiacal amatory tributes."

A treatise on cannabis usage in India includes the following citation (Chopra and Chopra 1957, p. 12): "It [cannabis resin] is considered a sovereign remedy for relieving pain in dysmenorrhea and menorrhagia, and against dysurea."

In Cambodia, mothers reportedly use hemp products extensively after birth (Martin 1975), making an infusion of ten flowering tops to a liter of water to provide a sense of well-being. When insufficient milk is present for nursing, female hemp flowers are combined with other herbs for ingestion. An alcoholic extract of cannabis and various barks is said to alleviate postpartum stiffness. Another hemp extract mixture is employed to cure hemorrhoids and polyps of the sex organs.

In Vietnam (Martin 1975), cannabis seed kernels in a preparation called sac thuoc are said to cure dysmenorrhea, or provide a feeling of wellness after childbirth. Citing Martin's work, Rubin noted the following usage in Vietnam (Rubin 1976, p. 3): "21 kernels boiled in water may be given to the expectant mother to reset the neonate in normal position at birth."

Hemp is of ancient use in China, but it was noted (Shou-zhong 1997, p. 148): "In modern clinical practice, Hemp Seeds are still in wide use. They are able to . . . promote lactation, hasten delivery, and disinhibit urination and defecation."

Perry and Metzger (1980) noted continued folk use of cannabis in China and Southeast Asia, where the seeds were specially prepared for treatment of uterine prolapse and as a birthing aid.

In South Africa, a Sotho herbalist used cannabis to facilitate childbirth (Hewat 1906, p. 98) and was "in the habit of getting his patient stupified by much smoking of dagga."

In modern times, urban Africans have also employed cannabis medicinally for a number of purposes (Du Toit 1980), as one informant related: "Pregnant women should always have some burnt for her so as to have a completely healthy child." But is particularly during childbirth that "pregnant women were given dagga to make them brave," and "so that they wouldn't feel pain" (p. 209).

In Brazil, it was observed (Hutchinson 1975, p. 180), "Such an infusion [of marijuana leaves] is taken to relieve rheumatism, 'female troubles,' colic and other common complaints."

In a twentieth-century English herbal, Grieve (1971) noted the following uses of hemp (p. 397): "The tincture helps parturition, and is used in senile catarrh, gonorrhoea, menorrhagia, chronic cystitis and all painful urinary affections. An infusion of the seed is useful in after pains and prolapsus uteri." Dosages were provided (p. 397): "Of tincture for menorrhagia, 5 to 10 minims. Three to four times a day (i.e., 24 grains of resinous extract in a fluid ounce of rectified spirit)."

Finally, this passage was offered (p. 397): "The following is stated to be a certain cure for gonorrhoea. Take equal parts of tops of male and female hemp in blossom. Bruise in a mortar, express the juice, and add an equal portion of alcohol. Take 1 to 3 drops every two to three hours."

Merzouki et al. (2000) have examined the usage of cannabis as part of herbal mixtures employed by Moroccan herbalists to induce therapeutic abortion, concluding that the cannabis component did not produce this effect, but rather other clearly toxic components were responsible. The herbal mixture is applied per vaginam, or alternatively, its smoke is fumigated in close proximity to the genitals (Merzouki 2001).

By the late 1960s, cannabis cures entered the scene in modern America. A popular treatise on marijuana noted medicinal effects (Margolis and Clorfene 1969, p. 26):

> You'll also discover that grass is an analgesic, and will reduce pain considerably. As a matter of fact, many women use it for dysmenorrhea or menorrhagia when they're out of Pamprin or Midol. So if you have an upset stomach, or suffer from pain of neuritis or neuralgia, smoke grass. If pains persist, smoke more grass.

Popular cannabis folklore, thus, did not escape American consciousness. Another example was noted by Thompson (1972, p. 3): "In the Jack's Creek area of Fayette County, Kentucky, poultices with hemp leaves are supposed to relieve hemorrhoidal pains and bleeding when applied in the appropriate area of the human body."

RECENT THEORY AND CLINICAL DATA

Solomon Snyder (1971, p. 14), the discoverer of opiate receptors, examined cannabis' pros and cons as an analgesic:

> For there are many conditions, such as migraine headaches or menstrual cramps, where something as mild as aspirin gives insufficient relief and opiates are too powerful, not to mention their potential for addiction. Cannabis might conceivably fulfill a useful role in such conditions.

In the mid-1970s, Noyes et al. wrote several articles on analgesic effects of cannabis. In case reports (Noyes and Baram 1974), one young woman successfully employed cannabis to treat the pain and anxiety after a tubal ligation, and another in dysmenorrhea (p. 533): "The relief she got from smoking was prompt, complete, and consistently superior to that from aspirin."

In 1993, Grinspoon and Bakalar published *Marihuana, the Forbidden Medicine,* and subsequently revised it (Grinspoon and Bakalar 1997). The book contains numerous "anecdotal" testimonials from patients and doctors documenting clinical efficacy of cannabis where other drugs were ineffective. An entire section with case studies was included on premenstrual syndrome (PMS), menstrual cramps, and labor pains, supporting excellent symptomatic relief at low doses without cognitive impairment.

Numerous surveys cite cannabis usage for obstetric and gynecological complaints, but in one Australian example, 51 percent of the women indicated indications for PMS or dysmenorrhea (Helliwell 1999).

Rätsch (1998) has observed (p. 162), "Several women who delivered their babies at home have told me that they smoked or ate hemp products to ease the painful contractions and the birth process in general."

Beyond direct effects mediated by the cannabinoid receptors, McPartland has proposed that therapeutic effects of cannabis in dysmenorrhea involve anti-inflammatory mechanisms (McPartland 1999, 2001).

It has been observed that women with PMS exhibit a fault in fatty acid metabolism that impedes the conversion of linoleic acid (LA) to gamma-linolenic acid (GLA) and prostaglandins. A daily dose of 150 to 200 milligrams of GLA over a twelve-week period significantly improved PMS-related symptoms (Horrobin and Manku 1989). As pointed out by Leson and Pless (2002), this amount of GLA can be supplied by only 5 mL of hemp seed oil daily.

Experimentally, Δ^9-THC inhibited herpes virus replication (HSV-1 and HSV-2) in vitro, even at low concentrations (Blevins and Dumic 1980), and was suggested for trials of topical usage.

An Italian group recently demonstrated the inhibition of proliferation of human breast cancer cells by anandamide in vitro (De Petrocellis et al. 1998); 2-arachidonylglycerol and the synthetic cannabinoid HU-210 acted similarly, while this activity was blocked by the CB_1 antagonist, SR 141716A. It was felt that these effects were mediated through inhibition of endogenous prolactin activity at its receptor. It is likely that THC acts similarly. Palmitylethanolamide has subsequently been demonstrated to inhibit expression of fatty acid amidohydrolase, thereby enhancing the anti-proliferative effects of anandamide on human breast cancer cells (Di Marzo et al. 2001).

Recent animal work has elucidated the role of endocannabinoids in mammalian fertility. Recently Das et al. (1995) detected CB_1 receptor mRNA in mouse uterus, thus suggesting that this organ is capable of anandamide production. Anandamide (arachidonylethanolamide, AEA) and Δ^9-THC inhibited forskolin-stimulated cyclic AMP production in mouse uterus, whereas cannabidiol did not, suggesting that the uterine site is active in endocannabinoid production.

Schmid et al. (1997) demonstrated very high levels of anandamide in the peri-implantation mouse uterus. Data suggest that down-regulation of AEA levels promote uterine receptivity, while up-regulation may inhibit implantation. It was surmised that aberrant AEA synthesis or expression may be etiological in early pregnancy failure or infertility. The corresponding role that THC or cannabis may have in human females at the time of fertilization and implantation is open to conjecture, but deserves further investigation.

Wenger et al. (1997) claimed similarity in effects of injected THC and AEA in pregnant rats, prolonging length of gestation, and increasing stillbirths, perhaps due to inhibition of prostaglandin synthesis. The same lead author posited cannabinoid influences on hypothalamic and pituitary endocrine functions in a subsequent paper (Wenger et al. 1999).

Paria et al. (2001) suggested the need for tight regulation of endocannabinoid signaling during synchronization of embryonic development and uterine receptivity. They demonstrated inhibition of implantation in wild-type mice with sustained high-level exposure to "natural cannabinoid" while not in CB_1 ($-/-$)/CB_2 ($-/-$) double knockout mutant mice.

Issues of cannabis use in human pregnancy remain a great concern. The topic is reviewed in (Fried 2002; Murphy 2001; Zimmer and Morgan 1997). A variety of studies have demonstrated transient effects of cannabis on endocrine hormone levels, but no consistent effects seem to occur in chronic settings (Russo et al. 2002). Certainly subtle changes at critical times of fertilization or implantation may be significant. A valid assessment was provided (Murphy 1999, p. 379): "the hormone milieu at the time of exposure may dictate a woman's hormonal response to marijuana smoking."

Studies are hampered by the obvious fact that laboratory animals are not human in their responses. Estrous cycles and behaviors in animals are not always analogous to menstrual cycles and other physiological effects in women. Nevertheless, animal data suggest that in female rats, at least, THC acts on the CB_1 receptor to initiate signal transduction with membrane dopamine and intracellular progesterone receptors to initiate sexual responses (Mani et al. 2001).

One available approach to the issues is provided by examining factors in spontaneous abortions. In a study of 171 women, 25 percent of pregnancies ended spontaneously within 6 weeks of the last menses. Cannabis exposure seemed to have no observable effect in these cases (Wilcox et al. 1990).

The population of Ottawa, Ontario, Canada, has been extensively examined over the last two decades with respect to cannabis effects in pregnancy. In a small study of cannabis using mothers versus abstainers (O'Connell and Fried 1984), ocular hypertelorism and "severe epicanthus" were only noted in children born to users.

In 1987, the Ottawa group compared effects of cannabis, tobacco, alcohol and caffeine during gestation (Fried et al. 1987). Whereas tobacco negatively affected neonatal birth weight and head circumference, and alcohol was associated with lower birth weight and length, no effects on any growth parameters were ascribable to maternal cannabis usage.

In a subsequent study (Witter and Niebyl 1990), examination of 8,350 birth records revealed that 417 mothers (5 percent) claimed cannabis-only usage in pregnancy, but no association was noted with prematurity or congenital anomalies. The authors suggested that previously ascribed links to cannabis were likely confounded by concomitant alcohol and tobacco abuse.

A group in Boston noted a decrease in birth weight of 79 g in infants born to 331 of 1226 surveyed mothers with positive using drug screen for cannabis ($p = 0.04$) (Parker and Zuckerman 1999), but no changes in gestation, head circumference or congenital abnormalities were noted.

The largest study of the issue to date evaluated 12,424 pregnancies (Linn et al. 1983). Although low birth weight, shortened gestation and malformations seemed to be associated with maternal cannabis usage, when logistic regression analysis was employed to control for other demographic and exposure factors, this association fell out of statistical significance.

Dreher has extensively examined prenatal cannabis usage in Jamaica (Dreher 1997; Dreher et al. 1994), wherein the population observations were not compounded by concomitant alcohol, tobacco, or polydrug abuse. This study is unique in that regard, no less due to the heavy intake of cannabis ("ganja"), often daily, in this cohort of Rastafarian women. No differences were seen between groups of cannabis-using and non-cannabis-using mothers in the weight, length, gestational age or Apgar scores of their infants (Dreher et al. 1994). Deleterious effects on progeny of cannabis smokers were not apparent; in fact, developmental precocity was observed in some measures in infants born to women who smoked ganja daily. The author noted (Dreher 1997, p. 168):

> The findings from Jamaica, however, suggest that prenatal cannabis exposure is considerably more complex than we might first have thought. Loss of appetite, nausea and fatigue compound the "bad feeling" that women in this study commonly reported. For many women, ganja was seen as an option that provided a solution to these problems, i.e., to increase their appetites, control and prevent the nausea of pregnancy, assist them to sleep, and give them the energy they needed to work. . . . The women with several pregnancies, in particular,

reported that the feelings of depression and desperation attending motherhood in their impoverished communities were alleviated by both social and private smoking. In this respect, the role of cannabis in providing both physical comfort and a more optimistic outlook may need to be reconceptualized, not as a recreational vehicle of escapism, but as a serious attempt to deal with difficult physical, emotional, and financial circumstances.

DISCUSSION AND CONCLUSIONS

This presentation supports the proposition that cannabis has been employed historically for legion complaints in obstetrics and gynecology. To list briefly, these include treatment of menstrual irregularity, menorrhagia, dysmenorrhea, threatened abortion, hyperemesis gravidarum, childbirth, postpartum hemorrhage, toxemic seizures, dysuria, urinary frequency, urinary retention, gonorrhea, menopausal symptoms, decreased libido and as a possible abortifacient.

It is only recently that a physiological basis for these claims has been available with the discovery of the endocannabinoid system. Limited research to date supports these claims in terms of cannabinoid analgesia, antispasmodic and anti-inflammatory activities, but requires additional study to ascertain mechanisms and confounding variables.

Recommendations for cannabis therapeutics have often supported only utilization for terminal, intractable, or chronic disorders (Joy et al. 1999). However, simple logic would indicate that side effects of any medicine would be less evident when the agent is employed sporadically. Generally, that situation prevails for many of the listed ob-gyn indications for cannabis. Available historical and epidemiological data supports very low toxicity, even in pregnancy, to mother or child. Professor Philip Robson of Oxford has summarized the situation with cannabis in obstetrics nicely (House of Lords 1998, p. 123):

If you could have an agent which both speeded labour up, prevented hemorrhage after labour and reduced pain, this would be very desirable. Cannabis is so disreputable that nobody would begin to think of that and yet that is really an obvious application that we should seriously consider with perhaps some basic research and pursue it.

A few intriguing issues remain. Is cannabis truly an abortifacient? Our four specific references are equivocal, one ancient (Darmesteter 1895), one old (Short 1751), and two modern (Merzouki et al. 2000; Merzouki 2001), but these and current epidemiological data would seem to indicate that cannabis does not produce this effect *sui generis*. Perhaps its actual role is one to mitigate side effects of the active components.

Numerous citations historically support the notion that cannabis is quite potent in its obstetric and gynecological actions, with specific attestation that medical benefits are frequently obtained at doses that are sub-psychoactive. The therapeutic ratio of cannabis with respect to cognitive impairment seems generous.

Another mystery worthy of additional study surrounds the very rapid activity claimed for cannabis extracts in promotion of labor (Grigor 1852; Christison 1851). Certainly modern anecdotal claims of a similar nature are legion when cannabis is smoked. Pharmacodynamically, oral administration of extracts would be unlikely to provide benefits within minutes. Perhaps these tinctures were demonstrating a sublingual or mucosal absorption akin to those in modern trials of cannabis-based medical extracts (Whittle et al. 2001).

In summary, the long history of cannabis in women's medicine supports further therapeutic investigation and application to a large variety of difficult clinical conditions. Cannabis as a logical medical alternative in obstetrics and gynecology may yet prove to be, in the words of Robson (1998), a phoenix whose time it is to rise once more.

REFERENCES

Alakbarov, F.U. 2001. Medicinal properties of cannabis according to medieval manuscripts of Azerbaijan. *J Cannabis Therapeutics* 1(2):3-14.

al-Baytar, ibn. 1291. *Kitab al-Yami' li-mufradat al-adwiya wa-l-agdiya.* Bulaq.

Aldrich, M.R. 1977. Tantric cannabis use in India. *J Psychedelic Drugs* 9(3):227-233.

al-Mayusi. 1877. *Kamil al-sina'a al-tibbiya.* Bulaq.

Anonymous. 1930. Effects of alcohol and cannabis during labor. *J Amer Med Assoc* 94(15):1165.

Aulde, J. 1890. Studies in therapeutics-Cannabis indica. *Therapeutic Gazette* 14:523-526.

Bartholow, R. 1903. *A practical treatise on materia medica and therapeutics,* Eleventh edition. New York: D. Appleton.

Batho, R. 1883. Cannabis indica. *Brit Med J* (May 26):1002.

Benet, S. 1975. Early Diffusion and Folk Uses of Hemp. In V. Rubin (ed.), *Cannabis and Culture* (pp. 39-49). The Hague, Paris: Mouton.

Blevins, R.D., and M.P. Dumic. 1980. The effect of delta-9-tetrahydrocannabinol on herpes simplex virus replication. *J Gen Virol* 49(2):427-431.

Brown, J. 1883. Cannabis indica; A valuable remedy in menorrhagia. *Brit Med J* 1(May 26):1002.

Budge, E.A.W. 1913. *The Syriac book of medicines.* London: Oxford University.

Chopra, I.C., and R.W. Chopra. 1957. The use of cannabis drugs in India. *Bull Narc* 9:4-29.

Christison, A. 1851. On the natural history, action, and uses of Indian hemp. *Monthly J of Medical Science of Edinburgh, Scotland* 13:26-45, 117-121.

Churchill, F. 1849. *Essays on the puerperal fever and other diseases peculiar to women.* London: Sydenham Society.

Commission, Indian Hemp Drugs. 1894. *Report of the Indian Hemp Drugs Commission, 1893-94.* Simla: Govt. Central Print. Office.

Cowperthwaite, A.C. 1891. *A text-book of materia medica and therapeutics,* Sixth edition. Chicago: Gross & Delbridge.

Crawford, V. 2002. A homelie herbe: Medicinal cannabis in early England. *J Cannabis Therapeutics* 2(2):71-9.

Darmesteter, J. 1895. *Zend-Avesta,* Part I, *The Vendidad.* London: Oxford University.

Das, S.K., B.C. Paria, I. Chakraborty, and S.K. Dey. 1995. Cannabinoid ligand-receptor signaling in the mouse uterus. *Proc Natl Acad Sci USA* 92(10):4332-4336.

Dastur, J.F. 1962. *Medicinal plants of India and Pakistan.* Bombay: D.B. Taraporevala Sons.

De Petrocellis, L., D. Melck, A. Palmisano, T. Bisogno, C. Laezza, M. Bifulco, and V. Di Marzo. 1998. The endogenous cannabinoid anandamide inhibits human breast cancer cell proliferation. *Proc Natl Acad Sci USA* 95(14):8375-8380.

Di Marzo, V., D. Melck, P. Orlando, T. Bisogno, O. Zagoory, M. Bifulco, Z. Vogel, and L. De Petrocellis. 2001. Palmitoylethanolamide inhibits the expression of fatty acid amide hydrolase and enhances the anti-proliferative effect of anandamide in human breast cancer cells. *Biochem J* 358(Pt 1):249-255.

Dixon, L.S. 1994. Beware the wandering womb–painterly reflections of early gynecological theory. *Cancer Invest* 12(1):66-73.

Dreher, M.C. 1997. Cannabis and pregnancy. In M.L. Mathre (ed.), *Cannabis in medical practice* (pp. 159-190). Jefferson, NC: McFarland.

Dreher, M.C., K. Nugent, and R. Hudgins. 1994. Prenatal marijuana exposure and neonatal outcomes in Jamaica: an ethnographic study. *Pediatrics* 93(2):254-260.

Du Toit, B.M. 1980. *Cannabis in Africa: A survey of its distribution in Africa, and a study of cannabis use and users in multi-et[h]nic South Africa.* Rotterdam: A.A. Balkema.

Dwarakanath, C. 1965. Use of opium and cannabis in the traditional systems of medicine in India. *Bull Narc* 17:15-19.

Dymock, W. 1884. *The vegetable materia medica of Western India.* Bombay: Education Society's Press.

Farlow, J.W. 1889. On the use of belladonna and Cannabis indica by the rectum in gynecological practice. *Boston Med Surg J* 120:507-509.

Felter, H.W., and J.U. Lloyd. 1900. *King's American dispensatory.* Cincinnati, OH: Ohio Valley Co.

Fishbein, M. 1942. Migraine associated with menstruation. *J Amer Med Assoc* 237:326.

Fried, P.A. 2002. Pregnancy. In F. Grotenhermen and E.B. Russo (eds.), *Cannabis and cannabinoids: Pharmacology, toxicology and therapeutic potential.* Binghamton, NY: The Haworth Press, Inc.

Fried, P.A., B. Watkinson, R.F. Dillon, and C.S. Dulberg. 1987. Neonatal neurological status in a low-risk population after prenatal exposure to cigarettes, marijuana, and alcohol. *J Dev Behav Pediatr* 8(6):318-326.

Ghalioungui, P. 1987. *The Ebers papyrus: A new English translation, commentaries and glossaries.* Cairo: Academy of Scientific Research and Technology.

Grieve, M. 1971. *A modern herbal.* New York: Dover Publications.

Grigor, J. 1852. Indian hemp as an oxytocic. *Monthly J of Medical Sciences* 14:124.

Grinspoon, L. and J.B. Bakalar. 1997. *Marihuana, the forbidden medicine,* Revised and expanded edition. New Haven: Yale University Press.

Hamilton, E. 1852. *The Flora Homoeopathica; or the medicinal plants used as homoeopathic remedies.* London: H. Bailliere.

Hare, H.A. 1922. *A text-book of practical therapeutics,* Eighteenth edition. Philadelphia: Lea & Febiger.

Helliwell, D. 1999. GPs are key informants in medicinal cannabis survey. *GP Speak, Newsletter of the Northern Rivers Division of General Practice.* (April):4.

Hewat, M.L. 1906. *Bantu folk lore.* Capetown, South Africa: Maskew Miller.

Hewitt, G. 1872. *The pathology, diagnosis and treatment of diseases of women, including the diagnosis of pregnancy,* Second American edition. Philadelphia: Lindsay & Blakiston.

Horrobin, D.F., and M.S. Manku. 1989. Premenstrual syndrome and premenstrual breast pain (cyclical mastalgia): Disorders of essential fatty acid (EFA) metabolism. *Prostaglandins Leukot Essent Fatty Acids* 37(4):255-261.

House of Lords. 1998. *Cannabis: the scientific and medical evidence: Evidence.* London: House of Lords Select Committee on Science and Technology, Stationery Office.

Hutchinson, H.W. 1975. Patterns of marihuana use in Brazil. In *Cannabis and culture,* edited by V. Rubin. The Hague: Mouton.

ibn Sina. 1294. *Al-Qanun fi l-tibb.* Bulaq.

Joy, J.E., S.J. Watson, and J.A. Benson Jr. 1999. *Marijuana and medicine: Assessing the science base.* Washington, DC: Institute of Medicine.

Kabelik, J., Z. Krejei, and F. Santavy. 1960. Cannabis as a medicament. *Bull Narc* 12:5-23.

Kahl, O. 1994. *Sabur ibn Sahl: Dispensatorium parvum (al-Aqrabadhin al-Saghir).* Leiden: E.J. Brill.

Kaplan, J. 1969. *Marijuana. Report of the Indian Hemp Drugs Commission, 1893-1894.* Silver Spring, MD: Thos. Jefferson.

Leson, G., and P. Pless. 2002. Hemp seed and hemp oil. In F. Grotenhermen and E.B. Russo (eds.), *Cannabis and cannabinoids: Pharmacology, toxicology and therapeutic potential* (pp. 411-425). Binghamton, NY: The Haworth Press, Inc.

Lewis, H.E. 1900. *Cannabis indica*: A study of its physiologic action, toxic effects and therapeutic indications. *Merck's Archives of Materia Medica and its Uses* 2:247-251.

Lewis, W. 1794. *The Edinburgh new dispensatory,* Fourth edition. Edinburgh: M. Lavoisier.

Lilly. 1898. *Lilly's handbook of pharmacy and therapeutics*. Indianapolis: Lilly and Company.

Linn, S., S.C. Schoenbaum, R.R. Monson, R. Rosner, P.C. Stubblefield, and K.J. Ryan. 1983. The association of marijuana use with outcome of pregnancy. *Am J Public Health* 73(10):1161-1164.

Lozano, I. 1993. Estudios y documentos sobre la historia del cáñamo y del hachís en el islam medieval. Doctoral dissertation, Departamento de Estudios Semíticos, Universidad de Granada, Spain.

Lozano, I. 1998. *Solaz del espíritu en el hachís y el vino y otros textos árabes sobre drogas*. Granada, Spain: Universidad de Granada.

Lozano, I. 2001. The therapeutic use of *Cannabis sativa* L. in Arabic medicine. *J Cannabis Therapeutics* 1(1):63-70.

Mani, S.K., A. Mitchell, and B.W. O'Malley. 2001. Progesterone receptor and dopamine receptors are required in Delta 9-tetrahydrocannabinol modulation of sexual receptivity in female rats. *Proc Natl Acad Sci USA* 98(3):1249-1254.

Mannische, L. 1989. *An ancient Egyptian herbal*. Austin: University of Texas.

Margolis, J.S., and R. Clorfene. 1969. *A child's garden of grass (The official handbook for marijuana users)*. North Hollywood, CA: Contact Books.

Martin, M.A. 1975. Ethnobotanical aspects of cannabis in Southeast Asia. In V. Rubin (ed.), *Cannabis and Culture* (pp. 63-75). The Hague, Paris: Mouton Publishers.

Mattison, J.B. 1891. Cannabis indica as an anodyne and hypnotic. *St. Louis Med Surg J* 61:265-271.

McConnell, J.F.P. 1888. Uses of Cannabis indica. *Practitioner* 40:95-98.

McMeens, R.R. 1860. Report of the Ohio State Medical Committee on *Cannabis indica*. White Sulphur Springs, OH: Ohio State Medical Society.

McPartland, J.M. 1999. Marijuana and medicine: The endocrine effects of cannabis. *Altern Ther Women's Health* 1(6):41-44.

McPartland, J.M. 2001. Cannabis and eicosanoids: A review of molecular pharmacology. *J Cannabis Therapeutics* 1(1):71-83.

Merzouki, A. 2001. El cultivo del cáñamo (*Cannabis sativa* L.) en el Rif, Norte de Marruecos, taxonomía, biología y etnobotánica. doctoral dissertation, Departamento de biología vegetal, Universidad de Granada, Spain.

Merzouki, A., F. Ed-derfoufi, and J. Molero Mesa. 2000. Hemp (*Cannabis sativa* L.) and abortion. *J Ethnopharmacol* 73(3):501-503.

Michel. 1880. Propriétés médicinales de l'Indian hemp ou du Cannabis indica. *Montpellier Medical* 45:103-116.

Mu'min, S.M. 1669. *Tuhfat al-Mu'minin* (Gift of religious believers). The manuscript of the Institute of Manuscripts (Baku). Code: M 243/3747 (in Persian).

Murphy, L. 1999. Cannabis effects on endocrine and reproductive function. In H. Kalant, W.A. Corrigall, W. Hall and R.G. Smart (eds.), *The health effects of cannabis* (pp. 377-400). Toronto, Canada: Centre for Addiction and Mental Health.

Murphy, L. 2001. Hormonal system and reproduction. In F. Grotenhermen and E.B. Russo (eds.), *Cannabis and cannabinoids: Pharmacology, toxicology and therapeutic potential* (pp. 289-297). Binghamton, NY: The Haworth Press, Inc.

Nadkarni, K.M. 1976. *Indian materia medica,* Third edition, Volume 1. Bombay: Popular Prakashan.

Noyes, R., Jr., and D.A. Baram. 1974. Cannabis analgesia. *Compr Psychiatry* 15(6): 531-535.

O'Connell, C.M., and P.A. Fried. 1984. An investigation of prenatal cannabis exposure and minor physical anomalies in a low risk population. *Neurobehav Toxicol Teratol* 6(5):345-350.

Oliver, J. 1883. On the action of *Cannabis indica. Brit Med J* 1:905-906.

O'Shaughnessy, W.B. 1842. *Bengal dispensatory and companion to the pharmacopoeia.* London: Allen.

Ott, J. 2002. Pharmaka, philtres, and pheromones. Getting high and getting off. *Bull Multidisciplin Assoc Psychedelic Stud* 12(1):26-32.

Paria, B.C., H. Song, X. Wang, P.C. Schmid, R.J. Krebsbach, H.H. Schmid, T.I. Bonner, A. Zimmer, and S.K. Dey. 2001. Dysregulated cannabinoid signaling disrupts uterine receptivity for embryo implantation. *J Biol Chem* 276(23): 20523-20528.

Parker, S.J., and B.S. Zuckerman. 1999. The effects of maternal marihuana use during pregnancy on fetal growth. In G.G. Nahas (ed.), *Marihuana for medicine* (pp. 461-466). Totowa, NJ: Humana Press.

Parkinson, J., T. Bonham, and M. de L'Obel. 1640. *Theatrum botanicum: The theater of plants.* London: Tho. Cotes.

Perry, L.M., and J. Metzger. 1980. *Medicinal plants of East and Southeast Asia: Attributed properties and uses.* Cambridge: MIT Press.

Pharmaceutical Society of Great Britain. 1934. *The British pharmaceutical codex.* London: Pharmaceutical Press.

Racime, H. 1876. Le Haschisch ou chanvre indien. *Montpelier Medical* 36:432-449.

Ratnam, E.V. 1916. *Cannabis indica. J Brit Med Assoc, Ceylon Branch* 13:30-34.

Rätsch, C. 1998. *Marijuana medicine: A world tour of the healing and visionary powers of cannabis.* Rochester, VT: Healing Arts Press.

Reynolds, J.R. 1890. Therapeutical uses and toxic effects of *Cannabis indica. Lancet* 1:637-638.

Riddle, J.M. 1997. *Eve's herbs: A history of contraception and abortion in the West.* Cambridge, MA: Harvard University.

Ringer, S. 1886. *A handbook of therapeutics,* 11th edition. New York: W. Wood.

Robson, P. 1998. Cannabis as medicine: time for the phoenix to rise? *Brit Med J* 316(7137):1034-1035.

Rubin, V. 1976. Cross-cultural perspectives on therapeutic uses of cannabis. In S. Cohen and R.C. Stillman (eds.), *The therapeutic potential of marihuana* (pp. 1-17). New York: Plenum Medical.

Rumpf, G.E., and E.M. Beekman. 1981. *The poison tree: Selected writings of Rumphius on the natural history of the Indies,* Library of the Indies. Amherst: University of Massachusetts.

Russo, E.B., M.L. Mathre, A. Byrne, R. Velin, P.J. Bach, J. Sanchez-Ramos, and K.A. Kirlin. 2002. Chronic cannabis use in the Compassionate Investigational New Drug Program: An examination of benefits and adverse effects of legal clinical cannabis. *J Cannabis Therapeutics* 2(1):3-57.

Sajous, C., and M. Sajous. 1924. *Cannabis indica* (Indian hemp: hashish). In *Sajous's analytic cyclopedia of practical medicine* (pp. 1-9). Philadelphia: Davis.

Schlimmer, J.L. 1874. *Terminologie medico-pharmaceutique et anthropologique francaise-persane.* Teheran: Lithographie d'Ali Goulikhan.

Schmid, P.C., B.C. Paria, R.J. Krebsbach, H.H. Schmid, and S.K. Dey. 1997. Changes in anandamide levels in mouse uterus are associated with uterine receptivity for embryo implantation. *Proc Natl Acad Sci USA* 94(8):4188-4192.

Scudder, J.M. 1875. *Specific medication and specific medicines.* Cincinnati, OH: Wilstach, Baldwin and Co.

Shoemaker, J.V. 1899. The therapeutic value of *Cannabis indica. Texas Medical News* 8(10):477-488.

Short, T. 1751. *Medicina Britannica: Or a treatise on such physical plants, as are generally to be found in the fields or gardens in Great-Britain,* Third edition. Philadelphia: B. Franklin and D. Hall.

Shou-zhong, Y. 1997. *The divine farmer's materia medica: A translation of the Shen Nong Ben Cao Jing.* Boulder, CO: Blue Poppy Press.

Silver, A. 1870. On the value of Indian hemp in menorrhagia and dysmenorrhoea. *Medical Times and Gazette* 2:59-61.

Snyder, S.H. 1971. *Uses of marijuana.* New York: Oxford University.

Solis-Cohen, S., and T.S. Githens. 1928. *Pharmacotherapeutics, materia medica and drug action.* New York: D. Appleton.

Stillé, A. 1860. *Therapeutics and materia medica: A systematic treatise on the action and uses of medicinal agents, including their description and history.* Philadelphia: Blanchard and Lea.

Stuart, G.A. 1928. *Chinese Materia Medica.* Shanghai: Presbyterian Mission.

Tibbnama. 1712. (The Book of Medicine). The manuscript of the Institute of Manuscripts (Baku). Code: C 331/1894 (medieval Azerbaijani).

Thompson, L.S. 1972. *Cannabis sativa* and traditions associated with it. *Kentucky Folklore Record* 18:1-4.

Thompson, R.C. 1924. *The Assyrian herbal.* London: Luzac and Co.

Thompson, R.C. 1949. *A dictionary of Assyrian botany.* London: British Academy.

Vriend, H.J. de. 1984. *The Old English Herbarium and, Medicina de quadrupedibus, Early English Text Society.* London: Oxford University.

Wenger, T., G. Fragkakis, P. Giannikou, K. Probonas, and N. Yiannikakis. 1997. Effects of anandamide on gestation in pregnant rats. *Life Sci* 60(26):2361-2371.

Wenger, T., B.E. Toth, C. Juaneda, J. Leonardelli, and G. Tramu. 1999. The effects of cannabinoids on the regulation of reproduction. *Life Sci* 65(6-7):695-701.

Whittle, B.A., G.W. Guy, and P. Robson. 2001. Prospects for new cannabis-based prescription medicines. *J Cannabis Therapeutics* 1(3-4):183-205.

Wilcox, A.J., C.R. Weinberg, and D.D. Baird. 1990. Risk factors for early pregnancy loss. *Epidemiology* 1(5):382-385.

Willis, I.P. 1859. *Cannabis indica. Boston Med Surg J* 61:173-178.

Witter, F.R., and J.R. Niebyl. 1990. Marijuana use in pregnancy and pregnancy outcome. *Am J Perinatol* 7(1):36-38.

Wood, G.B., and F. Bache. 1854. *The dispensatory of the United States.* Philadelphia: Lippincott, Brambo & Co.

Wright, T.L. 1862. Correspondence. *Cincinnati Lancet and Observer* 5(4):246-247.

Wright, T.L. 1863. Some therapeutic effects of *Cannabis indica. Cincinnati Lancet and Observer* 6(2):73-75.

Zargari, A. 1990. *Medicinal plants,* Fourth edition, Volume 4. Teheran: Teheran University Publications.

Zias, J., H. Stark, J. Sellgman, R. Levy, E. Werker, A. Breuer, and R. Mechoulam. 1993. Early medical use of cannabis. *Nature* 363(6426):215.

Zimmer, L.E., and J.P. Morgan. 1997. *Marijuana myths, marijuana facts: A review of the scientific evidence.* New York: Lindesmith Center.

Zotter, H. 1996. *Medicina antiqua: Codex Vindobonensis 93 der Österreichischen Nationalbibliothek: Kommentar, Glanzlichter der Buchkunst; Bd. 6.* Graz: Akademische Druck-u. Verlagsanstalt.

UPDATE

Ethan B. Russo

The role of the endogenous cannabinoid system and exogenous cannabis usage in pregnancy remains of critical interest. A recent critical review focused on animal studies (Park et al. 2004). Additional work on fertility and its regulation by endocannabinoids has been advanced in Italy (Maccarrone et al. 2004, 2005). Obvious caution is needed in contemplation of cannabinoid use in pregnancy, but therapeutic indications still may be apparent, particularly for hyperemesis gravidarum (see Chapter 14, plus accompanying update) (Curry 2002; Westphal et al. 2005). See Chapter 8 update for additional references.

REFERENCES

Curry, W.-N.L. 2002. Hyperemesis gravidarum and clinical cannabis: To eat or not to eat? *Journal of Cannabis Therapeutics* 2 (3-4):63-83.

Maccarrone, M., M. DeFelici, F. G. Klinger, N. Battista, F. Fezza, E. Dainese, G. Siracusa, and A. Finazzi-Agro. 2004. Mouse blastocysts release a lipid which activates anandamide hydrolase in intact uterus. *Mol Hum Reprod* 10 (4):215-221.

Maccarrone, M., E. Fride, T. Bisogno, M. Bari, M. G. Cascio, N. Battista, A. Finazzi Agro, R. Suris, R. Mechoulam, and V. Di Marzo. 2005. Up-regulation of the endocannabinoid system in the uterus of leptin knockout (ob/ob) mice and implications for fertility. *Mol Hum Reprod* 11 (1):21-28.

Park, B., J. M. McPartland, and M. Glass. 2004. Cannabis, cannabinoids and reproduction. *Prostaglandins Leukot Essent Fatty Acids* 70 (2):189-197.

Westphal, R., P. Janssen, P. Lucas, and R. Capler. 2006. Survey of medicinal cannabis use among childbearing women: Patterns of its use in pregnancy and retroactive self-assessment of tis efficacy against "morning sickness." *Complementary Therapies in Clinical Practice* 12:27-33.

Chapter 17

Crack Heads and Roots Daughters:
The Therapeutic Use of Cannabis in Jamaica

Melanie Dreher

There are only two illicit substances that are widely used in Jamaica: marijuana (or "ganja," as it is called locally) and crack cocaine. This chapter describes the use of cannabis as a cheap, available therapy for the treatment of cocaine addiction by working-class women in Kingston, Jamaica. The findings reported here are derived from an ethnographic study of crack-using women in Kingston (Dreher and Hudgins 1992). The purposes of this study were to identify the social and economic conditions that promote and reinforce cocaine use and generate implications for treatment and prevention. Complementing the earlier large-scale opinion survey that had influenced drug policy in Jamaica (Stone 1990), the ethnographic design was deployed to: (1) observe the actual drug-linked behavior of crack using women in the natural settings of home and community, (2) permit a longitudinal examination of the processes embedded in drug careers over several months, and (3) overcome the potential mistrust of investigators that often accompanies research on illegal and socially sensitive activities.

Participant observation in inner-city Kingston provided opportunities to witness, firsthand, the social interactions and behavior associated with crack consumption and procurement, the daily routine of crack users, the techniques of crack cocaine ingestion, and the role and status of crack users in their communities. In addition to the general observations in the homes, yards, and community establishments of a Kingston neighborhood, 33 women who had ever used cocaine and its derivatives were followed for a period of nine months, in which their drug use and life events were monitored and recorded. An unstructured interview schedule served as a guide for the investigators, ensuring the comparability of the data while not constraining the responses of informants. As their histories unfolded, probes by the investigator generated new factors that were added to the interview schedule and explored in repeat visits to all participants.

Handbook of Cannabis Therapeutics
© 2006 by The Haworth Press, Inc. All rights reserved.
doi:10.1300/5741_18

The data derived from both interviews and observations included: (1) socio-demographic characteristics such as age, place of birth, residence, transience, religion, education, employment, marital status, health status and ethnicity; (2) past and present social relationships including family of origin, conjugal unions, children, household composition, friends and recreational activities; (3) major life events; and (4) drug-use careers including the circumstances surrounding initiation to crack, current use patterns, perceived short-term and long-term effects of crack use and their opinions of crack as both a personal and social phenomenon. Their wealth of experience and their willingness to share it provided us with a window into the drug-related behavior of women in Jamaica.

GANJA

Although both the use and distribution of ganja (cannabis) are illegal in Jamaica, the substance has been part of Jamaican working-class culture for over a century (Rubin and Comitas 1975; Dreher 1982). There is a strong cultural tolerance for ganja, and for most of the working class it simply is not regarded as a "drug" (Dreher and Shapiro 1994). The Rastafarian community has adopted ganja as its sacrament—a substance "from the earth," in harmony with the environment, natural (or "ital") and indigenous. Even heavy cannabis users, such as Rastafarians, are accepted because they do not threaten the social fabric of the community.

The use of cannabis for therapeutic purposes is not new in Jamaica. For over a century, the health-rendering properties of cannabis have enjoyed widespread endorsement (Rubin and Comitas 1975; Dreher 1997). Ganja tonics, teas and other infusions are household medicines used both curatively and prophylactically by Jamaicans of all ages, of both sexes and in a wide range of socioeconomic levels. Believed to improve health, stimulate the appetite, enhance work, promote a calm, meditative approach to life, reduce violence and augment sexual performance, ganja is a substance that symbolizes and promotes enduring values about health and behavior in Jamaica. Over the years, socially generated rules have evolved regarding who can use ganja, when, where, in what form and how much, creating a "complex" of social institutions that have served to guide the use of ganja and inhibit its abuse.

For example, since its introduction to Jamaica in the midnineteenth century by indentured laborers from India, ganja smoking, either in a "spliff" (ganja cigarette that is sometimes mixed with tobacco) or a pipe (also called a "chillum" or "chalice"), has been almost universally a male-dominated activity. Indeed, the early anthropological studies of cannabis use in Jamaica, conducted in the late 1960s and early 1970s, focused on ganja smoking as a working-class, male social activity (Dreher and Rogers 1976, 1982; Rubin and Comitas 1975). The female ganja smoker was rare, except in a presexual context with their mates, and the few women that did smoke ganja outside of socially prescribed contexts were regarded as disreputable and often held in contempt by both men and women in their communities (Dreher 1984).

The organization of consumption based on sex was validated by the ethnophysiological explanation that ganja, when smoked, goes "directly to the brain," producing psychoactive effects that include the power to "reason" or engage in intellectual and philosophical discourse. In contrast, when drunk as teas or tonic, it goes "directly to the blood," where it promotes health, prevents disease, and makes the body strong and ready to work. According to the men who smoked ganja, women "do not have the brains" for smoking and were excluded from the adult recreational and work groups in which ganja was used and exchanged socially. At the same time, however, it was usual and acceptable for women to cultivate and sell ganja, and even more common for women to prepare and administer ganja in the form of medicinal teas and tonics to their families and household members (Dreher 1984).

The institutionalized social rules that comprise the ganja "complex," including the widespread sanctions against female smoking, have continued to limit use among women. Within the past twenty years, however, increasing numbers of women have begun to smoke ganja routinely, in a manner not unlike their male counterparts. Partly due to the increase in Rastafarianism, not only are such women tolerated, but many have been given the commendatory title of "roots daughter" (Dreher 1987). The term "roots" has become part of the Rastafarian and youth vernacular in Jamaica to signify that which is real, natural, original, perhaps African, or at least, non-Western. The appellation "roots daughter" is used to identify women who come from a fine, if humble, tradition, who have "good brains," who can "smoke hard as a man" and with whom men can "reason" (discuss and debate) as they would with other men.

The roots daughter is not simply a ganja smoker but also a clear thinker and a woman of dignity. She "must keep a standard" and "go about properly." If she is involved in a stable union, her partner can expect her to be helpful and sexually faithful. As one informant explained, "If your woman is roots and you see her talking to another man, there is no reason to be jealous." Roots daughters are dignified, conservative, independent, nonpromiscuous, hardworking and spiritual. They often are contemptuous of jewelry and makeup and may be recognizable by their hair, which frequently is styled in dreadlocks and covered. Finally, a roots daughter is a responsible, strict but nurturing mother who values education (both intellectual and moral) and who will forego her own ganja smoking to prepare ganja teas and tonics for her children to "make them smarter and stronger." Nevertheless, roots daughters are not the norm and the restrictions on female ganja use in the general population remain intact.

COCAINE

The presence of cocaine, especially in the form of crack, is relatively recent in Jamaica. Unlike the "ganja complex," with its institutionalized social rules that guide use, there is no "culture" for crack cocaine. Explosive rates of addiction have resulted in widespread social and economic dysfunction (Dreher and Hudgins 1992; Dreher 1995). Cocaine is chemically prepared, synthetic and not indigenous to Jamaica. Crack users, in general, are considered inherently "repulsive," straying from what is considered "normal" human behavior. For most Jamaicans, the use of crack cocaine is not only a violation of the law but indicative of an undisciplined, lazy and even unhygienic person. In a society that values "clear" skin, fleshiness, sexual vigor, self-control and family loyalty, the "mawga" (skinny), debauched, impotent crack user is seen as fundamentally "bad," violent, self-serving, and the antithesis of everything that is good and important in Jamaica.

In Jamaica, crack is consumed in two ways: either directly in a pipe, or ground and sprinkled on a ganja cigarette, called a "seasoned" or a "dust up" spliff. In a seasoned spliff, the rock (crack) is mashed and spread over the mixture of ganja and tobacco, which is then rolled and smoked. Some users sprinkle the ashes from the pipe on the seasoned spliff so as not to waste any part of the crack. The seasoned spliff is of particular interest because it is the form of drug consumption in which two opposing Jamaican metaphors intersect: ganja (the wholesome multipurpose herb) and crack (the noxious drug).

Opinions regarding the "seasoned spliff" are mixed and reflect the beliefs and behavior of the users. Rastafarians, with their ideological commitment to ganja as a sacrament, disdain the idea of mixing crack cocaine (a white man's poison, an unnatural substance) with a natural substance that is associated with physical and mental health and is considered indigenous to Jamaica. Almost universally, they regard the seasoned spliff as "defiled herb," alleging that it is the signature of "commercial Rastas" or "Rastatutes," who earned their livelihood by being the sexual partners of American and European female tourists.

Ironically, many crack pipe users were equally derisive of the seasoned spliff, claiming that herb (ganja) weakens the effects of the crack: "Real crack users aren't interested in the seasoned spliff." "Real crack addicts are not interested in ganja at all." "Wi' de pipe, you feel de effects instantly." "Me prefer de blow." According to one self-identified coke addict, she didn't like the seasoned spliff because when she smoked it, it made her feel like her "mind is beatin' [racing], but when you smoke it in a pipe it makes you feel numb."

Based on the results of his national survey, Stone (1990) attributed the increase in crack cocaine use to the seasoned spliff, asserting that ganja is the "gateway" to cocaine use. In the sense that ganja established inhalation as the primary mechanism by which to achieve a psychoactive experience (intravenous drug use is rarely, if ever, practiced in Jamaica), crack smoking clearly fit well into the existing Jamaican drug paradigm. The gateway explanation is further reinforced by reports of vendors "seasoning" ganja to create a more potent product and thus a market for cocaine. On the other hand, the almost universal presence of ganja smoking and the comparatively small percentage of crack cocaine users suggest that there is no direct or necessary relationship between ganja and crack and, at the very least, call for further analysis.

WOMEN AND CRACK

Unlike ganja, crack routinely is consumed with members of the opposite sex, and thus the most likely explanation for the higher proportion of women among crack smokers than that among ganja smokers. In some Jamaican communities women are reported to make up 25 percent of the crack users (Dreher and Shapiro 1994). Several women reported that they first were exposed to cocaine by "big men," such as entertainers, who allegedly are responsible for introducing literally hundreds of young women to cocaine. Women who are directly or indirectly associated with the tourist industry are most at risk (Broad and Feinberg 1995). As one study participant stated simply, "Tourists like to try different drugs when they are on vacation." Thus, women who are hotel workers or waitresses, as well as exotic dancers and prostitutes, are recruited to procure crack for tourists and are likely to be invited to join them in smoking it. Women who are associated with men who work in tourism and the entertainment industry also are at risk. Taxi drivers, for example, often are asked to obtain crack/cocaine and then are invited to partake with their female tourist customers. They, in turn, may take some home for their girlfriends to try and even turn to selling crack/cocaine themselves.

In contrast to roots daughters, women who smoke crack are considered drug addicts and held in the very lowest esteem. To support their dependency, the vast majority of crack addicts become street prostitutes and engage in sexual practices that are outside normative behavior for Jamaicans, including oral sex, anal sex, and performance sex with other women. Female crack users in Jamaica suffer a life of peril and degradation. Prostitutes reported being beaten, stabbed, and robbed by their clients. In addition they are exposed to HIV infection and other sexually transmitted diseases. Moreover, their exposure to danger is increased at the very time that their ability to avoid or manage high-risk situations is most impaired.

Of the 33 women who were followed in the study (Table 17.1), 17 were using crack in some form at the time of the study while 14 were former users. Of the 17 current users, 5 were exclusively pipe smokers, 11 smoked both the pipe and seasoned spliff and only 1 smoked seasoned spliffs exclusively. Of the 14 former users, only 1 had used the pipe exclusively, 7 were exclusively seasoned spliff users and 5 used both pipe and seasoned spliff. The remaining former user was the only woman in the study who "snorted" cocaine powder while she lived abroad but had not used cocaine since she had returned to Jamaica and became a Rastafarian. The 8 women who exclusively used the seasoned spliff typically defined themselves not as crack *addicts* but rather as crack *users,* for whom the seasoned spliff was enhanced herb, with an extra "kick" or "boost." In contrast, all the pipe smokers, whether they used it exclusively or in addition to a seasoned spliff, identified themselves as addicts.

All the women in the study agreed that the two modes of ingestion produced very different effects. As one woman stated, "The pipe makes you more high than dust spliff." She recounted how she likes to smoke a seasoned spliff and that her capacity to "reason" was facilitated by the mixing of crack with ganja. Another woman stated that the pipe made her feel "more drunk," "like a monster." She also said that it will make you "grow fine like a thread" (thin), if you continue to use it alone. The youngest user in the study, who smoked only seasoned spliffs, commented that the "pipe do you bad—make you want it more often." Both kinds of crack users believed the pipe is more addicting than a seasoned spliff or even "snorting."

TABLE 17.1. Crack/cocaine using women in Kingston, Jamaica, according to type of use.

	Current users	Former users	Total
Pipe	5	1	6
Seasoned spliff	1	7	8
Combined	11	5	16
Intranasal	0	1	1

Many of the women who had smoked crack in a seasoned spliff for several months or even years reported that when they were exposed to the pipe, it quickly became their predominant and preferred mode of use. One woman described how cocaine was pushed on her by a "guy who dust up a cigarette" and gave it to her. She said she refused it several times but he was persistent and finally she tried it. Because she had experienced little danger in the seasoned spliff, she started smoking the pipe, which she now uses exclusively. Thus while crack and ganja commonly are thought of as linked in both consumption and distribution, participants in this study saw them as quite distinct. "The difference between ganja and coke is that with the ganja you can still work, cook and clean up. . . . When you're high on ganja you want to eat but when you are high on coke you don't want to do anything. You are just afraid and want to hide."

The devastating impact of crack on their health and physical appearance, typical of crack users cross-culturally (Ratner 1993; Inciardi et al. 1993), was a consistent complaint of participating women. Not only does crack "rob" them of their strength and ability to work, it impairs their appearance with dry hair, dark blotches and sores on their skin, burned and stained fingers, and, perhaps most important for this Jamaican population, severe weight loss. In addition to the physical effects of crack, the women reported a disregard for personal hygiene and grooming, including hair, skin and clothing. Regardless of their family history or social status, they reported stealing from and lying to their friends and relatives and being referred to as "coke heads" or "crack heads," universally despised and disrespected. Many of the women in the study were banished from their home communities and one woman reported that her mother threw a pail of boiling water at her as she approached her family home, where her children were living with their grandmother. As prostitutes, they engaged in sexual practices that others found repulsive and it was not unusual for young boys to call them names, e.g., "suck hood," or "lick 'im batty" (referring to fellatio and oral-anal sex), or even to stone them. The combination of community distrust and repulsion reinforced their social isolation and self-loathing.

Both current and former crack-using women lamented their waste of money. Although they had the potential to generate comparatively large sums of money in a very short period of time through prostitution, they reaped no permanent benefits. They stated repeatedly that their need for crack supersedes all other needs, including food, clothing, housing and child support. Indeed, it is the impact on their children that was the most compelling source of guilt and remorse. Children had to be placed with other family members, friends or even neighbors because of the mother's inability to care for them. Women poignantly described having their children removed by police, subjected to ridicule by community members, neglected and abused both physically and sexually, often by their prostitution clients.

Consistent with the literature on women cocaine users in general (Pottieger and Tressell 2000), children were a primary motivation for these Jamaican women to discontinue cocaine use. One former crack user, for example, discontinued her habit one month before her first grandson was born because she did not want her grandchild to "come and find his granny a prostitute and a drug addict." During the interview, one of her children brought her grandchild in to her. As he sat on her lap during the interview, she caressed his head and smiled, "He's my drugs. I know I am not going back. I have control and I love my grandson and my kids." A few women reported that they had stopped smoking during their pregnancies because they heard that their addiction might kill the baby.

Also consistent with reports from other cultures (Labigalini et al. 1999), the drug histories of these women did not fall into a uniform trajectory, moving singly and consistently from nonuse to addiction and then, if they recovered, back to nonuse. It was not unusual, for example, to refrain from smoking for a few days, or even weeks, while they visited their families or when they felt that they were getting too thin. Many used a trip to their family home, usually outside of Kingston, as an opportunity to "stay clean" and "fatten up." Some women who had been ostracized by their families and thus could not go home reported actually trying to get arrested so that they would be incarcerated and could sleep and get three meals a day. A short jail sentence was a welcome relief from sex work and provided an opportunity to gain weight.

While their children, family members, and communities were powerful motivators for these women to discontinue crack cocaine, they also reported that such motivators were insufficient to maintain abstinence for long periods of time. In most cases, the return to crack use generally was triggered by a personal problem or simply because they were depressed and wanted to feel better. One participant, for example, reported that her boyfriend got her pregnant to get her off coke and she was clean for one year and three months but she started using it again when he returned to Jamaica with his wife. Another woman, working as a prostitute, said that she had stopped for four months and then started back when a client paid her with crack.

With the exception of the youngest participant in the study, who used only the seasoned spliff, all current users longed to discontinue smoking crack permanently and get their lives in order. Most were uninformed of any treatment facilities available to them. Four had tried to enroll in the University of West Indies Hospital drug intervention program but had been put on waiting lists of several months. In fact, treatment and counseling programs in which these women could avail themselves of professional assistance were almost nonexistent.

Given the unavailability of formal detoxification and recovery programs in Jamaica, the experience of the 14 former users is both important and cogent. Of the 14, 1 was an intranasal cocaine user while living abroad who became a Rastafarian on her return to Jamaica, gave up cocaine and now partakes of ganja as a religious sacrament. One was a woman who had never used ganja and was the only participant who had received professional assistance. Of the remaining 12, 7 had been exclusively seasoned spliff users and 5 were pipe users who also smoked seasoned spliffs. Of these last 5, 3 started using ganja for the express purpose of reducing the cravings, the paranoia and the loss of appetite associated with crack use.

Labigalini et al. (1999), reporting a similar folk therapy in Brazil, described the experience of several male patients in a treatment program who had used cannabis to reduce their craving for crack, thus helping them to overcome their addiction. According to these authors, the control of impulsive behavior and stabilization of the hunger mechanism is likely explained by the capacity of cannabis to increase the cerebral availability of serotonin that has been compromised by crack cocaine. Indeed, there were numerous reports from both ganja and crack users that ganja slows down the immediate effects of crack, and makes the overall high less intense but last longer and trail off more gradually. This avoids both the plummeting euphoria and subsequent paranoia that precipitate the need to smoke again. According to one woman:

> It makes me charged but not as strong as the pipe. It stays longer than the pipe—about twenty minutes to half an hour, while the pipe stays in your system for only ten minutes. The pipe is a killer. . . . I was always wanting the next pipe. The seasoned spliff is much better to me than the pipe. You can eat and drink at the same time because the herb opens the appetite. When it wears off, I feel like I want a fresh (bath) and sleep. When you smoke season spliffs, you don't feel "paro." It is a different meditation. Crack and coke are like demons and devils, they are not good and to how dem see de pipe mash up people, dem a turn to season spliff and some a dem nah touch de pipe.

The opinion of some of the users was that ganja simply reduces the volume of crack needed for a high while others claim it has a psychological role in counteracting the triggers in the environment that stimulate the need for crack cocaine:

> It mek you meditate an' have an interest away from crack.

> When you want crack you should smoke a spliff instead.

Nuff time me would use crack but (ganja) mek me t'ink twice.

Herb helps me not want to smoke.

If you're trying to stop and you smoke weed, you nah wan de rock.

With two spliff, I can resist crack.

The use of ganja as a vehicle for getting through the stress and urgency associated with the need for a "lick" of cocaine was reported by almost all of the women who were followed in this study.

Among the current users, the women who combined ganja consumption with their crack consumption were much more "successful" users in terms of physical health and lifestyle. In addition to reducing the need to smoke large quantities of crack, and thus engage in extensive and depleting prostitution, the role of ganja as an appetite stimulant was mentioned by several women. Even committed pipe smokers smoked ganja to compensate for the weight loss that accompanies cocaine use. Among the eight users (current and former) who smoked crack only in a seasoned spliff and did not consider themselves to be true addicts, all claimed that they were able to discontinue crack consumption easily and that they smoked a seasoned spliff because they enjoyed it, not because they needed it.

While the intriguing, preliminary evidence supports the physiological capacity of ganja to promote cocaine abstinence, its *cultural role* as a health rendering substance that induces thoughtfulness, meditation and communion with "Jah" (God) also warrants mention. Roots women, especially those with definitive Rastafarian affiliations, rejected a lifestyle requiring prostitution and culturally deviant sexual practices. Although there is no explicit injunction against crack in Rastafarian doctrine, the "roots" concept provides a comprehensive plan for living that includes responsibility, dignity and a family orientation. As the one Rasta woman in the study stated:

> Me nah trouble dat ting . . . me a roots. Now I am proud and happy to state that I am completely cured from that sin, and indeed, I am ever so thankful to Jah. Surely, God is good. . . . A very common saying is that cocaine addiction is uncurable. I have proved that saying to be completely wrong. My advice to all who want to quit using that garbage is to sincerely ask Jah for his help.

Being a roots daughter provides the motivation not only to discontinue the use of crack cocaine but to reduce exposure to the drug in the first place.

As such, Rastafarianism, with the ganja sacrament, has ideological value for prevention as well as treatment. The only roots daughter among the 33 women in the study was the 1 informant who had used cocaine intranasally when she lived abroad some years earlier. Since she became a Rastafarian, using ganja sacramentally, she speaks in great opposition to crack cocaine. The effectiveness of religious involvement in the treatment of alcohol and drug addiction has been long acknowledged (Buxton et al. 1987), and the notion that one substance can be used as a deterrent to, or replacement for, others is not new. Historical evidence suggests that peyotism, for example, provided an alternative substance as well as an alternative lifestyle, thus serving as a deterrent to alcoholism among Native American populations (Hill 1990). Even Sefaneck and Kaplan (1995) reevaluated their "stepping-stone" theory in the light of Dutch heroin users who succeeded in controlling the damaging effects by smoking cannabis.

CONCLUSIONS

Although the evidence is preliminary, the reported success rate of self-cure, using the cheapest and most available psychoactive substance, is persuasive. It lends credence to the reports of male crack users in Brazil and heroin users in the Netherlands and, at the very least, deserves further investigation. The data certainly suggest that ganja is neither a precondition nor a gateway to crack use. In fact, 9 of the 33 women had never used ganja at all and reported hating "even the smell of it." Although the majority of the participants in the study had smoked ganja prior to using crack cocaine, the number of years elapsing between initiating crack use ranged from 1 to 13, suggesting no automatic or direct linkage either physiologically or socially between ganja and crack. The youngest woman in the study (16 years old) said that she started using a seasoned spliff because her boyfriend wanted her to try it but spoke adamantly against pipe use. Moreover, for the women who were ganja users prior to becoming crack users, the number of years elapsing between initiating crack use ranged from 1 to 13 suggesting, again, no automatic or direct linkage.

Indeed, these findings indicate that rather than serving as a gateway to crack, cannabis may be instrumental in both the prevention and treatment of crack addiction. Of the 14 women who succeeded in discontinuing crack use, 13 attribute their success to the use of ganja, either because of its capacity to control the damage of crack cocaine use physiologically or, in one case, because of its religious value. Moreover, it is clear that the women who combined ganja and crack were at least able to maintain their weight and care for their children. At the very least, these findings beg the need to revisit the notion of multiple drug use in a more culture-specific context. Far from being the hedonistic multidrug users that present so many challenges to prevention and treatment programs, the women in this study were actually self-medicating, either to modify the effects of pipe smoking or to relinquish the habit all together.

IMPLICATIONS

Crack is a highly addictive form of cocaine with serious social consequences. The exponential increase in crack use worldwide has generated an urgent demand for treatment and prevention programs and international development agencies in the United States have invested considerable monetary and technical support to develop such programs in Jamaica as well as other countries. It is common knowledge, however, that health and social service programs are not automatically transferable from one society to another. Effectiveness requires that such programs be designed according to what is meaningful and important in the culture where it is to be applied. Thus the commitment to demand reduction and treatment programs by both the Jamaican and United States governments has created a need for continued monitoring of the knowledge, attitudes and practices surrounding substance consumption and distribution. Not only is ganja typically not thought of as a drug in Jamaica, it has assumed a positive value for limiting the ravages of cocaine as an appetite stimulant that counteracts the anorexia of cocaine addiction, and as an assistive substance in relinquishing cocaine addiction. Yet the tendency to include ganja, often as a starting point, for drug prevention and intervention in Jamaica continues to exist. Whether or not the use of ganja is a remedy for crack addition in the biological, psychological or sociological sense, programs that fail to acknowledge the different cultural meanings and experiences attached to these two illicit substances ultimately will lose credibility with the very population they need to serve. The experience of women who have managed to relinquish their cocaine habit without expensive professional intervention would appear to be highly consequential for the design of effective, low-cost, culture-specific treatment programs both in the United States and internationally.

REFERENCES

Broad, K. and B. Feinberg. 1995. Perceptions of ganja and cocaine in urban Jamaica. *J Psychoactive Drugs* 27(3):261-276.

Buxton, M., D. Smith, and R. Seymour. 1987. Spirituality and other points of resistance to the 12-step recovery process. *J Psychoactive Drugs* 19:275-286.

Dreher, M. 1982. *Working men and ganja*. Philadelphia: Institute for the Study of Human Issues.

Dreher, M. 1984. Marijuana use among women—An anthropological view. *Adv Alcohol Subst Abuse* 3(3):51-64.

Dreher, M. 1987. The evolution of a roots daughter. *J Psychoactive Drugs* 19(2): 165-170.

Dreher, M. 1995. Women and drugs: Case studies from Jamaica. *Drugs: Education, Prevention and Policy* 2(2):167-176.

Dreher, M. 1997. Cannabis and Pregnancy. In M.L. Mathre (ed.), *Cannabis in medical practice: A legal, historical and pharmacological overview of the therapeutic use of marijuana* (pp. 159-170). Jefferson, NC: McFarland & Co.

Dreher, M. and R. Hudgins. 1992. *Women and crack in Jamaica*. Report submitted to U.S. Department of State, United States Embassy. Kingston, Jamaica.

Dreher, M. and C. Rogers. 1976. Getting high: The ganja man and his socioeconomic milieu. *Caribbean Studies* 16(2):219-231.

Dreher, M. and D. Shapiro. 1994. *Drug consumption and distribution in Jamaica: A national ethnographic study*. Report submitted to U.S. Department of State, United States Embassy, Kingston, Jamaica.

Hill, T. 1990. Peyotism and the control of heavy drinking: The Nebraska Winnebago in the early 1900s. *Human Organization* 49(3):255-265.

Inciardi, J., Lockwood, D., and A. Pottieger 1993. *Women and crack cocaine*. New York: MacMillan.

Labigalini, E., Rodrigues, L.R. and D.X. DaSilviera. 1999. Therapeutic use of cannabis by crack addicts in Brazil. *J Psychoactive Drugs* 31(4):451-455.

Pottieger, A.E. and P.A. Tressell. 2000. Social relationships of crime-involved women cocaine users. *J Psychoactive Drugs* 32(4):445-460.

Ratner, M. (ed). 1993. *Crack pipe as pimp: An ethnographic investigation of sex-for-crack exchanges*. New York: Lexington Books.

Rubin, V., and L. Comitas. 1975. *Ganja in Jamaica*. The Hague: Mouton.

Sefaneck, S.J. and C.D. Kaplan. 1995. Keeping off: Stepping on and stepping off: The stepping stone theory reevaluated in the context of the Dutch cannabis experience. *Contemp Drug Problems* 22(8):483-512.

Stone, C. 1990. *National survey on the use of drugs in Jamaica*. Mona: University of West Indies.

UPDATE

Ethan B. Russo

The possibility of utilizing cannabis to treat other drug dependencies remains a tantalizing proposal. Such use for alcoholism was explored in the final article in the final issue of *Journal of Cannabis Therapeutics* (Mikuriya 2004), while the rational basis for use of cannabis-based medicines to treat cocaine addiction, as in this article, has received additional basic science support (Parker et al. 2004). While the "gateway effect" of cannabis leading to usage of other drugs has long been touted, a recent experiment has demonstrated that full CB_1 agonists restore heroin-seeking behavior in animals while THC, a partial agonist, does not (Fattore et al. 2003). The body of work by Cichewicz and her colleagues has amply demonstrated that THC effectively synergizes opioid analgesia, while ameliorating withdrawal and reducing tolerance (Cichewicz and McCarthy 2003; Cichewicz et al. 2003; Cichewicz and Welch 2003).

SR141716A (Rimonabant/Acomplia), a powerful CB_1-antagonist, has also been tested as a treatment for nicotine dependence and smoking cessation. It is eminently predictable that further clinical trials of cannabis-based medicines and cannabinoid antagonists will play important roles in this area of investigation.

REFERENCES

Cichewicz, D.L., and E.A. McCarthy. 2003. Antinociceptive synergy between delta(9)-tetrahydrocannabinol and opioids after oral administration. *J Pharmacol Exp Ther* 304 (3):1010-1015.

Cichewicz, D.L., A. Rubo, and S.P. Welch. 2003. Recovery of morphine- and codeine-induced antinociception by delta-9-tetrahydrocannabinol. Paper read at 2003 Symposium on the Cannabinoids, at NAV Centre, Cornwall, Ontario, Canada.

Cichewicz, D.L., and S.P. Welch. 2003. Modulation of oral morphine antinociceptive tolerance and naloxone-precipitated withdrawal signs by oral Delta 9-tetrahydrocannabinol. *J Pharmacol Exp Ther* 305 (3):812-817.

Fattore, L., M.S. Spano, G. Cossu, S. Deiana, and W. Fratta. 2003. Cannabinoid mechanism in reinstatement of heroin-seeking after a long period of abstinence in rats. *Eur J Neurosci* 17 (8):1723-1726.

Mikuriya, T.H. 2004. Cannabis as a substitute for alcohol: A harm-reduction approach. *Journal of Cannabis Therapeutics* 4 (1):79-93.

Parker, L.A., P. Burton, R.E. Sorge, C. Yakiwchuk, and R. Mechoulam. 2004. Effect of low doses of Delta(9)-tetrahydrocannabinol and cannabidiol on the extinction of cocaine-induced and amphetamine-induced conditioned place preference learning in rats. *Psychopharmacology (Berl)* 175(3):360-366.

Chapter 18

Cannabis in Multiple Sclerosis: Women's Health Concerns

Denis J. Petro

INTRODUCTION

Women's health issues have received attention as gender differences in disease expression and drug action are discovered. A gender-based approach recognizes the fundamental physiologic differences between men and women. The areas of difference between men and women in the nervous system are extensive including anatomy, cell numbers, neurotransmitter systems, response to hormones, sensation threshold and disease frequencies. Gender and multiple sclerosis (MS) has been the subject of several excellent reviews (Olek and Khoury 2000; Coyle 2000). Specific disorders such as migraine headache, depression and motor neuron disease also show clear gender preferences.

Multiple sclerosis is a disorder with important gender-associated differences in expression. Cannabis also interacts with the endocrine and immune systems of males and females with distinctions. As therapeutic cannabis use among MS patients has increased over the past generation, a review of the subject with attention to women's health concerns is warranted.

Multiple sclerosis is the most common cause of chronic neurological disability in young adults (Rusk and Plum 1998) and is more likely seen in women and in those who grew up in northern latitudes. In a summary of 30 incidence/prevalence studies, the cumulative female-to-male ratio was 1.77: 1.00 (Irizarry 1997). With 350,000 MS patients in the United States, the number of female MS patients is approximately 225,000. Gender is clearly a determinant of susceptibility to MS. The increased female incidence in MS is similar to other autoimmune diseases with onset of symptoms in adulthood such as myasthenia gravis, Hashimoto's thyroiditis, Sjögren's syndrome and systemic lupus erythematosus. The female preponderance in

Handbook of Cannabis Therapeutics
© 2006 by The Haworth Press, Inc. All rights reserved.
doi:10.1300/5741_19

MS lessens in those in whom presentation occurs later in life. MS attacks are less frequent during pregnancy while the postpartum period is one of higher risk (Whitaker 1998). While the postpartum increase in risk for MS attacks may discourage childbearing, women who have borne a child fare better in the long term than those women who have not (Runmarker and Anderson 1995). Interestingly, the occurrence of a first pregnancy may lead to some permanent change in immune status.

Recognizing that current MS treatment is less than optimal, the use of cannabis offers an opportunity to demonstrate the therapeutic potential of cannabinoids on a number of neurological symptoms. In a survey of health care in 471 people with MS in the United Kingdom, use of cannabis was acknowledged by 8 percent (Somerset et al. 2001). Extrapolating to the 60,000 MS patients in the United Kingdom provides an estimate of 4,800 MS patients who employ cannabis in the United Kingdom and 28,000 in the United States. In a publication commenting on the use of cannabis in South Africa, James (1994) reported the experiences of a female MS patient (p. 369):

> A few years ago I had started to eat small quantities of marijuana . . . the effects were immediate and remarkable. Control of bladder functioning which was a humiliating problem is restored to normal and has been a liberating influence in my life-style. I can now go out shopping, to the theater, etc., without anticipation of dread and panic. Painful and disturbing attacks of spasticity are relieved and now restful patterns of sleep are ensured where previously sleep was disrupted by urinary frequency or pain and discomfort not least I can laugh and giggle, have marvelous sex and forget that I have this awful, incurable, intractable disease.

The challenge for physicians is to evaluate patient observations using scientific methodology. Many authors have described individual patient experiences of therapeutic use of cannabis to treat symptoms of MS (Grinspoon and Bakalar 1997; Brown 1998; Iversen 2000). Additional support has been provided by single-patient clinical trials ($N = 1$) and prospective double-blind placebo-controlled studies.

TREATMENT OPTIONS: ACUTE EPISODES, DISEASE MODIFICATION AND SYMPTOM MANAGEMENT

Management of an acute episode of demyelination in MS is sometimes achieved to a limited extent with corticosteroids. Disease modification is difficult to assess because MS is a chronic, unpredictable disorder in which the burden of white matter involvement is highly variable and the clinical response to drug treatment is modest. Five drugs have been approved by regulatory authorities to modify the clinical course of MS. Avonex (interferon-beta-1a), Betaseron (interferon-beta-1b), Copaxone (glatiramer acetate/copolymer 1), and Rebif (interferon beta 1a) have demonstrated efficacy in relapsing-remitting MS and may slow the course of secondary progressive MS. Novantrone (mitoxantrone) is approved for secondary progressive and progressive relapsing MS. Immunosuppressants such as corticosteroids, methotrexate, and cyclophosphamide have been used to alter the natural history of MS with some success.

CANNABIS IN ACUTE TREATMENT AND DISEASE MODIFICATION

While patients may claim that cannabis can alter the natural history of MS, no clinical trials have been conducted in either acute treatment or disease modification. Data from animal research supports cannabinoids as a potential disease modifying treatment for MS. The immune-mediated disease, experimental autoimmune encephalomyelitis (EAE), is considered the laboratory model of MS. In a study in the Lewis rat and guinea pig, Lyman and colleagues (1989) demonstrated that the oral administration of Δ-9-tetrahydrocannabinol (THC) was effective in the prevention and suppression of EAE. The authors suggested that Δ-9-THC might prove to be a new and relatively innocuous agent for the treatment of immune-mediated diseases such as MS. Since Δ-9-THC is the cannabinoid associated with negative psychotropic actions, investigators used other cannabinoids to assess actions in EAE. Wirguin and colleagues (1994) studied the effect of Δ-8-THC on EAE in the rat. Orally administered Δ-8 THC significantly reduced the incidence and severity of neurological deficit while parenteral administration was not effective. The difference can be explained on first-pass metabolism in the liver, which produces the active metabolite. Additional support for beneficial effects of cannabinoids in EAE was reported by Achiron and coinvestigators (2000) using a synthetic nonpsychotropic cannabinoid, dexanabinol (HU-211). The authors suggested that dexanabinol may provide an alternate treatment of acute exacerbations of MS. Finally, Guzman et al. (2001) reviewed the experimental evidence showing the protective effects of cannabinoids from toxic insults such a glutamatergic over-stimulation, ischemia and oxidative damage. The authors described the potential of cannabinoids to downregulate inflammatory cytokine production.

If cannabinoid drugs are to be used in acute treatment of MS or in disease modification, then studies in female patients will be needed. These studies involve assessment of drug effects on fertility, pregnancy and in nursing mothers. Since inclusion of women in early clinical trials is usually insufficient to identify gender-based differences in response, animal models are used to identify potential pharmacologic and toxicological effects (Christian 2001). Unfortunately, current animal models do not consistently demonstrate gender-based differences seen in humans. The cannabinoid Δ-9-THC is marketed in the United States as Marinol and information concerning use in women is provided in the *Physicians' Desk Reference* (2002). Marinol is included in Category C (FDA designation for drugs with animal data showing harm to the fetus with no controlled human studies). The drug labeling states that Marinol should be used only if the potential benefit justifies the potential risk to the fetus. Likewise, its use in nursing mothers is not recommended since Marinol is concentrated in and secreted in human breast milk and is absorbed by the nursing baby.

Drug interaction studies would be needed to investigate the potential for significant interactions with drugs commonly used by women. Because cannabinoids are highly bound to plasma proteins and might displace other protein-bound drugs, dosage adjustment for other highly protein-bound drugs may be needed. In addition, drugs metabolized by hepatic mixed-function oxidase enzymes may be inhibited by cannabinoids (Benowitz and Jones 1977). In the PDR drug interaction section for Marinol, specific precautions are included regarding potential interactions with a number of drugs including sympathomimetic agents, antihistamines, tricyclic antidepressants, muscle relaxants, barbiturates and theophylline. Other drugs which may be important in female patients include birth control drugs, hormones administered to treat symptoms associated with menopause, steroids, and drugs used in the treatment of osteoporosis.

The effects of inhaled cannabis on fetal development have been studied extensively. In a study of six one-year-old infants exposed daily to cannabis prenatally and through breastfeeding, no malformations were found in cannabis-exposed infants (Tennes et al. 1985). A prospective study of the effects of prenatal exposure to cigarettes and cannabis on growth from birth to adolescence found no significant effects on growth measures at birth although a smaller head circumference observed at all ages reached statistical significance among the adolescents born to heavy marijuana users (Fried et al. 1999). Finally, the relationship between maternal use of cannabis and pregnancy outcome was investigated in a study of 12,000 women in the United Kingdom (Fergusson et al. 2002). Five percent of mothers reported smoking cannabis before and/or during pregnancy. The use of cannabis during pregnancy was not associated with increased risk of perinatal mortality or morbidity. The babies of women who used cannabis weekly before and during pregnancy were lighter than those of nonusers and had shorter birth lengths and smaller head circumferences. The findings of this study are consistent with earlier studies that have found an absence of statistical association between cannabis use and antenatal or perinatal morbidity and mortality. The reduced birth weight seen with regular or heavy cannabis use suggests that to optimize fetal growth and minimize the risk of an adverse pregnancy outcome, pregnant women should limit cannabis use during pregnancy. In female patients during the reproductive years, fertility and pregnancy are usually not affected by MS. While MS activity seems to decrease during pregnancy, exacerbation rates increase in the first six months postpartum (Birk and Rudick 1986). Since cannabinoids are secreted in human breast milk and absorbed by the nursing baby, cannabis use while breastfeeding should be avoided.

Special studies of cannabis in menopausal and post-menopausal women have been conducted. Mendelson and colleagues (1985) studied LH levels in menopausal women after marijuana smoking and found no significant difference in LH levels when compared to values for healthy menopausal women. In a study of the acute effects of marijuana smoking in postmenopausal women, Benedikt and colleagues (1986) noted statistically significant increases in pulse rate, intoxication levels and the confusion component of the Profile of Mood States Questionnaire (POMS). The finding of neuropsychological performance impairment in post-menopausal women is not unlike the findings in moderate cannabis users (Pope et al. 2001) and in heavy cannabis users (Solowij et al. 2002). The degree of impairment in memory and attention are not surprising in chronic heavy users. Pope (2002) presents the consensus opinion that some cognitive deficits persist for hours or days after acute intoxication with cannabis has subsided. Since cognitive impairment is associated with MS, the potential for significant adverse effect on memory and attention in MS patients using therapeutic cannabis should be a subject of future clinical research.

CANNABIS IN SYMPTOM MANAGEMENT

Manifestations of MS are protean and depend on the location of persistent central nervous system lesions. Since MS lesions have a predilection for certain anatomic locations, recognizable clinical syndromes are common in MS. Surveys of symptoms in MS have been carried out with the most common symptoms including fatigue, balance impairment, muscle disturbances (weakness, stiffness, pain and spasm), and bowel and bladder impairment (Compston 1999). In chronic MS, signs and symptoms of motor dysfunction are found in at least 75 percent of patients (Miller 2000) with sensory impairment noted in 50 percent. Cerebellar abnormalities (ataxia, tremor, nystagmus or dysarthria) are found in at least a third of MS patients. Autonomic symptoms including bowel, bladder or sexual dysfunction are found in at least 50 percent of patients.

A survey of cannabis-using MS patients in the United States and United Kingdom by Consroe and colleagues (1997) reported improvements after cannabis use in spasticity, chronic pain, acute paroxysmal phenomena, tremor, emotional dysfunction, anorexia/weight loss, fatigue, diplopia, sexual dysfunction, bowel and bladder dysfunction, vision dimness, dysfunction of walking and balance, and memory loss (descending rank order). While the authors of this study discuss the potential shortcomings of the survey design, this report suggests that cannabis may significantly relieve signs and symptoms of MS such as spasticity and pain along with a number of other complaints.

IMPAIRED MOBILITY: SPASTICITY

In the nineteenth century, O'Shaughnessy (1842) used hemp extract in treating muscle spasms associated with tetanus and rabies. Reynolds (1890) reported using cannabis to treat muscle spasms, as well as for epilepsy, migraine, and other indications. While medicinal cannabis use continued in the years after the work of O'Shaughnessy and Reynolds, little was published concerning cannabis and spasticity until the 1970s. A survey of ten spinal-cord injured males was published in 1974 in which five patients reported reduced spasticity, three patients noted no effect and two patients did not have significant spasticity (Dunn and Davis 1974).

The use of cannabis to treat spasticity associated with MS has been reported by a number of investigators over the subsequent interval. Petro (1980) reported one patient with MS who used cannabis to treat nocturnal leg fatigue and spasms associated with spasticity. Petro and Ellenberger (1981) conducted a double-blind clinical trial that demonstrated statistically significant reduction in spasticity following the oral administration of Δ-9-THC in doses of 5 and 10 mg. Investigators have confirmed the observation using Δ-9-THC (Hanigan et al. 1985; Ungerleider et al. 1988; Maurer et al. 1990), cannabis (Meinck et al. 1990) and nabilone (Martyn et al. 1995). Additional preclinical support for the benefit from cannabis in spasticity was provided by the report of Baker and colleagues (2000). In this study, cannabinoid receptor agonism improved tremor and spasticity in mice with chronic relapsing experimental allergic encephalomyelitis (CREAE) and indicated that the endogenous cannabinoid system may be active in control of spasticity and tremor. Further support for cannabinoid receptor involvement was provided in an animal study in which cannabinoid receptor (CB_1) changes were found in regions of the brain involved in the control of motor symptoms (Berrendero et al. 2001). The role of the endocannabinoid system in spasticity was demonstrated in CREAE mice in a further study, which manipulated tone using cannabinoid receptor agonists and antagonists (Baker et al. 2001).

Since a considerable body of scientific evidence supports the efficacy of cannabinoids in spasticity, review articles (Gracies et al. 1997; Consroe 1999) and medical texts (Compston 1999; Compston 2001) include cannabis as a treatment option in spasticity. In *Brain's Diseases of the Nervous System*, Eleventh Edition (Compston 2001), among the treatments for spasticity associated with MS, cannabinoids are listed along with baclofen, dantrium, benzodiazepines and tizanidine.

Gender issues are involved in MS-associated spasticity. Since females are more likely to experience demyelination at an earlier age than males, the burden of white matter disease over time may be greater in females. The earlier appearance of symptoms in females is somewhat counterbalanced by a greater prevalence of spinal MS seen in males and occurring later in life. The late occurring form of MS often involves progressive spinal lesions presenting with spasticity and pain.

TREMOR

Tremor in MS is treated with beta-blockers, anticonvulsants or, in rare cases, stereotactic procedures. Experimental evidence for benefit from cannabis is provided in a preclinical study by Baker and colleagues (2000) in which treatment with a CB_1 antagonist resulted in increased forelimb tremor. Since isolation of tremor from spasticity may be difficult in experimental animals, interpretation of such evidence may be questioned. In the survey of patients with MS by Consroe and associates (1997), 90 percent of subjects with tremor reported improvement after cannabis. In a study of eight MS patients with tremor and ataxia, oral THC was effective in two of eight subjects with both subjective and objective improvement (Clifford 1983).

NYSTAGMUS

Nystagmus is an eye movement abnormality often associated with MS. In an $N = 1$ clinical trial, a 52-year-old man with MS and pendular nystagmus was studied in the United Kingdom over 3 months before and after cannabis in the form of cigarettes, nabilone and cannabis oil-containing capsules (Schon et al. 1999). The investigators demonstrated improved visual acuity and suppression of the patient's pendular nystagmus after inhaled cannabis and were able to correlate the therapeutic effect with acute changes in serum cannabinoid levels. Nabilone and orally administered cannabis oil capsules had no effect. Because of the anatomical relationships involved in eye movement control, the authors suggest an effect at the level of the dorsal pontine tegmentum. In support of action at the level of the deep brainstem is the benefit seen with cannabis in intractable hiccups (Gilson and Busalacchi 1998) and evidence supporting cannabinoid analgesic actions mediated in the rostral ventromedial medulla (Meng et al. 1998). Responding to the report of benefit in nystagmus associated with MS, Dell'Osso (2000) reported an individual with congenital nystagmus whose oscillations dampened after smoking cannabis. Dell'Osso commented that while he had seen similar reports from patients, cannabis research is discouraged in the United States.

POSTURAL REGULATION

The complex integration of sensory and motor function required for postural regulation is impaired in many patients with MS. Impairment of posture is most disabling for patients, distressing for caregivers, and frustrating for physicians. Lesions of spinal, cerebral and cerebellar pathways result in loss of balance. In a study of ten MS patients, inhaled cannabis caused increased postural tracking error both in MS patients and in normal control subjects (Greenberg et al. 1994). The authors admitted in their publication that dynamic posturography "is not a measure of spasticity." Some authors have reported incorrectly that this study is a negative study in spasticity. Since cerebellar dysfunction is a common finding in MS seen in a third to 80 percent of patients, one can anticipate that many MS patients with both motor and cerebellar symptoms may find improved spasticity and impaired balance. Cannabinoids should be used with caution in patients with the combination of corticospinal (spasticity) and cerebellar (balance) deficits.

FATIGUE

Fatigue is one of the most frequently reported symptoms in MS and is clearly distinct from fatigue experienced in an otherwise healthy individual. The mechanism for fatigue in MS is unknown. No differences have been found in the level of MS-associated fatigue between men and women.

Clinical trials have demonstrated that amantadine may be beneficial; however, the supporting evidence is weak (Branas et al. 2000). In a single-blind trial of modafinil in patients with MS (Rammohan et al. 2002), fatigue scores were improved during treatment (200 mg/day). In the only study addressing the effect of cannabis on fatigue, Consroe et al. (1997) reported survey data which showed from 60 to 70 percent of subjects reported cannabis reduced fatigue states (tiredness, leg weakness). No controlled clinical trials of cannabinoids have investigated this condition.

PAIN

Because of the nature of MS as a disruption of transmission of nerve impulses, paroxysmal manifestations are commonly seen including tonic brainstem attacks, trigeminal neuralgia, and spasticity. Anticonvulsants and antidepressants are commonly used in MS pain syndromes, with some benefit. Cannabinoids have not been studied extensively in MS-associated pain. In other pain models, cannabinoids have demonstrated efficacy comparable to potent analgesics, such as the opioids (Campbell et al. 2001). Gender differences can affect pain via biological differences in the nociceptive and perceptual systems. In humans, women are, in general, more sensitive to painful stimuli when compared to men (LeResche 2001). The prevalence of pain syndromes in female patients with MS has not been studied.

BLADDER DYSFUNCTION

Bladder impairment in MS is seen in up to 80 percent of patients at some time during the course of the disease and can vary from slight inconvenience to potentially life-threatening when renal function is compromised. The complex interaction between bladder detrusor and sphincter function is disrupted with spinal cord lesions in MS. Drugs used in the treatment of spasticity such as baclofen and diazepam are effective in treating bladder symptoms in many MS patients by inhibiting the urethral sphincter. MS patients, as the example of the female patient from South Africa described earlier (James 1994), report improvements in bladder function after cannabinoid use. Based on the observations of improved urinary tract function, an open-label pilot study of cannabis based medicinal extract (CBME) has been reported by Brady and colleagues (2001). In this study sublingual CBME improved lower urinary tract function in ten patients with advanced MS and refractory urinary tract dysfunction over eight weeks of treatment.

SEXUAL DYSFUNCTION

Treatment of sexual dysfunction in male MS patients includes a range of options including pharmacological treatments such as sildenafil (Viagra), papaverine or phentolamine. No treatment other than local administration of artificial lubrication is available for treatment of sexual dysfunction in females. In the Consroe et al. survey of cannabis effects on MS signs and symptoms (1997), 51 subjects reported sexual dysfunction with 62.7 percent claiming improvement in sexual function after cannabis. No analysis by gender was reported. Based on previously reported survey data, the clinical study of cannabis as a treatment of sexual dysfunction in MS appears warranted.

DISCUSSION

Neurologists in practice in the 1970s noted two distinct patient groups using therapeutic cannabis. Military personnel injured in Vietnam claimed that cannabis was helpful in controlling symptoms associated with traumatic spinal injury. Female patients described beneficial effects from cannabis in treating spasticity, migraine headache or menstrual pain. These observations led to a number of small clinical trials supporting the claims of individual patients. Because of regulatory hurdles in conducting clinical research with cannabis, the total number of patients treated with cannabinoid drugs remains low.

Fortunately, interest in the subject has increased with the initiation of several large-scale cannabis studies in MS in the United Kingdom. The National Institute of Clinical Excellence (NICE), the UK regulatory authority, will assess the results of clinical trials scheduled be completed by the end of 2002.

Over the years, many patients have asked questions concerning the efficacy and safety of cannabis as a therapeutic agent. While cannabis remains as a prohibited drug in the United States, Δ-9-THC is marketed as Marinol without objection. One can contrast a potential package insert for cannabis with that for the antispastic drug, Lioresal Intrathecal. With the use of Lioresal via a spinal pump, the drug labeling states that in clinical trials, "13 deaths occurring among the 438 patients treated with Lioresal Intrathecal in premarketing studies." Interestingly, two MS patients died suddenly within two weeks of drug administration. Imagine the regulatory reaction if a single patient would die after cannabis use. A potential risk associated with cannabis is secondary to the inhalation of cannabis containing smoke. The evidence of significant health risk associated with cigarette smoking is overwhelming. While many patients avoid inhalation risks by using oral cannabis, the rapid action of an inhaled formulation is effective with symptoms such as flexor spasms or tonic brainstem attacks. One study noted an elevated risk of myocardial infarction (4.8 times baseline) in the 60 minutes after cannabis inhalation (Mittleman et al. 2001). While cannabis was considered a rare trigger of acute myocardial infarction, risk elevation was associated with obesity, current cigarette smoking and male gender.

Additional safety concerns associated with cannabis use in MS include the negative effects of cannabis on balance and cognition. While these negative effects may limit the potential usefulness of cannabis as a treatment of chronic symptoms in MS, many MS patients may yet benefit from cannabis.

While the interest in cannabis as a therapeutic agent for MS is high, many unanswered scientific questions remain, including the following:

1. How does cannabis compare with current standard treatments for MS symptoms?
2. Can alternative delivery systems be developed to provide rapid onset of action with greater safety when compared to inhaled cannabis?
3. Can specific cannabinoids be used more effectively to stimulate or block cannabinoid system receptor activity?
4. Can the immune-modulating actions of cannabis be used to alter the natural history of MS?
5. Can the long-term risks and benefits of cannabis be quantified to determine a useful risk/benefit ratio in treating the life-long disability in MS?

CONCLUSIONS

Evidence in support of cannabis treatment for spasticity associated with MS includes animal studies and a small number of clinical trials using cannabinoid drugs. Clinical reports of benefit in tremor and nystagmus have been published in MS patients. Potential other signs and symptoms in MS, which may be improved with cannabis, include fatigue, pain, bladder disturbances and sexual dysfunction. Women are twice as likely as men to develop MS. Gender specific concerns in female patients include use of cannabis during pregnancy, potential effects on the fetus, and risks associated with breast-feeding. Large-scale clinical trials may provide some answers concerning the potential of cannabis in treatment of MS.

REFERENCES

Achiron, A., S. Miron, V. Lavie, R. Margalit, and A. Biegon. 2000. Dexanabinol (HU-211) effect on experimental autoimmune encephalomyelitis: Implications for the treatment of acute relapses of multiple sclerosis. *J Neuroimmunol* 102(1): 26-31.

Baker, D., G. Pryce, J.L. Croxford, P. Brown, R.G. Pertwee, J.W. Huffman, and L. Layward. 2000. Cannabinoids control spasticity and tremor in a multiple sclerosis model. *Nature* 404:84-87.

Baker, D., G. Pryce, J.L. Croxford, P. Brown, R.G. Pertwee, A. Makriyannis, A. Khanolkar, L. Layward, F. Fezza, T. Bisogno, and V. Di Marzo. 2001. Endocannabinoids control spasticity in a multiple sclerosis model. *FASEB J* 15(2): 300-302.

Benedikt, R.A., P. Cristofaro, J.H. Mendelson, and N.K. Mello. 1986. Effects of acute marijuana smoking in post-menopausal women. *Psychopharmacol* 90:14-17.

Benowitz, N.L., and R.T. Jones. 1977. Effect of delta-9-tetrahydrocannabinol on drug distribution and metabolism: Antipyrine, pentobarbital and ethanol. *Clin Pharmacol* Ther 22(3):259-268.

Berrendero, F., A. Sanchez, A. Cabranes, C. Puerta, J.A. Ramos, A. Garcia-Merino, and J. Fernandez-Ruiz. 2001. Changes in cannabinoid CB_1 receptors in striatal and cortical regions of rats with experimental allergic encephalomyelitis, an animal model of multiple sclerosis. *Synapse* 41:195-202.

Birk, K., and R. Rudick. 1986. Pregnancy and multiple sclerosis. *Arch Neurol* 43:719-726.

Brady, C.M., R. DasGupta, O.J. Wiseman, K.J. Berkley, and C.J. Fowler. 2001. Acute and chronic effects of cannabis-based medicinal extract on refractory lower urinary tract dysfunction in patients with advanced multiple sclerosis— early results. *Congress of the IACM* Abstracts, p. 9.

Branas, P., R. Jordan, A. Fry-Smith, A. Burls, and C. Hyde. 2000. Treatment for fatigue in multiple sclerosis: A rapid and systematic review. *Health Technol Assess* 4(27):1-61.

Brown, D.T. 1998. The therapeutic potential for cannabis and its derivatives. *Cannabis: The genus* Cannabis. Amsterdam: Harwood Academic.

Campbell, F.A., M.R. Tramer, D. Carroll, D.J.M. Reynolds, R.A. Moore, and H.J. McQuay. 2001. Are cannabinoids an effective and safe treatment option in the management of pain? A qualitative systematic review. *Brit Med J* 323:13-16.

Christian, M.S. 2001. Introduction/overview: gender-based differences in pharmacologic and toxicologic responses. *Int J Toxicol* 20(3):145-148.

Clifford, D.B. 1983. Tetrahydrocannabinol for tremor in multiple sclerosis. *Ann Neurol* 13:669-671.

Compston, A. 1999. Treatment and management of multiple sclerosis. *McAlpine's multiple sclerosis*. New York: Churchill Livingstone.

Compston, A. 2001. Multiple sclerosis and other demyelinating diseases. In M. Donaghy (ed.), *Brain's diseases of the nervous system* (pp. 909-958). New York: Oxford University Press.

Consroe, P. 1999. Clinical and experimental reports of marijuana and cannabinoids in spastic disorders. *Marijuana and medicine*. Totowa, NJ: Humana Press.

Consroe, P., R. Musty, J. Rein, W. Tillery, and R. Pertwee. 1997. The perceived effects of smoked cannabis on patients with multiple sclerosis. *Eur Neurol* 38: 44-48.

Coyle, P.K. 2000. *Women's issues multiple sclerosis: Diagnosis, medical management, and rehabilitation* New York: Demos Medical Publishing.

Dell'Osso, L.F. 2000. Suppression of pendular nystagmus by smoking cannabis in a patient with multiple sclerosis. *Neurology* 54(11):2190-2191.

Dunn, M., and R. Davis. 1974. The perceived effects of marijuana on spinal cord injured males. *Paraplegia* 12:175.

Fergusson, D.M., L.J. Horwood, and K. Northstone. 2002. Maternal use of cannabis and pregnancy outcome. *Brit J Obstet Gyn* 109(1):21-27.

Fried, P.A., B. Watkinson, and R. Gray. 1999. Growth from birth to early adolescence in offspring prenatally exposed to cigarettes and marijuana. *Neurotoxicol Teratol* 21(5):513-525.

Gilson, I., and M. Busalacchi. 1998. Marijuana for intractable hiccups. *Lancet* 351:267.

Gracies, J.M., P. Nance, E. Elovic, J. McGuire, and D.M. Simpson. 1997. Traditional pharmacological treatments for spasticity. Part II: General and regional treatments. *Muscle & Nerve* 20 Suppl 6:S92-S120.

Greenberg, H.S., S.A.S. Werness, J.E. Pugh, R.O. Andrus, D.J. Anderson, and E.F. Domino. 1994. Short-term effects of smoking marijuana on balance in patients with multiple sclerosis and normal volunteers. *Clin Pharmacol Ther* 55:324-328.

Grinspoon, L., and J.B. Bakalar. 1997. Common medical uses: multiple sclerosis. *Marijuana, the forbidden medicine*. Revised and expanded editon. New Haven: Yale University Press.

Guzman, M., C. Sanchez, and I. Galve-Roperh. 2001. Control of the cell survival/death decision by cannabinoids. *J Mol Med* 78:613-625.

Hanigan, W.C., R. Destree, and X.T. Truong. 1985. The effect of Δ-9-THC on human spasticity. *Clin Pharmacol Ther* 35:198.

Irizarry, M.C. 1997. Multiple sclerosis. In M. Cudkowicz and M. Irrizarry (eds.), *Neurologic disorders in women* (pp. 85-98). Boston: Butterworth-Heinemann.

Iversen, L.L. 2000. *The science of marijuana*. New York: Oxford University Press.

James, T. 1994. The baby and the bathwater. *S Afr Med J* 84(6):369.

LeResche, L. 2001. Gender, cultural, and environmental aspects of pain. In J.D. Loeser, S.H. Butler, L.R. Chapma, and D.C. Turk (eds.), *Bonica's management of pain,* Third edition. Philadelphia: Lippincott Williams & Wilkins.

Lyman, W.D., J.R. Sonett, C.F. Brosnan, R. Elkin, and M.B. Bornstein. 1989. Delta-9 tetrahydrocannabinol: A novel treatment for experimental autoimmune encephalomyelitis. *J Neuroimmunol* 23:73-81.

Martyn, C.N., L.S. Illis, and J. Thom. 1995. Nabilone in the treatment of multiple sclerosis. *Lancet* 345:579.

Maurer, M., V. Henn, A. Dittrich, and A. Hoffmann. 1990. Delta-9 tetrahydrocannabinol shows antispastic and analgesic effects in a single case, double-blind trial. *Eur Arch Psych Clin Neurosci* 240(1):1-4.

Meinck, H.M., P.W. Schonle, and B. Conrad. 1990. Effect of cannabinoids on spasticity and ataxia in multiple sclerosis. *J Neurol* 236(2):120-122.

Mendelson, J.H., P. Cristofaro, J. Ellingboe, R. Benedikt and N.K. Mello. 1985. Acute effects of marijuana on luteinizing hormone in menopausal women. *Pharmacol Biochem Behav* 23:765-768.

Meng, I.D., B.H. Manning, W.J. Martin, and H.L. Fields. 1998. An analgesia circuit activated by cannabinoids. *Nature* 395:381-383.

Mittleman, M.A., R.A. Lewis, M. Maclure, J.B. Sherwood, and J.E. Muller. 2001. Triggering myocardial infarction by marijuana. *Circulation* 103(23):2805-2809.

Olek, M.J., and S.J. Khoury. 2000. Multiple sclerosis. In M.B. Goldman and M.C. Hatch (eds.), *Women and health* (pp. 686-703). San Diego: Academic Press.

O'Shaughnessy, W.B. 1842. On the preparation of the Indian hemp or ganjah *(Cannabis indica)*: The effects on the animal system in health, and their utility in the treatment of tetanus and other convulsive diseases. *Trans Med Phys Soc Bombay* 8:421-461.

Petro, D.J. 1980. Marijuana as a therapeutic agent for muscle spasm or spasticity. *Psychosomatics* 21(1):81-85.

Petro, D.J. and C. Ellenberger. 1981. Treatment of human spasticity with Δ-9-tetrahydrocannabinol. *J Clin Pharmacol* 21:413S-416S.

Physicians' desk reference, Fifty-sixth edition. 2002. Montvale, NJ: Medical Economics.

Pope, H.G. 2002. Cannabis, cognition, and residual confounding. *J Amer Med Assoc* 287(9):1172-1174.

Pope, H.G., A.J. Gruber, J.I. Hudson, M.A. Huestis, and D. Yurgelun-Todd. 2001. Neuropsychological performance in long-term cannabis users. *Arch Gen Psychiatry* 58:909-915.

Rammohan, K.W., J.H. Rosenberg, D.J. Lynn, A.M. Blumenfeld, C.P. Pollak, and H.N. Nagaraja. 2002. Efficacy and safety of modafinil (Provigil) for the treatment of fatigue in multiple sclerosis: A two centre phase 2 study. *J Neurol Neurosurg Psychiatry* 72(2):179-183.

Reynolds, J.R. 1890. On the therapeutic uses and toxic effects of *Cannabis indica*. *Lancet* 1:637-638.

Runmarker, B. and O. Anderson. 1995. Pregnancy is associated with a lower risk of onset and a better prognosis in multiple sclerosis. *Brain* 118:253-261.

Rusk, A. and F. Plum. 1998. Neurologic health and disorders. In *Textbook of women's health.* Philadelphia: Lippincott-Raven.

Schon, F., P.E. Hart, T.L. Hodgson, A.L.M. Pambakian, M. Ruprah, E.M. Williamson, and C. Kennard. 1999. Suppression of pendular nystagmus by smoking cannabis in a patient with multiple sclerosis. *Neurology* 53(9):2209-2210.

Solowij, N., R.S. Stephens, R.A. Roffman, T. Babor, R. Kadden, M. Miller, K. Christiansen, B. McRee, and J. Vendetti. 2002. Cognitive functioning of long-term heavy cannabis users seeking treatment. *J Amer Med Assoc* 287(9):1123-1131.

Somerset, M., R. Campbell, D.J. Sharp and T.J. Peters. 2001. What do people with MS want and expect from health-care services? *Health Expectations* 4:29-37.

Tennes, K., N. Avitable, C. Blackard, C. Boyles, B. Hassoun, L. Holmes, and M. Kreye. 1985. Marijuana, prenatal and postnatal exposure in the human. In Pinkert, T.M. (ed.), Current research on the consequences of maternal drug abuse. *NIDA Res Monogr* 59:48-60.

Ungerleider, J.T., T. Andyrsiak, L. Fairbanks, G.W. Ellison, and L.W. Myers. 1988. Delta-9-THC in the treatment of spasticity associated with multiple sclerosis. *Pharmacological Issues in Alcohol and Substance Abuse* 7(1):39-50.

Whitaker, J., 1998. Effects of pregnancy and delivery on disease activity in multiple sclerosis. *N Engl J Med* 339:339-340.

Wirguin, I., R. Mechoulam, A. Breuer, E. Schezen, J. Weidenfeld, and T. Brenner. 1994. Suppression of experimental autoimmune encephalomyelitis by cannabinoids. *Immunopharmacology* 28:209-214.

UPDATE

Ethan B. Russo

Despite the fact that this chapter nicely summarized the pertinent clinical literature available on the topic at the time, a genuine renaissance of activity has followed in the interim. Reviews of basic science include helpful works from Baker et al. (Baker 2004; Baker and Pryce 2003; Pryce et al. 2003; Pryce and Baker 2005), while clinical trial information also abounds (Carroll et al. 2004; Fox et al. 2004; Teare et al. 2005; Zajicek et al. 2003, 2004; Berman et al. 2004; Brady et al. 2004; Notcutt et al. 2004; Nicholson et al. 2004; Wade et al. 2004, 2005, 2003). See Update to Chapter 8 for additional details.

More entries are forthcoming in short order. Cannabis therapeutics portends to figure prominently in symptomatic treatment of spasticity, spasm, pain, sleep disturbance (Russo 2005) and intractable lower urinary tract symptoms (LUTS) in MS in the near future. It is also quite likely that such preparations will also demonstrate important neuroprotective effects that may supplement current immunotherapy.

REFERENCES

Baker, D. 2004. Therapeutic potential of cannabis and cannabinoids in experimental models of multiple sclerosis. In G. W. Guy, B. A. Whittle and P. J. Robson (eds.), *Medicinal uses of cannabis and cannabinoids* (pp. 141-164). London: Pharmaceutical Press.

Baker, D., and G. Pryce. 2003. The therapeutic potential of cannabis in multiple sclerosis. *Expert Opin Investig Drugs* 12 (4):561-567.

Berman, J.S., C. Symonds, and R. Birch. 2004. Efficacy of two cannabis based medicinal extracts for relief of central neuropathic pain from brachial plexus avulsion: Results of a randomised controlled trial. *Pain* 112 (3):299-306.

Brady, C.M., R. DasGupta, C. Dalton, O.J. Wiseman, K.J. Berkley, and C. J. Fowler. 2004. An open-label pilot study of cannabis based extracts for bladder dysfunction in advanced multiple sclerosis. *Multiple Sclerosis* 10:425-433.

Carroll, C.B., P.G. Bain, L. Teare, X. Liu, C. Joint, C. Wroath, S.G. Parkin, P. Fox, D. Wright, J. Hobart, and J.P. Zajicek. 2004. Cannabis for dyskinesia in Parkinson disease: A randomized double-blind crossover study. *Neurology* 63 (7): 1245-1250.

Fox, P., P.G. Bain, S. Glickman, C. Carroll, and J. Zajicek. 2004. The effect of cannabis on tremor in patients with multiple sclerosis. *Neurology* 62 (7):1105-1109.

Nicholson, A.N., C. Turner, B.M. Stone, and P.J. Robson. 2004. Effect of delta-9-tetrahydrocannabinol and cannabidiol on nocturnal sleep and early-morning behavior in young adults. *J Clin Psychopharmacol* 24 (3):305-313.

Notcutt, W., M. Price, R. Miller, S. Newport, C. Phillips, S. Simmonds, and C. Sansom. 2004. Initial experiences with medicinal extracts of cannabis for chronic pain: Results from 34 "N of 1" studies. *Anaesthesia* 59:440-452.

Pryce, G., Z. Ahmed, D.J. Hankey, S.J. Jackson, J.L. Croxford, J.M. Pocock, C. Ledent, A. Petzold, A.J. Thompson, G. Giovannoni, M.L. Cuzner, and D. Baker. 2003. Cannabinoids inhibit neurodegeneration in models of multiple sclerosis. *Brain* 126 (Pt 10):2191-2202.

Pryce, G., and D. Baker. 2005. Emerging properties of cannabinoid medicines in management of multiple sclerosis. *Trends Neurosci* 28 (5):272-276.

Russo, E.B. 2005. Sativex cannabis based medicine maintains improvement in sleep quality in patients with multiple sclerosis and neuropathic pain. In *American Academy of Neurology*. Miami, FL: American Academy of Neurology. Poster.

Teare, L.J., J.P. Zajicek, D. Wright, and L.J. Priston. 2005. What is the relationship between serum levels of cannabinoids and clinical effects in patients with multiple sclerosis and does it explain the differences between Δ9-tetrahydrocannabinol and whole extract of cannabis? Paper read at Conference on the Cannabinoids, at Clearwater, FL.

Wade, D.T., P.M. Makela, H. House, C. Bateman, and P.J. Robson. 2005. Long-term use of a cannabis-based medicine in the treatment of spasticity and other symptoms in multiple sclerosis. *Multiple Sclerosis* (in press).

Wade, D.T., P. Makela, P. Robson, H. House, and C. Bateman. 2004. Do cannabis-based medicinal extracts have general or specific effects on symptoms in multiple sclerosis? A double-blind, randomized, placebo-controlled study on 160 patients. *Mult Scler* 10 (4):434-441.

Wade, D.T., P. Robson, H. House, P. Makela, and J. Aram. 2003. A preliminary controlled study to determine whether whole-plant cannabis extracts can improve intractable neurogenic symptoms. *Clinical Rehabilitation* 17:18-26.

Zajicek, J., P. Fox, H. Sanders, D. Wright, J. Vickery, A. Nunn, and A. Thompson. 2003. Cannabinoids for treatment of spasticity and other symptoms related to multiple sclerosis (CAMS study): Multicentre randomised placebo-controlled trial. *Lancet* 362 (9395):1517-1526.

Zajicek, J., P. Fox, H. Sanders, D. Wright, J. Vickery, A. Nunn, and A. Thompson. 2004. The cannabinoids in MS study—Final results from 12 months follow-up. *Mult Scler* 10 (suppl.):S115.

PART V:
SIDE EFFECTS

Chapter 19

Cannabis and Harm Reduction: A Nursing Perspective

Mary Lynn Mathre

INTRODUCTION

Nursing is the art and science of caring. Since 1999 when nurses were included in the Gallup "Honesty and Ethics" poll, nurses have been rated as one of the most trusted professional groups by the American public (http://www.gallup.com/poll/releases/pro011205.asp). What is it about nurses that the public is willing to trust? Could it be that nurses often see people in their most vulnerable states and, during that time, treat them with respect and provide a safe environment to nurture them back to a more independent self-caring state? Nursing is much more than simply caring and providing comfort; it involves the art of knowing how to give the right kind of care and comfort to facilitate the healing process, and this knowledge is based in science. The goal of nursing care is to promote health and reduce the harm caused by injury, disease, or poor self-care.

Nurses are the largest group of health care professionals and are keenly aware of the potential risks related to medications. While pharmacists dispense medications and physicians prescribe medications, nurses administer them to countless numbers of patients and monitor the effects of the medications. Nurses are in a key position to see not only the beneficial effects of a particular medication but also the side effects or adverse reactions that can accompany medications even when used as recommended. Safe administration of medication is a critical skill all nurses must master because any error could cost a patient added suffering or organ damage, or could result in death.

Harm reduction is a public health approach to human behaviors, which involves helping persons learn to make better personal choices to minimize the potential risks associated with their behavior. Examples of harm reduction

Handbook of Cannabis Therapeutics
© 2006 by The Haworth Press, Inc. All rights reserved.
doi:10.1300/5741_20

practices include using condoms properly during intercourse to avoid STDs, wearing a seatbelt when traveling in a motor vehicle, or using a helmet when riding a motorcycle. Today, harm reduction is gaining popularity as a more effective and realistic modality for helping persons who use drugs to reduce negative consequences associated with their drug use. Such harm reduction strategies include needle exchange programs for intravenous drug users to prevent bloodborne infections, use of a designated driver for persons consuming alcohol away from home, overdose prevention education, and offering a variety of drug treatment options (www.harmreduction. org).

Harm reduction is based on the premise that people are responsible for their behavior, that they make personal choices which affect their health and well-being, and that they can make safer and better decisions if given useful and honest information. The harm reduction approach accepts the fact that individuals will use drugs for various reasons and offers to help them "where they're at." In contrast, the War on Drugs is based on the premise that certain drugs are "bad" and that the government has the paternal right and duty to prohibit the use of these drugs. This "zero tolerance" or "just say no" approach condemns the use of certain drugs and punishes those who use them. Acceptance comes after transgressors admit their wrongful ways and adhere to the abstinence option.

The underlying flaw in a war on drugs is the belief that some drugs are inherently bad and therefore deserve to be prohibited for the greater good of society. A drug is not simply good or bad, right or wrong, but rather the manner of use of a drug by an individual may be helpful or harmful. The harm reduction approach is based on science and the respect of others, while the war on drugs is based on moralistic ideology and the control of others. Drug use will always have the potential of causing sequelae. Harm reduction strives to minimize the harmful effects from drug use, while the drug prohibition creates more harmful effects from drug use.

Cannabis is an herbal agent that has been used as a medicine, a recreational drug, as well as a source of food and fiber. It is environmentally friendly and essentially nontoxic, yet currently forbidden by our federal government. U.S. citizens are prohibited from growing this plant or possessing any of its leaves, seeds, stems, or flowers. In most states, physicians are forbidden to prescribe it for medical use. When the cannabis plant is examined in a scientific and logical manner, its therapeutic value becomes apparent. From a nursing perspective, cannabis could be a useful harm reduction tool, yet the laws prohibiting its use present contrived risks that can cause more harm than the drug itself.

This chapter examines cannabis as a harm reduction agent from a nursing perspective. Cannabis as medicine is not a magic bullet that will work for everyone, and it is not without potential risks. Cannabis as a recreational drug is not enjoyable for everyone and is not harmless, but when put in the broader perspective and compared to standard medicines or common recreational drugs, cannabis offers greater benefit with fewer relative risks.

CANNABIS WAS A MEDICINE IN THE UNITED STATES

Prior to the prohibition of marijuana, cannabis products were widely used by American physicians. By the 1930s there were 23 pharmaceutical companies producing cannabis preparations. In 1937, the passage of the Marihuana Tax Act marked the beginning of the cannabis prohibition. The head of the Federal Bureau of Narcotics (now the Drug Enforcement Administration or DEA), Harry Anslinger, led this legislative effort using exaggerations and lies (Bonnie and Whitebread 1974). During the congressional hearings the American Medical Association (AMA) opposed the Act and supported cannabis as a therapeutic agent. The lawmakers won and the AMA has since given up the fight.

The Controlled Substances Act of 1970 furthered the cannabis prohibition when it called for a system to classify psychoactive drugs according to their risk potential. Five schedules were created, with Schedule I being the most restrictive category. Under the Act, cannabis was initially placed in Schedule I, but Congress called for a National Commission on Marihuana and Drug Abuse to determine whether that placement was appropriate. President Nixon appointed most of the commissioners, including a former Republican governor of Pennsylvania, Raymond Shafer, as the chairman. The Shafer Commission completed its study in 1972, and it remains the most comprehensive review of marijuana ever conducted by the federal government. In the end, the Shafer Commission concluded that cannabis did not belong in Schedule I and stated (National Commission on Marihuana and Drug Abuse 1972, p. 130), "Marihuana's relative potential for harm to the vast majority of individual users and its actual impact on society does not justify a social policy designed to seek out and firmly punish those who use it." The recommendations were ignored, and cannabis remained in Schedule I—a forbidden drug.

Now, thirty years later, the infamous Nixon tapes of Oval Office conversations from 1971 to 1972 have been declassified and made available to the public (transcripts available at www.csdp.org). It is clear that Nixon used his political power to influence the outcome of the Shafer Commission, and when that didn't work he simply dismissed their recommendations and launched the War on Drugs. Curiously, at the same time, the Bain Commission in the Netherlands (with a similar mission) issued its report with similar findings. The government of the Netherlands acted on the recommendations of the Bain Commission, and today the Dutch have half of the per capita cannabis use as the United States, with far fewer drug-related problems at much lower drug enforcement costs (Zeese 2002).

CANNABIS AS A HARM REDUCTION MEDICINE

Compared to standard medications, cannabis has a remarkably wide margin of safety. In 1988, after a lengthy legal battle to reschedule cannabis, the DEA Administrative Law Judge, Francis Young, ruled that marijuana should be assigned to Schedule II and thus available for physicians to prescribe. In his summary he noted that (p. 57), "Marijuana in its natural form is one of the safest therapeutically active substances known to man." Throughout the centuries of its use, there has never been a death from cannabis (Abel 1980). In contrast, there are more than 32,000 deaths per year associated with prescription medications in hospitalized patients (Lazarou et al. 1998). All opioids carry the risk of overdose. Even over-the-counter (OTC) medications can be lethal. There are approximately 120 annual deaths from aspirin.

Cannabis has been studied extensively in regard to determining its health risks. General McCaffrey called upon the Institute of Medicine (IOM) to study the therapeutic value of marijuana in 1997. In March of 1999 the IOM released its 18-month study, which concluded that cannabis does have therapeutic value and is safe for medical use (Joy et al. 1999). Concern was noted about the potential risks related to smoking medicine, but the study concluded that for patients suffering from cancer or AIDS, the potential pulmonary risks were minimal when compared to the benefits. The study also noted that while more research is warranted, cannabis is safe enough for physicians to conduct $N = 1$ studies on their patients who they believe could benefit from cannabis if other medications are not effective.

The IOM report put health risks associated with cannabis in perspective noting (p. 5), "except for the harms associated with smoking, the adverse effects of marijuana use are within the range of effects tolerated for other medications." A recent study of the chronic effects of cannabis on four of the seven federally provided medical marijuana patients showed minor bronchitis in two of the patients (Russo et al. 2002). These patients smoked from 5 to 10 low-grade (2 to 4 percent THC content) cannabis cigarettes on a daily basis for 10 to 20 years. No other attributable long-term problems were noted, but rather a reduction in their use of other medications and a feeling of well-being was experienced by the patients.

While smoking cannabis may cause lung damage after chronic use, there are various actions that can be taken to reduce the harm from smoking. Patients can smoke less if using a high potency product (THC content greater than 10 percent) and can easily adjust the dosage by decreasing the number of inhalations. Also, when smoking cannabis, patients should limit their breath holding to less than ten seconds to avoid lung damage (Tashkin 2000). Vaporizers are being developed that heat the plant material to the point of vaporization without combustion, thus avoiding smoke inhalation (Gieringer 2001; Whittle et al. 2001). Finally, patients may use cannabis in alternative delivery forms such as pills, sublingual spray, eye drops, suppository, dermal patch, or salve, thereby eliminating pulmonary risks.

The federal government claims that cannabis is harmful to the immune system. When reviewing the published animal studies that reported harm to the immune system the reader should note that most of the researchers used delta-9-tetrahydrocannabinol (THC) rather than natural cannabis and that extremely high doses were used. A review of the active ingredients in cannabis suggests that some of these constituents act synergistically to enhance the beneficial effects of THC, while others may mitigate the harmful side effects of THC, including possible immunosuppression (McPartland and Russo 2001). Given the thousands of immunocompromised patients who have used cannabis, there have been no reports of direct damage to the immune system from cannabis except when the patient has used a contaminated supply. Many AIDS patients who, by virtue of their disease, have a severely compromised immune system do not show any decline in their health status related to cannabis. In fact, a recent study of cannabis use by AIDS patients showed that cannabis did not interfere with protease inhibitors and helped increase weight gain for a significant number of patients (Abrams et al. 2000).

Another cannabis risk has been an allegation that it causes brain damage. Although the federal government continues to use this scare tactic, modern research has not confirmed such findings. A Johns Hopkins study examined cannabis' effects on cognition on 1,318 subjects over a 15-year period (Lyketsos et al. 1999). The researchers found no significant differences in cognitive decline between heavy users, light users, and nonusers of cannabis. They concluded that the results provided strong evidence of the absence of long-term residual effects of cannabis use on cognition.

Perhaps the most illogical argument the federal government uses to prohibit the therapeutic use of cannabis is that to allow its medical use would "send the wrong message to our youth." General Barry McCaffrey openly fought the growing popular opinion and scientific findings that cannabis has medical value. In response to the passage of state initiatives allowing the medical use of marijuana, McCaffrey dismissed its therapeutic value and declared that state laws allowing medical use of cannabis would increase the rate of drug use among teenagers. He stated, "While we are trying to educate American adolescents that psychoactive drugs are bad, now we have this apparent message that says 'No they're medicine. They're good for you'" (Substance Abuse Report 1996). That is nonsense. Teenagers don't think, "Insulin is medicine. It must be good for me." A persistent message that parents and health care professionals should demonstrate and reinforce with children and teenagers is that medicine is for sick people and that all medicine should be used with caution based upon an awareness of the risks and benefits.

Since nurses are advocates and health educators for patients, families, and communities, they have a key role in helping others learn to use medications safely. With more than 400,000 medication preparations available in the United States it is unlikely that any person can know everything about these medications. However, the user can reduce harm from medications by following some general guidelines designed to ensure that the risks are minimized. Mothers Against Misuse and Abuse (MAMA) has developed medication guidelines that persons may follow when using any OTC, prescribed medication, or recreational drug. The premise for these guidelines is that no medication is completely risk free, but harm can be minimized if the user has appropriate information to make an informed decision. MAMA seeks opportunities to teach these guidelines to parents to help them set a good example for their children when it comes to the use of medications or recreational drugs (www.mamas.org). This includes essential information that nurses include in their patient education, such as the name of the medication, desired effect, possible side effects or adverse reactions, proper dosage and route of administration, risk of tolerance, dependence, or drug interactions.

Pain is the most frequent symptom for patients seeking medical care. Cannabis analgesia provides a good example of its potential as a harm reduction medication. Innumerable chronic pain patients have found it difficult to find a balance between managing their pain and being able to function in daily life. Opiates are frequently used for management of severe pain, yet they sometimes leave the patient feeling "drugged" and come with the risk of overdose and side effects such as constipation, nausea and vomiting. Increasingly, patients are acting on the advice of others and are trying cannabis as an analgesic.

Per numerous reports (Mathre 1985; Corral et al. 2002; Russo et al. 2002; Rosenblum and Wenner, 2002), the introduction of cannabis into pain management regimens has been very helpful. Most patients report a significant reduction in the use of opioids or need them on occasion for acute exacerbations; this reduction in the use of opioids lessens the risk for physical dependence. Cannabis is an effective antiemetic and is not constipating. In summary, many chronic pain patients who use cannabis report that they feel better, experience fewer untoward side effects, are able to reduce their use of opioids and other medications, and are thereby able to eliminate additional side effects that may accompany those medications as well as the added risks from drug interactions.

Margo McCaffery (1968) has taught us that pain "is whatever the experiencing person says it is, existing whenever he says it does." Pain is a subjective experience and patient feedback is essential to effective pain management. Current national guidelines for pain management endorse McCaffery's standard (Jacox et al. 1994). Given patients' reports of pain control with cannabis and its relative safety, nurses recognize that cannabis should be an option for patients. To date 11 state nurses associations (Arkansas, California, Colorado, Hawaii, Mississippi, New Jersey, New Mexico, New York, North Carolina, Virginia, and Wisconsin) have passed formal resolutions supporting patient access to this medicine (www.medical cannabis.com). In addition, the American Nurses Association's Congress on Nursing Practice issued a statement in 1996 calling for the education of all RNs on evidence-based therapeutic indications for cannabis.

CANNABIS AS A SOCIAL/RECREATIONAL DRUG

While the federal government may be waging a war on certain drugs, it is clear to onlookers that America is a drug-using society. Americans are constantly bombarded with advertisements for drugs that can take care of any of life's problems. We have pills to help us sleep, to help us stay awake, to help us calm down, to help us feel better, to take away our pain, to regulate our bowels, and on and on. We tend to call these drugs *medications,* and that identifies them as "good" drugs. Americans don't even consider caffeine as a drug, but for many a cup of coffee in the morning is a must to start their day. Caffeinated drinks are even aggressively marketed to our youth—as though kids need any more energy. (For children with too much energy, we simply drug them with a "medication" such as Ritalin.) We also have regulated drugs that are acceptable for adult usage. Alcohol can be used for enjoyment. The tobacco industry is struggling with the mandated health warnings and their advertisement ploys: "Smoking may cause lung cancer" versus "You've come a long way, baby."

Psychoactive drug use has and will be a part of our society. In American culture, drug experimentation among adolescents is considered normative behavior (Newcomb and Bentler 1988; Shedler and Block 1990). Adolescence is a time of transition, when young people are trying to determine their identity. Testing limits is part of their developmental process and for many the "forbidden" drugs are a temptation too great to resist. A longitudinal study investigated the psychological characteristics and drug-use patterns in children studied from age 3 to 18 (Shedler and Block 1990). Those adolescents who experimented with drugs (primarily cannabis) were the "best adjusted" compared to abstainers and frequent users.

These children were tested prior to the initiation of drug use and there were notable antecedent personality differences. The frequent users were found to be relatively maladjusted as children, unable to form good relationships, insecure and showed signs of emotional distress. The abstainers were relatively over controlled, timid, fearful, and morose. Shedler and Block (1990) described (p. 617), "the picture of the frequent user that emerges is one of a troubled adolescent, an adolescent who is interpersonally alienated, emotionally withdrawn, and manifestly unhappy, and who expresses his or her maladjustment through uncontrolled, overtly antisocial behavior." In contrast, Shedler and Block noted (p. 618), "the picture of the abstainer that emerges is of a relatively tense, overcontrolled, emotionally constricted individual who is somewhat socially isolated and lacking in interpersonal skills." The experimenters were found to be psychologically healthy, sociable, and reasonably inquisitive individuals. Twenty years earlier Hogan et al. (1970) compared marijuana users with nonusers in a college population. They found that users "are more socially skilled, have a broader range of interests, are more adventuresome, and more concerned with the feelings of others" (p. 63). Nonusers were found to be "too deferential to external authority, narrow in their interests, and overcontrolled" (p. 61).

Shedler and Block (1990) also examined the quality of parenting the children received through direct observations of mother-child interactions when the children were five years old. Compared to the mothers of the experimenters, the mothers of the frequent users and abstainers "were perceived to be cold, critical, pressuring, and unresponsive to their children's needs" (p. 624). They found no noteworthy findings involving the fathers of frequent users. However, when compared to the fathers of experimenters, the fathers of abstainers were seen "as relatively unresponsive to their children's needs and as authoritarian, autocratic, and domineering" (p. 625).

The researchers caution readers not to misinterpret their findings as an encouragement for adolescents to use drugs. The findings do indicate that problem drug use is a symptom, not a cause, of personal and social maladjustment. It is also helpful to understand that experimentation with certain behaviors can be expected with healthy adolescents. When it comes to the potential risks of drug experimentation, cannabis is a relatively safer drug choice.

The federal government has historically used the stepping-stone hypothesis and gateway drug hypothesis as valid reasons for the marijuana prohibition. The stepping-stone hypothesis presumes that there are pharmacological properties in cannabis that lead the user to progress to other drugs, while the gateway theory presumes that as an illicit drug cannabis serves as an entry to access other illicit drugs. The premise of both theories is that cannabis use leads to harder, more dangerous drug abuse. There is no question that cocaine, methamphetamine, heroin, or other hard drug users may have used cannabis in their earlier stages of drug use, but there has never been a causal relationship established. In fact, most drug users begin with alcohol and nicotine, usually when they are too young to do so legally. The Shafer Commission noted, "No verification is found of a causal relationship between marihuana use and subsequent heroin use" (p. 88). The IOM report found that (Joy et al. 1999, p. 6), "There is no conclusive evidence that the drug effects of marijuana are causally linked to the subsequent abuse of other illicit drugs." More recently, a study by Jan van Ours of Tilberg University in the Netherlands, which will be published by the Centre for Economic Policy Research in London, also concluded that cannabis is not a gateway drug (*Sunday Times* 2001). It is not the cannabis that is associated with progression to other illicit drugs, but rather its illegal status that makes it a gateway drug.

When compared to the legal and regulated drugs such as alcohol and tobacco, cannabis is much less harmful. I have worked as a registered nurse for more than 25 years in acute care facilities and, during the past 10, I have served as the addictions consult nurse in a university hospital setting. During that time I have had the typical nursing experience of caring for persons who were hospitalized as a result of their drug use. Common reasons for admissions related to alcohol abuse include traumatic injuries secondary to acute intoxication (motor vehicle accidents, falls, fights, etc.), overdose with alcohol alone or in combination with other drugs/medications, life-threatening alcohol withdrawal, pancreatitis, liver disease, gastrointestinal bleeding, cardiomyopathy, cardiac arrhythmias secondary to acute intoxication, depression, suicide attempts, various cancers, and malnutrition. Common admissions related to tobacco dependence include heart attacks, vascular diseases, pulmonary problems, and various cancers. Hospital admissions for cannabis-related health problems are rare. Alcohol is responsible for more than 100,000 annual deaths, nicotine for more than 430,700 (Schneider Institute for Health Policy, 2001), while use of cannabis has never killed anyone due to toxicity.

Driving under the influence of alcohol is the second leading cause for motor vehicle accidents after fatigue. While driving under the influence of any psychoactive drug is not recommended, several studies have shown that cannabis use does not seem to significantly impair driving performance and thus is not associated with an increase in accidents (National Commission on Marihuana and Drug Abuse 1972; Hunter et al. 1998; Bates and Blakely 1999; Frood 2002). It seems that drivers on cannabis tend to be aware of their intoxicated state and therefore drive more cautiously to compensate. The new study by the Transport Research laboratory in England did find that drivers under the influence of cannabis showed impairment in their tracking ability (being able to hold a constant speed while following the middle of the road), but those with a blood alcohol level of 50 mg/dL (0.05 g) showed even more impairment (Frood 2002).

In 1996, two leading experts in psychoactive drugs rated six commonly used drugs (Hilts 1994) (Table 19.1). Henningfield and Benowitz ranked

TABLE 19.1. Ranking of risk of six commonly used drugs.

	Withdrawal		Reinforcement		Tolerance		Dependence		Intoxication	
	NIDA	UCSF	NIDA	UCSF	NIDA	UCSF	NIDA	UCSF	NIDA	UCSF
Nicotine	3	3	4	4	2	4	1	1	5	6
Heroin	2	2	2	2	1	2	2	2	2	2
Cocaine	4	3	1	1	4	1	3	3	3	3
Alcohol	1	1	3	3	3	4	4	4	1	1
Caffeine	5	4	6	5	5	3	5	5	6	5
Marijuana	6	5	5	6	6	5	6	6	4	4

Source: Reprinted from *Cannabis in Medical Practice: A Legal, Historical and Pharmacological Overview of the Therapeutic Use of Marijuana,* © 1997 Mary Lynn Mathre, by permission of McFarland & Company, Inc., Box 611, Jefferson, NC 28640 <www.mcfarlandpub.com>.

Note: Ranking scale: 1 = Most serious; 6 = Least serious.

Explanation of terms

Withdrawal—Presence and severity of characteristic withdrawal symptoms.

Reinforcement—Substance's ability, in human and animal tests, to get users to take it repeatedly, and instead of other substances.

Tolerance—Amount of substance needed to satisfy increasing cravings, and level of plateau that is eventually reached.

Dependence (addiction)—Difficulty in ending use of substance, relapse rate, percentage of people who become addicted, addicts self-reporting of degree of need for substance, and continued use in face of evidence that it causes harm.

Intoxication—Level of intoxication associated with addiction, personal, and social damage that substance causes. (By Dr. Jack E. Henningfield of the National Institute of Drug Abuse (NIDA) and Dr. Neal L. Benowitz of the University of California at San Francisco (UCSF), data from an article in the *New York Times,* August 2, 1994, p. C3.)

nicotine, heroin, cocaine, alcohol, caffeine, and marijuana according to their potential risks for withdrawal symptoms, reinforcement, tolerance, addiction, and intoxication. They rated marijuana as the least serious risk, except for intoxication in which they both ranked it above caffeine and nicotine.

In recent years, treatment programs have had an increase in admissions for "marijuana dependence." The reason for this increase seems to be due to the fact that individuals charged with marijuana offenses (usually simple possession) are offered a choice of incarceration or treatment. Most choose to stay out of prison and enter treatment for "marijuana dependence." Just recently, the current director of the Office of National Drug Control Policy (ONDCP), John Walters, spoke to 4,500 teens and adults at the Pride World Drug Prevention Conference in Cincinnati. He told the audience that 65 percent of drug-dependent people have a primary or secondary dependence on marijuana and that (Kranz 2002), "Marijuana is two-thirds of the addiction problem in America today. . . . We have too many people trapped in addiction to marijuana because they thought it couldn't happen, or they were told it couldn't happen." Where did these numbers originate? Drug experts Henningfield and Benowitz ranked marijuana as the least likely to lead to addiction or dependence. Inquiries made to the ONDCP asking for the source of these figures have remained unanswered. The IOM report (Joy, Watson, and Benson 1999) concluded that marijuana is not highly addictive. Hopefully the American public will not accept these gross exaggerations.

One must ask the question that given the health and social risks related to alcohol and tobacco, which are regulated drugs for adult use, why isn't cannabis regulated for adults to use as well? Politicians, such as Representative Barr and Senator Feinstein, have justified the continued marijuana prohibition by rationalizing that we simply shouldn't add another dangerous drug for adults. From a harm reduction perspective one would have to ask, why wouldn't it make sense to allow adults to choose to use cannabis, a drug that is much less harmful (this is not to say it is harmless) to individuals and society?

CANNABIS PROHIBITION CAUSES MORE HARM THAN THE DRUG

Cannabis is the most commonly used illicit recreational/social drug in the United States. Today, at least 76 million Americans have tried it (Substance Abuse and Mental Health Services Administration 2000, p. G-4). Many of those Americans who have risked "breaking the law" by using cannabis have suffered harsh consequences. In 2000, 46.5 percent (or 734,497) of the 1,579,566 total arrests for drug abuse violations were for cannabis. Of those, 88 percent (or 646,042 people) were arrested for possession alone (Federal Bureau of Investigation 2001). With mandatory minimums for drug offenses, the prison sentences for cannabis convictions can be as long as several decades to life. Why are we willing to spend so much on prison terms for nonviolent marijuana offenders? Are they truly such a danger to society that we are willing to take away their freedom and pay up to $40,000 per year per individual in prison costs? Would it not be wiser to allow them to continue to work and pay taxes? Couldn't this money be better spent by using it for drug addicts who are seeking treatment?

Children may be removed from their homes because a parent has been convicted of cannabis possession. Family members convicted of cannabis possession have been sent hundreds to thousands of miles away to serve time in overcrowded out-of-state prisons. These nonviolent cannabis prisoners are often at the mercy of hardened criminals and suffer rapes, assaults and even death while in prison. Are they such a danger to society that we are willing to destroy the lives of these individuals and break up their families?

The Shafer Commission was very clear in their conclusions that such punishment was unwarranted (p. 78): "Neither the marihuana user nor the drug itself can be said to constitute a danger to public safety," and (p. 96), "Most users, young and old, demonstrate an average or above average degree of social functioning, academic achievement, and job performance." The Commission concluded (p. 41), "The most notable statement that can be made about the vast majority of marihuana users—experimenters and intermittent users—is that they are essentially indistinguishable from their non-marihuana using peers by any fundamental criterion other than their marihuana use." Yet hundreds of thousands of Americans remain behind bars separated from their families because of the marijuana prohibition. Readers may consult the web site of Families Against Mandatory Minimums (FAMM) for more information (www.famm.org).

Drug testing in the workplace remains a controversial issue. Most government organizations and private companies that perform drug testing conduct urine drug screens. To many this testing is an invasion of privacy, especially when done as a pre-employment requirement or random on-the-job testing. Urine testing is not a screen for drug abuse, it only tests for past drug use. There are numerous issues associated with drug testing, but cannabis poses a particular problem. The metabolites from THC are fat soluble and can remain in the body for up to a month after the last use. Alcohol, in contrast, can be out of the system in a day (and is often not even included in the urine screen). Countless numbers of citizens have lost an opportunity for employment or been fired from their job based solely on a drug screen positive for cannabis.

There are waiting lists at many drug treatment facilities. Cannabis users who have been coerced into treatment by threat of incarceration or job loss are filling the openings that could and should be available for persons whose lives have been destroyed by their drug addiction. This is not to say that no cannabis users may be in need of help, but rather there are alcoholics, IV drug addicts, crack cocaine addicts and others who have lost all control and are desperate for help that are turned away because there is no room for them.

The policy of prohibition interferes with the procedures necessary for quality control of this medication/drug necessary to prevent the risks of infection or other untoward reactions resulting from a contaminated product. Patients (especially AIDS patients) can suffer from a respiratory tract infection if the cannabis becomes moldy with the *Aspergillus* fungus (Krampf 1997; McPartland et al. 2000). Patients/users can also suffer toxic effects of other contaminants such as Paraquat, a highly toxic herbicide that was used by the federal government to destroy marijuana crops (McPartland et al. 2000).

The therapeutic use of cannabis could greatly reduce the financial costs to patients when they are able to eliminate other medications. The cost of therapeutic cannabis should be minimal in a regulated environment. However, prohibition has inflated the price of cannabis to that of gold. More important than the financial costs, patients who could benefit from the therapeutic use of cannabis are denied this medicine that may help them when all other medications have failed. There is no excuse for denying them the option of trying this medicine.

Denying patients access to therapeutic cannabis does nothing to prevent substance use/abuse among adolescents. The government claims they are concerned about drug abuse among our children and that by acknowledging the therapeutic potential of cannabis they would be sending the wrong message to our youth. Rather, the continued prohibition sends other more chilling messages to our youth: Their government is willing to put patients in prison simply for taking a medicine to ease their suffering. Their government will ignore, try to cover up, or lie about scientific studies that do not support its unjust policies/laws. If their government is lying about cannabis, what else is it lying about?

Finally, cannabis prohibition interferes with open communication between patients and their healthcare providers (Mathre 1985). Patients fear talking to their primary care provider because of possible negative reactions. Patients don't want their use noted in their health record because they fear there may be legal consequences. This fear of admitting to cannabis use to their health care provider interferes with the development of a trusting relationship. Health care professionals cannot adequately monitor the effects of cannabis if they aren't aware of its use. Health care professionals cannot educate the cannabis user about the potential risks of cannabis if they are unaware of its use.

CONCLUSIONS

The possibility of a "drug free" society is unrealistic. People seek and use drugs to feel better. Medications/drugs are not risk free, but the risks can be minimized only with accurate and readily available information on the harmful effects prior to their use. Compared to most medications available today, cannabis is remarkably safe and effective and therefore should be available as an initial option to patients. As a social/recreational drug, the effects of cannabis are pleasant for many with little personal or societal risks and therefore may be the safer choice compared to other social/recreational drugs used by adults. While concern is justified about the dangers related to children and teenagers using drugs, the lies and cruelty of the marijuana prohibition are confusing to young people who learn not to trust their government. The harm resulting from the prohibition of cannabis costs individuals and our society as a whole much more than the drug itself.

When viewed from a nursing perspective, cannabis can be a useful therapeutic agent if it were legally available. Cannabis could be a useful harm reduction agent for substance abuse if it were regulated. The greatest harm from cannabis is the threat of legal consequences related to its illegal status. Nurses and other health care providers can play a vital role in reducing the harmful effects from medication/drug use. Health care professionals can teach patients and the public how to minimize the potentially harmful effects of cannabis when it is used as a medicine or social/recreational drug, but as long as cannabis remains in Schedule I, health care providers will be reluctant to talk with their patients about this drug. The role of the health care provider is severely compromised by cannabis prohibition and society suffers from this unjust, cruel, and costly policy.

REFERENCES

Abel, E.L. 1980. *Marihuana: The first twelve thousand years*. New York: Plenum Press.

Abrams, D.I., S.B. Leiser, S.B. Shade, J. Hilton, and T. Elbeik. 2000. Short-term effects of cannabinoids on HIV-1 viral load. Poster presentation at the 13th International AIDS Conference, Durban, South Africa. July 13, 2000.

Bates, M.N. and T.A. Blakely. 1999. Role of cannabis in motor vehicle crashes. *Epidemiol Rev* 21(2): 222-232.

Bonnie, R.J. and C.H. Whitebread. 1974. *The marihuana conviction: A history of the marihuana prohibition in the United States.* Charlottesville, VA: University Press of Virginia.

Corral, V.L., H. Black, and T. Dalotto. 2002. Medical cannabis providers. Panel presentation at The Second National Conference on Cannabis Therapeutics, Analgesia and Other Indications, Portland, Oregon, May 4, 2002.

Federal Bureau of Investigation. 2001. *Uniform Crime Reports for the United States 2000.* Washington, DC: U.S. Government Printing Office.

Frood, A. 2002. Alcohol impairs driving more than marijuana. *New Scientist (UK).* March 20.

Gieringer, D.H. 2001. Cannabis "vaporization": A promising strategy for smoke harm reduction. *J Cannabis Therap* 1(3/4):153-170.

Hilts, P.J. 1994. Is nicotine addictive? Depends on whose criteria you use. *New York Times.* August 2, p. C3.

Hogan, R., D. Mankin, J. Conway, and S. Fox. 1970. Personality correlates of undergraduate marijuana use. *J Consult Clin Psychol* 35:58-63.

Hunter, C.E., R.J. Lokan, M.C. Longo, J.M. White, and M.A. White. 1998. *The prevalence and role of alcohol, cannabinoids, benzodiazepines and stimulants in non-fatal* crashes. Adelaide, South Australia: Forensic Science, Department for Administrative and Information Services.

Jacox, A., D.B. Carr, R. Payne, C.B. Berde, W. Brietbart, J.M. Cain, C.R. Chapman, C.S. Cleeland, B.R. Ferrell, R.S. Finley et al. 1994. *Management of cancer pain: Clinical practice guideline #9.* AHCPR Publication No. 94-0592: Rockville, MD.

Jones, R.T., N.M. Benowitz, and J. Bachman. 1976. Clinical studies of cannabis tolerance and dependence. *Ann NY Acad Sci* 282:221-239.

Joy, J.E., S.J. Watson, and J.A. Benson, Jr. 1999. *Marijuana and medicine: Assessing the science base.* Washington, DC: Institute of Medicine, National Academy Press.

Krampf, W. 1997. AIDS and the wasting syndrome. In M.L. Mathre (ed.), *Cannabis in medical practice: A legal, historical and pharmacological overview of the therapeutic use of marijuana* (pp. 84-93). Jefferson, NC: McFarland & Company Publishers.

Kranz, C. 2002. U.S. drug chief waves the flag. *Cincinnati Enquirer,* April 11.

Lazarou, J., B.H. Pomeranz, and P.N. Corey. 1998. Incidence of adverse drug reactions in hospitalized patients: A meta-analysis of prospective studies. *J Amer Med Assoc* 279:1200-1205.

Lyketsos, C.G., E. Garrett, K. Liang, and J.C. Anthony. 1999. Cannabis use and cognitive decline in persons under 65 years of age. *Amer J Epidem* 149(9):794-800.

Mathre, M.L. 1985. *A survey on disclosure of marijuana use to health care professionals* (thesis). Cleveland, OH: Frances Payne Bolton School of Nursing, Case Western Reserve University.

McCaffery, M.1968. *Nursing practice theories related to cognition, bodily pain, and man-environment interactions.* Los Angeles: UCLA Students Book Store.

McPartland, J.M., R.C. Clarke, and D.P. Watson. 2000. *Hemp diseases and pests: Management and biological control.* New York: CABI Publishing.

McParland, J.M. and E.B. Russo. 2001. Cannabis and cannabis extracts: Greater than the sum of their parts? *J Cannabis Therap* 1(3/4):103-132.

National Commission on Marihuana and Drug Abuse. 1972. *Marihuana: A signal of misunderstanding.* Washington, DC: Government Printing Office.

Newcomb, M. and P. Bentler. 1988. *Consequences of adolescent drug use: Impact on the lives of young adults.* Newbury Park, CA: Sage.

Rosenblum, S. and W. Wenner. 2002. OR and HI clinical case studies. Panel presentation at The Second National Clinical Conference on Cannabis Therapeutics, Analgesia and Other Indications, Portland, Oregon, May 3, 2002.

Russo, E., M.L. Mathre, A. Byrne, R. Velin, P.J. Bach, J. Sanchez-Ramos, and K.A. Kirlin. 2002. Chronic cannabis use in the compassionate investigational new drug program: An examination of benefits and adverse effects of legal clinical cannabis. *J Cannabis Therap* 2(1):3-57.

Schneider Institute for Health Policy. 2001. *Substance abuse: The nation's number one health problem.* Princeton, NJ: Robert Wood Johnson Foundation.

Shedler, J. and J. Block. 1990. Adolescent drug use and psychological health: A longitudinal inquiry. *Amer Psychologist* 45(5):612-630.

Substance Abuse and Mental Health Services Administration. (2000). *Summary of findings from the 1999 National Household Survey on Drug Abuse.* Rockville, MD: Department of Health and Human Services.

Substance Abuse Report. December 1, 1996. Medical marijuana laws will increase teen drug use: Drug czar. Boston: Warren, Gorham & Lamont.

Sunday Times. December 16, 2001. Science: Cannabis no gateway drug. London.

Tashkin, D.I. 2000. Potential health risks of therapeutic cannabis–pulmonary effects. Oral presentation at The First National Conference on Cannabis Therapeutics, Medical Marijuana: Science Based Clinical Applications, University of Iowa, Iowa City. 8 April 2000.

Whittle, B.A., G.W. Guy and P. Robson. 2001. Prospects for new cannabis-based prescription medicines. *J Cannabis Therap* 1(3/4):183-205.

Wiesbeck, G.A., M.A. Schuckit, J.A. Kalmijn, J.E. Tipp, L.K. Bucholz, and T.L. Smith. 1996. An evaluation of the history of marijuana withdrawal syndrome in a large population. *Addiction* 91(10):1469-1478.

Wikler, A. 1976. Aspects of tolerance and dependence on cannabis. *Ann NY Acad Sci* 282:126-147.

Young, F.L. 6 September 1988. *In the matter of marijuana rescheduling petition* (Docket #86-22). Washington, DC: U.S. Department of Justice, Drug Enforcement Administration.

Zeese, K. 26 March 2002. Once secret "Nixon tapes" show why the U.S. outlawed pot. <AlterNet.org>. Story ID-12666.

Chapter 20

Chronic Cannabis Use in the Compassionate Investigational New Drug Program: An Examination of Benefits and Adverse Effects of Legal Clinical Cannabis

Ethan B. Russo
Mary Lynn Mathre
Al Byrne
Robert Velin
Paul J. Bach
Juan Sanchez-Ramos
Kristin A. Kirlin

The authors would like to dedicate this study to the loving memory of Robert Randall, the first patient in the Compassionate IND program.

The authors would like to acknowledge the generous financial support of John Gilmore, Preston Parish in memory of W. Erastus Upjohn, the Zimmer Family Foundation, and MAPS (Multidisciplinary Association for Psychedelic Studies).

William Bekemeyer, MD generously provided interpretation of pulmonary function tests.

Jennifer Moe and Donna Francisco typed dictated portions of the manuscript. Amy Shoales, administrator of Montana Neurobehavioral Specialists, provided a great deal of logistical support. Lola Goss and Jim Gouaux, MD of the St. Patrick Hospital/Community Medical Center Joint Investigational Review Board were most helpful in aiding study review.

The authors also thank Eve Wall, Janet Kenter, Barbara Pencek, and the many technicians and staff of Montana Neurobehavioral Specialists, St. Patrick Hospital and the Red Lion Inn in Missoula for their patience, understanding, service and hospitality shown to the study subjects. Most of all, the authors thank the patients themselves for their selfless contributions to the advancement of knowledge of clinical cannabis.

Handbook of Cannabis Therapeutics
© 2006 by The Haworth Press, Inc. All rights reserved.
doi:10.1300/5741_21

INTRODUCTION

The Missoula Chronic Clinical Cannabis Use Study was proposed to investigate the therapeutic benefits and adverse effects of prolonged use of "medical marijuana" in a cohort of seriously ill patients approved through the Compassionate Investigational New Drug (IND) program of the Food and Drug Administration (FDA) for legal use of cannabis obtained from the National Institute on Drug Abuse (NIDA), under the supervision of a study physician. The aim was to examine the overall health status of eight surviving patients in the program. Four patients were able to take part, while three wished to remain anonymous, and one was too ill to participate. Unfortunately, that person, Robert Randall, succumbed to his condition during the course of the study. Thus, seven surviving patients in the United States remain in the Compassionate IND program.

Despite the obvious opportunity to generate data on the use of cannabis and its possible sequelae in these patients, neither NIDA, other branches of the National Institutes of Health, nor the FDA has published an analysis of information from this cohort. An examination of the contents of the National Library of Medicine Database (PubMed) and search engines of NIDA employing multiple combinations of key words failed to retrieve a single citation. The Missoula Chronic Cannabis Use Study thus provides a unique and important opportunity to scrutinize the long-term effects of cannabis on patients who have used a known dosage of standardized, heat-sterilized quality-controlled supply of low-grade medical marijuana for 11 to 27 years.

The results are compared to those of past chronic use studies in an effort to gain insight into the benefits and sequelae of this controversial agent in modern health care.

PREVIOUS CHRONIC CANNABIS USE STUDIES

The first systematic modern study of chronic cannabis usage was the *Indian Hemp Drugs Commission Report* at the end of the nineteenth century (Kaplan 1969; Indian Hemp Drugs Commission 1894). The British government chose not to outlaw cultivation and commerce of the herb after ascertaining that it had negligible adverse effects on health, even in chronic application.

Similar conclusions were obtained in the LaGuardia Report (Mayor's Committee on Marihuana, Wallace, and Cunningham 1944), which was the first to employ clinical and scientific methods of analysis.

Three important systematic epidemiological studies undertaken by research teams in the 1970s exhaustively examined medical issues in chronic cannabis use, but remain obscure due to limited press runs and out-of-print status. The first of these was *Ganja in Jamaica: A Medical Anthropological Study of Chronic Marihuana Use* (Rubin and Comitas 1975). Therapeutic claims for cannabis were mentioned, but the focus of study was on "recreational use." Sixty men were included in a hospital study of various clinical parameters if they had maintained a minimum intake of three spliffs a day for a minimum of ten years. Jamaican ganja spliffs formed of unfertilized female flowering tops (sinsemilla) tend to be much larger than an American joint of 500 to 1,000 mg. The potency of the cannabis was analyzed with measures in 30 samples ranging from 0.7 to 10.3 percent THC, with an average of 2.8 percent.

In 1977, a detailed study was undertaken in Greece, titled *Hashish: Studies of Long-Term Use* (Stefanis, Dornbush, and Fink 1977). Once again 60 subjects smoking for more than 10 years were selected. Hashish potency was 4 to 5 percent THC and was generally mixed with tobacco. Alcoholics were excluded.

In 1980, *Cannabis in Costa Rica: A Study of Chronic Marihuana Use* was published (Carter 1980). Forty-one subjects smoking for ten years or more were recruited. Although 10 or more cigarettes per day were smoked, the weight of material was only 2 g with an estimated THC range of 24 to 70 mg per day. Thirteen samples were assayed with a range of 1.27 to 3.72 percent, and average of 2.2 percent THC. Claims of benefit for cough, asthma, headache, hangovers, anorexia, impotence, depression and malaise were mentioned, but once more the focus was on social use.

The current study is the first designed to examine clinical benefits and side effects of chronic clinical cannabis usage in which known amounts of quality-controlled material has been employed.

A BRIEF HISTORY OF THE COMPASSIONATE IND

Robert Randall was diagnosed with severe glaucoma at age 24 and was expected to become totally blind long before he turned 30. He soon began a fascinating medical odyssey that has been memorialized in his "personal reflection" co-authored by his wife, Alice O'Leary, titled *Marijuana Rx: The Patients' Fight for Medicinal Pot* (Randall and O'Leary 1998), and other books (Randall 1991a,b). Until the day he died on June 2, 2001, at age 52 of complications of AIDS, Randall retained his vision, and remained a vocal advocate for the benefits of clinical cannabis.

His own journey commenced when he independently discovered that smoking a certain amount of cannabis eliminated the annoying visual haloes produced by his glaucoma. A subsequent arrest in August 1975 for cannabis cultivation led in turn to his dogged pursuit of the right to a legal means to supply his medicine of choice. He subsequently learned of medical support for his treatment (Hepler and Frank 1971). D. Pate has published two more recent reviews (Pate 1999; Pate 2001).

Through painstaking documentation and experimentation, Randall subsequently confirmed the inability of medical science to control his intraocular pressure (IOP) by any legal pharmaceutical means. In contrast, smoked cannabis in large and frequent amounts was successful, where even pure THC was not. As Dr. Hepler observed in their experiments together (Randall and O'Leary 1998, p. 60), "clearly, something other than THC or in addition to THC is helping to lower your pressures. . . . It seems that marijuana works very, very well."

After a great deal of bureaucratic wrangling, Randall obtained his first government-supplied cannabis in November 1976, and the legal case against him was subsequently dismissed. The material he received from his study physician was cultivated in a five-acre plot at the University of Mississippi, mostly from seeds of Mexican origin, and was rolled and packaged at the Research Triangle Institute in North Carolina under the supervision of the National Institute on Drug Abuse (NIDA).

Randall was encouraged to be thankful, but silent, about his treatment. Instead, he chose a different path (Randall and O'Leary 1998, p. 134): "Having won, why go mum? There were souls to save. Better to trust my fellow citizens and shout in to the darkness than rely on a devious Government dedicated to a fraudulent prohibition." He chose to make it his mission to seek approval of clinical cannabis for other patients. He developed protocols for glaucoma, multiple sclerosis, chronic pain, and AIDS that he shared with prospective medical marijuana candidates. Randall proved to be a tireless and persistent researcher, ferreting out hidden facts useful to his cause. Through the Freedom of Information Act (FOIA), he discovered in 1978 that the government's cost of cannabis cultivation and production was 90 cents per ounce (28 g), with two-thirds of this cost attributable to security measures. Thus, the actual cost of production approximated 1 cent per gram (US $0.01/g).

Supply and quality control issues arose frequently, and Randall and other patients experienced delays in receipt of shipments or substitution of weaker strains that required doubling of smoked intake.

The AIDS epidemic and its subsequent involvement in the medical marijuana issue suddenly provided an unlimited supply of available patients for the Compassionate IND program, and Randall assisted them as well. Some succumbed before their supply was approved, or shortly thereafter. By 1991, 34 patients were enrolled in the program according to Randall (Randall and O'Leary 1998), while other sources cite the number as only 15. Facing an onslaught of new applications, the Public Health Service (PHS) in the first Bush administration closed the program to new patients in March 1992. A significant number had received medical approval but were never supplied. Randall sought to ascertain who signed the ultimate termination order through the FOIA but was never successful in this endeavor. At the time of this writing, seven patients survive in the program.

METHODS

The identities of six of eight of the original Compassionate IND program subjects were known to Patients Out of Time and were contacted in relation to participating in a study of the clinical parameters cited as concerns with chronic cannabis usage. Four subjects agreed to participate, and three traveled to Missoula, Montana, for testing at Montana Neurobehavioral Specialists, and Saint Patrick Hospital on May 3 and 4, 2001. One patient was tested to the extent possible in her local area due to physical limitations on travel (Patient Demographics: Table 20.1). Tests included the following (Tests Performed: Exhibit 20.1): MRI scans of the brain, pulmonary function tests (spirometry), chest X-ray (P-A and lateral), neuropsychological test battery, hormone and immunological assays (CD4 counts), electroencephalography (EEG), P300 testing (a computerized EEG test of memory), and neurological history and clinical examination.

TABLE 20.1. Chronic cannabis IND patient demographics.

Pt.	Age/ gender	Qualifying condition	IND approval/ cannabis usage	Daily cannabis/ THC content	Current status
A	62/F	Glaucoma	1988/25 years	8 g/3.80%	Disabled operator/ singer/activist/ vision stable
B	52/M	Nail-Patella syndrome	1989/27 years	7 g/3.75%	Disabled laborer/ factotum/ ambulatory
C	48/M	Multiple congenital cartilaginous exostoses	1982/26 years	9 g/2.75%	Full-time stock-broker/disabled sailor/ambulatory
D	45/F	Multiple sclerosis	1991/11 years	9 g/3.50%	Disable clothier/ visual impairment/ ambulatory aids

EXHIBIT 20.1.
Tests Performed: Chronic Cannabis IND Study.

I. MRI scan of the brain
II. Pulmonary function tests (spirometry)
III. Chest X-ray, P-A and lateral (Patients A-C)
IV. Neuropsychological tests
    A. Wechsler Adult Intelligence Scale, 3rd Edition (WAIS-III)
    B. Wechsler Memory Scale, 3rd Edition (WMS-III)
    C. California Verbal Learning Test (CVLT)
    D. Halstead-Reitan Battery
       1. Trail Making Test A and B
       2. Grooved Peg Board
       3. Finger Tapping and Category Subtests
    E. Controlled Oral Word Association Test
    F. Thurstone Word Fluency Test
    G. Category Fluency Test (animal naming)
    H. Wisconsin Card Sorting Test (WCST)
    I. Conner's Continuous Performance Test, 2nd Edition (CPT-II)
    J. Beck Depression Inventory, 2nd Edition (BDI-II)
V. Endocrine assays
    A. FSH, LH, prolactin, estradiol, estrone, estrogen, testosterone, progesterone
VI. Immunological assays
    A. CBC, CD4 count
VII. Electroencephalography (EEG) (Patients A-C)
VIII. P300 testing (Patients A-C)
IX. Neurological examination

Past medical records were reviewed insofar as possible and the histories were supplemented with additional information. All patients signed informed consent documents, and the St. Patrick Hospital/Community Hospital Joint Investigational Review Board (IRB) reviewed the protocol.

RESULTS AND DISCUSSION

Case Histories and Test Data
on Four Compassionate IND Program Patients

In the following section, case histories, clinical examinations and objective test results are presented.

Patient A

Medical History. This almost-62-year-old female was born with congenital cataracts in Cali, Colombia, and spent 13 years of her life there. There was a question of possible maternal exposure to malaria or quinine. Over time the patient required a series of 11 surgeries on the right eye and 3 on the left for the cataracts and had resulting problems with glaucoma. Her last surgery was complicated by hemorrhaging, leading to immediate and complete loss of vision OD.

By 1976, the patient's intraocular pressure was out of control with all available drugs, many of which caused significant side effects. At that time she started eating and smoking cannabis to treat the condition. She underwent extensive testing in that regard, measuring pressures to titrate the dosage of cannabis. She initially had personal issues with the concept of smoking. Without cannabis her intraocular pressures may run into the 50s, while with it, values are in the teens to 20s. In 1988, she was arrested for cultivation of six cannabis plants. Her ophthalmologist noted (Randall and O'Leary 1998, p. 303), "it's quite clear-cut this is the only thing that will help her." At her trial, she stated in her own defense (Randall and O'Leary 1998, p. 305), "Marijuana saved my sight. I don't think the law has the right to demand blindness from a citizen." She was acquitted on the basis of "medical necessity," but her approval for the Compassionate IND program took six months. She had smoked cannabis on her own from black market sources for 12 years previously.

At present, she also uses Timoptic (timolol, beta-blocker) eye drops daily in the morning, but has concerns about resulting bronchoconstriction.

She normally uses cannabis 3 to 4 grams smoked and 3 to 4 grams orally per day. She feels that the amount that she receives legally from NIDA is insufficient for her medical needs. At times she accepts donations from cannabis buyers' clubs. She admits that the results of these outside cannabis samples on her intraocular pressure are unclear. She has had occasion to go to Amsterdam where intraocular pressures were measured in the teens simply employing cannabis available there. She has used Marinol on an emergency basis, such as on traveling to Canada, in doses of up to 5 to 10 mg qid. She reports that it lowers intraocular pressure for one day, but within 3 to 5 days becomes useless for that purpose.

The patient has a history of cigarette smoking as well, one to two packs a day. She quit in 1997, but subsequently went on a "binge" of cigarette smoking for 13 months, finally quitting on New Year's Day 2001. She feels that past pulmonary function has been normal.

She also notes lifelong insomnia that is alleviated by eating cannabis. Without such treatment, she feels she would sleep four hours, whereas with it she sleeps six to seven. She also feels that the drug produces antidepressant and antianxiety effects for her. She has a history of scoliosis, but notes no symptoms from this and feels that muscle relaxant effects of cannabis have made her quite limber.

The patient had a history of delirium associated with malaria as a child. She had some hardware in her foot from a 1980 surgery after a fall from platform shoes. She had a hysterectomy for fibroids. The patient was menopausal at age 48 and has had no hormone replacement treatment. There is no known history of specific meningitis, encephalitis, head trauma, seizures, diabetes, or thyroid problems. She is on no medicine save for cannabis and timolol eye drops. There are allergies to penicillin and tetracycline. She completed the equivalent of high school, and is right-handed.

Family history is largely negative, although her two children had some cataract involvement.

Social history revealed that the patient has worked in the past as a switchboard operator. She is currently disabled due to legal blindness from her condition. She supports herself on Social Security Disability Income (SSDI). She has been an activist with respect to clinical cannabis. The patient drinks alcohol at a rate of about a bottle of wine a week. She had past heavy use of caffeine, but now drinks decaf only. The patient walks for exercise about an hour a day.

Medical test results. Objective: Weight: 132 lbs. OFC (Occipitofrontal Circumference): 55.5 cm. BP: 104/62. General: Very pleasant, cooperative 62-year-old female. Head: normocephalic without bruits. ENT: noteworthy as below. Neck: supple. Carotids: full. Cor: S1, S2 without murmur. On auscultation of the chest, there seemed to be a prolonged expiratory phase, but no wheezing. Mental Status: The patient was alert and fully oriented. Fund of knowledge, right-left orientation, praxis and naming skills were normal. She was unable to read a grade 6 paragraph with large type due to visual blurring. When it was read to her, memory of the contents was within normal limits. She performed serial three's well. She remembered three objects for five minutes. On a word list task she named 15 animals in 30 seconds (normal 10 to 12). Speech and affect were normal.

Cranial nerves. I: Intact to coconut scent. II: Acuity had recently been measured. There was no vision OD, 20/200 OS corrected. Visual fields OS intact to confrontation. Optokinetic nystagmus (OKNs) was present in that eye in all fields. The patient is aphakic with an irregular eccentric pupil OS and clouding OD. The disk on the left appeared normal. There was prominent horizontal nystagmus resembling a congenital pattern. External extraocular movements were normal. Remaining cranial nerves V and VII-XII appeared intact in full.

Motor. The patient had normal tone and strength with no drift. Sensation was intact to fine touch, sharp/dull, vibration, position and graphesthesia. Romberg was negative. The patient performed finger-to-nose and heel-to-shin well. Rapid alternating movements of the hands were slightly clumsy and fine finger movements slightly deliberate. Gait including toe and heel were normal with tandem gait normal, but very carefully done. Reflexes were 2 to 3+, symmetric with downgoing toes.

The patient underwent a battery of tests. On pulmonary function tests (Table 20.2), a Functional Vital Capacity (FVC) was 103 percent predicted.

Forced Expiratory Volume in 1 second (FEV₁) was 84 percent of predicted and the FEV₁/FVC ratio was 0.67. This was read as showing a mild obstructive defect based on the above ratio and flow volume curve morphology. No restrictive abnormality was noted. A CBC was wholly within normal limits (Table 20.3). Absolute lymphocyte count was 4.0, CD4 61.6 percent and absolute CD4 count 2465, all within normal limits. A full endocrine battery was performed (Table 20.4), including FSH, LH, prolactin, estradiol, estrone, estrogen, testosterone, and progesterone, all within normal limits for age and gender.

An EEG was performed during wakefulness and early stages of sleep (read by EBR). A normal alpha background was identifiable at 12 hertz, along with a great deal of beta activity. Occasional left frontal phase reversing sharp waves were seen with rare episodes of slight slowing in the same area.

The patient had a P300 test performed with a latency of 355 milliseconds, within normal limits for a normed population in this laboratory (Figure 20.1).

The patient had an MRI brain study without contrast. This was read as showing a mild, symmetric, age-consistent cerebral atrophy. A small focus of T2 hyperintensity and increased signal was noted on the FLAIR sequence in

TABLE 20.2. Pulmonary function tests.

Parameter	Patient A	Patient B	Patient C	Patient D
FVC (percent predicted)	103	107	108	79
FEV₁ (percent predicted)	84	95	67	76
FEV₁/FVC	0.67	0.78	0.51	0.86
Interpretation	Mild obstructive defect	WNL; slightly prolonged forced expiratory time	Moderate obstructive defect	No obstructive defect; minor changes not excluded

TABLE 20.3. Hematological/immunological parameters.

Parameter	Patient A	Patient B	Patient C	Patient D
CBC	WNL	Polycythemia	WNL	WNL
Lymphocytes, absolute count (K/μL)	4.0	3.4	1.8	2.3
CD4 percent	61.6	68.7	49.1	58
CD4 absolute count (/μL)	2465	2324	911	1325

TABLE 20.4. Endocrine parameters.

Parameter	Patient A	Patient B	Patient C	Patient D
FSH (mIU/mL)	32.8	5.4	3.0	12.4
LH (mIU/mL)	20.6	3.8	4.1	16.2
Prolactin (ng/mL)	7.2	7.8	5.1	4.1
Estradiol (pg/mL)	8.0	10.0	10.0	212
Estrone (pg/mL)	15.0	20.0	22.0	146
Estrogen, total (pg/mL)	23.0	30.0	32.0	538
Testosterone (ng/dL)	7.0	505.0	296.0	34
Progesterone (ng/mL)	0.61	0.42	0.68	2.1
Interpretation	WNL for age and gender (meno-pausal)	WNL for age and gender	WNL for age and gender	WNL for age, gender and cycle (pre-menopausal)

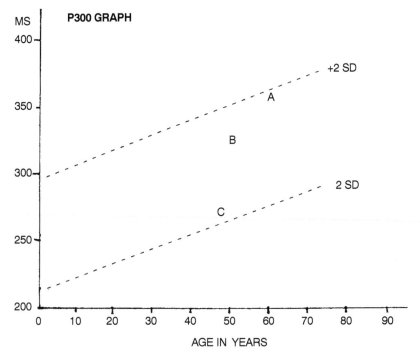

FIGURE 20.1. P300 latency graph.

the mid-pons to the left of midline with no surrounding mass effect or edema. This was felt to be a nonspecific finding representing gliosis most likely from microvascular ischemic change. No corresponding signal abnormality was seen in the same area on a diffusion-weighted sequence.

A chest x-ray showed slight hyperinflation of the lung fields with no other findings.

Patient A was very pleasant and cooperative throughout the neuro-psychological assessment and appeared to put forth very good effort. She did have very significant visual deficits and, as a result, several instruments were dropped from the battery, including Grooved Peg Board, Picture Arrangement, Symbol Search, and the Faces and Family Pictures Subtests from the Wechsler Memory Scale, 3rd Edition (WMS-III). She was able to complete the Trail-Making Test A & B from the Halstead-Reitan Neuro-psychological Battery, Spatial Span from the Wechsler Memory Scale, 3rd Edition (WMS-III), and the Wechsler Adult Intelligence Scale, 3rd Edition (WAIS-III)—Picture Completion, Digit Symbol, and Matrix Reasoning, but these were not used in interpretation secondary to the very probable interfering effects of her limited sight.

Review of the WAIS-III revealed a Verbal IQ in the upper end of the Average Range (VIQ = 108), and a Performance IQ in the Extremely Low Range, at only the second percentile (PIQ = 69). This latter, however, is secondary to visual deficits as she had extremely low scores on the Digit Symbol and Picture Completion subtests. She obtained an age scaled score of 7 on Block Design; this performance was also adversely impacted by her visual defects to a mild degree.

Assessment of attention and concentration revealed that these abilities are mildly to moderately impaired relative to age-matched controls. She demonstrated an abnormally high number of omission errors on the Conner's Continuous Performance Test, 2nd Edition (CPT-II) as well as significant variability of reaction time.

Formal assessment of learning and memory revealed that this subject's ability to acquire new verbal material on the WMS-III is within the Average Range relative to age-matched peers. Her Auditory Immediate Index score was in the average range as was her Auditory Delayed Index. She obtained index scores of 97 and 108 on these two indices, respectively. Recognition memory for auditory material was actually in the High Average range, the seventy-fifth percentile (Index Score = 110). In contrast she did much more poorly on visual measures secondary to very significant visual defects.

On the California Verbal Learning Test (CVLT), the subject generally performed within normal limits. Although initial learning trials were two standard deviations below expected limits, her ultimate acquisition at Trial 5 was one standard deviation above normative data sets. Short Delay Free Recall was perfectly normal and long delay recall was only one standard deviation below expected levels. This loss of recalled items from short delay to long delay free recall represented a loss that is approximately one standard deviation more than expected. Thus, she appeared to have mild difficulties with initial acquisition of very complex verbal material and also appeared to have minimal-to-mild difficulty retaining it in memory relative to age-matched peers.

Higher-level executive functions appear to be entirely normal in this patient. The Wisconsin Card Sorting Test (WCST) yielded a T-score of 63, while she obtained a T-score of 42 on the Category Test. Thus, she is still within the parameters seen in a normative data set of age and education-matched peers.

This subject's performance on the Thurstone Word Fluency Test was also entirely normal with a T-score of 51. Likewise, on the Controlled Oral Word Association Test, she obtained an overall score placing her at the 78th percentile. She produced 26 items on the Animal Naming Test over a 60-second period. This is within normal limits.

On the Beck Depression Inventory, 2nd Edition, she obtained an overall score of 6, arguing against significant depressive symptoms.

In summary, Patient A appears to have mild-to-moderate difficulty with attention and concentration, and minimal-to-mild difficulty with the acquisition and storage of very complex new verbal material. General learning, however, as measured on the Wechsler Memory Scale, 3rd Edition (WMS-III) appears to be within normal limits. Higher-level executive functions and verbal fluency abilities are well within normal limits.

Patient B

Medical history. This 50-year-old white male carries the diagnosis of the nail-patella syndrome, also known as hereditary osteo-onychodysplasia, a rare genetic disorder producing hypoplastic nails and kneecaps and renal insufficiency. Information was obtained from the patient, a published affidavit (Randall 1991b), and submitted medical records.

He first smoked cannabis in 1970, but did not become "high." Rather, he felt more relaxed, without his customary muscle spasms and pain. He first actually used clinical cannabis in a different manner. At the time he was mining, and he developed chemical burns in his hands. A Mexican lady gave him a tincture of cannabis flowering tops in grain alcohol to apply. This reduced his hand swelling and burning.

He has been smoking cannabis regularly for medical purposes since about 1974. During a medical crisis in 1985, he suffered a decrease in supply of available cannabis. His recollection is that all the various analgesics he received during this time were ineffective and produced dangerous side effects including sedation and incapacity.

By 1988, he pursued regular usage of cannabis, about 1/8 of an ounce (3.5 to 4 g/d) a day when available. He initiated inquiries with the FDA to obtain legal cannabis. Ultimately, with the assistance of Robert Randall, he received approval from the government in March 1990.

He related a history of deformities from birth including missing fingernails, loose finger joints, and small patellae. He was frequently ill as a child, and at age ten suffered a progression from conjunctivitis to varicella, strep throat and rheumatic fever. He was hospitalized for six months, and required another three months of bed rest. Subsequently, he underwent four right knee surgeries, reconstructions and rotations, including three arthroscopies. He had had a right wrist graft with nonfusion. He had had right elbow surgery and had a "nicked" ulnar nerve. In the late 1960s he developed both hepatitis A and B with prolonged hospitalizations. Despite this, he pursued heavy manual labor in mining, construction, auto bodywork and aircraft repair. He lost all his teeth by age twenty-one. In 1972 he dislocated his knee and had three subsequent surgeries. In 1976 he had a wrist fracture with subsequent surgery and later fusion. In 1978 he was hospitalized after a nail wound in his foot failed to heal. In 1983, he injured his back in a fall. Pain continued.

After a 1985 chiropractic session, he became acutely ill with severe back pain. He was given narcotics, and suffered renal failure. He was transferred to a university center. Lithotripsy sessions were followed by transurethral procedures in attempts to clear his nephrolithiasis. Eventually an open procedure was performed for perinephric abscess, but the flank wound failed to heal over the course of a year. Ultimately, it was determined that he was suffering a tubercular nephritis. He took triple therapy with isoniazid (INH), rifampin and pyridoxine regularly for 18 months. Eventually, a massive debridement was necessary, before the flank wound eventually healed. His prolonged convalescence forced him to close his business.

On September 3, 1987, he complained of persistent flank pain and low back discomfort increasing over the preceding two years treated with multiple modalities, including TENS unit. He also was using an abdominal binder. Pain radiated to the buttocks and posterior thighs. X-rays of the lumbar spine showed spondylolisthesis grade 1 in the lumbar area with no significant motion of flexion extension views.

On April 8, 1988, the patient was seen for right knee pain after a twisting injury and fall. An effusion developed. X-rays showed a micropatella consistent with nail-patella syndrome, but no evidence of fracture. He was treated conservatively. In October 1988, chest x-ray showed a diffuse nodular infiltrate unchanged since September 1985.

By June 7, 1989, the patient was in a wheelchair, but was able to ambulate with a cane. Previous x-rays showed bilateral iliac spurs. His chart notes included an FDA consent form in relation to the patient's use of cannabis (Figure 20.2). On subsequent visits, he had been approved for the Compassionate IND program, and was smoking ten cannabis cigarettes a day.

On April 1, 1991, some cough was noted attributed to cigarettes. As a baseline, very severe pain was noted in the extremities, but this was reduced to slight to moderate on subsequent visits. By April 17, 1991, the patient was on no medicines except for cannabis. By January 18, 1993, he was said to have only slight to moderate problems with a cane for support. There were some abdominal spasms.

On the May 14, 1996, visit, he was smoking ten cannabis cigarettes a day. He used occasional aspirin for increased pain. He had resumed smoking .5 to 1 pack of cigarettes a day. Examination was fairly unremarkable save

FD 1571 Atachment 10(b)

PATIENT CONSENT FORM

I, _____, understand that this study will evaluate marijuana's use in the treatment of symptoms of chronic pain and muscle spasticity caused by severe spinal cord injuries. As a patient who suffers from intense pain and uncontrollable spasticity, I am interested in marijuana's potential medical uses and I volunteer to participate in this study of marijuana's effect on my symptoms.

I realize that in addition to marijuana's possible benefits in controlling pain and reducing spasticity, the drug may also cause various side effects including, but not limited to, alterations in consciousness and mood, anxiety, euphoria, drowsiness, depression, disorientation, paranoia, confusion, rapid pulse, pounding of the heart, dizziness, fainting, bloodshot eyes and dryness of the mouth. Although not validated by clinical studies, I understand some researchers believe marijuana may cause damage to the lungs and brain, changes in hormone levels, personality changes and/or reduce the body's ability to fight infection. However, I also understand marijuana, at the dosages I will receive, has been well tolerated by other patients who smoke marijuana to reduce intraocular pressures, control nausea and vomiting and ease spasticity. Due to marijuana's reported side effects I agree not to operate a car or other motor vehicle if I become intoxicated while smoking marijuana.

During this study I will be under the care of my doctor. I understand that if I experience any adverse effects while smoking marijuana I should report these effects to my physician. If I leave my doctor's care I understand my access to marijuana will be terminated unless another physician responsible for my care receives FDA approval to provide me with marijuana. I also understand that if for any reason I decide to leave this program, my doctor will notify the FDA of my decision and marijuana will be unavailable to me for this purpose.

Signed _____ _____ Date _____, 1989

Witness _____ Date _____, 1989

Witness _____ Date _____, 1989

FIGURE 20.2. Informed consent document, Patient B.

for orthopedic deformities. He was able to walk on his toes and heels. The patient was given 2 more packages of 300 marijuana cigarettes.

On July 16, 1996, the patient was seen for disability examination. It was noted the patient had suffered for many years from lack of strength, mobility and range of motion, and persistent episodes of nausea and muscle spasms. The note indicated, "The marijuana helps the patient function better in the sense that he has increased flexibility, increased strength and range of motion. He has less nausea and less muscle spasm." He needed to shift into different positions at home to get comfortable and could do a sit-down type job for an hour or two at most before experiencing spasms, pain and nausea. He had limited backward flexion, and limited right hand strength. He was unable to kneel. He could walk 50 feet before needing to rest, used a cane and sometimes a wheelchair for longer distances. It was felt he could not be a traveling salesman, and any prospective job would require frequent rests. Overall, he was assessed as having a significant functional impairment due to nail-patella syndrome, and was judged unemployable in the short or long term, with little rehabilitation potential.

A May 9, 1997, letter indicates, "continues to smoke about 8-10 marijuana cigarettes per day and still continues to benefit from that medication. He has less pain, less spasms, he is able to ambulate better. His nausea is improved, he is able to sleep better. He is making some slow deterioration of this disease process." It goes on to say, "I personally do feel that [Patient B] continues to benefit from marijuana and hope that we can continue providing this unfortunate man with marijuana medication."

On May 10, 2000, a letter to FDA noted the patient continued to do well on the therapy, smoking eight to ten cigarettes per day without other medication. He continued to function well using a cane and occasionally a wheelchair when bothered by spasms and nausea.

At present, he utilizes about 7 grams a day or .25 ounce of NIDA material that is 3.75 percent THC, and was processed in April 1999. The patient cleans the cannabis to a minimal degree first, estimating a loss of about 25 percent of material. He indicates that he has been short on his supply three times in ten years, generally for one to two weeks, secondary to lack of supply or paperwork problems. When this occurs he suffers more nausea and muscle spasms and is less active as a consequence. He was never allowed to try Marinol and points out that he could not afford it in any event.

The patient reports continued problems with pain in the back, hips and legs, also in the upper extremities, right greater than left. When he undergoes spasms the pain rises to a 10 on a 10-point scale and is associated with projectile emesis. His baseline level of pain is 6 to 7/10. He notes that this pain was never helped by prescription medicines. Morphine sulfate produced a minimal decrement in pain for up to two hours, but caused inebriation. By the third day of application it would become totally ineffective. Without cannabis he feels that he would need very high doses of narcotics. He previously had dependency issues and took heroin for two years in the mid-1960s. Eventually he had become allergic to most pharmaceutical preparations or had side effects of nausea. The latter continues, particularly in static positions, which without cannabis treatment he rates as a 10/10. In 1985, he was without cannabis for some 30 days and lost 57 pounds when his supply ran out at the same time that he had TB nephritis.

In relation to the spasms, these can occur anywhere in his body. He feels the medicine eliminates them or substantially reduces nocturnal manifestations. Without it he would be "running" at night.

He has no history of diabetes, thyroid problems, meningitis, encephalitis or head trauma. He may have had seizures associated with fever. The patient has taken rare antibiotics for staph infections of the skin. He feels that he has had lots of reactions to synthetic chemicals of various types, which he considers quite serious. The patient left school at age 14 originally but attained a GED and had some junior college experience. He is left-handed.

Family history is noteworthy for nail-patella syndrome in mother, niece, two sisters, nephew and daughter. One sister died of the disease at age 44. He has two unaffected children. His affected daughter does not receive legal cannabis. His father died of TB and tumors at age 40.

Social history. He currently smoked cigarettes about 1/2 pack a day, but as high as a pack a day in the past. The patient drinks beer about one a month, with little alcohol use in ten years. The patient last worked full-time in 1985, and part-time in 1990. He is on SSDI, but does volunteer and activist work. The patient is able to walk very little due to pain, but bikes when he can a short distance (about four miles every other day). The patient sleeps from 10 p.m. to 6 a.m., but this is disrupted due to pain or nausea.

Medical test results. Weight: 173 lbs. Height: 69 inches (BMI: 25.6). OFC: 60 cm. BP: 122/80. General: Very pleasant, cooperative 50 YOM who appears somewhat wizened. Head: normocephalic without bruits. ENT was noteworthy for edentulous state. Neck: supple. Carotids: full, without bruit. Cor: S1, S2 without murmur. The patient has a large indentation scar in the right flank. Palpation to the spine was unremarkable. Chest auscultation revealed a prolonged expiratory phase without wheezing. Abdominal examination was unremarkable. He had dysplastic nails.

Mental status. The patient was alert and fully oriented. Fund of knowledge, right-left orientation, praxis and naming skills were normal. He read a grade 6 paragraph well with good recall. Serial threes were well done. Signature was normal. He remembered two of three objects after five minutes with hesitation, failed the third with hint, but got it with choice of three. He had a hoarse voice. He named 11 animals in 30 seconds (normal). Affect was normal. Cranial Nerves: I: intact. II: acuity was measured as 20/25 OD, 20/50 OS uncorrected. Fields and OKNs were normal. Fundi were benign. Pupils equally reactive with full EOMs and no nystagmus. Remaining cranial nerves V and VII-XII were unremarkable. On motor examination, the patient had hypotonicity but decreased bulk. The patient lacked full elbow extension on the right. His strength was generally 4+ secondary to limitations and pain. There was no arm drift. Sensation was intact to fine touch, vibration, position and graphesthesia, but there was some slight vibratory loss in the feet. Romberg was negative. The patient performed finger-to-nose well. Heel-to-shin required partial assist of the hands. Rapid alternating movements of the hands were very slow on the right secondary to mechanical problems. Fine finger movements were normal. The patient had a stiff, bent gait, but toe gait appeared more normal. On heel gait he favored the left leg. Tandem gait was difficult due to back pain and he wavered some. I was unable to ascertain reflexes at the biceps on the right, but responses elsewhere were 1-2+ with downgoing toes.

The patient underwent the prescribed battery of tests. Pulmonary function tests revealed an FVC of 107 percent of predicted, FEV_1 of 95 percent of predicted, and FEV_1/FVC of 0.75. This was interpreted as within normal limits, but with a slightly prolonged forced expiratory time (Table 20.2). A complete blood count showed some mild polycythemia, probably due to tobacco smoking. An absolute lymphocyte count was 3.4 with CD4 count 68.7 percent and absolute count of 2324 (Table 20.3). The patient had a full endocrine battery. Measurement of FSH, LH, prolactin, estradiol, estrone, estrogen, testosterone and progesterone were wholly within normal limits for age and gender (Table 20.4). An EEG was performed during wakefulness and was within normal limits, but did demonstrate some low voltage fast activity in the beta range, with no focal or epileptiform activity. The patient had a P300 response with a latency of 338 milliseconds, within normal limits for the laboratory (Figure 20.1). An MRI of the brain without contrast was read as normal. A PA and lateral chest was read as normal.

Patient B was friendly and cooperative and appeared to put forth very good effort on neuropsychological testing. On the WAIS-III, he obtained Verbal and Performance IQ Scores in the Average Range (VIQ = 105 and PIQ = 92). In terms of overall intellectual functioning, he obtained an overall score placing him at the 50th percentile (Full Scale IQ = 100). Assessment of attention and concentration with the CPT-II revealed that these abilities tended toward mildly-to-moderately impaired relative to the normative data set. He made an abnormally high number of omission errors and also demonstrated substantial variability in his reaction time. He also became more variable as time progressed over this 14-minute measure.

On the WMS-III, he obtained Auditory Immediate and Auditory Delayed Index scores of 89 and 86, placing him in the low average range. His Auditory Recognition Delayed Index was in the average range with an index score of 90. Visual Immediate and Visual Delayed abilities were also in the low average range with index scores of 88 on both. Overall, these performances are within normal limits, albeit it in the low average range.

On the CVLT, this patient's initial acquisition of items after the first trial was one standard deviation below expected levels, and his recall after five learning trials was two standard deviations below. Short Delay Free Recall and Long Delay Free Recall were essentially at the same level. Thus, his acquisition of very complex verbal material does appear at least mildly impaired. Interestingly, he does not lose this information from memory after a delay.

Assessment of higher level executive functions yields an overall performance on the WCST at a mildly impaired level relative to age and education matched peers, with a T-score of 38. His overall performance on the Category Test was in the borderline range with a T-score of 40. He also had difficulty following new complex sequences with a T-score of 40 on the Trails A Subtest and a T-score of 32 (mildly-to-moderately impaired) on the Trails B component.

Simple motor testing reveals that Tapping Speed was within normal limits, but he had difficulty with fine motor coordination on the Groove Pegboard Test with his dominant left hand. He obtained a T-score of 36 on this particular measure with his left hand, a T-score of 42 with his right hand.

On the Thurstone Word Fluency Test, he obtained a T-score of 54 and a T-score of 40.2 on the Controlled Oral Word Association Test. Animal naming was within normal limits with a total score of 22.

In summary, Patient B does appear to have a mild-to-moderate impairment of attention and concentration, and his ability to acquire new, complex detailed verbal material also appears to be mildly-to-moderately impaired. There is quite some variability in this regard, however, with performances on the Wechsler Memory Scale, 3rd Edition (WMS-III) being generally within normal limits, and his California Verbal Learning Test (CVLT) performance falling approximately two standard deviations below expected levels. He had difficulty on motor tasks. His performances may have been adversely affected by peripheral pain as he complained of such during the assessment process. His overall score of 0 on the Beck Depression Inventory (BDI) argues against significant depressive symptoms.

Patient C

Medical history. This 48-year-old male carries a diagnosis of multiple congenital cartilaginous exostoses, an autosomal dominant disorder. History was obtained from the patient, a published affidavit (Randall 1991b), and submitted progress notes dating from December 5, 1996.

He recalls few medical problems until age ten, when he threw a baseball and his arm became paralyzed for a few hours. Radiographs revealed what was interpreted as an old fracture that had healed with jagged bone fragments. Multiple referrals ensued, and ultimately 250 bony tumors were found throughout his body. He was diagnosed as having multiple congenital cartilaginous exostoses. Each was capable of growth, massive tissue disruption, pain, and malignant transformation. By age 17, he underwent multiple surgical procedures on the left leg and right wrist. By age 12, constant pain and frequent hemorrhages severely limited his gait along with other basic functions. He required a home tutor by grade 7. By age 14, he required ongoing narcotics for analgesia, escalating to Dilaudid (hydromorphone), and Sopor (methaqualone, now Schedule I in USA) for sleep. He reports resultant fatigue, ennui, and disorientation as side effects.

At age 20, he developed a large bone spur on the right ankle, which recurred dramatically after one surgery. Amputation was recommended, but refused. At age 22, a fist-sized tumor was removed from the pelvis. A medical odyssey ensued, which failed to identify better therapies and he required massive doses of hydromorphone, methaqualone, and muscle relaxants.

He described himself as a conservative young man who was against drugs but in college acquiesced to try marijuana. He enjoyed chess but was normally able to sit for only 5 to 10 minutes without pain. One day, he smoked cannabis and an hour into a chess match he remained pain free. After discussion with his doctor, he experimented by smoking it regularly for six months. He noted a marked enhancement of his analgesia and a reduction on his dependence on hydromorphone (taken intravenously for some time), Demerol (meperidine), and hypnotics. Cannabis analgesia exceeded that of any prescription drugs.

He began to investigate possible legal avenues to obtain cannabis, and met Robert Randall in 1978. By 1979, he was spending $3,000 annually on therapeutic cannabis through the black market, an unsustainable burden. A Byzantine bureaucratic process ensued over several years, with final FDA approval of his IND application in November 1982. Weekly monitoring sessions including needle electromyography (EMG) were deemed necessary to assess the effects of treatment in his protocol.

Subsequently, he described numerous instances of delayed shipments of cannabis, or exhaustion of supplies of higher potency product. Substitution of 1 percent THC cannabis required a doubling of dosage to 20 cannabis joints a day.

He was once arrested in Florida despite documentation, handcuffed and jailed overnight, sustaining an ankle hemorrhage in the process. Only four of seven confiscated joints were ultimately returned. Beyond this, he describes cannabis as much safer than prescribed medicine, and free of serious adverse effects except chest pain with prolonged usage of inferior product.

In 1992, Patient C had occasion to try Marinol during a stockholders meeting in Canada due to his legal proscription from traveling with cannabis. Although he had no side effects on a dose of 10 mg, it was without any benefits, and left his muscles very tight and painful.

Detailed progress notes from the last several years were obtained and will be summarized. December 5, 1996, the patient was using 10 to 20 mg of baclofen and 10 to 15 cannabis cigarettes a day. Assessment was of multiple congenital cartilaginous exostoses with hepatitis C, and GE reflux. He was prescribed diazepam 5 mg for spasm. An EKG was read as showing normal sinus rhythm. February 28, 1996, the patient had pulmonary functions with FVC 112 percent of predicted, FEV_1 of 79 percent of predicted, read as indicating mild obstruction.

January 24, 1997, he had episodic spasm with pain affecting both arms and legs. It was noted at the time that the patient had a malunion of the right radius. He was down to two to three cannabis cigarettes a day, as he had received no supply from NIDA since September 1996, due to logistical problems in seeing his study physician. A transfer of providers was recommended.

September 4, 1997, he remained on baclofen 10 mg p.m., 5 mg a.m. and Prilosec (omeprazole) for epigastric discomfort that had been going on for 7 years, and cannabis 12 cigarettes a day. September 9, 1997, the patient had a chest x-ray with no findings. September 9, 1997, the patient had laboratory tests done, including a CBC, nonreactive hepatitis A and B tests, and normal thyroid functions. Glucose was low at 24, potassium high at 5.4, SGOT 79 with other parameters negative. September 17, 1997, the patient was said to be doing well smoking 10 to 12 cannabis cigarettes a day with dramatic decreases in frequency and intensity of flexor spasms. He was also taking baclofen. It was noted that with strong spasms the patient would bruise his skin and sometimes even bleed. His weight was constant, appetite normal. Neurological exam was fairly unremarkable. He was asked to slowly decrease the baclofen to 2.5 mg bid.

May 13, 1998, the patient was said to be doing quite well. In the interim, a liver biopsy demonstrated minimal changes secondary to hepatitis C. Chest x-rays were said to show no changes. The prior December the patient had twisted his left knee with a lot of swelling, and an MRI revealed a minor crack in the tibial head. Pain was under good control with 12 cannabis cigarettes a day with only occasional muscle spasms. Exam was unremarkable. He was said to be doing quite well off of the baclofen and was asked to continue 12 cigarettes of cannabis a day. May 26, 1999, the patient related no difficulty breathing. Weight was constant. There was dull pain in the ankles and some sharp shooting also in the knees. There was minor weakness in the right hand with no other deficits. The remainder of the exam was normal. The patient was felt to be doing well and advised to continue 12 cannabis cigarettes a day. October 6, 1999, the patient was seen in follow up, was on omeprazole, Vitamin C, and cannabis. The patient had some congestion and mildly productive cough. He was felt to have acute bronchitis and was given cough syrup. January 5, 2000, the patient had pulmonary functions done with an FVC 118 percent of predicted, FEV_1 82 percent of predicted. This was felt to indicate borderline obstruction. January 13, 2000, glucose was 126, BUN 26, SGOT 71 with other parameters normal, including CBC. Hepatitis C antibody was reactive with other titers negative. Thyroid functions were normal. An SGPT was 181.

May 4, 2000, the patient was occasionally playing softball and had no complaints of shortness of breath. Again there was mild weakness of the hand with other muscles normal. It was felt that the patient was doing well without aches, pains or spasms on his cannabis.

November 21, 2000, the patient had noticed some increased discomfort following a motor vehicle accident the prior month wherein he was rear-ended and had neck pain. Subsequently, he noted persistent pain in the right thigh. An x-ray was negative. He tried physical therapy, heat and electrical stimulation. He noted more muscle tension with weather change. No neurological changes were observed.

December 28, 2000, the patient was on his omeprazole and cannabis. January 6, 2001, SGOT was 50, SGPT 94 with normal CBC and PSA. A cholesterol total was 221 with LDL 136.

At the time he was examined in Missoula, he noted constant baseline pain of 9 to 10 on a 10-point scale without cannabis. At rest, with cannabis this fell to a 4/10. He was smoking 9 grams a day of 2.7 percent THC NIDA cannabis, or 11 ounces every 25 days. At times he has had to cut back due to an inadequate supply. He would sometimes have to use street cannabis at a cost $110 per quarter ounce (circa $16/g) of an estimated 4 to 5 percent THC content. Interestingly, although he found the flavor was an improvement over the government supply, he noted little difference in analgesic effect except perhaps greater relaxation effect. Interestingly, even with extensive cannabis use there are only two times he thinks that he ever may have been "high." One time he left his coat somewhere in freezing weather, which is extremely uncharacteristic, and the other he had been without cannabis for a long time and briefly felt euphoric while smoking. However, once he advanced to a second joint, this feeling was gone.

The patient has the most problems with the left arm where pain is a 7 to 8/10 when there are flare-ups despite medicine. This decreases after he takes rofecoxib (Vioxx) for a week. He experiences pain in both knees, but usually minimal (1 to 2/10) with his cannabis. He may periodically pull a muscle or hemorrhage, especially in the ribs. He has occasional problems in the wrist.

The patient's sleep remains disrupted, rarely attaining six hours total. Typically, he is up every 45 to 60 minutes with stiffness and needs to have pillows to position himself. He once got eight hours of sleep with methaqualone (now illegal in the United States), waking only twice.

He feels that his hepatitis C is asymptomatic and was probably due to a transfusion in his teens. Although he did use hydromorphone intravenously for a long period of time, he feels that he pursued a scrupulous aseptic technique. Besides surgeries noted above, he has dental caps due to bruxism, and tonsillectomy. He has had past hypertension, which he feels was work related. There is no history of diabetes, thyroid problems, meningitis, encephalitis, head trauma or seizures. He uses only omeprazole 30 mg a day regularly in addition to his cannabis. He is allergic to barbiturates. The patient had three semesters of college. He is primarily right-handed, somewhat ambidextrous.

Family history is negative for other known involvement, but his father was adopted. His mother has migraine.

Social history. The patient works full-time as a stockbroker. He is also a very decorated disabled sailor. He plays softball once a week. He may use a stationary bike about ten minutes at a time, but this is subject to weather effects. He does not smoke tobacco. The patient drinks about 1.75 liters of

Jack Daniels whiskey every 10 to 14 days, which helps him sleep. He does not drink coffee.

Medical test results. Weight: 153 lbs. Height: 5′ 4 1/2″. General: Very pleasant, cooperative 48-year-old white male who is somewhat obese (BMI: 25.5). Head: normocephalic without bruits. ENT: unremarkable. Neck: supple. Carotids: full, without bruits. Cor: S1, S2 without murmur. The patient had very slight gynecomastia. He has prominent exostoses of the left shoulder, left wrist, right shoulder, and right calf. Auscultation of the chest revealed a prolonged expiratory phase without wheezing. Abdominal palpation was negative.

Mental status. The patient was alert and fully oriented. He knew the president and had normal right-left orientation, praxis and naming skills. He read a grade six paragraph well with good recall. Serial threes were done very rapidly. He remembered three objects for five minutes. He named 15 animals in 30 seconds, which is well above the average of 10 to 12. Speech and affect were normal.

Cranial nerves. I: intact. II: fields and OKNs were normal. Fundi were benign. Pupils were equally reactive with full EOMs and no nystagmus. Remaining cranial nerves V and VII-XII were unremarkable. On motor exam, the patient had some limitation due to pain, but seemed to have good strength throughout except for 4+/5 foot dorsiflexion on the right. There was no drift. Sensation was intact to fine touch, vibration, position and graphesthesia, but there was decrease in sharp/dull discrimination at the top of the right foot secondary to post-operative changes. Romberg was negative. Finger-to-nose and rapid alternating movements of the hands were normal. Heel-to-shin was incomplete on the right, better on the left. Fine finger movements were minimally decreased. On gait testing the patient slightly favored the right leg at the ankle. Toe gait looked better. Heel gait was barely possible due to pain on the right side. Tandem gait was minimally hesitant. Reflexes were 1+, symmetric with downgoing toes.

Medical test results. On pulmonary function tests, an FVC was 108 percent of predicted and FEV_1 67 percent of predicted. A FEV_1/FVC was 0.51 felt to be indicative of a moderate obstructive defect based on the latter ratio and flow volume curve morphology. No restrictive abnormality was noted (Table 20.2).

A CBC was wholly within normal limits. An absolute lymphocyte count was 1.8 with CD4 49.1 percent and CD4 absolute count of 911 (Table 20.3). An endocrine battery, including FSH, LH, prolactin, estradiol, estrone, estrogen, testosterone and progesterone, was wholly within normal limits for age and gender (Table 20.4).

An EEG was performed during wakefulness and early stages of sleep, which was within broad normal limits. There was a good bit of low voltage fast activity in the beta range. No focal nor epileptiform activity was appreciated. A P300 showed a latency of 262 milliseconds felt to be within normal limits for the lab (Figure 20.1).

An MRI was performed without contrast. There was felt to be no definite abnormality of an acute nature. There were some minor changes in the right parietal area suggestive of a mild degree of gliosis with associated dilated perivascular spaces of doubtful significance. There was a small area of abnormal signal in the right parotid gland overlying the right masseter muscle felt to be probably benign.

A P-A and lateral chest x-ray were performed. This was read as showing a pulmonary nodule in the left upper lobe with minimal airway changes. One examiner (EBR) reviewed those films and felt that the lesion was actually located in a rib. As a result, the patient underwent a CT scan of the chest after returning home. This showed no evidence of mass, lymphadenopathy, or pulmonary nodules. A small amount of pleural calcification was noted. An exostosis was noted in the right anterior third rib, accounting for the false-positive chest x-ray.

On neuropsychological testing, Patient C was pleasant, cooperative, and appeared to put forth very good effort. His attention was noted to be quite poor at times and many instructions had to be repeated.

On the WAIS-III, he obtained Verbal and Performance IQ Scores in the Average Range with a Verbal IQ of 103 and a Performance IQ of 104. In terms of overall intellectual functioning, he is currently performing at a level equal to or above 58 percent of the general population (Full Scale IQ = 103).

Assessment of attention and concentration with the CPT-II revealed that immediate attentional abilities were within normal limits. His ability to concentrate, however, did appear mildly impaired, as he tended to lose efficiency with the passage of time. Thus, vigilance appeared to be mildly decreased relative to a normative data set.

On the WMS-III, Patient C obtained an Auditory Immediate Index in the Average Range at the 70th percentile. His Auditory Immediate Index was 108. Auditory Delayed Index was also 108, placing him in the Average Range, and his Auditory Recognition Delayed Index was 115, placing him in the High Average Range. The Visual Immediate Index was 115 with a Visual Delayed Index of 122, performances in the High Average and Superior Ranges, respectively.

On the CVLT, this patient's initial acquisition on Trial One was two standard deviations below expected levels and his acquisition of only ten items by Trial 5 was one standard deviation below expected levels. Short Delay Free Recall was also one standard deviation below expected levels but he performed within normal limits if provided cues. His ultimate free recall after a 20-minute delay was also one standard deviation below expected levels. There was not a substantial loss of information between Long Delay and Short Delay Free Recall trials. Thus, his ability to acquire very complex and detailed new verbal material does appear minimally-to-mildly decreased relative to age matched peers, well below his ability to acquire new thematically organized verbal material, which was in the above average range. Memory, however, appears normal.

Assessment of higher level executive functions yielded a T-score of 45 on the WCST and a T-score of 44 on the Category Test from the Halstead-Reitan Neuropsychological Battery. His ability to follow new complex sequences was entirely within normal limits as indicated by T-scores of 52 and 62 on Trail Making Test A and B, respectively.

Simple motor speed measured by Finger Tapping was within normal limits, bilaterally, as was fine motor coordination measured by the Grooved Pegboard Test.

His performance on the Thurstone Word Fluency Test yielded a T-score of 56, which is entirely within normal limits relative to age and education-matched peers. Likewise, his overall performance on the Controlled Oral Word Association Test yielded a T-score of 52.52, and Animal Naming Fluency also was within normal limits. His overall score on the Beck Depression Inventory-2nd Edition (BDI-II) was 0.

Overall, Patient C appears to have mild difficulty sustaining attention and also minimal to mild difficulty with the acquisition of very new, complex verbal material. Overall, however, he appears to be functioning quite well.

Patient D

Medical history. This 45-year-old female carries a diagnosis of multiple sclerosis (MS). The patient was interviewed by telephone (EBR) in lieu of the possibility of contemporaneous examination. The patient feels her first problem may have occurred at age 18 when her vision sequentially went completely black for two months with slow improvement over a subsequent four months. A possible attribution to oral contraception was hypothesized. She was subsequently evaluated at a quartenary referral center and diagnosed as having retro-bulbar neuritis. She was prescribed nicotinic acid. On reevaluation in 1983, no active disease was noted. On May 29, 1986, best corrected vision was 20/30 OD, 20/25 OS. By May 19, 1988, values fell to 20/200 OD, and 20/70 OS. The patient was formally diagnosed as having MS April 1 of that year with associated bilateral optic neuropathy. She had had symptoms for perhaps six months with blurring in both eyes and leg spasms that interfered with walking. The patient had never used cannabis recreationally and began it only because of her symptoms.

She has been followed in her local area by a psychiatrist and neurologist. Extensive, well-documented notes commencing December 20, 1989, were provided, and will be summarized. When first seen on that date the patient was married for the second time. It was noted that she had been diagnosed with MS about a year and a half previously and had been on diazepam from time-to-time. She was taking 10 mg tid to cope with stress. She had previously tried trazodone and buspirone, had become paralyzed with her MS, and was consequently very frightened of these medicines. On examination she was felt to be quite anxious and was provisionally diagnosed as having a dysthymic disorder.

On March 20, 1990, she seemed to be suffering from more depression, although she managed to smile. She described difficulty with self-esteem and hopelessness. She had only been taking diazepam intermittently and was rather prescribed Prozac (fluoxetine) 20 mg and Xanax (alprazolam) 0.25 mg up to 3 times a day. She was felt to have recurrent major depression. On subsequent visits the patient had slight adjustments of medicine and was feeling better by May 2, 1990. By August 6, 1990, the patient was having greater difficulties with insomnia. She was given trazodone 50 mg at bedtime on a trial basis. August 24, 1990, the patient was only sleeping until 4 a.m., which was about 2 hours better than without medicine. This was increased to 75 mg.

The patient had heard about some studies of using cannabis in MS as a relaxing agent. She indicated that she had tried this with a good relaxation response. There was a discussion of possible effects on the lungs, and her expected diminished life expectancy because of MS. She was given a prescription for Marinol (dronabinol, synthetic THC) 10 mg to be tried q 4 hours prn to see if this would help with relaxation and nausea. When seen September 5, 1990, she had found that the Marinol had reduced the nausea considerably and had even helped her vision. She continued on fluoxetine.

September 27, 1990, the patient was not sleeping well, possibly due to fluoxetine, and was given a benzodiazepine. October 17, 1990, the patient was seen in follow-up and was on Xanax (alprazolam). It was noted that she had improvement with Marinol, but the patient noted she actually had a better response to smoked cannabis. They began to look into obtaining a legal supply.

December 3, 1990, the patient reported increased depression and was increased to 40 mg a day of fluoxetine. December 5, 1990, the patient had recurrent depression even on the fluoxetine two a day and low dose alprazolam. Apparently, her doctor had received notification that he could no longer prescribe Marinol "off label" unless a Schedule I permit for cannabis was being pursued. December 19, 1990, the patient reported nausea, for which some of her remaining Marinol had helped. January 16, 1991, the patient complained of spasticity spells and episodes of nausea. She had run out of Marinol and had no cannabis supply. She indicated she had tried other medications without success and was resistant to try others due to side effects.

February 20, 1991, the patient had purchased illicit cannabis in the interim. April 16, 1991, the patient continued on fluoxetine 20 mg bid. More jerkiness was noted with increased spasticity. She had not smoked cannabis before coming in. It was felt that she would need six cannabis cigarettes a day to reduce symptoms. May 10, 1991, she was taking alprazolam about every two weeks. She was continuing to have some spasms. She continued to try cannabis illicitly but had not yet obtained it legally. June 14, 1991, she had lost her driver's license due to visual problems associated with MS. During this interval there were more marital issues. July 2, 1991, it was indicated the patient was legally blind and there were no possible corrective measures. Plans were in place to obtain legal cannabis for spasticity and nervous problems. It was noted that cannabis seemed to be very effective for her clinically. August 7, 1991, the patient was still without a supply and complained of her legs jerking at night and increased difficulty walking. The patient requested Marinol, but this could not be prescribed. She was given baclofen 5 mg tid to try.

August 30, 1991, she received her fist shipment of NIDA cannabis, seven months after approval of the Compassionate IND. The patient was advised that she should confine her use to government cannabis. She was having problems with her gait, able to walk only with a cane. There were continued vision problems. She complained of left-sided weakness. The patient smoked a cannabis cigarette in front of the doctor, which led to her feeling better. It was suggested she try three cannabis cigarettes a day. September 3, 1991, the patient reported that the government supply of cannabis did not have the "punch" that street-bought material had. Her dose was increased to five joints a day. It was indicated that her spasticity responded positively to the dose increase. September 11, 1991, the patient was on five NIDA cigarettes a day. This was helping her spasticity. She was unclear as to whether her vision was helped. September 20, 1991, it was felt that seven cigarettes a day would be necessary. The patient reported increased muscular activity, uncontrollable at times. October 2, 1991, the patient had run out and was noticeably more spastic on examination. Her dose was increased to ten a day. October 9, 1991, the patient was on ten cannabis cigarettes a day of the strongest available dosage, which seemed to help her spasticity. She was walking without a cane. It was not felt that her depression was improved. November 4, 1991, she had been out of her supply for ten days. Spasticity increased and she complained of pain in the left leg. Increased tone was noted throughout the body. December 5, 1991, apparently a supply came in of lower potency cannabis. December 19, 1991, it was felt she had continued improvement of her spasticity with better gait. February 14, 1992, she was using 1 can of cannabis a month, equal to 300 cigarettes. The patient reported she had not been falling. March 13, 1992, she continued the cannabis at the same rate, plus 40 mg of fluoxetine and no alprazolam. The patient reported she was able to walk, swim better, and do all of her ADLs much easier than she could prior to the cannabis. There was no observable gait disturbance on exam.

April 14, 1992, it was felt that she got a lot of relief from her medicine and that it "probably offers her greater efficacy in her spasticity, also, than Valium would." May 19, 1992, the patient continued to be stable with no exacerbations of her MS and the spasticity under good control. There were concerns about periodontal disease from her dentist. It was thought she might do better with less smoking of a higher potency supply. The patient was also smoking cigarettes and was subsequently advised to avoid tobacco. By July 17, 1992, she continued to respond to cannabis. September 18, 1992, reflexes were equal and not hyperactive. November 16, 1992, there was an increase of depression slowly and insidiously. December 9, 1992, the patient had been off of her treatment for a week and was very shaky. Smoking a joint in front of her doctor caused her to become calm, less shaky and better able to walk. January 19, 1993, she got her first cans of the stronger cannabis, which the patient felt more effective after smoking one joint. March 22, 1993, she was smoking six to seven a day. She seemed better after smoking one in the office. April 22, 1993, the patient was smoking ten cigarettes a day. Smoking produced a decrease in spasticity as observed. There were no adverse effects that were noted in the office. May 24, 1993, the patient was tried on lorazepam. June 24, 1993, the patient was upset with financial issues and was placed on Mellaril (thioridazine). July 22, 1993, when she was examined, no tremor or spasticity was noted. Again cannabis was smoked with no adverse effects noted. August 30, 1993, the patient requested a decrease in her fluoxetine. She felt that spasticity and depression were both helped by the cannabis. September 29, 1993, the patient reported that on a lower fluoxetine dose she was getting tearful. Reflexes were not hyperactive. November 2, 1993, the patient had some paresthesias on the left side, but was maintaining good motor control. December 28, 1993, she was tried on bupropion. January 4, 1994, problems had been noted on bupropion and it was not as effective. She was tried on sertraline. She reported that the cannabis helped her to not think about her MS. She was having fewer spasticity problems.

February 4, 1994, when the patient smoked cannabis in the office, she seemed to be a little more talkative and relax significantly with less spasticity and no adverse effects. February 28, 1994, again significant relief from spasticity was noted upon smoking. March 30, 1994, the patient had some numbness and tingling in the limbs. The patient reported the new material was stronger and had a better effect. May 9, 1994, some increase in emotional lability was noted. The patient was taken off of sertraline and put on Effexor (venlafaxine). May 25, 1994, she was unable to tolerate the latter and was started back on fluoxetine. August 29, 1994, she continued on fluoxetine and cannabis. Smoking a joint calmed her and limited tremor. September 28, 1994, it was indicated in relation to cannabis "it seems to have a positive effect on her mental status overall." October 31, 1994, the patient was felt to be without signs of depression. She actually lowered her dose on a higher potency material. February 1, 1995, the patient was on diazepam again. February 14, 1995, she was increasingly shaky and tearful. March 29, 1995, she was hardly able to walk due to an exacerbation. May 2, 1995, she still needed support. At the same time the patient was having marital difficulties. August 4, 1995, the patient reported she could see much better with the cannabis. By September 6, 1995, she was walking quite well and was no longer on diazepam, merely the fluoxetine and cannabis. October 4, 1995, she continued to walk well with no problems.

January 17, 1996, an MRI revealed multiple bilateral periventricular and diffuse white matter changes in the cerebrum and cerebellum, but seemingly fewer than on a April 4, 1995, study.

April 19, 1996, the patient had been out of cannabis for a week and was experiencing more spasticity and ambulation difficulties. She was more depressed. May 17, 1996, the patient had been tried on a stimulant. July 10, 1996, the patient reported that cannabis was the only thing that had helped her with her symptoms over the course of her illness.

By September 25, 1996, the patient had been without medicine for a month and had to buy it on the street. She had lost weight and her condition had reportedly decompensated to some degree. The patient reported a ten-pound weight loss. November 13, 1996, the patient was having difficulty sleeping, but did not wish to take trazodone. November 27, 1996, the patient had fallen and had a brief loss of consciousness. December 5, 1996, she had had an episode of spasticity that was the worse she had ever had, starting in the neck and going down her back. January 8, 1997, cannabis came in after a summer drought since September 25. An emergency supply was requested. January 22, 1997, the patient remained concerned about lack of cannabis supply. February 5, 1997, she continued with this concern. February 19, 1997, there was discussion of difficulty the patient had experienced with the authorities in an airport. April 2, 1997, it was felt the patient continued to get a great deal of relief from smoking 10 joints a day without any adverse effects. July 2, 1997, the patient was observed to become more loquacious and interactive after dosing.

January 29, 1998, the patient was not complaining of spasticity, seeming to have considerable relief with cannabis. Her fluoxetine was lowered to 20 mg a day. March 24, 1998, it was felt that she had a very slow progression of her MS helped by her consumption of cannabis. September 22, 1998, the patient said that the medicine took away her fear of the disease and when she would get a pain she would be able to smoke and take it away.

October 27, 1998, she apparently had been out of her supply for six weeks, but had gotten by smoking only four cigarettes a day instead of the usual ten. January 24, 1998, the patient was doing relatively well and was walking with a cane. December 22, 1998, she was having increasing problems. January 26, 1999, the patient indicated that medicine helped her maintain her weight. March 24, 1999, it was observed, "I think her spasticity is being helped with the cannabis." April 23, 1999, she continued to get good relief with ten cigarettes a day. June 24, 1999, the patient reported some increasing difficulty with walking in the heat and hot weather. July 20, 1999, she was said to have no tremor or spasticity. September 1, 1999, she was having some exacerbation and difficulty walking and limping because her right leg was not working as well. October 20, 1999, the patient reported the only bad side effect would be when she smoked too much she would tend to go to sleep. She discussed alternative treatments for multiple sclerosis with her doctor and they agreed not to pursue them. November 19, 1999, the patient was walking on a wide base felt to be the result of a mild exacerbation. November 24, 1999, neurological examination confirmed greater ataxia. Methylphenidate was prescribed.

December 1, 1999, an MRI of the brain was said to reveal multiple focal white matter changes in bilateral cerebral areas especially in the basal ganglia and in the cerebellar peduncle, compatible with MS.

January 12, 2000, the patient was tried on Ritalin (methylphenidate). She was switched to Remeron (mirtazapine) from fluoxetine. February 22, 2000, the patient reported that her eyes were improved. March 9, 2000, visual acuity was 20/200 OD and 20/80 OS. April 6, 2000, it was felt that she had no declines in function from cannabis use.

June 27, 2000, her cannabis had been late coming in and she had cut from ten to six or seven cigarettes a day, feeling that that had hurt her physically and that she was not walking as well. January 31, 2001, the patient was a little bit down and labile, but by February 28, 2001, she was not depressed or hyper. April 11, 2001, she was having some trouble walking due to a flare of symptoms, which had been present for a month, but she noted no changes in vision.

When the patient was interviewed by EBR (June 2001), she reported that her vision was currently clear with cannabis. She was able to ambulate without aids, but has to stop after a block or less due to weakness. She swims a few days a week. She feels that there is no nystagmus in her vision and no diplopia. She characterizes her MS as mildly progressive.

The patient indicated that she received the cannabis legally in 1991 and continues to smoke ten cigarettes a day. She currently receives material of 3.5 percent THC content that was processed April 1999. Her study physician requests the highest potency material available, which has recently varied between 2.9-3.7 percent THC. When she uses outside cannabis of higher potency, she feels that she gets twice the relaxation. There is no chronic cough or other difficulties. The patient feels that Marinol at 10 mg was too strong. She used it for six months before the cannabis. Customarily she splits each of her supplied cigarettes in two, and manicures it slightly. When she is not on cannabis she has had no withdrawal symptoms, but has had increase in movement problems.

The patient has had a tubal ligation. She continues to menstruate on a regular monthly basis. Her main problems have been depression and some degree of anxiety. I asked about other diagnoses and she replied that she had "ten personalities and they are all feeling fine!" She denied history of diabetes, thyroid problems, meningitis, encephalitis, head trauma or seizures. The patient remains on fluoxetine 40 mg a day. She is allergic to penicillin. The patient had one year of college. She is right-handed.

Family history is noteworthy for father having narcolepsy and a sister who is bipolar.

Social history. She had one child by choice. The patient is a retired clothier and is unable to work at this time. She is currently smoking 1/2 pack of cigarettes a day, previously 1 pack a day, and has smoked since age 20. The patient does not drink at all, has not for five years, nor has she ever had a problem with alcohol. She does not drink coffee. She customarily sleeps eight hours.

Medical test results. The patient is 5 feet tall and 97 pounds (BMI: 19). On pulmonary function tests, an FVC was 79 percent of predicted, and FEV_1 76 percent of predicted. The FEV_1/FVC was 86 (Table 20.2). There was felt to be no obstruction based on this ratio or analysis of the F/V curve morphology. Early small airway disease and borderline restrictive disease (e.g., due to MS) were not excluded.

A CBC was wholly within normal limits. An absolute lymphocyte count was 2.3 with CD4 of 58 percent and CD4 absolute count of 1325 (Table 20.3). An endocrine battery was performed, with values of FSH, LH, prolactin, estradiol, estrone, estrogen, testosterone and progesterone, all within normal limits for age an gender (pre-menopausal female) (Table 20.4).

Neuropsychological tests were performed in her home on June 17, 2001. Some confusion was noted throughout the evaluation and significant fatigue over the course of the day was also apparent. She did not have significant difficulty with instructions, however, and effort and cooperation were sufficient to obtain what is believed to be valid data. As a result of significant visual deficits, many visually based tests were omitted and interpretations from those requiring significant visual input were provided in a very cautious manner. For example, this patient required a magnifying glass in order to accomplish the Picture Completion and Trails subtests that very likely had a significant negative impact on her overall performance.

On the WAIS-III, the patient obtained a Verbal IQ of 93. A Performance IQ was not calculated secondary to significant visual deficits that interfered with assessment in this realm. On the WMS-III, the patient performed, on verbal measures, in the Low Average Range. Immediate auditory memory was at the eighteenth percentile, with an auditory delayed index in the Average Range. Her ability to acquire non-thematically-organized verbal material was in the mildly impaired range relative to age-matched peers, but her retention was actually very good. Also, she did very well on a test measuring her ability to acquire verbal paired associates with a learning slope actually in the above average range, and excellent retention. Her ability to acquire more detailed and non-thematically-organized verbal information was moderately-to-severely impaired relative to age-matched peers. Overall performances on the CVLT ranged from two to five standard deviations below expected levels. Numerous intrusions during both free and cued recall were noted at levels above and beyond what is generally seen in the normative population. She made eight false-positive errors on recognition testing, which are also an abnormally high number of errors.

Concentration was noted to be markedly impaired in this patient, following the mildly to moderately impaired range overall. Assessment of Executive Functions reveals that abstract concept formation and logical analysis abilities were significantly reduced, falling in the moderately impaired range overall. The patient was also noted to be quite perseverative, having difficulty shifting cognitive strategies. In slight contrast, flexibility of thought as measured by the Similarities Subtest from the WAIS-III, was within normal limits. Verbal Fluency was within normal limits relative to age and education-matched peers.

In summary, this patient appears to have decrements in concentration, low average learning, and memory efficiency for new thematic material and verbal paired associates. Her ability to acquire more detailed and non-thematically-organized verbal information is at least moderately impaired. Memory functions, however, appear to be normal in the sense that once she acquires information, she seems to hold it quite effectively. Higher level executive functions are reduced at a moderate level despite a very remarkable psychiatric history. Responses to the BDI-II were well within normal limits.

Patient D thus demonstrates numerous neurocognitive impairments. The general pattern is not particularly uncommon in the context of multiple sclerosis and significant psychiatric dysfunction. This profile, when combined with the others from the data set do not provide any consistent pattern that one could reasonably ascribe to the therapeutic use of cannabis.

Review of Neuropsychological and Cognitive Data

The scientific study of the effects of chronic cannabis on cognition has remained problematical since such concerns were first raised. Despite intensive effort in this regard, little in the way of "hard findings" or consistent results has emerged. A complete review of alleged problems is beyond the scope of this article, but a few citations are meritorious.

In the Jamaican studies (Rubin and Comitas 1975), 19 neuropsychological tests were administered to chronic cannabis users and controls with no major significant differences between groups. In fact, ganja smokers scored the highest on Wechsler Adult Intelligence Scale (WAIS) Digit Span performance ($p < 0.05$). The authors concluded (p. 119), "in a wide variety of human abilities, there is no evidence that long-term use of cannabis is related to chronic impairment."

In Greece (Kokkevi and Dornbush 1977), no differences were noted between hashish users and age and socio-economically matched controls in total or Performance IQ (PIQ) scores on the WAIS. Controls performed better on three subtests: Comprehension ($p < 0.01$), Similarities ($p < 0.005$), and Digit Symbol Substitution ($p < 0.05$). Control Verbal IQ (VIQ) surpassed that of users ($p < 0.05$). However, these results must be viewed in light of the fact that normal population studies in Greece revealed PIQ:VIQ differences of 7 points. Thus, the authors concluded (p. 46), "These observations do not provide evidence of deterioration of mental abilities in the hashish users."

In Costa Rica, an extensive battery of neuropsychological measures showed no pathological changes (Carter 1980). It was observed (p. 188), "we failed to uncover significant differences between user and nonuser groups—even in those subjects who had consumed cannabis for over eighteen years."

Subsequently follow-up studies were performed on some of this cohort, and certain significant differences were claimed, including learning of word lists and selective and divided attention tasks (Fletcher et al. 1996). However, a detailed critical analysis of those results in *Marijuana Myths, Marijuana Facts* (Zimmer and Morgan 1997) seems to deflate any such claim.

Lyketsos et al. (1999) studied effects of cannabis on cognition in 1318 adults over a period of 12 years. No differences were noted in the degree of decline between heavy, light, and non-users of cannabis on the Mini-Mental State Examination (MMSE). Critics have indicated that the latter represents too crude a tool to measure the issue properly.

In a series of studies in the 1990's summarized in a book, *Cannabis and Cognitive Functioning* (Solowij 1998), Nadia Solowij studied subjects employing cannabis at least twice a week on average for a period of three years. After a review of data, the author stated (p. 227), "the weight of the evidence suggests that the long-term use of cannabis does not result in any severe or grossly debilitating impairment of cognitive function." She did note more subtle difficulties in attention parameters including distraction, loose associations and intrusion errors in memory tasks. In a recent review of cognitive effects of cannabis (Solowij and Grenyer 2001), it was observed (p. 275), "the long term risks for most users are not severe and their effects are relatively subtle."

Results from the current study seem to indicate similar findings. As part of a Comprehensive Neuropsychological Evaluation, all subjects were administered a battery of instruments including the WAIS-III, the WMS-III, the CVLT, the Trail Making Test A and B, Grooved Peg Board, Finger Tapping, and Category Test, the Controlled Oral Word Association Test, the Thurstone Word Fluency Test, a Category Fluency Test (Animal Naming), the WCST, the CPT-II, and the Beck Depression Inventory, 2nd Edition (BDI-II).

Comparing Patients A-D, it appears that all four do have at least mild difficulty with attention and concentration, and verbal acquisition of varying complex new verbal material (as measured on the CVLT), which is at least minimally impaired. Importantly, however, higher-level executive functions generally appear to be within normal limits in two of the subjects.

Difficulties in attention and concentration as well as new complex verbal learning may be directly related, and must be understood in the context of not only these subjects' chronic cannabis use, but also their underlying chronic diseases and clinical syndromes, with attendant fatigue and preoccupation. Interestingly, depressive symptoms are not currently noted at a clinical level in any of the subjects despite their chronic medical conditions or long-term cannabis use. None displayed evidence of social withdrawal or apathy characteristic of the alleged "amotivational syndrome." Rather, all were animated, engaging in conversation and demonstrating an active involvement with their ongoing care and the current research.

Overall, once more, no significant attributable neuropsychological sequelae are noted due to chronic cannabis usage.

Review of Neuroimaging

In 1971, it was reported that "consistent cannabis smoking" of 3 to 11 years in 10 patients produced evidence for cerebral atrophy employing air encephalography (Campbell et al. 1971), an excruciatingly painful and long-abandoned technique. Subsequent study by Kuehnle et al. (1977) employing CT scans on 19 men with long durations of heavy cannabis usage failed to show any changes in the ventricles or subarachnoid spaces. They criticized the prior study for lacking controls on antecedent head trauma or other causes of neurological damage. In the same issue of the *Journal of the American Medical Association,* Co et al. (1977) studied an additional 12 heavy cannabis smokers who displayed no CT abnormalities.

In 1983, an additional 12 subjects who smoked more than 1 g of cannabis daily for 10 years were studied by CT scans of the brain, and only one with concomitant history of alcoholism showed any abnormalities compared to controls (Hannerz and Hindmarsh 1983).

Most recently, Block et al. (2000) employed automated imaging analysis with MRI to examine 18 young heavy users of cannabis. No abnormalities were ascertained. The authors stated (p. 495), "frequent marijuana use does not produce clinically apparent MRI abnormalities or detectable global or regional changes in brain tissue volumes of gray or white matter, or both combined." It was recently noted (Solowij and Grenyer 2001, p. 270), "There is no evidence from human studies of any structural brain damage following prolonged exposure to cannabinoids."

Despite this additional documentation, the claim of brain damage and cerebral atrophy remains a popular myth in prohibitionist rhetoric.

Current MRI studies on Patients A-C with a General Electric Sigma LX MR 1.5 Tesla magnet system reveal no clear abnormalities. Patient A had age-compatible atrophy, and Patient C had minor tissue changes of a non-specific nature, commonly seen in middle-aged populations. Patient D has previously demonstrated MRI brain lesions consistent with MS, with possible improvement observed during the period of clinical cannabis usage.

Review of Neurophysiology Tests

In discussing the issue of cannabis and cerebral effects, Homer Reed observed (Reed 1975, pp. 122-123), "The association between many of the

EEG measures used to indicate CNS changes and the clinical condition of the patient is approximately zero." That not withstanding, various researchers have advanced numerous claims of pertinent EEG changes due to cannabis. Cohen (1976) noted differences in computerized EEG measures of delta band power and theta band phase angle (lead/lag) relationship. No mention was made of the alleged significance of these tests, or of the results of standard EEG.

All the Jamaican subjects had EEG examinations (Rubin and Comitas 1975). As previously noted in other studies, 9 of 30 cannabis smokers had significant low voltage fast activity in the beta range. Although this finding may indicate sedative effects of medication, it is often ascribed to a normal variant. Three of the 30 were said to have unequivocal focal abnormalities, but 4 of 30 controls had similar findings, and another had diffuse abnormalities. Overall, no significant differences were noted between ganja smokers and controls.

Similarly, in Greece (Panayiotopoulos et al. 1977), 8.8 percent of 46 hashish smokers had abnormal EEGs, while 15 percent of 40 normal controls were so characterized. The authors stated (p. 62), "We failed to find either an abnormality or an particular EEG change in the resting EEG records of chronic hashish users."

Current results, performed on a 21-channel Nicolet Voyageur digital EEG system and read by EBR, confirm the presence of low voltage fast activity in Patients A-C, and intermittent sharp waves and rare subtle slowing in the left frontal area in Patient A. Age appropriate atrophy was seen in the same patient on MRI, but she has no history of seizures or CNS insults. There are no corresponding abnormalities on neurological examination. Similar abnormalities are identified on EEGs of 6 percent of patients, whereas there is only a 0.5 percent prevalence of seizure disorders in the general population. In essence, no EEG pathology of an attributable nature seems apparent in the study group on the basis of cannabis usage.

With respect to P300 responses, a type of electrophysiological event related potential, even greater caution is necessary. This parameter is offered as an electrophysiological measure of memory, inasmuch as prolongation of its latency occurs with age. The test was popular in the 1980s as an objective test for dementia. Amplitude differences have also been noted in different clinical conditions (Carillo-de-la-Pena and Cadaviera 2000), but were termed (Spehlmann 1985, p. 370), "of uncertain diagnostic importance because of the great normal variability of the P300 amplitude." Overall, these issues and significant incidence of false positives and false negatives have largely relegated use of this technique to the sidelines as a clinical tool.

Solowij (1998) studied the P300 in chronic cannabis users vs. controls, and noted results felt to be indicative of (p. 150), "inefficient processing of information and impaired selective attention." These consisted of reduced processing negativity to relevant attended stimuli, inappropriately large processing negativity to a source of complex irrelevant stimuli, and reduced P300 amplitude to attended target stimuli to that of controls.

In contrast, Patrick et al. (1995) examined the P300 in psychologically normal chronic cannabis users and controlled the data for age. Results showed no amplitude differences.

More recent studies have shown significant reductions in P300 ampli-tude in schizophrenia (Martin-Loeches et al. 2001), but also in cigarette smokers (Anokhin et al. 2000), with notable effects according to motiva-tional instructions (Carrillo-de-la-Pena and Cadaveira 2000), and even di-urnal variations (Higuchi et al. 2000).

Our study employed a Nicolet Viking 3P 4-channel system with a P300 oddball paradigm. Patients A-C displayed P300 latencies that were well within norms for age-matched controls (Figure 20.1).

Review of Pulmonary Issues

Pulmonary concerns remain paramount in relation to chronic cannabis smoking. Excellent recent reviews are available (Zimmer and Morgan 1997; Tashkin 2001a,b). In brief, cannabis smoking produces an increase in cough and bronchitis symptoms, but to a lesser degree than in tobacco smokers (Sherrill et al. 1991). Daily cannabis smokers seek medical care for smoking-associated health concerns at a slightly higher rate than nonsmok-ers (Polen et al. 1993). In a large epidemiological study, cannabis use was associated with little statistical association on total mortality in women, and non-AIDS mortality in men (Sidney et al. 1997).

One of the primary associated risks of tobacco smoking is the develop-ment of emphysema and lesser declines in bronchial function over time. A careful longitudinal study of chronic smokers has demonstrated a longitudi-nal decline in the FEV_1 in tobacco smokers, but not heavy cannabis smokers (Tashkin et al. 1997).

Some association of cannabis smoking has been observed to head and neck cancers (Zhang et al. 1999), and pre-cancerous cytological changes have been noted in the lungs in bronchoscopy studies (Fligiel et al. 1988), but to date, no cases of pulmonary carcinoma have been noted in cannabis-only smokers.

In examining the data from chronic cannabis use studies, in Jamaica, a slight downward trend not attaining statistical significance was noted on forced vital capacity (FVC) values (Rubin and Comitas 1975). A similar downward trend was observed on FEV_1 without statistical significance. No differences between cannabis smokers, occasional smokers and non-smokers were observed on FEV_1/FVC ratios. Results of all tests may have been affected by concomitant tobacco usage.

The Greek studies did not closely examine pulmonary function, and although an increase in bronchitis symptoms was noted in hashish smokers over abstainers, the former group also smoked more tobacco. Differences were not statistically significant in any event (Boulougouris, Antypas, and Panayiotopoulos 1977).

In the Costa Rican studies, no spirometry measures were significantly different between cannabis users and non-users. However, statistical trends were, in fact, positive with respect to cannabis usage. Cannabis smokers displayed larger indices of small-airway patency. The authors suggested that in concomitant smoking of tobacco, cannabis seemed to counteract the expected effects of tobacco on small airways. The author stated (Carter 1980, p. 171), "at least it cannot be said of the users that they have suffered an additive of [*sic*-"or"] synergistic decrement in pulmonary function over that attributable to tobacco alone."

In our Patients A-C, no ultimate chest radiographic changes of significance were noted, despite a false-positive reading of pulmonary nodule in Patient C. It is of particular note that he has had a previous bronchoscopy procedure with no reported cytological changes.

Observed pulmonary function values in this cohort reveal no clear trends except a slight downward trend in FEV_1 and FEV_1/FVC ratios, and perhaps an increase in FVC (Patients A-C) (Table 20.2). Concomitant tobacco smoking (Patients A, B, and D) complicates analysis. It is particularly interesting that Patient B, a current concomitant smoker of tobacco displayed the best spirometry values, while those in Patient C, a never-smoker of tobacco were the worst. His underlying connective tissue disease may have played an active role in this finding. His use of the lowest grade cannabis and highest amount per day are the more likely explanation.

Significant questions remain as to the role of low-grade NIDA cannabis as a contributor to the above findings, which will subsequently discussed.

Review of Hematological Studies

No effects on complete blood counts or hemoglobin were observed in the LaGuardia Commission report (Mayor's committee on marihuana, Wallace and Cunningham 1944). In the Jamaican studies, slight increases were observed in hematocrit and hemoglobin readings in cannabis smokers over controls, but results were affected by concomitant tobacco use (Rubin and Comitas 1975). No hematological data was obtained from the Greek studies.

In Costa Rica, a downward trend was observed in hematocrit readings of cannabis smokers, but this was not statistically noteworthy (Carter 1980).

In our studies (Table 20.3), Patient B, a concomitant tobacco smoker, displayed a mild degree of polycythemia and slightly elevated WBC. No other hematological changes of any type were evident in the other three patients.

Review of Immunological Parameters

Immune system damage remains an area of contention with respect to cannabis usage (Zimmer and Morgan 1997), but one in which there is considerably more heat than light. A closer examination of the available literature may allay concern.

In the chronic use studies in Jamaica, no decrement was observed in cannabis smokers versus controls in either lymphocyte or neutrophils counts (Rubin and Comitas 1975). Neither were significant changes noted in the data in Costa Rica (Carter 1980).

In the 94-Day Cannabis Study, initial acute low values were observed in T cell counts, but these returned to normal over the course of the testing (Cohen 1976).

A closer examination of the pertinent literature raises concerns on theoretical levels to a greater degree than practical ones. Excellent reviews are available (Klein, Friedman, and Specter 1998; Hollister 1992; Cabral 2001a,b).

Early reports of inhibition of cell mediated immunity in cannabis smokers (Nahas et al. 1974) were refuted by later studies in which no impairment of lymphocytic response to phytohemagglutinin in hashish smokers was observed (Kaklamani et al. 1978).

A seminal review of the topic was undertaken by Hollister (1992), who stated (p. 159), "evidence of altered immune functions is derived mainly from in vitro tests or ex vivo experiments, which employed doses of cannabinoids far in excess of those that prevail during social use of marijuana." More recently, Klein, Friedman and Specter (1998) have similarly noted (p. 102), "Although cannabinoids modulate immune cell function, it is also clear that these cells are relatively resistant to the drugs in than many effects appear to be relatively small and totally reversible, occur at concentration higher than needed to induce psychoactivity (> 10 μM or > 5 mg/kg), and occur following treatment with nonpsychoactive cannabinoid analogues." They added (p. 102), "The public health risk of smoking marijuana in terms of increased susceptibility to infections, especially opportunistic infections, is still unclear." Finally, despite concerns raised by THC effects on immunity in animals and in vitro, Cabral and Dove Pettit (1998) admitted (p. 116), "Definitive data which directly link marijuana use to increased susceptibility to infection in humans currently is unavailable."

A particular public health concern surrounds cannabis effects on HIV/AIDS. Four studies among others may reduce related concern. Kaslow et al. (1989) demonstrated no evidence that cannabis accelerated immunodeficiency parameters in HIV-positive patients. Di Franco et al. (1996) ascertained no acceleration of HIV to full-blown AIDS in cannabis smokers. Whitfield, Bechtel and Starich (1997) observed no deleterious effects of cannabis usage in HIV/AIDS patients, even those with the lowest CD4 counts. Finally, Abrams et al. (2000) studied the effects of cannabis smoking on HIV-positive patients on protease inhibitor drugs in a prospective randomized, partially blinded placebo-controlled trial. No adverse effects on CD4 counts were observed secondary to cannabis.

In our studies of four subjects (Table 20.3), Patient B had an elevated WBC count, probably attributable to the stress of phlebotomy, but without accompanying disorders of cell count differential. All patients had CD4 counts well within normal limits.

Review of Endocrine Function

Topical reviews of this topic are contained in two recent publications (Murphy 2001; Zimmer and Morgan 1997). As with other physiological systems, much data is based on animal studies, and early claims of deleterious effects on acute endocrine function are not necessarily supported by subsequent investigations or chronic use studies.

One long-held claim is the production of gynecomastia in males associated with cannabis use. A case study or three cannabis smokers with this malady was reported by Harmon and Aliapoulios (1972). A more thorough investigation a few years later failed to show any differences in cannabis use in affected males between users and controls (Cates and Pope 1977).

Similarly, Kolodny et al. (1974) reported decreased testosterone levels in chronic marijuana smokers, while no differences in testosterone or luteinizing hormone (LH) levels were identified in a three-week trial of smokers versus nonsmokers (Mendelson et al. 1978).

LH levels in menopausal women showed no significant changes after cannabis usage (Mendelson et al. 1985), but the next year, a similar group noted a 30 percent suppression of LH in women by smoking a single cannabis cigarette during the luteal phase (Mendelson et al. 1986).

Subsequently, a more in-depth study of both sexes was undertaken to assess multiple hormone effects comparing subjects with different levels of cannabis usage versus controls (Block, Farinpour, and Schlechte 1991). No significant effects were noted on testosterone, LH, FSH, prolactin or cortisol in young women and men.

Jamaican chronic use studies were confined to examinations of thyroxine and steroid excretion with no significant findings observed due to cannabis use (Rubin and Comitas 1975).

In the 94-Day Cannabis Study, acute drops in testosterone and LH levels were noted after smoking a cannabis cigarette (Cohen 1976). Subsequent drops in testosterone levels were noted after the fifth week of daily usage. LH levels fell after the fourth week and FSH after the eighth week to unspecified degrees.

In Costa Rica, no differences were noted in male testosterone levels between abstainers and cannabis smokers stratified according to amount of use (Carter 1980). Similarly, fertility was unimpaired, with both groups having identical numbers of progeny. The author stated (p. 172), "These findings cast serious doubt on cause-and-effect relationship between marihuana smoking and plasma testosterone level in long-term use."

Zimmer and Morgan (1997) summarized their observations by stating (p. 92), "There is no scientific evidence that marijuana delays adolescent sexual development, has a feminizing effect on males, or a masculinizing effect on females."

The latter statement would seem to be borne out by our findings. While one male subject had a minor degree of gynecomastia associated with obesity, none of the Patients A-D displayed any abnormal values in any endocrine measure (Table 20.4).

Patient A has two children, Patient B has three, and Patient D had one by choice.

Problems in the Compassionate IND Program

All four patients described varying degrees of logistical difficulties in obtaining their medicine. All have to travel or make special arrangements with their study physician, who is the arbiter of the potency of received material. All described incidents of inadequate supply or provision of inferior quality cannabis. All have had to supplement their supplies of cannabis from illegal black market sources at times.

All have experienced inconveniences or security concerns when traveling. One, Patient C, was arrested, detained, and had some of his medicine permanently confiscated without replacement.

Patients A through C decried the lack of an official identity card that might be readily recognized and accepted by law enforcement and security personnel. Rather, all used combinations of letters and other documents to convey their legal status to interested authorities, often to the accompaniment of much doubt and suspicion. All describe significant worry and anxiety about their medicine supplies, and whether official promises of continuation of the program will be honored.

A paramount issue affecting the Compassionate IND patients revolves around cannabis quality. It has been well established that recreational cannabis smokers prefer higher potency materials (Herning, Hooker, and Jones 1986; Chait and Burke 1994; Kelly et al. 1997). The same pertains for most clinical cannabis patients.

Chait and Pierri (1989) published a detailed analysis of NIDA marijuana cigarettes that is worthy of review in this context. NIDA marijuana is grown outside, one crop per biennium, harvested from a five-acre facility at the University of Mississippi. Average yield of "manicured material" is 270 g per plant at 9 square feet of canopy per plant, or 30 g per square foot (letter from NIDA, Steven Gust to Chris Conrad, August 18, 1999). Material is shipped to the Research Triangle Institute in North Carolina where it is chopped and rolled on modified tobacco cigarette machines, then stored partially dehydrated and frozen. Cigarettes average 800 to 900 g in weight. Material requires rehydration before usage, which the IND patients usually achieve by storage overnight in a refrigerated plastic bag with leaves of lettuce.

As of 1999 (letter, Steven Gust to EBR, June 7, 1999), NIDA had available cannabis cigarettes of 1.8, 2.8, 3.0, and 3.4 percent THC, and bulk cannabis of up to 5 percent THC content. Other cannabinoid components were not quantitated. It was further stated that the strongest material was not provided to patients in their cigarette shipments because it was too sticky and would interfere with the rolling machine's functioning (Personal Communication to EBR, Steven Gust, December 1999).

Static burn rates of NIDA cannabis cigarettes were inversely related to potency (Chait and Pierri 1989), while the number of puffs that could be drawn from each cigarette averaged 8.8. While total particulate matter increased with potency, arguably less smoked material is necessary for medicinal effect. Of more concern, carbon monoxide levels were highest in the lower potency material; that is, CO was inversely proportional to THC content. Finally, test subjects in their study of NIDA cannabis reported (pp. 66-67), "that the marijuana is inferior in sensory qualities (taste, harshness) than the marijuana that they smoke outside the laboratory. Some have stated that it was the worst marijuana they had ever sampled, or that it tasted 'chemically treated.'"

All the study patients criticize the paper employed to roll the cannabis cigarettes as harsh and tasting poorly. NIDA cannabis cigarettes resemble Pall Mall brand tobacco cigarettes without the logo (Figure 20.3).

All study patients clean their cannabis and reroll the material to varying degrees, although at least one former IND patient, now deceased, used the NIDA cigarettes unaltered.

NIDA cannabis is shipped to patients in labeled metal canisters containing 300 cigarettes (Figure 20.4), and material is frequently two or more years old upon receipt. Even under optimal storage conditions, a certain degree of oxidation of cannabinoids can be expected (Grotenhermen 2001b). Most consumers prefer a supply of cured cannabis that is as fresh as possible.

A close inspection of the contents of NIDA-supplied cannabis cigarettes reveals them to be a crude mixture of leaf with abundant stem and seed components (Figures 20.5 and 20.6). The odor is green and herbal in character. The resultant smoke is thick, acrid, and pervasive.

In contrast, a typical sinsemilla "bud" is seedless, covered with visible glandular trichomes, and emits a strong lemon or pine terpenoid scent. The smoke is also less disturbing from a sensory standpoint to most observers.

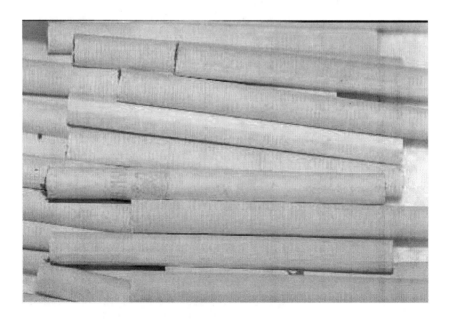

FIGURE 20.3. NIDA joints/Pall-Mall.

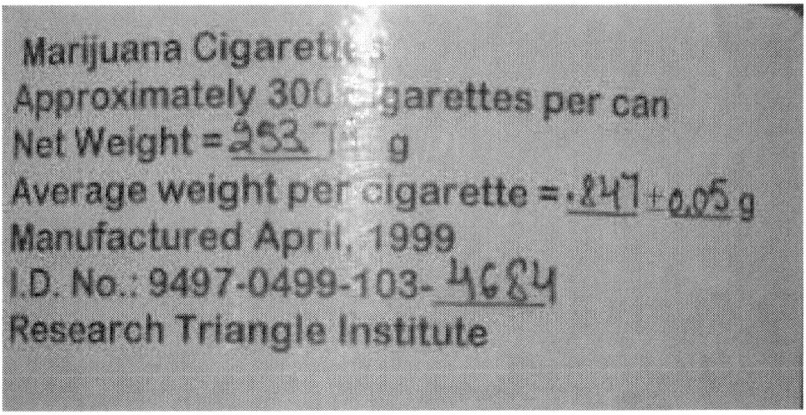

Marijuana Cigarett. .
Approximately 300 garettes per can
Net Weight = 253.7 : g
Average weight per cigarette = .847 ± 0.05 g
Manufactured April, 1999
I.D. No.: 9497-0499-103- 4684
Research Triangle Institute

FIGURE 20.4. Steel canister with label.

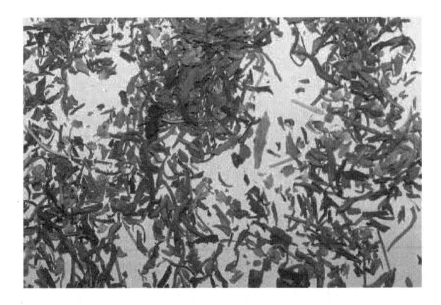

FIGURE 20.5. Loose NIDA cannabis as provided to compassionate IND patients.

Whittle, Guy, and Robson (2001) describe in detail the markedly contrasting steps undertaken in a government approved clinical cannabis program in the United Kingdom. Their material is organically grown in soil with no chemical treatment under controlled indoor conditions. All male

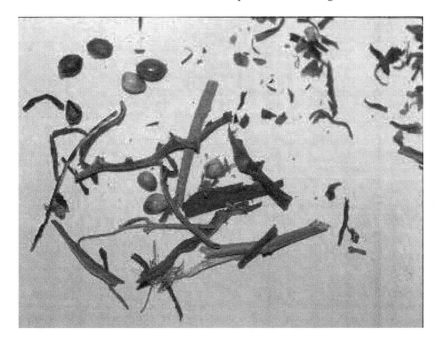

FIGURE 20.6. Close-up of debris from three NIDA cannabis cigarettes.

plants are eliminated, and only unfertilized female flowering tops are harvested for further processing. This material is assayed for cannabinoid and terpenoid content, with controlled ratios through genetic selection of seed strains before extraction. THC yields obtained are routinely 15 to 20 percent (personal communication, GW Pharmaceuticals, 2000).

Harm reduction techniques in relation to clinical cannabis consumption are well advanced (Russo 2001; Grotenhermen 2001a,b). Particular attention is merited toward vaporization techniques that provide cannabinoid and terpenoid component administration to prospective clinical cannabis patients without pyrolysis (Gieringer 1996a,b; Gieringer 2001). Sublingual administration of cannabis extracts is another most promising technique of clinical cannabis administration (Whittle, Guy, and Robson 2001).

Three of the four study subjects have employed Marinol, and found it inadequate or a poor substitute for cannabis in symptomatic relief of their clinical syndromes.

CONCLUSIONS AND RECOMMENDATIONS

1. Cannabis smoking, even of a crude, low-grade product, provides effective symptomatic relief of pain, muscle spasms, and intraocular pressure elevations in selected patients failing other modes of treatment.
2. These clinical cannabis patients are able to reduce or eliminate other prescription medicines and their accompanying side effects.
3. Clinical cannabis provides an improved quality of life in these patients.
4. The side effect profile of NIDA cannabis in chronic usage suggests some mild pulmonary risk.
5. No malignant deterioration has been observed.
6. No consistent or attributable neuropsychological or neurological deterioration has been observed.
7. No endocrine, hematological or immunological sequelae have been observed.
8. Improvements in a clinical cannabis program would include a ready and consistent supply of sterilized, potent, organically grown unfertilized female flowering top material, thoroughly cleaned of extraneous inert fibrous matter.
9. It is the authors' opinion that the Compassionate IND program should be reopened and extended to other patients in need of clinical cannabis.
10. Failing that, local, state and federal laws might be amended to provide regulated and monitored clinical cannabis to suitable candidates.

REFERENCES

Abrams, D., R. Leiser, T. Mitchell, J. Aberg, S. Deeks, and S. Shade. 2000. Short-term effects of cannabinoids in human immunodeficiency virus (HIV) infection: Clinical safety results. Paper read at 2000 Symposium on the Cannabinoids, June 23, 2000, at Hunt Valley, MD.

Anokhin, A. P., A. B. Vedeniapin, E. J. Sirevaag, L. O. Bauer, S. J. O'Connor, S. Kuperman, B. Porjesz, T. Reich, H. Begleiter, J. Polich, and J. W. Rohrbaugh. 2000. The P300 brain potential is reduced in smokers. *Psychopharmacology (Berl)* 149(4):409-413.

Block, R. I., R. Farinpour, and J. A. Schlechte. 1991. Effects of chronic marijuana use on testosterone, luteinizing hormone, follicle stimulating hormone, prolactin and cortisol in men and women. *Drug Alcohol Depend* 28(2):121-128.

Block, R. I., D. S. O'Leary, J. C. Ehrhardt, J. C. Augustinack, M. M. Ghoneim, S. Arndt, and J. A. Hall. 2000. Effects of frequent marijuana use on brain tissue volume and composition. *Neuroreport* 11(3):491-496.

Boulougouris, J., E. Antypas, and C. P. Panayiotopoulos. 1977. Medical studies in long-term hashish users: I. Physical and neurological examinations. In C. N. Stefanis, R. Dornbush, and M. Fink (eds.), *Hashish: Studies of long-term use* (pp. 55-58). New York: Raven Press.

Cabral, G. 2001a. Immune system. In F. Grotenhermen and E. B. Russo (eds.), *Cannabis and cannabinoids: Pharmacology, toxicology and therapeutic potential* (pp. 279-287). Binghamton, NY: The Haworth Press, Inc.

Cabral, G. A. 2001b. Marijuana and cannabinoids: Effects on infections, immunity and AIDS. *J Cannabis Therap* 1(3-4):61-85.

Cabral, G. A., and D. A. Dove Pettit. 1998. Drugs and immunity: Cannabinoids and their role in decreased resistance to infectious disease. *J Neuroimmunol* 83(1-2): 116-123.

Campbell, A. M., M. Evans, J. L. Thomson, and M. J. Williams. 1971. Cerebral atrophy in young cannabis smokers. *Lancet* 2(7736):1219-1224.

Carrillo-de-la-Pena, M. T., and F. Cadaveira. 2000. The effect of motivational instructions on P300 amplitude. *Neurophysiol Clin* 30(4):232-239.

Carter, W. E. 1980. *Cannabis in Costa Rica: A study of chronic marihuana use*. Philadelphia: Institute for the Study of Human Issues.

Cates, W., Jr., and J. N. Pope. 1977. Gynecomastia and cannabis smoking. A nonassociation among US Army soldiers. *Am J Surg* 134(5):613-615.

Chait, L. D., and K. A. Burke. 1994. Preference for high-versus low-potency marijuana. *Pharmacol Biochem Behav* 49(3):643-647.

Chait, L. D., and J. Pierri. 1989. Some physical characteristics of NIDA marijuana cigarettes. *Addict Behav* 14(1):61-67.

Co, B. T., D. W. Goodwin, M. Gado, M. Mikhael, and S. Y. Hill. 1977. Absence of cerebral atrophy in chronic cannabis users. Evaluation by computerized transaxial tomography. *J Amer Med Assoc* 237(12):1229-1230.

Cohen, S. 1976. The 94-day cannabis study. *Ann N Y Acad Sci* 282:211-220.

Di Franco, M. J., H. W. Sheppard, D. J. Hunter, T. D. Tosteson, and M. S. Ascher. 1996. The lack of association of marijuana and other recreational drugs with progression to AIDS in the San Francisco Men's Health Study. *Ann Epidemiol* 6(4):283-289.

Fletcher, J. M., J. B. Page, D. J. Francis, K. Copeland, M. J. Naus, C. M. Davis, R. Morris, D. Krauskopf, and P. Satz. 1996. Cognitive correlates of long-term cannabis use in Costa Rican men. *Arch Gen Psychiatry* 53(11):1051-1057.

Fligiel, S. E., H. Venkat, H. Gong, Jr., and D. P. Tashkin. 1988. Bronchial pathology in chronic marijuana smokers: A light and electron microscopic study. *J Psychoactive Drugs* 20(1):33-42.

Gieringer, D. 1996a. Waterpipe study. *Bull Multidisciplinary Assoc Psychedelic Stud* 6:59-63.

Gieringer, D. 1996b. Why marijuana smoke harm reduction? *Bull Multidisciplinary Assoc Psychedelic Stud* 6:64-66.

Gieringer, D. H. 2001. Cannabis "vaporization": A promising strategy for smoke harm reduction. *J Cannabis Therap* 1(3-4):153-170.

Grotenhermen, F. 2001a. Harm reduction associated with inhalation and oral administration of cannabis and THC. *J Cannabis Therap* 1 (3-4):133-152.

Grotenhermen, F. 2001b. Practical hints. In F. Grotenhermen and E. B. Russo (eds.), *Cannabis and cannabinoids: Pharmacology, toxicology and therapeutic potential* (pp.345-353). Binghamton, NY: The Haworth Press, Inc.

Hannerz, J., and T. Hindmarsh. 1983. Neurological and neuroradiological examination of chronic cannabis smokers. *Ann Neurol* 13(2):207-210.

Harmon, J., and M. A. Aliapoulios. 1972. Gynecomastia in marihuana users. *N Engl J Med* 287(18):936.

Hepler, R. S., and I. R. Frank. 1971. Marihuana smoking and intraocular pressure. *J Amer Med Assoc* 217(10):1392.

Herning, R. I., W. D. Hooker, and R. T. Jones. 1986. Tetrahydrocannabinol content and differences in marijuana smoking behavior. *Psychopharmacology* 90(2): 160-162.

Higuchi, S., Y. Liu, T. Yuasa, A. Maeda, and Y. Motohashi. 2000. Diurnal variation in the P300 component of human cognitive event-related potential. *Chronobiol Int* 17(5):669-678.

Hollister, L. E. 1992. Marijuana and immunity. *J Psychoactive Drugs* 24(2):159-164.

Indian Hemp Drugs Commission. 1894. *Report of the Indian Hemp Drugs Commission, 1893-94*. Simla: Govt. Central Print. Office.

Kaklamani, E., D. Trichopoulos, A. Koutselinis, M. Drouga, and D. Karalis. 1978. Hashish smoking and T-lymphocytes. *Arch Toxicol* 40(2):97-101.

Kaplan, J. (ed.) 1969. *Marijuana Report of the Indian Hemp Drugs Commission, 1893-1894*. Silver Spring, MD: Thos. Jefferson Pub. Co.

Kaslow, R. A., W. C. Blackwelder, D. G. Ostrow, D. Yerg, J. Palenicek, A. H. Coulson, and R. O. Valdiserri. 1989. No evidence for a role of alcohol or other psychoactive drugs in accelerating immunodeficiency in HIV-1-positive individuals. A report from the Multicenter AIDS Cohort Study. *J Amer Med Assoc* 261(23): 3424-3429.

Kelly, T. H., R. W. Foltin, C. S. Emurian, and M. W. Fischman. 1997. Are choice and self-administration of marijuana related to delta 9-THC content? *Exp Clin Psychopharmacol* 5(1):74-82.

Klein, T. W., H. Friedman, and S. Specter. 1998. Marijuana, immunity and infection. *J Neuroimmunol* 83(1-2):102-115.

Kokkevi, A., and R. Dornbush. 1977. Psychological test characteristics of long-term hashish users. In C. N. Stefanis, R. Dornbush and M. Fink (eds.), *Hashish: Studies of long-term use* (pp. 43-47). New York: Raven Press.

Kolodny, R. C., W. H. Masters, R. M. Kolodner, and G. Toro. 1974. Depression of plasma testosterone levels after chronic intensive marihuana use. *N Engl J Med* 290(16):872-874.

Kuehnle, J., J. H. Mendelson, K. R. Davis, and P. F. New. 1977. Computed tomographic examination of heavy marijuana smokers. *J Amer Med Assoc* 237(12): 1231-1232.

Lyketsos, C. G., E. Garrett, K. Y. Liang, and J. C. Anthony. 1999. Cannabis use and cognitive decline in persons under 65 years of age. *Am J Epidemiol* 149(9):794-800.

Martin-Loeches, M., V. Molina, F. Munoz, J. A. Hinojosa, S. Reig, M. Desco, C. Benito, J. Sanz, A. Gabiri, F. Sarramea et al. 2001. P300 amplitude as a possible correlate of frontal degeneration in schizophrenia. *Schizophr Res* 49(1-2):121-128.

Mayor's Committee on Marihuana, G. B. Wallace, and E. V. Cunningham. 1944. *The marihuana problem in the city of New York: Sociological, medical, psychological and pharmacological studies.* Lancaster, PA: Jaques Cattell Press.

Mendelson, J. H., P. Cristofaro, J. Ellingboe, R. Benedikt, and N. K. Mello. 1985. Acute effects of marihuana on luteinizing hormone in menopausal women. *Pharmacol Biochem Behav* 23(5):765-768.

Mendelson, J. H., J. Ellingboe, J. C. Kuehnle, and N. K. Mello. 1978. Effects of chronic marihuana use on integrated plasma testosterone and luteinizing hormone levels. *J Pharmacol Exp Ther* 207(2):611-617.

Mendelson, J. H., N. K. Mello, J. Ellingboe, A. S. Skupny, B. W. Lex, and M. Griffin. 1986. Marihuana smoking suppresses luteinizing hormone in women. *J Pharmacol Exp Ther* 237(3):862-866.

Murphy, L. 2001. Hormonal system and reproduction. In F. Grotenhermen and E. B. Russo (eds.), *Cannabis and cannabinoids: Pharmacology, toxicology and therapeutic potential* (pp. 289-297). Binghamton, NY: The Haworth Press, Inc.

Nahas, G. G., N. Suciu-Foca, J. P. Armand, and A. Morishima. 1974. Inhibition of cellular mediated immunity in marihuana smokers. *Science* 183(123):419-420.

Panayiotopoulos, C. P., J. Volavka, M. Fink, and C. N. Stefanis. 1977. II. Clinical electroencephalography and echoencephalography in long-term hashish users. In C. N. Stefanis, R. Dornbush and M. Fink (eds.), *Hashish: Studies of long-term use* (pp. 59-62). New York: Raven Press.

Pate, D. 1999. Anandamide structure-activity relationships and mechanisms of action on intraocular pressure in the normotensive rabbit model. Department of Pharmaceutical Chemistry, University of Kuopio, Finland.

Pate, D. 2001. Glaucoma and cannabinoids. In F. Grotenhermen and E. B. Russo (eds.), *Cannabis and cannabinoids: Pharmacology, toxicology and therapeutic potential* (pp. 215-224). Binghamton, NY: The Haworth Press, Inc.

Patrick, G., J. J. Straumanis, F. A. Struve, F. Nixon, M. J. Fitz-Gerald, J. E. Manno, and M. Soucair. 1995. Auditory and visual P300 event related potentials are not altered in medically and psychiatrically normal chronic marihuana users. *Life Sci* 56(23-24): 2135-2140.

Polen, M. R., S. Sidney, I. S. Tekawa, M. Sadler, and G. D. Friedman. 1993. Health care use by frequent marijuana smokers who do not smoke tobacco. *West J Med* 158(6):596-601.

Randall, R. C. 1991a. *Marijuana & AIDS: Pot, politics & PWA's in America*. Washington, DC: Galen Press.

Randall, R. C. (editor). 1991b. *Muscle spasm, pain & marijuana therapy: Testimony from federal and state court proceedings on marijuana's medical use in the treatment of multiple sclerosis, paralysis, and chronic pain*. Washington, DC: Galen Press.

Randall, R. C., and A. M. O'Leary. 1998. *Marijuana Rx: The patients' fight for medicinal pot*. New York: Thunder's Mouth Press.

Reed, H. B. C., Jr. 1975. Marijuana and brain dysfunction: Selected research issues. In J. R. Tinklenberg (ed.), *Marijuana and health hazards: Methodological issues in current research* (pp. 121-123). New York: Academic Press.

Rubin, Vera D., and Lambros Comitas. 1975. *Ganja in Jamaica: A medical anthropological study of chronic marihuana use*. The Hague: Mouton.

Russo, E. B. 2001. Role of cannabis and cannabinoids in pain management. In R. S. Weiner (ed.), *Pain management: A practical guide for clinicians* (pp. 357-375). Boca Raton, FL: CRC Press.

Sherrill, D. L., M. Krzyzanowski, J. W. Bloom, and M. D. Lebowitz. 1991. Respiratory effects of non-tobacco cigarettes: A longitudinal study in general population. *Int J Epidemiol* 20(1):132-137.

Sidney, S., J. E. Beck, I. S. Tekawa, C. P. Quesenberry, and G. D. Friedman. 1997. Marijuana use and mortality. *Am J Public Health* 87(4):585-590.

Solowij, N. 1998. *Cannabis and cognitive functioning, International research monographs in the addictions*. Cambridge; New York: Cambridge University Press.

Solowij, N., and B. F. S. Grenyer. 2001. Long term effects of cannabis on psyche and cognition. In F. Grotenhermen and E. B. Russo (eds.), *Cannabis and cannabinoids: Pharmacology, toxicology and therapeutic potential* (pp. 299-311). Binghamton, NY: The Haworth Press, Inc.

Spehlmann, Rainer. 1985. *Evoked potential primer: Visual, auditory, and somatosensory evoked potentials in clinical diagnosis*. Boston: Butterworth.

Stefanis, C. N., R. L. Dornbush, and M. Fink. 1977. *Hashish: Studies of long-term use*. New York: Raven Press.

Tashkin, D. P. 2001a. Effects of smoked marijuana on the lung and its immune defenses: Implications for medicinal use in HIV-infected patients. *J Cannabis Therap* 1(3-4):87-102.

Tashkin, D. P. 2001b. Respiratory risks from marijuana smoking. In F. Grotenhermen and E. B. Russo (eds.), *Cannabis and cannabinoids: Pharmacology, toxicology and therapeutic potential* (pp. 325-335). Binghamton, NY: The Haworth Press, Inc.

Tashkin, D. P., M. S. Simmons, D. L. Sherrill, and A. H. Coulson. 1997. Heavy habitual marijuana smoking does not cause an accelerated decline in FEV_1 with age. *Am J Respir Crit Care Med* 155(1):141-148.

Whitfield, R. M., L. M. Bechtel, and G. H. Starich. 1997. The impact of ethanol and Marinol/marijuana usage on HIV+/AIDS patients undergoing azidothymidine,

azidothymidine/dideoxycytidine, or dideoxyinosine therapy. *Alcohol Clin Exp Res* 21(1):122-127.

Whittle, B. A., G. W. Guy, and P. Robson. 2001. Prospects for new cannabis-based prescription medicines. *J Cannabis Therap* 1(3-4):183-205.

Zhang, Z. F., H. Morgenstern, M. R. Spitz, D. P. Tashkin, G. P. Yu, J. R. Marshall, T. C. Hsu, and S. P. Schantz. 1999. Marijuana use and increased risk of squamous cell carcinoma of the head and neck. *Cancer Epidemiol Biomarkers Prev* 8(12): 1071-1078.

Zimmer, L. E., and J. P. Morgan. 1997. *Marijuana myths, marijuana facts: A review of the scientific evidence.* New York: Lindesmith Center.

UPDATE

Ethan B. Russo

Despite due diligence by all, and the incredible capabilities of Haworth copy editors, mistakes are occasionally and inevitably apparent. Chris Conrad has pointed out to us one such error in the original publication in relation to a letter from Steven Gust regarding yields of cannabis from the farm at the University of Mississippi in Oxford. The actual figures should be 270 grams of cannabis harvested per plant at 9 square feet of canopy per plant, or 30 grams per square foot. Specifically, no distinction was made between the yield of cannabis leaf versus flower bud. The entire topic is clarified quite nicely in Chris Conrad's publication, *Cannabis Yields and Dosage,* available online at http://www.safeaccessnow.net/pdf/sanhandbook04.pdf.

All four patients discussed in this study remain on U.S.-government-supplied cannabis as of May 2005 and are basically stable with respect to their medical status.

Afterword

We hope that the preceding offering has proven valuable to its readers. We are proud that the *Journal of Cannabis Therapeutics* served in some small capacity to promote cognizance and recognition of the role of cannabinoids in current and future medical practice.

I would like to thank our many editorial board members and our contributors for their efforts in this regard, and add my admiration for Dr. Shrikrishna Singh and other staff members of the Journal Division of The Haworth Press for their incredible dedication and support to scholarship and the advancement of knowledge over the last several years.

The future of cannabis therapeutics is extremely promising in offering a better quality of life for millions of people with a wide variety of heretofore recalcitrant diseases and syndromes. We are pleased to be witness to its further development.

Ethan Russo

Handbook of Cannabis Therapeutics
© 2006 by The Haworth Press, Inc. All rights reserved.
doi:10.1300/5741_22

Index

Page numbers followed by the letter "b" indicate boxed material; those followed by the letter "i" indicate illustrations; those followed by the letter "t" indicate tables.

0-Archidonyl-ethanolamine
(virodhamine), 122
1,8 Cineole, 180t, 185-186
2-Arachidonylglycerol (2-AG)
biosynthesis pathways, 211, 212i,
213
chemical structure, 208i, 209
distinctive qualities, 211
as endocannabinoids, 122, 123,
123i, 208, 208i
in food substances, 230
and mammalian development, 231
physiopathological conditions,
213-215
recent research, 166
suckling response, 233-234
THC clinical studies, 130, 132
weight regulation, 229
2-Archidonylglyceryl ether (noladin
ether), 122
11-Hydroxy-Δ^9-tetrahydrocannabinol
(11-0H-THC)
first-pass metabolism, 171-172
metabolite, 133-134, 134i
11-nor-9-carboxy-THC (THC-COOH),
metabolite, 134, 134i

α-aminobutyric acid (GABA), 128-129,
129t
α-Pinene, 180t, 186
α-Terpineol, 181t, 186
Abortifacient, 338-339
Abortion, and HG, 284

Abrams, Donald, 308
Abscesses, 9
Absorption
cannabinoids, 190
of Δ^9-THC, 75-80, 76t, 77i, 78i
dermal administration, 80
eye drops, 79
inhalation route, 76t, 76-77, 77i, 103
of Nabilone, 100
oral administration, 75, 76t, 78i,
78-79, 103
and passive smoking, 77
rectal administration, 76t, 79
sublingual administration, 79, 103
Accomplia. See Rimonabant
(SR141716)
Acetylcholine, 128, 129t
Acetylsalicylic acid, 144
Acquired immunodeficiency syndrome
(AIDS)
brief history of, 303-304
cannabis impact studies, 436
Compassionate IND program,
402-403
ELISA test, 303
standard treatment of, 304-305
AIDS wasting syndrome
appetite enhancement, 1, 227-228,
249
indicator diseases, 304
Marinol treatment, 305
steroid treatments, 306
and testosterone enanthate, 250
Actuarius, John, 18
Ad Eunapium, 36, 38

Handbook of Cannabis Therapeutics
© 2006 by The Haworth Press, Inc. All rights reserved.
doi:10.1300/5741_23

Administration routes, modes of, 95-96, 97i, 97-98
Adolescents, drug experimentation, 389-390
Adverse effects. *See also* Side effects
  Levonantradol, 54
  Nabilone, 53
  Rimonabant (SR141716), 56
Aëtius, 25, 29, 35, 36-38
Africa, medical cannabis, 292
Agamenoi ôruontai, 26
AIDS. *See* Acquired immunodeficiency syndrome (AIDS)
Ajulemic acid (CT3)
  mechanism of action, 119
  metabolite activity, 134
  pharmacological effects, 136, 136i, 145
  synthetic cannabinoid, 54, 64
Al-Aqrabadhin A-Saghir, 317
Alakvarov, Farid, 318
Alcohol dependency
  harm of, 391, 392
  medical cannabis, 360
  risk of, 392t, 392-393
  and synthetic derivatives, 117
  withdrawal, 244b
Alexis I Comnenus, Emperor of Byzantium, 17
Allodynia, 56
Alpinus, Prosper, 47
Alzheimer disease, 57, 139, 166
AM-404, 137
Amenhotep I, Pharaoh of Egypt, 316
American Medical Association, 385
American Nurses Association, 389
American Society of Clinical Oncology, 247-248
Aminobutyric. *See* α-aminobutyric acid (GABA)
Amyotrophic lateral sclerosis, 57
Analgesic
  medical cannabis, 334
  medical marijuana, 244b, 252-253
Anandamide. *See* N-arachidonylethanolamide (anandamide)
"Anatolian hemp," 7
Anatomy of Melancholy, 47

Anglo Saxons
  cannabis cultivation, 45
  ob/gyn use, 318
Anorexia, 227
Anslinger, Harry, 385
Anti-inflammatory, 182, 244b
Anticonvulsant, 244b, 254-255
Antiemetic properties
  hemp, 10
  and HG symptoms, 284-285, 286
  medical marijuana, 244b, 245-248
Antiepileptic properties, 9
Antihypertensive, 244b
Antinausea preparation, 53
Antineoplastic properties
  basic research, 142
  drug interactions, 143
  medical marijuana, 244b
Antiparasitic properties, 10
Antipsychotic medications
  drug interactions, 143, 144
  metabolic interactions, 102-103
Antipsychotic properties, CBD, 173, 174t
Antipyretic properties
  ancient Arab practice, 10
  medical marijuana, 244b
Antiretroviral medications
  drug interactions, 143
  metabolic interactions, 103
Antispasmodic properties, 244b, 250-252
Antitussive properties, 244b
Anxiety disorders, 165
Apigenin, 187, 188t, 189
Appetite studies, 131, 139
Appetite enhancement
  and AIDS wasting, 1, 227-228, 249
  endocannabinoid system, 234-235
  and hypothalamus, 228-229
  of medical marijuana, 244b, 248-250
Arabia, medical studies, 5, 6-10, 316-317
Archarnians, The, 23, 27
Aristophanes, 23, 27
Aromatherapy, 309
Artemisia absinthium, 48, 179
Arthritis, 54, 141
Arvinil, 218, 219i

Ashurbanipal, King of Assyria,
315-316
Asia Minor, medicinal studies, 5
Aspergillus fungus, 395
Aspergillus flavus, 183, 184
Aspergillus parasiticus, 183, 184
Assyria, medical cannabis, 292,
315-316
Asthma, 255
Astrion, 23
Attention deficit hyperactivity disorder
(ADHD), 59, 166
Australia, 335
Autoimmune disease, 141
"Autotitrate," 297
Aversive events extinction, 56
Avicenna, 8, 317
Avonex, 365
Ayurvedic medicine, 316. *See also*
India
Azallû (hemp seeds), 316
Azerbaijan, 318

β-Caryophyllene, 180t, 183
β-Myrcene, 180t, 182-183, 184
β-Sitosterol, 188t, 190
Bacillus subtilis, 183, 186
Bain Commission, Dutch drug policy,
385-386
Balzac, Honoré, 13
Banckes, Richard, 46
Banga, 316
Bāsil, Istifān b., 5
Baudelaire, Charles, 13
Beck Depression Inventory (BDI-II)
Compassionate IND program, 404b,
430
patient A, 410
patient B, 416
patient C, 422
patient D, 428
Bencao Gang Mu, 318
Betaseron, 365
Bioavailability, cannabis compounds,
191
Bioavailability
CBD, 99
CBN, 100
Δ⁹-THC, 75-80, 76t, 77i, 78i

Birth, rites of, 298-299
Bladder dysfunction, 367, 368, 371,
373
Blood pressure, 142, 143
Body temperature, 126b
Bones, 132
"Bongs," 310
Booke of Simples, 48
Borneol, 181t, 187
Botanical studies, early Arabian, 5, 6
Boyd, Susan, 291
Brain
and anandamide/2-AG, 214-215
marijuana safety, 387
THC distribution, 81, 82
*Brain's Diseases of the Nervous
System,* 369
Brainstem, anandamide/2-AG, 215
Brazil, medical cannabis, 333
Breast cancer, medical cannabis, 335
Breast milk, THC distribution, 83
Breasts, medical cannabis, 318, 331
British Medical Journal, 324
British Pharmaceutical Codex, 331
Bronchodilator, 244b
Bullein, William, 47-48
Burn treatment, 30
Byzantine empire, dietary literature, 17

Caffeine, 392t, 392-393
California
chemotherapy studies, 272-273,
273t
medical cannabis, 288
California NORML (National
Organization to Reform
Marijuana Laws), 309
California Research Advisory Panel,
272
California Verbal Learning Test
(CVLT)
Compassionate IND program, 404b,
430
patient A, 409
patient B, 415-416
patient C, 421
patient D, 428
Cambodia, medical cannabis, 292, 333
Canada, pregnancy study, 336-337

Cancer
  chemotherapy, 305
  inhalation route, 310-311
  THC clinical studies, 126b
  THC research, 1
Candida albicans, 186
Cannabichromene type (CBC)
  pharmacological effects, 135
  phytocannabinoid research, 174t, 177
  properties of, 70
  subtype, 117-118
Cannabicyclol type (CBL), 70
Cannabidiol type (CBD),
  antibacterial action, 131
  current research, 145
  mechanism of action, 119, 120i,
    120-121
  medical marijuana studies, 252, 255
  medicinal value, 202
  newborn mice study, 231, 233
  phytocannabinoid research, 173,
    174t, 175-176
  properties of, 70, 71i, 99, 100t
  subtype, 117-118
  and weight loss, 238
Cannabielsoin type (CBE), 70
Cannabigerol type (CBG)
  antibacterial action, 131
  pharmacological effects, 135
  phytocannabinoid research, 174t,
    177
  properties of, 70, 71i
  subtype, 117-118
Cannabinodiol type (CBDL), 70, 74
Cannabinoid acids, 70, 71i, 72i
Cannabinoid receptors
  resent research, 165
  types of, 121-122
Cannabinoids. *See also*
    Endocannabinoid system,
    Endocannabinoids
  administration routes, 69, 74-75, 75i
  basic research findings, 141-143
  benefits of, 145
  compounds in, 172, 173, 174t-175t,
    175-178
  drug interactions, 143-144
  elimination of, 88-93, 91t, 92i, 93i
  mechanism of action, 119i, 119-121,
    120i

Cannabinoids *(continued)*
  metabolic interactions, 69, 101-103,
    101i
  metabolism of, 84i, 84-85, 85i,
    86t-87t, 104
  as neuroprotection, 57
  pharmaceuticals, 53-55
  pharmakinetic properties, 74-75
  plasma concentration, 97-88
  recent research, 117, 118i
  spasmodic disorders, 58
  therapeutic effects hierarchy,
    140-141
  therapeutic potential of, 1
  time effect relationship, 94-98, 94i,
    96i, 97i
  tissue distribution, 80-83, 103
  types of, 70-71, 71i, 72i, 72t, 73,
    73i, 117-118
Cannabinol type (CBN)
  phytocannabinoid research, 174t,
    176-177
  properties of, 70, 71i, 74, 100
  subtype, 117-118
Cannabis
  antiemetic properties, 1
  British investigation of, 44
  British prohibition of, 43-44
  chronic use studies, 400-401, 429,
    432
  cognitive impact, 429-431
  compounds found in, 172
  criminalization of, 385
  Greek names for, 23-24
  harm of prohibition, 393-396
  as harm reduction medicine,
    386-389
  harm reduction strategies, 308-309
  herbal versus synthetic, 171-172
  HG use, 288-290
  introduction to Europe, 44
  MS symptom management, 368-372
  multiple uses of, 384
  nursing organizations, 389
  pharmacokinetic properties, 69
  during pregnancy, 302
  recreational use, 389-390, 393
  Syntagma, 18-19
  versus alcohol use, 391-392
Cannabis agria (wild), 45

Cannabis and Cognitive Functioning, 430
"Cannabis baby," 293
Cannabis based medicinal extract (CBME), 371
Cannabis in Costa Rica: A Study of Chronic Marihuana Use, 401
Cannabis in Medical Practice, 295
Cannabis indica
    HG symptoms, 296
    obstetric/gynecological use, 322, 323, 324, 325-327, 332
    plant genus, 44
Cannabis ruderalis, 44
Cannabis sativa
    during Classical era, 45
    English cultivation, 45-46
    HG symptoms, 296
    obstetric/gynecological use, 332
    phenolic acids, 70-71
    plant genus, 44
Cannabis seeds
    food lists, 36
    and impotence, 28-29
    for tapeworms, 34-35
Cannabis smoke, side effects, 172, 176, 184. *See also* Inhalation
Cannabis sylvestris, 45
Cannabis Yields and Dosage, 447
Cannabitriol type (CBTL), 70
Cannflavin A, 188t, 189-190
Cardiovascular system, 126b
Carene. *See* Δ-3Carene, essential oil
"Carl" hemp, 45-46
Carminative properties, 9
Cartilage, 166
Caryophyllene. *See* β-Caryophyllene
Causalgia, 56
CB_1 receptor
    "atypical distribution of," 230-231
    as cannabinoid receptor, 121, 122, 124, 145
    and CBN, 176
    endogenous agonists, 207-208, 208i, 209-211
    food ingestion, 228
    newborn mice study, 231, 232i, 233
    and suckling response, 233, 234
    THC clinical studies, 130-131, 132, 135

CB_2 receptor
    as cannabinoid receptor, 121, 122, 124
    endogenous agonists, 207-208, 208i, 209-210
    THC clinical studies, 132
CD4+T lymphocytes, immune damage, 304
Cell metabolism studies, 132
Celsus, A. Cornelius, 24
Center for Disease Control and Prevention (CDC), AIDS deaths, 303
Center for Medicinal Cannabis Research (CMCR), 1
Central nervous system studies, 128-130
Centre for Economic Policy Research, 391
Cerebellar abnormalities, 368
Chemotherapy studies
    antiemetic properties, 245-248, 305
    in California, 272-273, 273t, 274t
    in Georgia, 268-270, 270t
    in Michigan, 267-268, 269t
    multi-state study, 265-266
    in New Mexico (1983), 270-271, 271t
    in New Mexico (1984), 271-272
    in New York, 273-274
    in Tennessee, 266-267, 267t
Chest X-ray
    Compassionate IND program, 403, 404b
    patient A, 409
    patient C, 421
Children, Jamaican cocaine study, 353-354
China
    HG symptoms, 290
    medical cannabis, 292, 333
    medicinal studies, 5
    obstetric/gynecological use, 318
Chocolate, 229-230
Christison, Alexander, 321-322
Chronic relapsing experimental autoimmune encephalomyelitis (CREA), 125, 368-369
Cineole. *See* 1,8 Cineole

Circulation system
  basic research, 142
  THC clinical studies, 130-131
Classical era use
  ear disease, 29, 31
  gonorrhea, 36-38
  gout treatment, 29-30
  Greek contraceptives, 315
  hemp use, 24
  horse treatments, 24
  mosquito repellent, 34
  recreational hemp use, 33-34
  "snacks," 33
  tapeworm treatment, 34, 41
  veterinary medicine, 24, 41
Clinical endogenous cannabinoid
      deficiency (CECDD), 56, 64
Clinical examination, Compassionate
      IND program, 403, 404b
Cocaine
  drug risk, 392t, 392-393
  Jamaican study, 347-348, 352-357
Codex Vindobonensis 93, 318, 319i
Cognition
  cannabis impact, 429-431
  THC clinical studies, 126b, 128
Colic, 58-59
"Collapsed digestive system," 286
Collectiones medicae, 36
Columbia Memorial Hospital (CMH),
      273, 274
Commercial Rastas, 350
Compassionate Investigation New Drug
      (IND) program
  brief history, 401-403
  cognitive impact, 429-431
  conclusions/recommendations, 442
  demographic information, 403t
  endocrine function, 404b, 408t,
      436-437,
  hematological studies, 404b, 407t,
      434-435
  immunological parameters, 404b,
      407t, 435-436
  medical marijuana study, 400
  methods, 403t, 403-404, 404b
  neuroimaging evidence, 404b, 408i,
      431
  neurophysiology tests, 404b, 431-433
  patient consent form, 412i

Compassionate Investigation New Drug
      (IND) program *(continued)*
  program problems, 437-441
  pulmonary tests, 404b, 407t, 433-434
  results/discussion, 404-441
Compassionate Use Act of 1996, 288,
      294
Compazine, 284, 285
Congress on Nursing Practice, 389
Conner's Continuous Performance Test
      (CPT-II)
  Compassionate IND program, 404b,
      430
  patient A, 409
  patient B, 415
  patient C, 421
Conrad, Chris, 447
Constantine VIII, Emperor of
      Byzantium, 17
Contraceptives, 315
Controlled Oral Word Association Test
  Compassionate IND program, 404b,
      430
  patient A, 410
  patient B, 416
  patient C, 422
Controlled Substance Act of 1970,
      schedules, 385
Controlled Substance Analogue
      Enforcement Act of 1986
  and synthetic THC, 257
  and THCV, 178
Copaxone, 365
Corticosteroids, MS, 364, 365
Cost
  Nabilone, 54
  Ondansetron (Zofran), 291
Costa Rica, chronic use study, 401,
      429-430, 434, 435, 437
Crack cocaine
  Jamaican consumption, 347,
      352-353, 352t
  Jamaican procurement, 347, 351
  Jamaican use, 350-351
  Jamaican user status, 347, 351-352,
      353-354
Cranial nerves examination
  patient A, 406
  patient B, 414
  patient C, 420

Crohn's disease, 141
Cryptococcus neoformans, 182, 186
Culpeper, Nicolas, 46, 47
Curry, Wei-Ni Lin, 288-290, 293, 298
Cyclooxygenase inhibitors, 144
Cyclophosphamide, 365
Cymene. *See* ρ-Cymene
Cystic fibrosis, 59
Czechoslovakia, ob/gyn use, 331

Δ-3Carene, essential oil, 181t, 187
d-Limonene, essential oil, 180t,
    183-184, 190-191
Datura stramonium (L. Solonaceae), 13
Dawamesk, 13
de Meijer, Etienne, 202
De Alimentorum Facultatibus (On the
    properties of food), 33, 35-36
De Historia Stirpium Commentarii, 20
De Remediis Parabilibus (On ready
    remedies), 34, 41
*De Simplicium Medicamentorum
    Temperamentis et
    Facultatibus* (On the
    temperaments and properties
    of simple medications), 32, 36
*De Simplicium Medicamentorum
    Temperamentis ac
    Facultatibus Liber VII,* 5
De Victu Attenuante (On the thinning
    regimen), 39
Deakle, David, 318
Death rituals, Scythian, 25-26
Dependency, THC, 139
Depression
    cannabinoids, 57
    and gender, 363
    synthetic derivatives, 117
Dermal administration, 80
Detoxification programs, Jamaica, 355
Detroit Metropolitan Comprehensive
    Cancer Center, 267
Dexanabinol (HU-211)
    EAE management, 365
    pharmacological effects, 135-136,
        136i
    properties, 101
    synthetic cannabinoid, 54-55, 64, 74

Di Marzo, Vincenzo, 225
Diarrhea, 29
Didi, HG symptoms, 294-295, 296,
    297
Digestive tract, 132
Dioscorides
    in Arabic medical tradition, 6-7
    Arabic translation of, 5
    and Byzantine science, 18
    on cannabis, 23-24, 30-32
    on gout, 29-30, 40
    on *khylos,* 29
    later use of, 46, 47
    Materia Medica, 5, 27-28, 30, 40
Dispensatory of the United States, 322
Diterpenoids, 178
Diuretic properties, 8
Dopamine, 128-129, 129t
Dreher, Melanie, 292, 337
Dronabinol, administration, 74, 75
Dronabinol
    AIDS wasting syndrome, 305
    antiemetic properties, 247, 250
    appetite stimulant, 227
    drug interactions, 143
    legal use of, 305-306
    and prochlorperazine, 246-247
    PWAs study, 308
    Tourette syndrome, 128
    use of, 129, 140
    weight stimulant, 249
Drug detection, 69, 103-104
Drug Enforcement Administration
    (DEA)
    chemotherapy studies, 266
    and dronabinol, 303
Drugs
    criminalization of, 291
    risks of, 392-393, 392t
Dumas, Alexandre, 13
*Durham Glossary of the Names of
    Worts,* 45
Dyskinesia, 53
"Dysmenine," 327, 329i
Dysmenorrhea
    medical cannabis, 292, 327-328,
        330, 331, 332-333, 334,
        335
    medical marijuana, 244b

Ear disease
　Arabic use, 7
　Classical era, 29, 31
"Eating for two," 281
Ebers Papyrus, 49, 316
Edinburgh New Dispensatory, 320
Egypt
　cannabis source, 44
　early cannabis use, 49
　medical cannabis, 292
　medical studies, 5
　ob/gyn use, 316
Electric shock, 253
Electroencephalography (EEG)
　cannabis impact, 431-432
　Compassionate IND program, 403,
　　404b
　patient A, 407
　patient B, 415
　patient C, 420
Elimination
　Dexanabinol (HU-211), 101
　Nabilone, 100
Empiricus, Marcellus, 24, 36
Endocannabinoid system
　degradation research, 165, 213
　discovery of, 207
　mammalian development, 230-231
　tonic activity, 124-125
　transporter research, 165
　weight regulation, 229
Endocannabinoids
　drug development, 216i, 216-219,
　　217i, 219i
　fertility research, 335-336
　in food substances, 229-230
　pharmacological effects, 135
　potential therapeutic agents, 56-57,
　　209
　receptors, 122-125, 123i, 207-208
Endocrine assays
　cannabis impact, 436-437
　Compassionate IND program, 403,
　　404b
　patient A, 407, 408t
　patient B, 408t, 415
　patient C, 408t, 420
　patient D, 408t, 428
Endocrine system, 363
Endogenous ligands, 117, 144

England. *See also* Great Britain; United
　　Kingdom
　early hemp history, 45, 46
　ob/gyn use, 320-322, 333
"Enhanced diffusion," 123-124
Enzyme-linked immunosorbent assay
　　(ELISA), 303
Ephippus, 34
Epilepsy
　Arab practice, 9
　and synthetic derivatives, 117
Escherichia coli, 183, 186
Esquirol, Jean-Étienne Dominique, 13
Essential oils, 179, 180t-181t
Ethnobotany
　herbal remedies, 305
　ob/gyn use, 331-334
Eugenia dysenterica, 182
Euporista, 40
Eve's Herbs, 315
Exceretion
　CBN, 100
　CBD, 99
　Nabilone, 100
　THC elimination, 90-93, 91t, 93i
Experimental autoimmune
　　encephalomyelitis (EAE), 365
Extended Glasgow Coma Scale, 64
Eye(s), clinical studies, 126b, 132
Eye drops, 75, 79

Families Against Mandatory
　　Minimums (FAMM), 394
Farm animals, 29
Fat, 82
Fatigue, 367, 368, 370-371, 373
Fatty acid amide hydrolase (FAAH)
　and endocannabinoids, 123, 124,
　　213, 217, 217i
　pharmacological effects, 137, 145
Febris quartana, 10
Feces, 90-91, 91t, 93
Federal Bureau of Narcotics, 385
Feinstein, Diane, 393
Fertility, 56, 133
Ferula galbaniflua, 7
Fetal development
　maternal cannabis use, 366-367
　THC clinical studies, 126b

Fetus, 81, 82-83
Fibromyalgia, CECDD, 56
"Fimble" hemp, 45-46
Finger Tapping and Category Test
    Compassionate IND program, 404b,
        430
    patient B, 416
    patient C, 422
"First-pass metabolism," 171-172
Fishbein, Morris, 331
Five Hundred Points of Good
        Husbandrie, 46
Flavonoids, 118,172, 187, 188t,
        189-190
Food, cannabis as, 27
Food and Drug Administration,
        Compassionate IND program,
        400
France, ob/gyn use, 324
Fuchs, Leonhart, 19-20
Furor uterinus, 320

GABA. *See* α-aminobutyric acid
        (GABA)
Galen
    in Arabic medical tradition, 6-7, 9
    Arabic translation, 5
    and Byzantine science, 18
    De Simplicium Medicamentorum
        Temperamentis ac
        Facultatibus, 5
    and Greek medicine, 35
    on cannabis seeds, 27, 32-34, 39,
        331
    on *khylos,* 29
    later use of, 46-47
Gamma-linolenic acid (GLA), 335
Ganja
    Jamaican cocaine study, 355-356
    Jamaican experience, 358
    in Jamaican tradition, 348-350
"Gangja complex," 349, 350
Ganja in Jamaica: A Medical
        Anthropological Study of
        Chronic Marihuana Use, 401
Gas chromatography-tandem mass
        spectrometry (GC-MS), 83
Gastrointestinal function, 56

Gastrointestinal tract, 126b
Gateway drug, 391
Gautier, Théophile, 13
Gender
    AIDS, 303
    cannabis interactions, 363
    MS prevalence, 363-364
    MS symptoms, 369
    nervous system differences, 363
Genetic research, 126b, 202
Geoponica, 41
Georgia, chemotherapy studies,
        268-270, 270t
German folk medicine, ob/gyn use,
        331, 332
Gina, HG symptoms, 294, 296-297,
        298
Ginkgo biloba, 185
Glaucoma
    drug interactions, 143
    medical marijuana, 253-254,
        401-402
Glutamate, 128-129, 129t
Glycine, 129t
Gonorrhea
    Classical era, 36-38
    folk medicine, 333-334
Gout, 29-30
Great Britain. *See also* United
        Kingdom
    medicinal cannabis, 43-44
    ob/gyn use, 320-321, 324-327, 331
Greece
    absence of cannabis use, 24-25
    ancient medicinal studies, 5
    Arabic use of, 6-7
    cannabis terms, 23-24
    cannabis use, 24, 27-28
    chronic hashish use study, 401, 429,
        432
Greece literature, cannabis in, 25
Grinspoon, Lester, 288, 298, 335
Grooved Peg Board
    Compassionate IND program, 404b,
        430
    patient B, 416
    patient C, 422
Gust, Steven, 447
Gynecology, 58, 315-331

Hachisch et de l'Alientation Mentale:
    Études Psychologiques, 13-14
"Haenep," 45
Hair growth, 8
Haloperidol versus marijuana, 246
Halstead-Reitan Battery
    Compassionate IND program, 404b
    patient A, 409
    patient C, 422
Harm reduction
    cannabis safety, 386-389
    cannabis use, 384-385
    clinical cannabis, 441
    principle of, 383-384
Harrison's Principles of Internal
    Medicine, 306
Harvard Guide to Women's Health,
    The, 282
Hashimoto's thyroiditis, 363
Hashish and Mental Illness, 14
Hashish
    chronic use study, 401, 429
    Moreau investigations, 13-15
Hashish: Studies of Long-Term Use,
    401
Health care system, 395-396
Hematological studies
    cannabis impact, 434-435
    Compassionate IND program, 403,
        404b
    patient A, 407, 407t
    patient B, 407t, 415
    patient C, 407t, 420
    patient D, 407t, 428
Hemp *(Cannabis sativa)*
    in Arabic literature, 6-10
    Classical use of, 24
    indigenous English use, 45-46
    indigenous European use, 44, 45
    medical cannabis, 333
    medicinal properties, 5, 45, 46
    vernucidal/vermifugal properties,
        7-8
Herbal (Culpeper), 47
Herbal (Dodoens), 46-47
Herbal (Grieves), 44, 333
Herbalism, Britain, 43
Herbarium, 23-24, 38, 45
Herodotus, 25-26, 33, 45
Heroin, 392t, 392-393

Herpes simplex viruses, 131, 335
Hesychius, 23, 26-27, 33
Hewitt, Grailey, 323
Hill equation, 96-97
Hillig, Karl, 202
Hippiatrica, 41
Hippocrates, 25
Hippocratic Corpus, 25
Histamine, 128
Historia Naturalis, 27-30
HIV. *See* Human immunodeficiency
    virus (HIV)
Hollister, Leo, 263-264, 306
Holmstedt, Bo, 15
Hormonal system, 126b, 133
Hormone regulation, 56
Horses, hemp use, 24
Hospice de Bicêtre, 15
Hôtel Pimodan, 13
HU-308, 55
Human growth hormone, 306
Human immunodeficiency virus (HIV),
    303, 306
Humors
    Arab practice, 9
    hemp properties, 6
Huntington disease, 57, 175
Hydrastina, 23
Hydroxylation, 84
Hyoscyamus niger, 48
Hyperemesis gravidarum (HG)
    definition of, 282
    description of, 281
    medical cannabis, 288, 345-346
    patient frustration, 288
    prevalence of, 284, 293
Hypothalamus
    anandamide/2-AG, 215
    weight regulation, 228, 229

Iatrica, 36-38
Ibn Baytār, al, 7, 9, 10
Ibn Buklāriš, 9
Ibn Habal, 9
Ibn Jatīb, al, 7
Ibn Māsawayah, 7, 8
Ibn Qurra, Tābit, 317
Ibn Sahl, Sabur, 317
Ibn Wafid, al-Lajimi, 317, 318

Idiopathic bowel syndrome (IBS),
    CECDD, 56
Immune system
    cannabis interactions, 363
    marijuana safety, 387
    THC clinical studies, 126b, 133
Immunological assays
    cannabis impact, 407t, 435-436
    Compassionate IND program, 403,
        404b
    patient A, 407, 407t
    patient B, 407t, 415
    patient C, 407t, 420
    patient D, 407t, 428
'Imrān, Ishāq b., hemp properties, 8
India
    in vivo research, 44
    medical studies, 5
    ob/gyn use, 332-333
    psychotropic cannabis, 44-45
*Indian Hemp Drugs Commission
    Report,* 327, 400
Indomethacin, 144
Ingall, John R., 267
Inhalation
    absorption rate, 76t, 76-77, 77i
    administration route, 69, 74-75, 75i
    cannabis smoke, 172, 176, 184
    chemotherapy cancer study, 305
    chemotherapy studies, 265, 266,
        276. *See also* Marijuana
        cigarettes
    harm reduction strategies, 309
    herbal cannabis, 172
    marijuana efficacy, 247, 248
    marijuana safety, 386-387
    plasma concentration, 87-88
    PWAs study, 308
    THC distribution, 81
    THC elimination, 88-89
    THC metabolism, 87t
    time effect relationship, 94i, 94-95,
        96i
Insomnia, 405
Institute for Clinical Research, 1
Institute of Medicine (IOM)
    gateway theory, 391
    medical marijuana, 258, 386
International Association for Cannabis
    As Medicine (IACM), 1

Internet, 295
Intravenous administration
    plasma concentration, 87
    THC elimination, 88, 90, 91t, 91-93
    THC metabolism, 86t
    time effect relationship, 94, 94t
Ishāq, Hunayn b., 5
Isoproterenal aerosol, 255
Israel, ob/gyn use, 316, 317i
Italy, breast cancer research, 335

Jamaica
    crack cocaine study, 347-348,
        352-357
    crack cocaine study conclusions,
        357-358
    ganja chronic use study, 401, 429,
        432, 433-434, 435, 437
    medical cannabis, 292-293, 337-338
Jamestown (VA), 45-46
Jamestown General Hospital (JGH),
    273-274
*Jeffrey's Journey: A Determined
    Mother's Battle for Medical
    Marijuana for Her Son,* 59
*Journal of Cannabis Therapeutics:
    Studies in Endogenous,
    Herbal, and Synthetic
    Cannabinoids*
    alcohol dependence withdrawal, 360
    "Marijuana (Cannabis) as
        Medicine," 306
    research support, 1, 2
*Journal of the American Medical
    Association* (JAMA)
    CT review, 431
    medical cannabis, 331
Judea, medical cannabis, 292

Kaloi, 24
Kama Sutra, 332
Kannabides, 27
Kannabion, 23
Kannabís, 27
Kannabos, 27
Kaposi's sarcoma, 304
Karpos (fruit), 24

Kesey, Ken, 263
Khylizein, 31
Khylos, 29, 31
"Killer weed," 292
Kräuterbuch, 318

LaGuardia Report, 400, 434
Lamivudine (3TC), 304
Langkavel, Bernhard, 18-19, 20
Laos, 292
Le Club des Hachichins, 13
Learning studies, 128
Leprosy, 8
Leptin, 131, 228-229
Levonantradol, 53-54, 136-137
Lexicon on the Properties of Food,
    17-21
Li Shih-Chen, 318
Lichen, 8
Limonene. *See* d-Limonene, essential
    oil
Linalool, 180t, 184-185
Linoleic acid (LA), 335
Lioresal Intrahecal, 372
Lipoproteins, 80, 81
Liver, 84
Liver cirrhosis, 166
Liverwort, 117
Lozano, Indalecio, 317, 318, 331
Lucilius, 29
Lupus erythematosus, 363
Lynn Pierson Therapeutic Research
    Program, 270, 271
Lypemania, 14
Lysophosphatidic acid (LPA), 233-234
Lyte, Henry, 46-47

Magnetic resonance imaging (MRI)
    scan
    cannabis impact, 431
    Compassionate IND program, 403,
        404b
    patient A, 407-408
    patient B, 415
    patient C, 421
Makhzan-ul-Adwiya, 318

Mammals
    cannabinoid receptors, 117
    endocannabinoid system, 230-231
    fertility research, 335-336
Marihuana, the Forbidden Medicine,
    335
Marijuana. *See also* Ganja, Medical
    marijuana
    bias against, 244
    drug risk, 392t, 392-393
    effects of, 69
    medical use, 243, 244b
"Marijuana (Cannabis) as Medicine,"
    306
Marijuana cigarettes
    California chemotherapy study, 272,
        273, 273t, 274t
    chemotherapy studies, 265
    Georgia chemotherapy study, 268,
        270, 270t
    Michigan chemotherapy study, 268,
        269t
    New Mexico (1983) chemotherapy
        study, 271, 271t
    New Mexico (1984) chemotherapy
        study, 272, 272t
    New York chemotherapy study,
        273-274
    Tennessee chemotherapy study, 266,
        267, 267t
    therapeutic use reviews, 243-244,
        244b
"Marijuana dependence," 393
"Marijuana Does Not Appear to Alter
        Viral Loads of HIV Patients
        Taking Protease Inhibitors,"
    308
*Marijuana Rx: The Patients' Fight for
        Medicinal Pot,* 401
Marijuana Tax Act, 385
Marinol
    AIDS wasting syndrome, 305
    antiemetic properties, 247
    Compassionate IND program, 405,
        413, 417
    inadequacy of, 441
    legal status, 366, 372
    oncologist survey, 275
    PWAs study, 308
    synthetic cannabis, 74, 75, 140, 171

Mary, HG symptoms, 287, 288
Materia medica
  Arabic, 317
  Classical use, 5, 27-28, 30, 31, 40
  Chinese, 318
  early European use, 48
Materia Medica and Drug Action, 330
Matricaria recutita, 187
Mattison, J. B., 327
McCaffrey, Barry, 386, 387-388
McCaffrey, Margo, pain standard, 389
Mechoulam, Raphael, HU-308, 55
Medical marijuana
  analgesic properties, 244b, 252-253
  anticonvulsant properties, 244b,
    254-255
  antiemetic properties, 244b, 245-248
  antispasmodic properties, 244b,
    250-252
  appetite stimulant, 244b, 248-250
  bias against, 244
  as bronchodilator, 244b, 255-256
  in Classical world, 27-39
  in early England, 45, 46-49
  glaucoma treatment, 253-254
  insomnia, 256
  in modern England, 49-50
  therapeutic use reviews, 243-244,
    244b
  term, 400
Medicina Britannica, 49, 320
MEDLINE, search engine, 172
Megace, 306
Megestrol acetate, 227
Melancholia, 14, 244b
Memory, 56, 128
Menopause, 330, 367
Mesopotamia, 5, 315-316
Metabolic system
  THC distribution, 81
  THC metabolism, 84i, 84-85, 85i,
    86t-87t, 104
Metabolism
  cannabinoid interactions, 101i,
    101-103
  CBD, 99, 100t
  Nabilone, 100
Metabolites, 133-134
Metaclopramide (Reglan), 284, 285
Metered dose inhaler (MDI), 75, 309

Methotrexate, 365
Metoclopramide, 246, 247
Metyrapone, 144
Michael VII Ducas, Emperor of
    Byzantium, 17
Michigan Cancer Foundation, 267
Michigan, chemotherapy studies,
    267-268, 269t
Mifepristone, 144
Migraine, 56, 363
Milk, 230
Mini-Mental State Examination
    (MMSE), 430
"Minor components," 201
Missoula Chronic Clinical Cannabis
    Use Study, 400. *See also*
    Compassionate IND program
Monoterpenoids, 178, 182-187
Moreau, Jacques-Joseph, 13-15, 14i
Morning sickness, 283-284
Morocco, 334
Mosquito repellent, 34
Mothers Against Misuse and Abuse
    (MAMA), 388
Mothers and Illicit Drug Use:
    Transcending the Myths, 291
Motor examination
  patient A, 406
  patient B, 414-415
  patient C, 420
Motor neuron disease, 363
Mount Olympus, 17, 18
Muller-Vahl, K. R. U., 14-15
Multidisciplinary Association for
    Psychedelic Studies (MAPS),
    309
Multiple sclerosis (MS)
  acute episodes management, 364
  basic research, 141
  cannabinoid therapeutics, 364,
    365-367
  and cannabinoids, 58
  common symptoms, 367-368
  Compassionate IND program, 403t,
    407t, 408i, 408t, 422-429
  Dexanabinol, 54-55
  disease modification, 364-365
  gender differences, 363-364, 373
  medical marijuana, 251-252
  Nabilone, 53, 63-64

Multiple sclerosis (MS) *(continued)*
  neuropathic pain, 1
  pregnancy/postpartum periods, 367
  recent research, 377
  U.K. cannabis use, 364
Muscle relaxants, 143
Myasthenia gravis, 363
Myocardial infarction, 373
Myrcene. *See* β-Myrcene

N-arachidonylethanolamide
    (anandamide)
  analogues/carriers, 216, 216i, 217i
  appetite stimulant, 228
  biosynthesis pathways, 211, 212i,
    213
  breast cancer research, 335
  chemical structure, 208i, 209
  distinctive qualities, 209-211
  endocannabinoids, 122, 123, 123i,
    124, 208, 208i
  hybrids, 218, 219i
  in food substances, 229-230
  mammalian development, 231
  pharmacological effects, 130
  physiopathological conditions,
    213-215
  recent research, 166
  THC clinical studies, 130
  weight regulation, 229
N-archidonyl-dopamine (NADA), 122,
    123, 124
Nabilone
  pharmacological effects, 135, 136i
  properties of, 100
  synthetic cannabinoid, 53-54, 63-64
  therapeutic effects, 140
Nail-patella syndrome, 403t, 410-411,
    413-414
Naringenin, 187
Nasha, 332
National Commission on Marijuana
    and Drug Use, 385
National Institute of Clinical
    Excellence (NICE), 372-373
National Institute on Drug Abuse
    (NIDA)
  chemotherapy studies, 266

National Institute on Drug Abuse
    (NIDA) *(continued)*
  Compassionate IND program, 400,
    402
  marijuana cigarette quality,
    438-439, 439i, 440i, 441i
National Library of Medicine Database
    (PubMed), 400
National Organization to Reform
    Marijuana Laws (NORML),
    309
Nausea
  antiemetic drugs, 286
  California chemotherapy study, 273,
    273t
  chemotherapy cancer study, 305
  chemotherapy studies, 265
  Georgia study, 268-269, 270
  HG symptoms, 282-283, 287-288
  Michigan study, 269t
  New Mexico (1983) study, 271, 271t
  New Mexico (1984) study, 272, 272t
  Tennessee study, 267t
Neonatal impact, Rimonabant
    (SR141716), 56
Nervous system
  and gender differences, 363
  THC clinical studies, 126b, 128-130
Netherlands
  cannabis availability, 1
  drug policy, 385-386
Neuralgia, 244b
Neuroimaging examination, 431
Neuropathic pain, 1, 53
Neuropeptides, 129t
Neuroprotection, 130, 141
Neuropsychological test battery
  cannabis impact, 429-431
  Compassionate IND program, 403,
    404b
  patient A, 409
  patient B, 415
  patient C, 421
  patient D, 428
Neurotransmitters, 128-130, 129t
New Mexico
  chemotherapy study (1983),
    270-271, 271t
  chemotherapy study (1984),
    271-272

New York, 273-274
"New-wort," 320
Nicandrus, 18
Nicotine, 392t, 392-393
Night vision, 56-57
94-Day Cannabis Study, 435, 437
Nitric oxide, 213
Nitrogenous compounds, 118
Nixon, Richard, 385
Noladin ether. *See* 2-
    Archidonylglyceryl ether
    (noladin ether)
Nonnus, Theophanies, 18
Nora, HG symptoms, 285-286
Noradrenaline, 129t
Norespinephrine, 128
North Shore Hospital (NSH), 273, 274
Novantrone, 365
Nurses
    harm reduction perspective, 384-385
    marijuana exposure, 69
    medication role, 388
    role of, 383
    and therapeutic cannabis, 389
    as trusted profession, 383
Nystagmus, 369-370, 373

O'Leary, Alice, 401
Obesity, 56, 238
Obsessive-compulsive disorder
    CECDD, 56
    hashish treatment, 14-15
    medical marijuana, 244b
Obstetrics, 58, 315-331
Office of National Drug Control Policy
    (ONDCP), 393
Ointments, 7
Old English Herbarium, 318
Ondanestron (Zofran)
    chemotherapy cancer study, 305
    cost of, 291
    HG symptoms, 284, 285
Ophthalmic administration, 79
Opiate withdrawal, 244b
Opioid peptides, 128
Opium dependency, 117
Oral administration
    absorption rate, 75, 76t, 78i, 78-79
    administration route, 69, 74-75, 75i,
        78i

Oral administration *(continued)*
    Arabic practice, 7
    chemotherapy studies, 265
    harm reduction strategies, 309
    plasma concentration, 88, 89i
    THC distribution, 81
    THC metabolism, 86t-87t
    time effect relationship, 94t, 95, 96i
"Organic mischief," 323
Oribasius, 35, 36, 38, 40-41
Oxandrolone, 306

p-Cymene, 181t, 187
P300 test
    cannabis impact, 432-433
    Compassionate IND program, 403,
        404b
    patient A, 407, 408i
    patient B, 408i, 415
    patient C, 408i, 420
Pain
    ancient Arab practice, 10
    and cannabinoids, 56
    and Levonantradol, 54
    and medical marijuana, 250
    MS symptom management, 368,
        371, 373
    recent research, 166-167
Pain management/regulation, 56,
    388-389
Palestine, 316, 317i
Palmitylethanolamide, 335
"Paramedical" use, 34
Paraquat, 395
Parasites, 10
Parkinson disease, 57
Parkinson, John, 46
Passive smoking, 69, 77
Patient A
    demographic information, 403t
    medical history, 405-406
    test data, 406-407, 407t, 408i, 408t,
        409-410
Patient B
    demographic information, 403t
    medical history, 410-411, 413-414
    test data, 407t, 408i, 408t, 414-416

Patient C
  demographic information, 403t
  medical history, 416-420
  test data, 407t, 408i, 408t, 420-422
Patient Consent Form, 412i
Patient D
  demographic information, 403t
  medical history 422-427
  test data, 407t, 408i, 408t, 427-429
Patient Qualification Review Board,
  266
Paulus of Aegina, 36
Pediatric use, 58-59
Pen T'sao Kang Mu, 318
Perception studies, 126b
Periaqueductal grey (PAG) area, 215
Perrot, E., 15
Persia, 5, 317-318
Persons with AIDS (PWAs)
  cannabinoid research, 308,
    313-314
  cannabis administration, 306
  cannabis experience, 306-307
  Compassionate IND program,
    402-403
  demographic information, 303-304
Pettit, Cabral, 435-436
Pettit, Dove, 435-436
Pfizer, Levonantradol, 54, 136-137
Phalis, 23
Pharmacotherapeutics, 330
Phenergan, 284, 285
Physicians' Desk Reference, 366
Phytocannabinoids
  characterization of, 117
  definition of, 173
  pharmacological effects, 135
  recent research, 173, 174t-175t,
    175-176
  THC effects, 119
Phytosterol, 172
Pinene. *See* α-Pinene
Pipe use
  cocaine, 350-351, 352-353, 352t
  ganja, 348
Piper nigrum, 182
Pityriasis, 8
Plasma
  THC distribution, 80-81
  THC elimination, 88-90

Plasma clearance rate
  CBD, 99
  CBN, 100
  Dexanabinol (HU-211), 101
  THC metabolism, 84, 87
Plasmodium falciparum, 183, 186
Pliny the Elder
  on cannabis, 24, 27-30
  later use of, 46
Pneumocystis carinii pneumonia, 304
Postural regulation, 370
Pregnancy
  anandamide/2-AG, 213
  ideal, 281
  and medical cannabis, 292, 336, 345
  U.K. cannabis use, 366-367
Premenstrual syndrome (PMS), 335
Prenatal exposure, 69
Pride World Drug Prevention
  Conference, 393
Prochlorperazine
  chemotherapy study, 305
  HG symptoms, 284, 285
  and marijuana, 246-247
Profile of Mood States Questionnaire
  (POMS), 367
Progesterone megestrol acetate
  (Megace), 306
"Prohibition tariff," 309
Promethazine (Phenergan), 284, 285
Propionibacterium acnes, 186
Prostaglandin, 128, 335
Prostitution, crack study, 351-352, 353
Protease inhibitors, 304, 308
Psellos, Michael, 18
Pseudo-Apuleius, 38, 42
Pseudo-Theodorus, 24, 36
Pseudomonas aeruginosa, 183
Psyche studies, 126b, 127-128
Psychoactive plants, 43
Psychological effects studies, 128
Psychomotor performance studies,
  126b, 128
Psychotropic effect
  cannabinoids, 104
  drug interactions, 143
  Indian hemp, 44-45
  time effect relationship, 94, 94i, 96i,
    97i
Public Health Service (PHS), 403

Pulegone, 180t, 185
Pulmonary function test
    cannabis impact, 433-434
    Compassionate IND program, 403, 404b
    patient A, 406-407, 407t
    patient B, 407t, 415
    patient C, 407t, 420
    patient D, 407t, 427-428
Purging, 8, 9

Quercetin, 188t, 189
Quinpirole, 214

Race, AIDS statistics, 303
Radula marginata, 117
Radula perrottetii, 117
Randall, Robert, 400, 401-403, 410, 417
Rastafarians
    Jamaican cocaine study, 355, 356-357
    Jamaican tradition, 348, 349
    medical cannabis, 292-293, 337-338
"Rastatutes," 350
Rebif, 365
Recreational use
    cannabis, 389-390, 393
    hemp, 33-34
Rectal administration
    absorption rate, 76t, 79
    administration route, 69, 75, 75i
    and dronabinol, 228
Reed, Homer, 431-432
"Reefer madness," 26
Reglan, 284
Research Triangle Institute of North
        Carolina, 402, 438
Respiratory system studies, 126b
Reynolds, Sir John Russell, 327
Riddle, John, 315
Rimonabant (SR141716)
    narcotic dependence treatment, 360
    newborn mice study, 231, 232i, 233
    pharmacological effects, 137i,
        137-138, 211
    Phase III trials, 166, 238
    synthetic cannabinoid, 55, 131
    weight reduction, 228

Ringer, Sydney, 325
Risks, commonly used drugs, 392-393, 392t
Ritual of denial, 298-299
Ritual of isolation, 298
Ritual of sacrifice, 298
Ritual of silence, 299
Ritual of suffering, 299
Romain III, Emperor of Byzantium, 17
Rome, 24-25
"Roots daughter," 349-350, 356
Rumpf, Georg Eberhard, 320
Russo, Ethan, 1, 49

S. epidermidis, 186
Saliva, 83
Salvia lavandulaefolia, 186
Sarah, HG symptoms, 282
Sativex, 1, 278
Scythians, 25 -26, 33, 45
Seasoned spliff, 350, 352-353, 352t
Sedative properties
    CBD, 173
    medical marijuana, 244b, 256
Self-medication, 44
Sensory impairment, 367-368
Septic shock, 213-214
Serenoa repens, 190
Serotonin studies, 128, 129t
Sesquiterpeoids, 178, 183
"Set," 295-296
Seth, Simeon, 17, 18-21
    William Turner's use of, 46
Sexual dysfunction, 368
Shafer Commission
    conclusions of 385
    on gateway theory, 391
    on punishments, 393
Shafer, Raymond, 385
Shirwani, Muhammad Riza, 318
Short-term memory research, 142-143
Side effects. *See also* Adverse effects
    AIDS treatment, 304-305
    California chemotherapy study, 274t
    chemotherapy studies, 275
    herbal cannabis, 171-172
    medical marijuana, 256

Side effects *(continued)*
  Michigan chemotherapy study, 268,
    269t
  Tennessee chemotherapy study, 267,
    267t
"Silver bullet," 171
Sitosterol. *See* β-Sitosterol
Sjögren's syndrome, 363
Skhoenostrophion, 23
Skin diseases, 8
Slow virus diseases, 57
"Smokers' cough," 310
Smoking. *See* Inhalation
Snack food
  appetite stimulant, 227, 228
  Classical era, 27, 33
Snyder, Solomon, 334
Sofia, HG symptoms, 282, 284, 285,
    286-288, 297-298
Soranus, 25
South Africa, 333, 364
Spasticity
  medical marijuana, 250-252
  MS symptom management, 367,
    368-369
  recent research, 166, 167
Sperm, 133
Sperma (seed), 24
Sphendamnos, 23
Spinal cord injury
  cannabinoids, 59
  cannabis use, 372
  medical marijuana, 250
Spleen, THC distribution, 82
Spliff
  cocaine use, 350-351, 352-353, 352t
  ganja use, 348, 401
SR141716. *See* Rimonabant
    (SR141716)
St. Joseph's Hospital, 273-274
Staphylococcus aureus, 183, 186
Starvation, HG, 281, 282, 283
"Stepping stone" theory, 357, 391
Stigma, medical cannabis, 292
Sublingual administration
  absorption rate, 79
  administration route, 69, 75, 75i
Sucus, 29
Suicidal ideation, HG symptoms,
    283-284, 298

Sulaymān, Ishāq b., 7, 8, 9
*Summary of Data on Hyperemesis
    Gravidarum,* 285
Sweat, 83
Sylphion, 315
"Synergetic shotgun," 171
Synhexyl (parahexyl) studies, 242
Synopsis ad Eustathium filium, 36,
    40-41
Syntagma de alimentorum facultatibus,
    17, 18-21
Syria, 5, 316

Tachycardia studies, 128, 130-131
Tapeworms
  Arab practice, 8
  Classical era, 34, 41
Target Problem Rating Scale, New
    Mexico (1983), 271, 271t
Tennessee, chemotherapy studies,
    266-267, 267t
"Terminal," 23-24
Terpenes, 118
Terpenoids, 172, 178-179, 180t-181t,
    182-187
Terpenophenolic metabolites, 44-45
Terpineol. *See* α-Terpineol
Terpineol-4-01, essential oil, 181t
Testis, 81
Testosterone enanthate, 250, 306
Tetrahydrocannabinol (Δ^8-THC)
  EAE experiments, 365
  phytocannabinoid research, 175t,
    178
Tetrahydrocannabinol (Δ^9-THC)
  absorption rate, 75-80, 76t, 77i, 78i
  analgesic properties, 252-253
  antibacterial action, 131
  anticonvulsant properties, 254-255
  antiemetic properties, 244b, 245-248
  antispasmodic, 250-251
  appetite stimulant, 248-250
  as bronchodilator, 255-256
  chemotherapy studies, 265-274
  degradation of, 74
  dependency, 139
  EAE experiments, 365
  elimination of, 88-93, 91t, 92i, 93i
  fetal ingestion, 290

Tetrahydrocannabinol *(continued)*
  glaucoma treatment, 253-254
  immune system safety, 387
  insomnia, 256
  isolation of, 243
  marijuana studies, 244
  mechanism of action, 119i,
      119-120
  metabolic interactions, 101-103,
      101i
  metabolism, 84i, 84-85, 85i, 86t-87t,
      104
  metabolite pharmacology, 133-134
  pharmacological effects, 125, 126b
  pharmakinetics of, 74-75, 75i
  physiochemical properties of,
      73-74
  phytocannabinoid research, 173,
      174t
  phytocannabinoids, 70-71, 71i, 72i,
      72t, 73, 73i
  plasma concentration, 97-88
  stereochemically defined, 117
  subtype, 117-119
  therapeutic use, 139-140
  time effect relationship, 94-98, 94i
  tissue distribution, 80-83, 103
  tolerance, 138-139
  toxicity, 125, 127
Tetrahyrocannabivarin (THCV)
  phytocannabinoid research, 175t,
      178, 202
  weight loss, 238
Thailand, 292
THC capsules
  California chemotherapy study, 272,
      273, 273t, 274t
  chemotherapy cancer study, 305
  chemotherapy studies, 265, 266
  Georgia chemotherapy study, 268,
      270, 270t
  New Mexico (1983) chemotherapy
      study, 271, 271t
  New Mexico (1984) chemotherapy
      study, 272, 272t
  Tennessee chemotherapy study, 266,
      267, 267t
Theatrum Botanicum, 46, 320
Theiler murine encephalomyelitis, 165
Thiethylperazine, 267-268

Thurstone Word Fluency Test (animal
      naming)
  Compassionate IND program, 404b,
      430
  patient A, 410
  patient B, 416
  patient C, 422
Tissue distribution
  CBN, 100
  Dexanabinol (HU-211), 101
  endocannabinoids, 211, 212i,
      213-215
Tobacco use
  Compassionate IND program, 405
  drug interactions, 143
  harm of, 391
  metabolic interactions, 102
  narcotic dependence treatment, 360
  patient B, 414
  patient D, 427
  withdrawal reduction, 182
Tolerance, 138-139
Topical antibiotic, 244b
Tourette syndrome
  cannabinoids, 139
  Dronabinol, 128
Tragemata (snacks), 27
Trail Making Test
  Compassionate IND program, 404b,
      430
  patient A, 409
  patient C, 422
Traité du Chanvre, 49
Treatise on Hemp, A, 49
Tremor, 368, 369, 373
Trichophyton mentagrophytes, 186
Triterpenoids, 178
Tumors, 9
Turner, William, 46
Tusser, Thomas, 46

U. S. Pharmacopoeia, medical
      marijuana, 243
U'Umdat al-tabīb, 8
United Kingdom. *See also* Great
      Britain
  cannabis use, 364
  clinically available cannabis,
      440-441

United Kingdom. *See also* Great
     Britain *(continued)*
  NICE study, 372-373
  pregnant cannabis use, 366-367
United States
  drug/medication culture, 389
  legal cannabis use, 385
  ob/gyn use, 322-325, 330-331, 334
University of Mississippi, 402, 447
University of West Indies Hospital, 354
Upstate Medical Center, 273-274
Urine, 90-93, 91t, 92i, 92i, 93i
Urtica dioica, 190
Uterus, 9

van Ours, Jan, 391
Vanilloid receptors, 122-123
Vapor bath, Scythian, 25, 26-27, 33, 45
Vaporizers
  cannabis compounds, 190
  harm reduction strategies, 309-310
Vermifuge, 7-8
Vernucide, 7-8
Vertuous Boke of Distillacioun, The, 46
Veterinary medicine, 24, 41
Viagra, 103
Victoria, Queen of England, 49
Vietnam, 292, 333
Viral load, 304
Virodhamine. *See* 0-Archidonyl-
     ethanolamine (virodhamine)
Vitiligo, 8
Volatile oils, 179
Voltatizer, 310
Vomiting
  antiemetic drugs, 286
  California chemotherapy study, 273,
     273t
  chemotherapy cancer study, 305
  chemotherapy studies, 265
  Georgia chemotherapy study,
     268-269, 270
  HG symptoms, 282, 287-288
  Michigan chemotherapy study, 269t
  New Mexico (1983) chemotherapy
     study, 271, 271t
  New Mexico (1984) chemotherapy
     study, 272, 272t
  Tennessee chemotherapy study, 267t

Walters, John, 393
War on Drugs, 384-385
Water pipes, 310
Wechsler Adult Intelligence Scale
     (WAIS-III)
  Compassionate IND program, 404b,
     430
  patient A, 409
  patient B, 415
  patient C, 421
  patient D, 428
Wechsler Memory Scale (WMS-III)
  Compassionate IND program, 404b,
     430
  patient A, 409, 410
  patient B, 415, 416
  patient C, 421
  patient D, 428
Westberg, Daniel, 318
Wisconsin Card Scoring Test (WCST)
  Compassionate IND program, 404b,
     430
  patient A, 410
  patient B, 416
  patient C, 422
Withdrawal, THC, 139
Women
  cannabis impact, 366-367
  early medical cannabis, 315-318
  early Western medical cannabis,
     318-331
  ganja tradition, 349-350
  Jamaican crack cocaine users,
     351-357
  modern ethnobotany, 331-334
  MS cannabis use, 364
  MS occurrence, 363-364, 373
  MS symptom management, 367-372
  recent clinical data, 334-338
Workplace drug testing, 394-395
Worms
  ancient Arab practice, 7, 8
  Classical era, 34, 41

Young, Francis, 386

Zend-Avesta, 316
Zidovudine (AZT/ZVD), 304

Zofran
  chemotherapy cancer study, 305
  cost of, 291
  HG symptoms, 284, 285
Zoroastrianism, 316